HANDBOOK OF CHILD AND ADOLESCENT TUBERCULOSIS

There are many contributions which the pediatrician can make to the tuberculosis control program. First the negativism about the tuberculosis so prevalent in pediatrics must be overcome. . . . Wherever there are tuberculous adults, there are infected children. No one is immune.

—Edith M. Lincoln, "Eradication of Tuberculosis in Children," *Archives of Environmental Health*, 1961

HANDBOOK OF CHILD AND ADOLESCENT TUBERCULOSIS

Edited By

Jeffrey R. Starke and Peter R. Donald

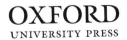

OXFORD
UNIVERSITY PRESS

Oxford University Press is a department of the University of Oxford. It furthers
the University's objective of excellence in research, scholarship, and education
by publishing worldwide. Oxford is a registered trade mark of Oxford University
Press in the UK and certain other countries.

Published in the United States of America by Oxford University Press
198 Madison Avenue, New York, NY 10016, United States of America.

© Oxford University Press 2016

First Edition published in 2016

Library of Congress Cataloging-in-Publication Data
Handbook of child and adolescent tuberculosis/edited by Jeffrey R. Starke and Peter R. Donald.
p. ; cm.
Includes bibliographical references and index.
ISBN 978–0–19–022089–1 (alk. paper)
I. Starke, Jeffrey R., editor.   II. Donald, P. R. (Peter Roderick), 1943– , editor.
[DNLM: 1. Tuberculosis, Pulmonary.   2. Adolescent.   3. Child. WF 300]
RC314
616.99′500835—dc23
2015022385

3 5 7 9 8 6 4

Printed by Sheridan, USA

This book is dedicated to Katherine H.K. Hsu, M.D., Dr. Starke's mentor and one of the many unsung pioneers of the modern study of childhood tuberculosis who dedicated their careers to understanding, treating and preventing this disease.

CONTENTS

PREFACE

TUBERCULOSIS (TB) in childhood arises almost exclusively as result of infection from an adult suffering from pulmonary tuberculosis. Consequently, the occurrence of tuberculosis in a child reflects the presence of infectious cases of tuberculosis in adults within a community. Once a child is infected, the development of disease is to a large extent determined by the age of the child. During the first two to three years of life, disease will more frequently follow infection, and the consequences of infection are much more likely to be serious, in the form of tuberculous meningitis and disseminated tuberculosis and marked by a high morbidity and mortality. Between three years of age and puberty, children enjoy a period of relative protection from disease following infection. With puberty, the picture again changes, and a higher risk of disease is experienced, which is manifested by typical "adult" tuberculosis, characterized by involvement of the upper lobes of the lungs and cavitation that is likely to contribute to the further spread of tuberculosis.

It can thus be easily understood that in economically developed communities, with fewer children and fewer adults to infect children, the proportion of tuberculosis disease occurring in children will be relatively low, and it will tend to be less serious than in a developing community. It is, perhaps, a lack of appreciation of these facts, and the fact that children will usually not contribute to the spread of tuberculosis, that created the perception that tuberculosis in children was not a serious problem and that efforts towards the treatment and control of tuberculosis must be concentrated solely on sputum microscopy smear-positive adults. With luck, the problem of childhood tuberculosis would just go away in due course! The events of the last two decades and the spread of human immunodeficiency virus (HIV) infection have finally dispelled these misconceptions, and the burden that tuberculosis infection and disease among children imposes on a community, particularly a developing community and its health services, is becoming clearer. The unique features of childhood tuberculosis—that young children can become seriously ill in a very short time, that childhood tuberculosis is often associated with malnutrition, that children absorb and metabolize many drugs differently from adults, that many cases can be prevented—require a different approach to case-finding and management than that used for adults. It also is apparent from recent epidemiological studies that childhood tuberculosis is far more common than recognized previously.

As a consequence of the above developments, there is now a greater interest in childhood tuberculosis than has existed since the days of the preventorium movement in the late nineteenth and early twentieth centuries. With many health service practitioners entering the field of tuberculosis for the first time, there is now, more than ever before, a great need for practical advice, guidance, and knowledge relating to childhood tuberculosis. It is our hope that this book, written by clinicians and researchers with great experience in childhood tuberculosis, will contribute to a greater understanding of the facts related to childhood tuberculosis and thus to the better management of the disease.

We hope that readers will also notice in this book the great spectrum of disease encompassed by childhood tuberculosis: from disseminated manifestations such as miliary tuberculosis and tuberculous meningitis, to pulmonary tuberculosis indistinguishable from that occurring in adults; it could be argued that the understanding of childhood tuberculosis contains many more scientific questions that are yet to be answered than does adult tuberculosis. These questions are of fundamental importance to our understanding of tuberculosis and its treatment, management, and prevention in both adults and children. The response of the body to tuberculosis undergoes continual change, if the changes in manifestations are any measure to go by, and these imply underlying changes in the immune system. In constructing new vaccines for tuberculosis, we are therefore aiming at a continually moving target, and the consequences of this continual change have yet to be fully understood.

An issue we have attempted to address in the book is the confusing language of tuberculosis. We have used the term "tuberculosis infection" rather than "latent tuberculosis infection (LTBI)" because the word "latent" is unnecessary and actually confusing when applied to child patients, many of whom were infected recently. As a result, we use the phrase "treatment of tuberculosis infection" rather than "preventive therapy" or "chemoprophylaxis" because the latter terms do not properly emphasize the importance of treating an established infection. We think this is important, both for accuracy and to better motivate physicians and families to make treatment of tuberculosis infection a priority. Equally confusing is the language associated with tuberculosis disease. We have not used the phrase "active tuberculosis" because the meaning of "active" is both unclear and redundant. As a result, we have simplified the language to "tuberculosis infection" and "tuberculosis disease."

Finally, we would like to thank the authors who generously gave of their time and experience to write the chapters in this book. We also want to thank the army of health care workers who care for the children afflicted with tuberculosis: who find them, get them through treatment, and support their many needs. Most importantly, we want to thank the children we have cared for and the families who have allowed us to learn from them so we know how to better prevent this disease and care for the children afflicted with it in the future.

—*Jeffrey R. Starke and Peter R. Donald*

ABOUT THE EDITORS

JEFFREY R. STARKE has been the director of the Children's Tuberculosis Clinic at Ben Taub General Hospital and Texas Children's Hospital for 30 years. He has published over 110 articles and 40 chapters on childhood tuberculosis. He has served on numerous advisory and guideline writing groups for the American Academy of Pediatrics, American Thoracic Society, Infectious Disease Society of America and the World Health Organization. He is a former chairman and current member of the U.S. Centers for Disease Control and Prevention (CDC) Advisory Council for the Elimination of Tuberculosis. His wife, Joan Shook, is also a pediatrician, and all three of their children are in various stages of medical training.

PETER R. DONALD is emeritus professor in the Department of Pediatrics and Child Health of the Faculty of Health Sciences, Stellenbosch University, South Africa. Professor Donald has served as a mentor to many of the authors in this book. He has been actively involved in the assessment of antituberculosis agents in children and adults for more than twenty years and was principal investigator in 12 studies of the early bactericidal activity (EBA) of antituberculosis agents that assisted in establishing the EBA technique as a reliable, objective manner of assessing an antituberculosis agent. He retired from a full-time university appointment in 2004, but remains active in various tuberculosis research activities focused on antituberculosis drug assessment in adults and children, and various aspects of the management and treatment of childhood tuberculosis. He was awarded the gold medal of the International Union Against Tuberculosis and Lung Disease for his contribution to child lung health, and obtained an A2 rating from the National Research Foundation of South Africa in 2008 that was renewed in 2013.

ABBREVIATIONS

ANTITUBERCULOSIS DRUGS

Amikacin   AMK
Bedaquiline   BDQ
Capreomycin   CAP
Ciprofloxacin   CIP
Clofazamine   CFZ
Cycloserine   CLS
Delamanid   DLM
Ethambutol   EMB
Ethionamide   ETH
Isoniazid   INH
Kanamycin   KM
Levofloxacin   LEV
Linezolid   LNZ
Moxifloxacin   MOX
Para-aminosalicylic acid   PAS
Pretonamid   PTO
Ofloxacin   OFL
Pyrazinamide   PZA
Rifabutin   RIF
Rifampin [rifampicin]   RMP
Rifapentine   RPT
Streptomycin   SM
Terizidone   TZD
Thiacetazone   THI

OTHER TERMS

Antiretroviral therapy   ARV
Bacille Calmette Guerin   BCG
Computerized tomography   CT
Deoxyribonucleic acid   DNA
Directly observed therapy short course   DOT
Disseminated BCG   dBCG
Drug susceptibility test[ing]   DST
Extensively drug-resistant tuberculosis   XDR
Human immunodeficiency virus   HIV
Immune reconstitution inflammatory
syndrome   IRIS
Interferon-¥ release assay   IGRA
International Union Against Tuberculosis
and Lung Disease   IUATLD

Magnetic resonance imaging   MRI
Multidrug-resistant tuberculosis   MDR-TB
Nontuberculous mycobacteria   NTM
Polymerase chain reaction   PCR
Pulmonary tuberculosis   PTB

Recombinant BCG   rBCG
Tuberculin skin test   TST
Tuberculous meningitis   TBM
World Health Organization   WHO

CONTRIBUTORS

Amina Ahmed
Department of Pediatrics
Levine Children's Hospital
Charlotte, North Carolina

Savvas Andronikou
Bristol Children's Hospital
University of Bristol
Bristol, England;
Department of Radiology
University of Cape Town
Cape Town, South Africa

Adrie Bekker
Department of Pediatrics and Child Health
Stellenbosch University
Cape Town, South Africa

Mark F. Cotton
Department of Pediatrics and Child Health
Division of Infectious of Diseases
Stellenbosch University
Cape Town, South Africa

Andrea T. Cruz
Department of Pediatrics
Baylor College of Medicine
Houston, Texas

Anne-Marie Demers
Desmond Tutu TB Center
Department of Pediatrics and Child Health
Faculty of Medicine and Health Sciences
Stellenbosch University
Cape Town, South Africa

Anne Detjen
Childhood TB
UNICEF
New York, New York

N. Poorana Ganga Devi
Department of Clinical Research
National Institute for Research in
Tuberculosis
Chennai, Tamil Nadu, India

Andrew R. DiNardo
Department of Internal Medicine
Baylor College of Medicine
Houston, Texas

Kathleen D. Eisenach
Department of Pathology
University of Arkansas for Medical Sciences
Little Rock, Arkansas

Katherine Floyd
Global TB Program
World Health Organization
Geneva, Switzerland

Anthony J. Garcia-Prats
Desmond Tutu TB Center
Department of Pediatrics and Child Health
Faculty of Medicine and Health Sciences
Stellenbosch University
Cape Town, South Africa

Philippe Glaziou
Global TB Program
World Health Organization
Geneva, Switzerland

Stephen M. Graham
Center for International Child Health
University of Melbourne
Murdoch Children's Research Institute
Royal Children's Hospital
Melbourne, Australia

Malgosia Grzemska
Global TB Program
World Health Organization
Geneva, Switzerland

Beate Kampmann
Pediatric Infection, Immunity and International
Child Health
Theme Leader Vaccines and Immunity
MRC Unit–The Gambia
Department of Pediatrics
Imperial College London
London, England

Tracy N. Kilborn
Red Cross War Memorial Children's Hospital
Department of Radiology
University of Cape Town
Cape Town, South Africa

Anna M. Mandalakas
Department of Pediatrics
Baylor College of Medicine
Houston, Texas

Ben J. Marais
Department of Pediatrics and Child Health
The Children's Hospital at Westmead
University of Sydney
Sydney, Australia

Helen McIlleron
Division of Clinical Pharmacology
Department of Medicine
University of Cape Town
Cape Town, South Africa

Mark P. Nicol
Division of Medical Microbiology
University of Cape Town and National Health
Laboratory Service
Cape Town, South Africa

Ian M. Orme
Department of Microbiology, Immunology, and
Pathology
Colorado State University
Fort Collins, Colorado

Carlos M. Perez-Velez
Division of Infectious Diseases
Banner–University Medical Center
University of Arizona College of Medicine
Phoenix, Arizona

Helena Rabie
Division of Infectious Diseases
Department of Pediatrics and Child Health
Tygerberg Hospital
Stellenbosch University
Cape Town, South Africa

Mario C. Raviglione
Global TB Program
World Health Organization
Geneva, Switzerland

H. Simon Schaaf
Desmond Tutu TB Center
Department of Pediatrics and Child Health
Faculty of Medicine and Health Sciences
Stellenbosch University
Cape Town, South Africa

James Seddon
Department of Pediatrics
Imperial College London
London, England

Charalambos Sismanidis
Global TB Program
World Health Organization
Geneva, Switzerland

Kim Connelly Smith
Department of Pediatrics
The University of Texas Health Science Center at Houston
Houston, Texas

Soumya Swaminathan
National Institute for Research in Tuberculosis
Chennai, Tamil Nadu, India

Ronald van Toorn
Pediatrics and Child Health
Stellenbosch University
Cape Town, South Africa

Andrew C. Whitelaw
Division of Medical Microbiology
Department of Pathology
Faculty of Medicine and Health Sciences
Stellenbosch University
National Health Laboratory Service
Tygerberg Hospital
Cape Town, South Africa

Elizabeth Whittaker
Pediatric Infection, Immunity and International Child Health
MRC Unit
The Gambia
Imperial College of London
London, England

Heather J. Zar
Department of Pediatrics and Child Health
MRC Unit on Child and Adolescent Health
Red Cross War Memorial Children's Hospital
University of Cape Town
Cape Town, South Africa

1

A BRIEF HISTORY OF CHILDHOOD TUBERCULOSIS

Peter R. Donald

TUBERCULOSIS IN childhood is an inevitable consequence of the presence of tuberculosis in any community, and archeological evidence of the occurrence of tuberculosis in children in early societies of Europe, Africa, and the Americas is provided by the skeletons of children that show signs of osteo-articular tuberculosis.[1] In some instances, molecular biology has detected the presence of specific DNA in these skeletal remains, confirming the role of *Mycobacterium tuberculosis*.[2,3] Despite many references in ancient texts to probable tuberculosis occurring in different populations throughout the world,[4] it was only relatively recently that tuberculosis in children was comprehensively studied and its clinical features and epidemiology shown to differ, in many respects, from findings in adults.

THE AGE OF POST-MORTEMS

From approximately the sixteenth century, an epidemic of tuberculosis engulfed Europe, then started to decline, as evidenced by data from European cities, from approximately the middle of the eighteenth century. Other industrializing cities in the Americas, Asia, and Australasia were similarly affected.[5] Under these conditions, primary infection nearly always occurred early in childhood, and mortality as a result of tuberculosis in the very young was higher than at any other period of life[6]; it was the conduct of post-mortem studies in these children dying of tuberculosis, coupled with the astute observations of clinicians, that first broadened our understanding of the pathogenesis of tuberculosis in children, but also in adults.

From 1800, in the aftermath of the French revolution, Paris emerged as a center of scientific medical research underpinned by regular post-mortems, allowing clinical findings and experience to be coupled to post-mortem findings. Foremost amongst the researchers regarding tuberculosis was René Laénnec (1781–1826), who is best known for his invention of the stethoscope, which assisted him in correlating clinical observations with post-mortem findings. He described his experience in a treatise "De L'Auscultation médiate" and stated that the basic lesion of tuberculosis was the tubercle, and that this was "the true anatomical character of consumption."[7] He demonstrated that tuberculosis could take many forms, but that all these manifestations in different organs were essentially the same disease. He was also well aware of the features of tuberculosis in children and stated, "The tuberculous matter is more often found (in children) in the bronchial glands and sometimes when there are no tubercles in the lungs or other serious involvement of these organs. This is particularly so in scrofulous children." Thus he was aware of the main features of primary tuberculosis in children, but he incorrectly attributed disease in the lungs to spread of disease from the mediastinal nodes.

In 1868, Jean-Antoine Villemin (1827–1892) in a treatise, "Etudes sur la tuberculosis," demonstrated that, whatever its cause, tuberculosis was infectious, and he described the successful production of tuberculosis lesions in rabbits with material from tuberculosis patients and cattle, and was then able to transfer the disease from rabbits to rabbits.[8] A major turning point was reached in 1882, when Robert Koch astounded the world with the announcement that he had discovered the cause of tuberculosis—a specific micro-organism, *Mycobacterium tuberculosis*.[9]

Joseph Marie-Jules Parrot (1829–1883) (Figure 1.1) was the son of a physician and qualified in medicine in Paris in 1857. He made a point of relating clinical experience to pathology findings. After gaining experience at the Hospice des Enfants-Assistés, he concentrated on the diseases of children and became one of the pioneers of pediatrics.[10] A significant step forward in the understanding of the pathogenesis of childhood tuberculosis was made on October 28, 1876, when Parrot's findings, following a series of 145 post-mortems carried out on children aged one to seven years with tuberculosis, were presented at the Societé de Biologie in Paris. Claude Bernard presided over the meeting, and the official report of Parrot's findings appeared in *Comptes Rendus de la Societé de Biologie (Paris)*[10]:

M. Parrot communicated the results of his researches into the relationship between the pulmonary lesions and those in the tracheo-bronchial glands . . . whenever a bronchial gland is the site of a tuberculous lesion there is an analogous lesion in the lung. . . . The pulmonary lesion may be very difficult to find and this is the reason why it's existence has been denied; there are cases in which it is no larger than a pin's head.[11]

Parrot was later appointed professor of child health, but he never published a formal scientific report of his experience. His name is perpetuated in Parrot's Law: "The nodes are the mirror of the lungs."

Parrot's work was continued by a pupil, Victor-Henri Hutinel (1849–1933), and it was one of Hutinel's pupils, George Küss (1867–1936) who in 1898 published an extensive monograph, "De L'Hérédité parasitaire del la tuberculose humaine."[12] Küss focussed on the question of whether tuberculosis was hereditary, or acquired following infection, but his findings left little doubt about the association between the tuberculosis focus in the lungs and the lymph nodes draining the relevant lung area. The relationship between the pulmonary focus, which he identified as being usually sub-pleural, and the tracheobronchial nodes demonstrated that tuberculosis probably resulted from an aerogenous infection by *M. tuberculosis* and was not the consequence of a congenital infection that had been lurking in the mediastinal lymph nodes.

In Vienna in the early twentieth century, as in most major European cities, tuberculosis was very common, and it is not surprising that Viennese researchers provided a more complete view of the pathology of childhood tuberculosis. Heinrich Albrecht (1866–1922) worked at St. Anne's Hospital in Vienna and published his findings following a series of post-mortems carried out on 3,213 children, of whom 1,060 (33%) had active tuberculosis.[13] On the basis of his findings, he agreed that tuberculosis infection was aerogenous and found a primary focus on post-mortem in nearly every case of childhood tuberculosis. Albrecht discussed his findings and their implications with his colleague Anton Ghon (1866–1936), who became, probably, the person best known in the English-speaking world regarding the pathogenesis of childhood tuberculosis. Ghon studied medicine at the University of Graz and in 1902 became Professor Extraordinarius in Pathology in Vienna. In 1903, he began the studies that have entrenched his name in the medical literature.[14] Between July 1907 and December 1909, he participated in 747 autopsies on children dying at St. Anne's Hospital, conducting 644 (86%) of these autopsies himself.

Among these children, 184 had tuberculosis, and Ghon divided the cases into two groups:

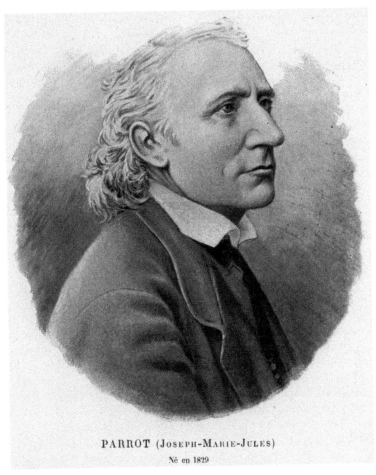

FIGURE 1.1   Joseph Marie-Jules Parrot (1829–1883). French pediatrician responsible for the first comprehensive description of the primary tuberculosis focus and complex in children.

Group A consisted of 170 children in whom a respiratory primary focus was found, and Group B of 14 in whom no respiratory focus was evident. Three of these latter children had obvious tuberculosis of the tracheobronchial nodes but no respiratory focus; in four children, intestinal tuberculosis was found, but also involvement of the mediastinal nodes; in five children, a focus outside of the respiratory system was identified and two children were tuberculin-positive, but no focus was found. Ghon concluded: "I saw no case in which the changes [in the lungs] from a patho-anatomical point of view were in a later stage of development than those of the adjoining lymphatic glands ... the lung focus cannot have originated in any retrograde sense from the lymphatic glands."[15]

In all of his writings, Ghon was at considerable pains to draw attention to the work of his predecessors and colleagues, and he made no claims that his findings were in any sense original. "The conception of the primary complex in tuberculosis originated with Ranke,[16] who designated by this term the 'definitely circumscribed' picture consisting of the primary focus of infection and the changes in the regional lymph nodes." Ghon added,

The basis for the teaching of the primary tuberculous focus lies in the law of Parrot, according to which every lung infection in the virgin body of the child shows itself likewise in the regional lymph nodes. It was Küss, chiefly, who made a detailed study of the law of Parrot and established thereby the relationship between the site of the primary lung focus and the lymph node change.[17]

Ghon's monograph was translated into English by Dr. David Barty-King and published in London in 1916. This brought Ghon's work to the attention of a large English-speaking audience and, ironically, despite Ghon's disclaimers, the primary tuberculous focus and the complex now carry Ghon's name. In 1910, Ghon became Professor of Anatomical Pathology at the German University of Prague. He retired in 1935 and died shortly afterwards, in 1936. Ghon's studies of the pathology of tuberculosis were continued in Buffalo, New York, by a pupil, Dr. K. Terplan, who published an extensive monograph, "Anatomical Studies on Human Tuberculosis," in the *American Review of Tuberculosis* in 1940.[18]

Despite the work of Parrot that culminated in the studies of Anton Ghon, there were influential researchers still of the opinion that the route of tuberculosis infection was gastro-intestinal.[19,20] Part of the confusion arose from the significant presence of *Mycobacterium bovis* in many European countries that was responsible for gastrointestinal infections in many cases, but that could also, in a minority of cases, cause pulmonary tuberculosis (PTB) and disseminated forms of tuberculosis. Thus Still (1899), working in London, recorded that in 20.5% of 259 post-mortems of children dying of tuberculosis, the portal of entry was gastrointestinal[21]; in Edinburgh, Shennan (1909) reported similar findings in 28.1% of 316 children dying of tuberculosis.[22] One of the last major post-mortem studies devoted exclusively to the pathology of childhood tuberculosis was undertaken by John Blacklock, and this assisted greatly in resolving the differing roles of *M. tuberculosis* and *M. bovis* in causing disease in children.[23]

Between 1924 and 1931, Blacklock carried out 1,800 consecutive post-mortems on children at the Royal Hospital for Sick Children, Glasgow, and tuberculosis was identified in 283 (16%) cases. One of Blacklock's main aims was to identify the causative mycobacterial strain. This had particular relevance in the west of Scotland, where bovine tuberculosis was a serious problem. Of the infecting organisms identified, 63% were *M. tuberculosis*, and 37% were *M. bovis*. In contrast to many other series, 101 of the post-mortems (36%) indicated that the primary focus was abdominal; 82% of these were associated with *M. bovis* infection. Conversely, only 3% of respiratory primary infections were due to *M. bovis*, and, although the lymph nodes were shown to be tuberculous, no primary focus could be demonstrated in the lungs. Of the respiratory infections due to *M. tuberculosis*, 86% were associated with miliary spread and 71% with cerebral tuberculosis. In the case of *M. bovis* abdominal infections, only 40% were associated with miliary tuberculosis and 46% with cerebral tuberculosis. Thus it was clear that, although *M. bovis*, entering the body via the alimentary tract, could cause respiratory tuberculosis, this was unusual; however, miliary spread accompanied by tuberculous meningitis (TBM) was a common cause of death. Conversely, there was a minority of cases where *M. tuberculosis* had undoubtedly entered the body via the alimentary tract, accompanied by involvement of the mesenteric lymph nodes, confirming the occurrence of a primary infection.

In the context of post-mortem studies, mention must also be made of the Lübeck tragedy, as a result of which an interesting perspective was provided on the consequences of infection in infants. In Lübeck in 1930, live, virulent *M. tuberculosis* was inadvertently given to 251 newborn infants instead of the vaccine Bacillus Calmette-Guérin (BCG). The bacilli were administered orally on three separate occasions, and on each occasion, the children received a very large dose of virulent bacilli. Within the next four years, 72 infants (27%) died, but 175 were alive with arrested lesions. Primary lesions in the gastrointestinal tract were found in all of those who died. These were present in the small intestine in 98% of children, but nodal enlargement was also present in the cervical area in 78% of children. In only 15% of children were primary lesions present in the lungs, and in each of these cases, it was thought that bacilli had been aspirated from lesions in the mouth or pharynx.[24,25] Arnold Rich observed that these findings indicate that, although usually considered very susceptible to tuberculosis disease following infection, the infant does possess a considerable degree of native resistance.[26] It is also noteworthy that the mortality of these heavily infected children was similar to that reported by Miriam Brailey for a group of very young, infected household contacts with parenchymal lung lesions during her studies conducted at the Harriet Lane Home in Baltimore; these infants were presumably infected by very low-dose droplet infection within their homes.[27]

TRANSMISSION OF TUBERCULOSIS INFECTION

Following his demonstration that *M. tuberculosis* caused tuberculosis, Koch speculated in 1884 regarding the manner of infection transmission and stated that, when a previously healthy individual was briefly in close contact with a tuberculosis patient, expectorated sputum might be inhaled, leading to infection. He noted, however, that it was likely that such infections did not occur easily, as the sputum drops were not small and so did not remain suspended in the air for long.[28] A number of researchers then took up the challenge of establishing exactly how infection occurred. Foremost among these early researchers were the German bacteriologist and hygienist Carl Flügge (1847–1923)[29,30] and the French veterinary surgeon P. Chaussé.[31,32] Very early it was shown that the largest sputum drops containing the most bacilli fell rapidly to the ground, but that the smallest droplets containing as few as one to three bacilli dried rapidly and could remain suspended in room air for up to five hours. These droplets became known as "Flügge droplets." When guinea pigs were placed in close proximity to coughing tuberculosis patients, they could become infected, even after only a short period of exposure, and typical primary foci were found on post-mortem.[31,32] It was also considered likely that, to negotiate the multiple twists and turns of the bronchi and bronchioli lined with a damp mucosa, only the smallest droplets would be able to penetrate as far as the alveoli to establish an infection.

In 1931, Bruno Lange, working in Berlin, published in a series of papers, the results of investigations in different animal models, including guinea pigs, mice, rabbits, and sheep, regarding their susceptibility to aerogenous infection with *M. tuberculosis*.[33,34,35] Infections were established by tracheal intubation with very low numbers of bacilli, and on later post-mortem, only a single primary focus was found in infected animals, which accorded with the findings of many post-mortem studies in children. He stated emphatically that the airways constitute a complicated filter, and that only very small expectorated drops could be inhaled to the very ends of the airways; it was thus unlikely that infectious particles could contain more than one to three bacilli. Arnold Rich, in his classic tome *The Pathogenesis of Tuberculosis*, discusses this subject at length[36]; he conceded that reference to "massive infection" is inappropriate, but had little doubt that droplets containing as many as 300 bacilli could readily pass into the terminal bronchioles, thus disputing Bruno Lange's claim that only the finest droplets containing no more than three bacilli are responsible for aerogenous tuberculosis infection.[34] As Rich points out, this is a very relevant matter regarding pathogenesis as, if only one bacillus is inhaled, four cell divisions will produce a population of 16 bacilli, whereas an infecting dose of 100 bacilli would produce a population of 1,600 bacilli, constituting a much stronger challenge to the innate immune system. A long series of subsequent studies has supported Lange's claims that only very small particles containing no more than three bacilli are capable of reaching the alveoli.[37,38,39] More recent animal studies have again replicated the process of low-dose infection and the establishment of typical primary infections followed by hematogenous spread of mycobacteria.[40,41]

THE DISCOVERY OF TUBERCULIN AND X-RAYS

Following his demonstration in 1882 that *M. tuberculosis* was the cause of tuberculosis,[9] Robert Koch attempted to develop a cure for tuberculosis. This led him to the evaluation of tuberculin, which he extracted from heat-concentrated cultures of *M. tuberculosis*.[42] Although tuberculin failed to cure tuberculosis, Clemens von Pirquet recognized its potential as a diagnostic test and described the cutaneous scratch test.[43] In 1908, Charles Mantoux refined the tuberculin test further by administering the tuberculin at first subcutaneously, and later by intradermal injection.[44] With the aid of the tuberculin test, it now became possible to detect not only tuberculosis disease, but also tuberculosis infection.

In 1895, Röntgen announced his discovery of X-rays,[45] and by 1898, Theodore Escherich, Professor Extraordinaire and director of St. Anne's Hospital in Graz, had gathered sufficient funds to buy one of the new radiology machines and gained sufficient experience with this revolutionary technique and its use in children to write a monograph on the subject.[46] In this he drew attention to the difficulty of interpreting the mediastinal shadows in young children, something that still troubles even the most experienced clinicians and radiologists. In 1902, Escherich was appointed director of St. Anne Children's Hospital in Vienna and established the use of radiology in pediatrics. One of Escherich's pupils in Vienna was Clemens von Pirquet, who in

1907 published the results of an evaluation of tuberculin sensitivity in children admitted to Escherich's clinic in Vienna.[47] At that time socioeconomic conditions in Vienna were particularly poor, and by the age of 10 years, close to 80% of children were already tuberculosis-infected.

Testing all children admitted to the clinic, von Pirquet showed that in very young hospitalized children, a positive tuberculin test was nearly always associated with disease, but that among the older age groups, there were increasing numbers of children who were tuberculosis-infected, but only a minority were diseased (Figure 1.2). He used the term *latent tuberculosis* to describe the children infected, but disease-free. The availability of chest radiographs and findings similar to those of von Pirquet made a dramatic impact on perceptions of childhood tuberculosis. Whereas the prognosis of childhood tuberculosis was previously regarded as dismal, it was now apparent that the components of the primary complex and its complications were radiologically visible in the great majority of children following primary infection, and that these children had minimal symptoms and clinical signs, if any. Nonetheless, it was also evident that very young children and adolescents were subject to a considerable risk of disease following infection. Radiology and tuberculin testing also enabled a number of observations documenting the finer details of the pathogenesis and natural history of tuberculosis.

Herbert Assman (1882–1950), a clinician working in Leipzig, was frequently consulted by adolescents and young adults complaining of an upper respiratory infection, cough, sweating, and loss of appetite with, sometimes, acid-fast bacilli in their sputum.[48] On chest radiology they had a round, well defined, sub-apical shadow (The Assman Focus), while the apices where free of any visible lesion. The great majority of these lesions were transitory and followed by full recovery with a generally good prognosis; the lesion became known as "Fruhinfiltrat" in the German literature. Very often the infiltrates disappeared completely, but they might leave a residue of radiologically visible markings or progress rapidly to cavitation followed by extensive lung involvement. Arnold Rich, discussing this entity, concedes the undoubted existence of these lesions as a radiological entity, but added that pathology suggests several options for their origins, and after experience with post-mortem findings concluded, "infection of the sub-apical region of the lung in adult PTB may arise (a) by continuous, downward extension of an apical lesion (not visible on chest radiology); (b) by aspiration of bacilli from a small apical lesion; or (c) by direct exogenous or hematogenous infection of the subapical region in the absence of apical involvement."[49] From the perspective of childhood tuberculosis, these lesions would be seen in adolescents as a form of "adult-type" tuberculosis.

Closely associated with the concept of the Assman Focus were foci in the lung apices described by George Simon that became known as Simon Foci.[50] Simon considered that these lesions, single, or in many cases multiple, were probably of hematogenous origin as they often appeared shortly after primary infection, but unlike primary foci were nearly always localized in the apices. These could, of course, reactivate at any time, and could constitute one source of adult-type disease arising in adolescence.

French clinicians were probably the first to describe the spontaneous resolution of lung

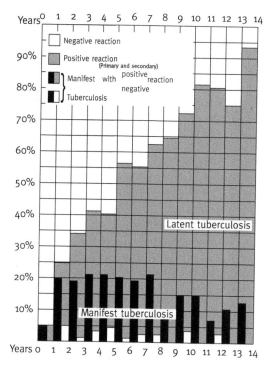

FIGURE 1.2   The results of cutaneous tuberculin testing by Clemens von Pirquet in 1,407 children admitted to the clinic of Theodore Escherich in Vienna, 1907–1908.

Reproduced from the *Journal of the American Medical Association*, 1907;52:675–678.

consolidation in patients with tuberculosis.[51] In 1919, Kleinschmidt described the resolution of extensive "exudates" seen on chest radiography in children with tuberculosis.[52] Shortly afterwards, Helène Eliasberg and Willy Neuland, working in Berlin, reported their finding of extensive lung shadowing in several tuberculin-positive children.[53] More important, and mystifying, was the apparent good health of these children and the fact that these extensive lesions, which often involved the upper or middle lobes, tended to regress spontaneously. They coined the term *epituberculosis* for this entity, being unwilling to accept that there was a real tuberculous process present in these children. A vigorous controversy followed as to the true nature of these exudates, some favoring atelectasis as their basis, others advocating a non-tuberculous pyogenic infection. It soon became apparent that, although atelectasis might have a role in certain cases, atelectasis alone could not explain all of the features of this condition. Following an extensive review of the then-existing literature, Reichle (1933) came to the conclusion that these lesions were "probably tuberculous pneumonias which have stopped short of caseation."[54] Pathologically, the common features of epituberculosis were summarized as (1) the presence of "cells of types characteristic of a tuberculous lesion (granuloma), that is to say, epithelioid cells and typical Langhans giant cells and (2) tubercle bacilli [that] were either absent or very few in number in the affected tissue.". Arnold Rich stated in this respect, "The tubercle may resolve and be completely absorbed leaving no trace. This can only occur before connective tissue appears, but that it can and does occur is unquestionable. We have frequently observed this remarkable phenomenon. This resolution is apparently neither preceded by, nor accompanied by necrosis."[55] Experimental work summarized by Fish and Pagel (1938) threw more light on the pathogenesis of this condition.[56] When tuberculin-sensitive rabbits were inoculated intratracheally, a radiological appearance similar to epituberculosis resulted. When the organisms used were alive, a fatal caseous pneumonia followed; when dead organisms were used, the infiltration still developed, but resolved spontaneously. They concluded: "Epituberculosis might therefore be regarded as a tuberculin reaction of the allergic lung tissue." The present-day importance of an understanding of "epituberculosis" lies, perhaps, in the field of the therapeutic trial where, even

more so than for adult tuberculosis, one should be reluctant to ascribe the resolution of tuberculosis lesions in children to a particular therapy, without the use of adequate controls.

THE "PRE-TUBERCULOUS" CHILD AND THE PREVENTION OF CHILDHOOD TUBERCULOSIS

Against the background of the developments described above, considerable concern developed towards the end of the nineteenth century and the early twentieth century among pediatricians and those concerned with child health regarding the fate of children infected with *M. tuberculosis*, exposed to infection or at risk of tuberculous infection and disease by virtue of poor home circumstances and malnutrition. In the introduction to a 1908 comprehensive review of tuberculosis in infancy and childhood, the editor Theophilus Kelynack drew attention to the toll exacted by childhood tuberculosis and the lack of attempts to arrest and control tuberculosis among children.[57] Evidence of tuberculosis was present in as many as 40% of children coming to post-mortem in various European countries and the United States of America. In England and Wales in 1902, deaths as result of tuberculosis in children under five years of age were 3.06/1,000; deaths as result of TBM numbered 5,961, and 68% of these occurred in children less than age five. While the importance of the "tuberculosis seed" was acknowledged, the relevance of predisposing factors was also highlighted, in particular, defective "hygienic" conditions and the proximity of open tuberculosis cases in a child's home. From these considerations, it was a short step to the development of a variety of interventions in the form of "preventoria," open-air schools and holiday camps or convalescent homes for "pretuberculous" children living in poor home circumstances or malnourished and for children already suffering from tuberculosis. In a manner similar to the alpine sanatoria developed for the management of adult tuberculosis, precise details of the structure of these institutions for the prevention and management of tuberculosis in children are provided in the compendium of Kelynack by representatives of many countries in Europe and elsewhere. Open-air classes were advised for those of school age, regular exercise and a location on the coast was to be preferred, and recommendations were even provided for where trees should be planted to keep too much wind at bay. Connoly provides graphic details of the involvement of nurses in these many and varied interventions.[58]

As time passed, skepticism emerged about the value of these measures for the treatment of "resolving parenchymal tuberculosis of first infection" in infants and children.[59] It was also pointed out that, if not properly controlled, conditions in some institutions could promote the epidemic spread of other respiratory forms of viral or bacterial infections, including tuberculosis, leading to a considerable mortality, and that the "collective care of infants is hazardous". The boarding out of eligible children in foster homes was still considered potentially advantageous and this was exemplified by the work of Prof. Jacques-Joseph Grancher (1843–1907) and his successors in France.[60] Later, Myers reported that children whose parents refused institutional care for the management of uncomplicated primary tuberculosis fared no worse in the long term than children receiving such care.[61] Despite these reservations, there can be little doubt that the emphasis on nutrition and health education of many of these interventions must have played some role in improving child health.

THE PLACE OF CHILDREN IN THE EPIDEMIOLOGY OF TUBERCULOSIS

Although it is possible to trace the presence of tuberculosis in many prehistoric and historic communities from skeletal remains and from ancient texts, these give no clues to the extent to which the disease might have influenced the relevant peoples. From the late seventeenth century, fragmentary documentation from European cities makes possible an estimation of the numbers of people dying from what was probably tuberculosis.[5] However, these estimates seldom provide an indication of the effects of tuberculosis regarding children. Towards the end of the nineteenth century, official notification of infectious diseases such as tuberculosis became policy in many countries, and for the first time, a more detailed picture began to emerge of the toll exacted by tuberculosis, the different forms of tuberculosis that affect young children as opposed to adults, and the influence of gender.

It was immediately obvious that age had a significant effect upon mortality, and this is, perhaps, best illustrated by the work of Wade Hampton Frost. In a classic paper, Frost explored the epidemiology of tuberculosis making use of the tuberculosis mortality rates for Massachusetts for 1880 through 1930.[6] In the introduction, he refers to the well-established age-related curve of tuberculosis mortality and points out that, for every shift in the mortality rate, there is probably a shift in balance between host resistance and "the destructive forces of the invading tubercle bacillus". In his conclusion, he highlights the consistency of the picture of relative mortality that emerges, of high susceptibility in the very young declining to low levels in the school-age child, but then increasing in adolescents and peaking in young adults, which suggests "rather constant physiological changes in resistance (with age) as the controlling factor."

From a pediatric viewpoint, it is significant that, in the earliest data that Frost presented, up to approximately 1900, tuberculosis mortality in the very young was higher than at any other time of life. A similar high annual mortality in the very young was reported from England and Wales for the period from 1891 to 1900, where close to 400/100,000 deaths occurred in children under five years of age as result of tuberculosis[62] (Figure 1.3). Under these epidemic conditions, there was also a noticeable predominance of males dying from tuberculosis

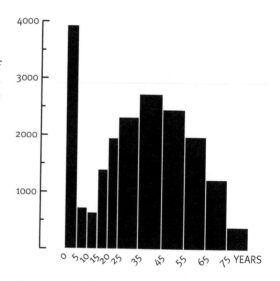

FIGURE 1.3   The average annual mortality from tuberculosis, per million living at each age period, in England and Wales, 1891–1900. (Cobbet 1910; from figures published in the "Supplement to the Sixty-fifth Annual Report of the Registrar-General, 1907," part I, cxciii.)

Reproduced from the *Journal of Pathology and Bacteriology*, 1910;14:563–604.

amongst the very young, but of females during adolescence. When these statistics are viewed from the perspective of a particular cohort, these tendencies are even more pronounced; thus, the mortality for males 0–4 years for Frost's cohort of 1880 was 760/100,000, declining to 43 for the group 5–9 years old; and then rising to 115 and 288 for the groups 10–19 and 20–29 years of age; before declining for those 30–39 and 40–49, to 253 and 175, respectively; and finally to 127 for the age group 50–59 years old. The large proportion of children in the affected populations, combined with the close household contact resulting from poor socioeconomic conditions and the exquisite susceptibility of the very young to disseminated serious forms of tuberculosis such as miliary tuberculosis and tuberculous meningitis, no doubt played a role in this distressing picture. As socioeconomic conditions improved and family sizes declined, these prominent features of the age-related incidence curve of tuberculosis changed dramatically; by 1930, the annual mortality of tuberculosis in young children in Massachusetts was lower than at any other time in life, although the peak for young adults of approximately 25 years of age remained at just below 100/100,000.

Accurate data are also available from New York for the period from 1898 to 1923 and sketch a picture of the ravages of tuberculosis among the very young, unfortunately a picture that is still all too familiar to practitioners in the cities of developing countries.[63] In 1898, tuberculosis mortality among children under age 15 years was 136/100,000; the major causes of death were TBM with a rate of 78/100,000, and PTB with a rate of 31/100,000. When one looks at infants only, however, a much a higher death rate for all forms of tuberculosis of 609/100,000 is seen, with a rate for TBM of 353/100,000. In this, and in many subsequent analyses of childhood tuberculosis mortality, TBM remains responsible for more than 50% of childhood tuberculosis deaths, irrespective of socioeconomic circumstances; thus, by 1959, in the United States, Great Britain, and France, 55%, 61%, and 68% of tuberculosis deaths in children, respectively, resulted from TBM.[64]

In the Netherlands, not only was accurate tuberculosis mortality data available from 1900–1945, but regular tuberculin testing of groups of young children allowed calculation of the annual risk of infection.[65] These data were then combined with mortality data and the annual risk of infection correlated with the causes of tuberculosis mortality in different age groups; importantly, in children, TBM was the major cause of death, particularly in the very young and was closely correlated with the annual risk of infection. More recent experience produced very similar findings in the Western Cape Province of South Africa.[66]

CONCLUSION

By approximately 1920, the broad facts underlying the manner of infection and anatomical features of tuberculosis in children and its epidemiology were established, and it now remained for concerned and persistent clinicians to make use of the tools of chest radiology and tuberculin testing to establish more precisely the natural history of tuberculosis infection in children and its long-term consequences. This subject is dealt with in Chapter 5.

REFERENCES

1. Zimmerman MR. Pulmonary and osseous tuberculosis in an Egyptian mummy. *Bull NY Acad Med.* 1979;55:604–608.
2. Salo W, Aufderheide AC, Buikstra J, Holcomb TA. Identification of *Mycobacterium tuberculosis* DNA in a pre-Columbian Peruvian mummy. *Proc Natl Acad Sci.* 1994;91:2091–2094.
3. Hlavenková L, Teasdale MD, Gábor O, et al. Childhood bone tuberculosis from Roman Pécs, Hungary. *Homo.* 2015 Feb;66(1):27–37 doi: 10.1016/j.jchb.2014.10.001.
4. Daniel TM. The history of tuberculosis. *Resp Med.* 2006;100:1862–1870.
5. Grigg ERN. The arcana of tuberculosis. *Am Rev Tuberc Lung Dis.* 1958;78:151–172, 426–453, 583–603.
6. Frost WH. The age selection of mortality from tuberculosis in successive decades. *Am J Hyg.* 1939;30:91–96.
7. Sakula A. Laënnec RTH 1781–1826. His life and work: a bicentenary appreciation. *Thorax.* 1981;36:81–90.
8. Villemin JA. *Etudes sur la tuberculosis.* Paris: J. B. Baillière et Fils, 1868.
9. Koch R. Die Aetiologie der Tuberkulose. *Berl Klin Wchnschr.* 1882;19:221–230.
10. Werner EG, Haage BD, Keil G, Wegner W. Parrot, Joseph Marie Jules. In: *Enzyklopädie Medizingeschichte.* Berlin: Walter de Gruyter, 2005.
11. Anonymous. Tuberculosis eponyms. *Ipsissima verba*—Parrot's nodes—Parrot's law. *Tubercle.* 1948;29:136.

12. Küss G. *De L'Hérédité parasitaire de la tuberculose humaine*. Paris, Asselin et Houzeau, 1898.

13. Albrecht H. Ueber Tuberkulose des Kindesalters. *Wien Klin Wchnschr*. 1909;22:327–334.

14. Ober WB. Ghon but not forgotten: Anton Ghon and his complex. *Pathol Annual* 1983;2:79–85.

15. Ghon A. *Der primäre Lungenherd bei der Tuberkulose der Kinder*. Berlin & Vienna: Urban & Schwarzenberg; 1912.

16. Ranke KE. Primare, sekundare and tertiare Tuberkulose des Menschen. *Münch Med Wchnschr* 1917;64:305–308.

17. Ghon A. *The Primary Lung Focus of Tuberculosis in Children*. London: Churchill; 1916.

18. Terplan K. Anatomical studies on human tuberculosis. *Am Rev Tuberc*. 1940;42 (Suppl 2):3–176.

19. Calmette A. *Tubercle Bacillus Infection and Tuberculosis in Man and Animals*. Baltimore, MD: Williams and Williams Co.; 1923.

20. von Behring E. Ueber Lungenschwindsuchtenstehung und Tuberkulose kampfüng. *Deutsche Med Wchnschr*. 1903;29:689.

21. Still GF. Observations on the morbid anatomy of tuberculosis in childhood, with special reference to the primary channels of infection. *Brit Med J*. 1899;2:455–458.

22. Shennan T. Tuberculosis in children. A statistical examination. *Edin Hosp Rep*. 1900;6:130–145.

23. Blacklock JWS. Tuberculous disease in children. Its pathology and bacteriology. Medical Research Council Special Report Series No. 172. London: His Majesty's Stationery Office; 1932.

24. Schürmann P. Die anatomischen Befunde bei den in Lübeck verstorben Saügglingen. *Verh D Deutsch Path Gesellsch*. 1931;26:265–272.

25. Schürmann P. Beobachtungen bei den Lübecker Säuglingstuberkulosen. *Beitr z Klin Tuberk*. 1932;81:294–300.

26. Rich AR. *The Pathogenesis of Tuberculosis*. 2nd ed. Springfield: Charles Thomas; 1951:119–148.

27. Brailey M. Mortality in tuberculin-positive infants. *Bull Johns Hopkins Hosp*. 1936;59:1–10.

28. Koch R. Die Aetiologie der Tuberkulose. *Mittheilungen aus dem Kaiserlichen Gesundheitsamte*. 1884;2:1–88.

29. Fluegge C. Ueber Luftinfection. *Ztschr f Hyg*. 1897;25:179–224.

30. Fluegge C. Die Bedeutung der Verstreuung von husten Tröpfchen fur die Verbreitung der Phthise. *Ztschr f Tuberk*. 1921;34:212–228.

31. Chaussé P. Teneur bacillaire et conditions de pulvérisabilité de la salive et des crachats tuberculeux, par les courants aériens. *Ann Inst Pasteur*. 1914a;28:608–638.

32. Chaussé P. Le tuberculeux: peut-il émettre des particules liquides respirables? *Ann Inst Pasteur*. 1914b;28:720–745.

33. Lange B. Tierexperimentele Untersuchungen über die Bedeutung von Infektionsdosis, naturlicher Resistenz und erworbener Immunität für Entstehung und Verlauf der Tuberkuloser 1. *Zeitschr Tuberkulose*. 1931;61:44–55.

34. Lange B. Tierexperimentele Untersuchungen über die Bedeutung von Infektionsdosis, naturlicher Resistenz und erworbener Immunität für Entstehung und Verlauf der Tuberkuloser. 2. *Zeitschr Tuberkulose*. 1931;61:97–112.

35. Lange B. Tierexperimentele Untersuchungen über die Bedeutung von Infektionsdosis, naturlicher Resistenz und erworbener Immunität für Entstehung und Verlauf der Tuberkuloser. Schluss. *Zeitschr Tuberkulose*. 1931;61:177–188.

36. Rich AR. *The Pathogenesis of Tuberculosis*. 2nd ed. Springfield, IL: Charles Thomas; 1951:823–896.

37. Wells WF. On air-borne infection. II. Droplets and droplet nuclei. *Am J Hyg*. 1934;20:611–618.

38. Ratcliffe HL, Palladino VS. Tuberculosis induced by droplet nuclei infection: initial homogenous response of small mammals (rats, mice, guinea pigs, and hamsters) to human and to bovine bacilli and patterns of tubercle development. *J Exper Med*. 1953;97:61–68.

39. Riley RL, Mills CC, Nyaka W, et al. Aerial dissemination of pulmonary tuberculosis. A two year study of contagion in a tuberculosis ward. *Am J Hyg*. 1959;70:185–196.

40. Balasubramian V, Wiegeshaus EH, Taylor BT, Smith DW. Pathogenesis of tuberculosis: pathway to apical localization. *Tubercle Lung Dis*. 1994;75:168–178.

41. McMurray DN. Hematogenous reseeding of the lung in low-dose, aerosol-infected guinea pigs: unique features of the host-pathogen interface in secondary tubercles. *Tuberculosis*. 2003;83:131–134.

42. Koch R. Weitere Mittheilungen uber ein Heilmittel gegen Tuberkulose. *Deutsch Med Wschr*. 1891;17:101–102.

43. von Pirquet C. Demonstration zur Tuberculin diagnose durch Hautimpfung. *Berl Med Wchsr*. 1907;48:699.

44. Mantoux C. Intra-dermo-réaction de la tuberculine. *Comptes rendus de l'Académie des Sciences*. 1908;147:355–357.

45. Röentgen W. Ein neue Art von Strahlen. *Sitzungsberichte d Physikalish-medizinischen Gessellschaft zu Wurzburg*. 1895;9:132–141.

46. Escherich T. La valeur diagnostique de la radiographie chez les enfants. *Rev de mal de l'enf.* 1898;16:233–242.

47. Von Pirquet C. Frequency of tuberculosis in childhood. *JAMA.* 1907;52:675–678.

48. Assman H. Uber eine typische Form isolierter tuberkulöser Lungenherde im klinische Begin der Erkrankung. *Beitr Klin Tuberk.* 1925;60:522–539.

49. Rich AR. *The Pathogenesis of Tuberculosis.* 2nd ed. Springfield, IL: Charles Thomas; 1951:119–148.

50. Simon G. Die Tuberkulose der Lungenspitzen. *Beitrage klin Tuberk.* 1927;67:467–476.

51. Neumann W. Die kliniese Auffasung der Tuberkulose im Lichte der französichen Forschung. *Ergebn d ges Tuberk.* 1931;2:253–273.

52. Kleinschmidt H. Zur differential Diagnose der Lungentuberkulose beim kinde. *Zschr artz Fortbild.* 1919;16:217–223.

53. Eliasberg H, Neuland W. Zur Klinik der epituberkülosen Infiltration der kindlichen Lunge. *Jahrb für Kinderheilkunde.* 1920;93:102–118.

54. Reichle HS. Resolving exudates in pulmonary tuberculosis of childhood. *Am J Dis Child.* 1933;45:307–330.

55. Rich AR. *The Pathogenesis of Tuberculosis.* 2nd ed. Springfield, IL: Charles Thomas; 1951.

56. Fish RH, Pagel W. The morbid anatomy of epituberculosis. *J Path Bact.* 1938;47:593–601.

57. Kellynack TN, ed. *Tuberculosis in Infancy and Childhood.* New York: William Wood and Company; 1908.

58. Connoly C. Pale, poor, and "pretubercular" children: a history of pediatric antituberculosis efforts in France, Germany, and the United States, 1899–1929. *Nurs Inq.* 2004;11:138–147.

59. Stewart CA. The prognosis and treatment of resolving parenchymal tuberculosis of first infection in infants and children. *Am Rev Tuberc.* 1932;26:597–613.

60. Kayne GG. The prevention of tuberculosis in childhood by methods of separation. *Tubercle.* 1935;16:541–560.

61. Myers JA. The natural history of tuberculosis in the human body. 1. The demonstrable primary pulmonary infiltrate. *Am Rev Tuberc.* 1959;79:19–30.

62. Cobbet L. The portals of entry of the tubercle bacilli which cause phthisis. *J Path Bact.* 1910;14:563–604.

63. Drolet GJ. Tuberculosis in children. *Am Rev Tuberc.* 1925;11:292–303.

64. Drolet GJ, Lowell AM. Tuberculosis mortality among children: last stage. *Dis Chest.* 1962;42:364–371.

65. Styblo K, Sutherland I. The epidemiology of tuberculosis in children. *Bull Int Union Tuberc.* 1982;57:133–139.

66. Berman S, Kibel MA, Fourie PB, Strebel MP. Childhood tuberculosis and tuberculous meningitis in the Western Cape of South Africa. *Tubercle Lung Dis.* 1992;73:349–355.

2

MICROBIOLOGY AND PATHOLOGY OF TUBERCULOSIS

Anne-Marie Demers, Andrew C. Whitelaw, and Kathleen D. Eisenach

HIGHLIGHTS OF THIS CHAPTER

- Caseating granulomas are the hallmark of the histopathological response to *M. tuberculosis*, especially in lymph nodes, which are usually a prominent part of the disease complex.
- Transport and handling of clinical specimens is particularly important for children because the bacilli are usually sparse.
- Because most forms of tuberculosis in children are paucibacillary, acid-fast stains of clinical samples are usually negative, and positive stains can be caused by nontuberculous mycobacteria.
- Gene Xpert MTB/RIF (rifampicin) is more sensitive than acid-fast microscopy when performed on respiratory samples from children, but both are less sensitive than culture.
- Both phenotypic and genotypic drug susceptibility testing are available, but discordance between them may occur because less-common mutations that confer resistance are detected only by phenotypic testing.

MYCOBACTERIOLOGY/ TAXONOMY

The genus *Mycobacterium* is the sole member of the family *Mycobacteriaceae*, which in turn is part of the order *Actinomycetales*. Mycobacteria are aerobic, non-spore-forming, nonmotile, and slightly curved or straight rods (0.2 to 0.6 μm by 1.0 to 10 μm). Compared to other bacteria, mycobacteria are characterized by their complex cell wall containing mycolic acids, and a genome with a high guanine plus cytosine (G+C) content.[1] Their high-lipid cell wall structure makes them hard to stain with dyes routinely used in bacteriology, such as the Gram stain. When stained with special procedures (e.g., Ziehl-Neelsen staining), they are not easily decolorized, even by acid alcohol, hence they are referred to as acid-fast or acid/alcohol-fast.[1]

More than 120 mycobacterial species have now been recognized, and more are constantly described.[2,3] Mycobacteria are grouped into members of the *Mycobacterium tuberculosis* complex (MTBC) and the nontuberculous mycobacteria (NTM) (also previously referred to as mycobacteria other than TB [MOTT] or atypical mycobacteria). *M. leprae* and *M. ulcerans* are often considered separately because of their distinct clinical and laboratory characteristics. Members of the MTBC include *M. tuberculosis*, *M. africanum*, *M. bovis*, *M. bovis* BCG, *M. microti*, *M. caprae*, *M. pinnipedii*, the dassie bacillus, and more recently *M. mungi*, *M. orygis*, and *M. suricattae*.[3-6] *M. canettii* is closely related to the complex but grows as smooth colonies instead of the typical rough colonies of the other MTBC members. The members of the MTBC display greater than 99.95% nucleotide sequence similarity at the genome level.[3] Of the MTBC, most human disease is due to *M. tuberculosis*, and the reservoir for *M. tuberculosis* is humans. All members of the MTBC have a doubling time close to 24 hours, compared to 20–45 minutes for most bacteria, and thus take three to four weeks to form colonies on solid media. Mycobacteria are aerobic and grow best in an atmosphere enriched with 5–10% carbon dioxide (CO_2) when using conventional solid media.[1] Their growth is also enhanced by fatty acids, which may be provided in the form of egg yolk or oleic acid. Although optimal growth temperatures vary widely among different mycobacterial species, *M. tuberculosis* grows best at 35–37°C.[1]

PATHOGENESIS

M. tuberculosis is almost invariably transmitted via the respiratory tract. Bacilli become aerosolized in droplet nuclei (1–5 µm airborne particles) generated after people who have pulmonary or laryngeal disease cough, sneeze, shout, or sing,[7] and these droplet nuclei may then be inhaled by a child or adult in the vicinity of the infectious index case. Inhaled mycobacteria enter the alveoli and are ingested by alveolar macrophages. Complex immunological events follow, which may result in either (1) complete elimination of the mycobacterium; (2) containment of the primary infection in a granuloma for a prolonged period, known as tuberculosis infection (which may persist for the individual's lifetime, or until progression to disease occurs); or (3) immediate progression to disease, usually in the context of impaired immunity or in young children (under 5 years of age)[8] (Figure 2.1).

The primary infection consists of a small parenchymal focus (Ghon focus), associated with bacilli that have spread via local lymphatics to regional lymph nodes. The Ghon focus, together with affected regional lymph nodes (with/without overlying pleural reaction), is called the primary (Ghon) complex.[9] The characteristic lesion of the primary infection is a caseating granuloma, which is a localized lesion in tissue consisting of a central area of caseous necrosis bordered by epithelioid macrophages and lymphocytes.[10] Caseating granulomas may enlarge and progress, or may calcify and heal with fibrosis and scarring. While the organisms are

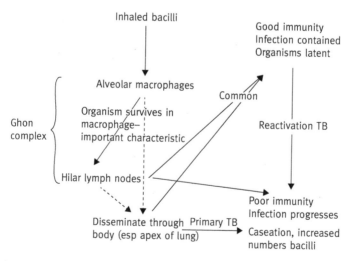

FIGURE 2.1   Pathogenesis of tuberculosis.

contained and constrained within caseating granulomas, not all are killed.

Primary infection may be associated with complications, especially in children under five years of age.[11] The parenchymal lesion may enlarge and caseate, or nodes may enlarge and compress or erode through a bronchus, causing pneumonia, atelectasis, or, more rarely, lung tissue destruction and cavity formation, invasion of the pericardium or pleural space.[12] The primary infection is usually accompanied by an occult, subclinical bacteremia that can seed distant sites, including the apices of the lungs, and cause extrapulmonary disease, particularly in the lymph nodes and the central nervous system (CNS) of children.[11] This may rapidly lead to severe forms of disease, including miliary and CNS tuberculosis. Extrapulmonary tuberculosis is more common in children than in adults.[13]

The histological aspect of caseating granulomas is similar for the primary infection in the lung as well as the secondary spread as tuberculomas in bones, brain, kidneys, lymph nodes, or other organs, in miliary tuberculosis, and in late stages of post-primary tuberculosis.[10] In most cases, the primary focus heals, and the bacteria continue to survive in a dormant state that is referred to as tuberculosis infection. Much is still unknown about the mechanisms that allow *M. tuberculosis* to survive in the host.[6,14] In a recent study using specific probes on tissue, *M. tuberculosis* was found to persist in multiple locations in the majority of persons without known tuberculosis disease. None of the organisms demonstrated was associated with granulomas, inflammatory infiltrates, or fibrosis, which challenges the traditional assumption that *M. tuberculosis* persists largely in isolated granulomatous foci.[15] In the same vein, small populations of bacilli may persist for months in a host being treated with effective drug therapy to which those bacilli are both phenotypically and genetically susceptible. Persistence seems tied to the bacilli's entering a slowly replicating or non-replicating state, but the host and bacterial conditions that enable or push a bacterium into this state are only beginning to be elucidated.[16–18]

The concentration of bacilli in the sputum depends on the type and number of tuberculous lesions from which the bacilli originate.[19,20] A 2 cm diameter cavity opening into a bronchus may contain 100 million bacilli, whereas a non-cavitated nodular lesion of the same size may contain only 100–1,000 bacilli.[21] Sputum from patients with cavitary tuberculosis have high bacillary loads, which are easier to detect in the laboratory (as detailed later). In contrast, sputum from patients with nodular or encapsulated lesions, such as those observed in childhood tuberculosis, discharge only small amounts of bacilli (hence referred to as paucibacillary) and detection of the organisms in the laboratory is much more difficult. Cavities do occur in children[12,22] but are not observed as frequently as in adults.[23]

MICROBIOLOGICAL DIAGNOSIS OF TUBERCULOSIS IN CHILDREN

Laboratory tests to diagnose tuberculosis can be grouped in two main categories[24]: (1) detection of organisms or components of organisms, which is the subject of this chapter, and (2) detection of the immune response to the organism, which is discussed in other chapters. Microbiological confirmation of tuberculosis in children is challenging for two main reasons. First, collecting specimens such as sputum from young children is typically more difficult than from adults. Second, even when sputum or other specimens are collected, they are usually paucibacillary (as described earlier), which makes detection of the organism more difficult. The high expectations that sensitive liquid culture methods and nucleic acid amplification tests (NAATs) would improve the ability to detect *M. tuberculosis* in childhood tuberculosis have not yet been met. The specimens collected are habitually of lower volumes, which can also compromise the yield: in an adult tuberculosis study, the sensitivity of an acid-fast smear from >5 ml of sputum was significantly greater than the sensitivity of a smear processed from a lower volume, as would normally be obtained from a small child.[25] Culture yield is also lower than in adults because investigations are often performed in the presence of nonspecific signs and symptoms.[26] Furthermore, a large proportion of true tuberculosis cases in children will be missed by culture.[27,28] Intrathoracic tuberculosis cases in children are rarely confirmed microbiologically,[27] defined recently for research purposes as at least one positive culture (with confirmed *M. tuberculosis* speciation) which could be sampled from expectorated sputum, induced sputum, nasopharyngeal aspirates, gastric aspirates, or string tests (or other relevant intrathoracic specimens).[26]

Notwithstanding the above concerns regarding the difficulty of confirming the diagnosis of tuberculosis in children microbiologically, there is still value in submitting specimens for microbiological testing.

- Some children with tuberculosis who have not yet been started on therapy will still be identified using laboratory tests.
- Drug susceptibility testing (DST) is becoming more important and (for the most part) requires isolation of the organism.
- Microbiological confirmation, for all its limitations, is still a vital part of research activities in tuberculosis, such as vaccine trials, treatment trials, and epidemiological surveys.

Nosocomial transmission of *M. tuberculosis* from patients or specimens is of major concern to health care workers and laboratory personnel.[1] Even if children with tuberculosis disease may be less contagious than adults, the same cannot be said for their adult caregivers if they are the source of the child's infection.[13] High-risk areas for tuberculosis transmission include spaces reserved for aerosol-generating procedures such as sputum collection areas.[7] In the laboratory, infection with *M. tuberculosis* is acquired by inhalation of *M. tuberculosis* produced by aerosols, which may be generated during processing of clinical or pathological tissue specimens, or during handling of cultured live *M. tuberculosis* for DST or other purposes.[29] A detailed discussion of infection control practices is beyond the scope of this chapter; however, infection control guidelines to minimize the risk of tuberculosis transmission are available for health-care facilities[7,30] and tuberculosis laboratories.[31]

Specimen Collection and Transport

One of the most important parameters affecting the performance of a microbiological diagnostic test is the quality of the specimen. Clinicians and pediatricians have tried to collect a broad variety of specimen types to improve the microbiological diagnosis of intrathoracic tuberculosis in children (Table 2.1). References on the most common methods of obtaining clinical specimens from children are available.[30,32,33] Specimens need to be representative of the site of infection, preferably collected aseptically, and stored and transported rapidly to the laboratory to minimize multiplication of contaminating organisms.[24] Ideally, specimens should arrive in the laboratory on the day of collection. If transport to the laboratory is delayed more than one hour, specimens should be refrigerated at 4°C as well as upon arrival in the laboratory until they are processed.[1] One study in adults showed that mycobacterial load and culture time to positivity were not significantly affected by refrigerated storage up to three days.[34] If prolonged storage or transport is unavoidable, preservatives can be added to the specimens to inhibit growth of contaminant bacteria and thus improve the yield from culture. Examples of these preservatives include sodium carbonate, cetylpyridinium chloride, and sodium borate. There are concerns that some of these compounds may not be compatible with some of the newer liquid-based culture systems such as the Bactec Mycobacteria Growth Indicator Tube (MGIT) system (Becton Dickinson Diagnostic Systems, Sparks, Md.), and they may also reduce the sensitivity of microscopy.[24] Fine-needle aspirates can be submitted in a culture medium (Middlebrook 7H9, glycerol, and Tween), which allows them to be stored for up to seven days prior to inoculation with no significant reduction in culture yield.[35] Gastric aspirates are commonly neutralized by the addition of sodium bicarbonate when collected[1,36]; however, one study has cast some doubt on this practice, finding a significant reduction in culture yield on neutralized gastric specimens.[37] More research is needed to confirm these findings. The laboratory should be contacted ahead of time for details regarding optimum collection and transport of specimens.

Processing

Processing specimens for mycobacterial culture is a complex process. Many specimens received for mycobacterial culture are viscous (particularly respiratory specimens), and some form of digestion is required, both to release mycobacteria that may be trapped in the specimen as well as to improve the decontamination process. Digestion and liquefaction of the specimen also facilitate concentration of the specimen. Since mycobacteria are usually slow growing and require long incubation times, other microorganisms (such as commensal or colonizing bacteria and fungi) can overgrow cultures of specimens obtained from non-sterile sites.[1] Specimens for microbiological investigations can be grouped according to the level of likely contamination (Table 2.2).[24] To eliminate contaminants as much as possible without affecting the viability of mycobacteria, specimens from non-sterile sites (Table 2.2, Groups 2 and 3) need to be decontaminated. This processing step is a delicate procedure: if it is too harsh, the yield is affected, as mycobacteria are also killed; if too mild, specimens will be overgrown

Table 2.1. Specimens used in the diagnosis of intrathoracic tuberculosis in children for microbiological tests

TYPE OF SPECIMEN	DESCRIPTION/FINDINGS
Gastric lavage/ aspiration	Traditionally diagnostic procedure of choice in young children unable to produce sputum. During sleep, the mucociliary mechanism of the respiratory tract sweeps mucus which may contain tubercle bacilli into the mouth. These secretions are swallowed and can be recovered in the gastric content, especially if the stomach has not emptied. Children are often hospitalized for the procedure, but it has also been successfully performed in outpatients.[36]
Expectorated sputum	Usually collected in older children who can cooperate.
Induced sputum	Another option to collect respiratory specimens in children unable to produce sputum. Sputum is collected after nebulization with hypertonic saline followed by nasopharyngeal suction. The technique has been safely performed in infants as young as 1 month of age.[93] Both ultrasonic and jet nebulizers have been used. Chest physiotherapy can also be performed to induce coughing and sputum production.[33]
Broncho-alveolar lavage (BAL) with bronchoscopy	Rarely performed in resource-poor countries. The diagnostic yield from bronchoscopy is no higher than that of gastric aspirates or induced sputum but may be useful to detect possible tracheobronchial obstruction or alternative diagnoses.[94]
Laryngeal swabs	Specimen used in older studies[95,96] but rarely if ever used in children anymore.
Nasopharyngeal aspirate	Suctioning of the nasopharynx collects upper respiratory tract secretions; stimulation of cough reflex may include lower respiratory secretions.[49]
String test	A weighted gel capsule containing a coiled nylon string is swallowed, with the trailing string held at the mouth and then taped to the cheek. Peristalsis carries the weighted capsule, which later dissolves, into the duodenum while the string unravels, extending from the mouth to stomach/duodenum. The string is left in situ for 4 hours during which it traps sputum along its length as lower respiratory tract secretions are carried up by the mucociliary escalator and spontaneously swallowed. Trapped secretions are retrieved upon withdrawal of the string and processed similar to a sputum specimen for AFB smear and culture.[97]
Fine-needle aspiration biopsy of peripheral lymphadenopathy	Children with pulmonary tuberculosis may have extrapulmonary disease manifestations in 10–30% of cases. Tuberculous lymphadenitis is the most common form of extrapulmonary disease in endemic areas, where up to 50% of extrapulmonary cases manifest as peripheral lymphadenopathy.[98] Fine-needle aspiration is a very useful adjunct to culture of respiratory specimens. The procedure may be performed safely on an outpatient basis by appropriately trained staff in a resource-limited setting.[49]
Stool	Collected on the rationale that young children tend to swallow rather than expectorate sputum, M. tuberculosis has been recovered in stool cultures after surviving the transit through the gastrointestinal tract. Stool cultures have been insensitive in general, but molecular techniques are promising.[99–102]

(continued)

Table 2.1. Continued

TYPE OF SPECIMEN	DESCRIPTION/FINDINGS
Urine	*M. tuberculosis* can be found in the urine of patients with active pulmonary tuberculosis, but the sensitivity of smear and culture is low. New diagnostic methodologies such as urine mycobacterial lipoarabinomannan (LAM) and urine mycobacterial DNA are being evaluated.[103] *M. tuberculosis* bacilli from infective foci in the lungs are destroyed by the immune response, releasing cell-free nucleic acids in plasma. The smaller sized cell-free nucleic acids pass through the kidney during filtration to produce transrenal DNA, which can be measured in urine by nucleic acid amplification techniques.[104]
Blood culture	Mycobacteremia due to *M. tuberculosis* is a common cause of bloodstream infections among HIV-infected adults in sub-Saharan Africa. However, the yield was low in among an ill, HIV-infected pediatric patient population in an area with a high tuberculosis burden, possibly due to the volume of blood collected being insufficient to recover mycobacteria.[105]
Bone marrow aspiration/biopsy	Not recommended routinely. It may assist in confirming an uncertain diagnosis of disseminated mycobacterial disease, establish an alternative diagnosis, or help rule out underlying malignancy.[106]
Cerebrospinal fluid (CSF)	A lumbar puncture should be performed in cases of suspected congenital or neonatal tuberculosis and in infants with disseminated disease.[107]

by other microorganisms, making the recovery of *M. tuberculosis* difficult. Of the various methods, the most frequently used is the NALC (N-acetyl L-cysteine)-NaOH (sodium hydroxide) method,[24] where NALC acts to digest the specimen, and NaOH decontaminates it. Briefly, an equal volume of NALC-NaOH is added to each specimen, then mixed by vortexing and left to stand for 15 minutes. Specimens are then neutralized by the addition of distilled water or phosphate buffer to reduce the continued action of the NaOH and lower the viscosity of the mixture.[38] Specimens are concentrated by centrifugation for another 15 minutes; the supernatant is discarded, and the remaining sediment (pellet) is resuspended in phosphate buffer. This resuspended pellet is then used for culture inoculation, smear microscopy, and NAATs. It has been estimated that up to one-third of the mycobacteria present in a specimen may be killed by this process, and it is possible that the NaOH concentrations used for processing specimens from adults may be inappropriate for paucibacillary specimens, such as those from children.[39] As a general rule, contamination rates of between 3% and 5% are accepted (up to 8% for broth-based culture).[40,41] Lower rates imply over-decontamination, and higher contamination rates indicate that the decontamination process is suboptimal.

Direct Tests: Smear Microscopy

Although used for more than 100 years, acid-fast bacilli (AFB) smear microscopy still plays an important role in the diagnosis of tuberculosis: (1) It can detect mycobacteria rapidly compared to culture results, which become available only after weeks of incubation; (2) it can identify the patients who are most likely to transmit *M. tuberculosis* to others; (3) it is still used in the identification work-up of positive cultures; and (4) it is often the only available diagnostic method in many developing countries. Smear microscopy is rapid, simple, inexpensive, and can be performed directly on clinical specimens. Two techniques are mainly used: carbol fuchsin stains (Ziehl-Neelsen or Kinyoun) for bright-field microscopy, and the fluorochrome stains (e.g., auramine O or auramine-rhodamine) for fluorescence microscopy (Figure 2.2).[42] Smear microscopy can detect a minimum of 5,000 to 10,000 bacilli per milliliter of sputum specimen. Given the paucibacillary nature

Table 2.2. Specimens according to level of contamination (adapted from[24])

GROUP	DESCRIPTION/EXAMPLES	DECONTAMINATION PROCEDURE
Group 1: Specimens collected aseptically from a site without commensal organisms	Specimens obtained by aspiration, biopsy, or surgical excision, and include cerebrospinal fluid, lymph node aspirates, aspirates from abscesses, bone marrow and joint aspirates, as well as tissue biopsies	These specimens do not require a decontamination procedure: they are inoculated directly onto the culture media (after centrifugation if necessary)
Group 2: Specimens are secretions from parts of the body with no or minimal commensal organisms, but connected to the body's surface by means of an open connection that harbors commensal organisms. These commensal organisms will be mixed with the secretions from the infected site as they pass through the opening to the surface	Specimens include those from the respiratory tract, gastric aspirates, urine, as well as uterine specimens	These specimens can usually be effectively decontaminated before culture is performed
Group 3: Specimens from parts of the body colonized with commensal and/or environmental organisms. They include normally colonized areas like the skin, oropharyngeal cavity, colon, and vagina, and secondarily colonized areas like ulcers and open wounds	Specimens like stool, skin specimens, as well as draining lymph nodes or abscesses belong to this group	These specimens are more heavily contaminated, which can affect the accuracy of microscopy and increases the chances of an unsuccessful mycobacterial culture

of childhood tuberculosis, this threshold explains why microscopy is of limited value in the diagnosis of childhood tuberculosis. Concentration of the specimen in the processing procedure (as described above)[43] and fluorescent microscopy (FM) increase smear microscopy sensitivity[43-45] by approximately 10%. FM implementation is limited by its high cost due to expensive mercury vapor light sources and the need for regular maintenance and a darkroom.[46] An alternative to FM is light-emitting diode (LED) microscopy, which is less expensive, requires less power, and can run on batteries, making it practical in resource-limited settings.[45] LED microscopy is marginally more sensitive (5% [95% confidence interval (CI), 0–11%]) with specificity similar to that of conventional fluorescence microscopy.[46] The World Health Organization (WHO) recommends that conventional fluorescence microscopy be replaced by LED microscopy, and that LED microscopy be phased in as an alternative for conventional Ziehl-Neelsen

light microscopy.[46] Reporting of smears is done using a semi-quantitative scale (Table 2.3). Due to an historical inaccuracy, the FM reporting scale for positive smears has been revised; the actual field observed is larger, and therefore more AFB are visible per field than previously calculated.[42] The American Thoracic Society and Centers for Disease Control and Prevention use a different scale, graded from negative to 4+.[47] Confirmation of FM low-positive smears by re-staining with Ziehl-Neelsen should not be done.[42] It is not possible to differentiate the various species of mycobacteria on microscopy.

Direct Tests: Nucleic Acid Amplification Tests (NAATs), Including GeneXpert

With the development of new molecular diagnostic tools, the rapid diagnosis of tuberculosis has made significant progress in recent years. These assays are based

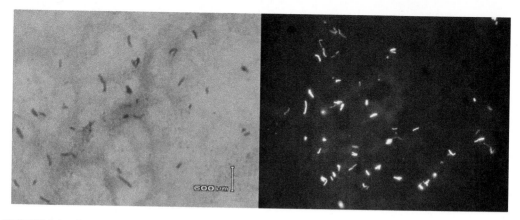

FIGURE 2.2   Smear microscopy: Ziehl-Neelsen staining at 1000X magnification (left side) and auramine staining at 200X magnification (right side).

on the detection of specific nucleotide sequences (DNA or RNA) and/or mutations in the *M. tuberculosis* genome, indicative of the presence of *M. tuberculosis* and/or associated drug-resistance mutations.[48] While detection of the nucleic acids is probably most often accomplished using the polymerase chain reaction (PCR), other nucleic acid amplification technologies also exist, such as loop mediated isothermal amplification (LAMP), ligase chain reaction (LCR), transcription mediated amplification (TNA), and strand displacement amplification (SDA), and all have been used in various assays to detect *M. tuberculosis*. In addition, after amplification of the nucleic acid, different methods can be used to detect the presence of specific mutations or polymorphisms in the amplified DNA—either to further speciate the isolate, or to detect mutations responsible for drug resistance. These techniques included hybridization to immobilized probes (as used in the Genotype MTBDR*plus* [Hain Lifescience, Nehren, Germany] line probe assays), or molecular beacons (as used in the GeneXpert MTB/RIF, Cepheid, Sunnyvale, Calif.).

Many of the NAATs can be performed directly on clinical specimens or on the resuspended sediments (pellets) after processing. Advantages of NAATs are numerous: (1) They are theoretically highly sensitive and able to detect very low copy numbers of nucleic acid; (2) they have a rapid turnaround time (<24 hrs. usually); (3) they may not require biosafety level 3 facilities; and (4) they are relatively easy to automate.[49] Disadvantages are:

(1) For many tests, NAATs require sophisticated laboratory infrastructure and highly skilled technicians.

(2) The risk of contaminating the test site with amplified DNA requires stringent quality-control procedures and a specific infrastructure to limit contamination.

(3) Although the sensitivity of commercial NAATs to detect *M. tuberculosis* is high in sputum acid-fast smear-positive specimens, it is lower in smear-negative and in extrapulmonary specimens and not as sensitive as culture.

(4) Rapid molecular assays for identification and detection of drug resistance in primary patient specimens do not replace culture-based methods, which remain the gold standard for diagnosis and phenotypic DST.

Newer NAAT methods have been developed to overcome some of the limitations outlined above. At the present time, the best-studied is the GeneXpert MTB/RIF test, which is completely automated and self-contained, and not dependent on reference laboratories or a high degree of technical expertise.[50] Multiple NAAT platforms and technologies are now available and described in detail elsewhere.[51]

Culture

Culture remains the gold standard for the laboratory diagnosis of tuberculosis disease. It has higher sensitivity than smear microscopy but a much longer turnaround time. Mycobacterial culture can be performed on solid egg-based media (e.g., Lowenstein-Jensen [LJ]), on solid agar-based media (e.g., Middlebrook 7H11) or on liquid media (e.g., Middlebrook 7H9). Liquid media

Table 2.3 Reporting of smear microscopy (from [42]). **(A)** Using a bright field microscope, Ziehl-Neelsen smears are examined with the 100X oil objective (10X eyepiece for a total of 1000X magnification). **(B)** With a fluorescent microscope, the smear is scanned with the 20X objective (with 10X eyepiece for a total of 200X magnification), occasionally using the 40X objective to see more detailed bacterial morphology

(A) GRADING SCALE FOR CARBOL FUCHSIN STAINS FOR BRIGHT-FIELD MICROSCOPY

WHAT YOU SEE	WHAT TO REPORT
No AFB in 100 fields	No AFB observed
1–9 AFB in 100 fields	Record exact number of bacilli
10–99 AFB in 100 fields	1+
1–10 AFB per field, check 50 fields	2+
More than 10 AFB per field, check 20 fields	3+

(B) GRADING SCALE FOR FLUOROCHROME STAINS

WHAT YOU SEE (200X)	WHAT YOU SEE (400X)	WHAT TO REPORT*
No AFB in one length	No AFB in one length	No AFB observed
1–4 AFB in one length	1–2 AFB in one length	Confirmation required**
5–49 AFB in one length	3–24 AFB in one length	Scanty
3–24 AFB in one field	1–6 AFB in one field	1+
25–250 AFB in one field	7–60 AFB in one field	2+
>250 AFB in one field	>60 AFB in one field	3+

*The number of AFB indicates how infectious the patient is. It is important to record exactly what you see.
**Confirmation required by another technician; or prepare another smear, stain and read.

are more sensitive than solid media for culture,[1,52] which is an advantage for the paucibacillary disease observed in children. The WHO recommends the use of liquid medium for culture and DST, emphasizing the need for rapid diagnostic tools facilitating species identification.[53] These liquid culture systems, however, are more prone to contamination by other non-mycobacterial organisms or NTM, even in experienced laboratories.[45] Commercial liquid culture systems (such as MGIT, the most widely used of these) are also more expensive, and many resource-poor countries still depend on LJ egg-based solid medium for the detection of growth of MTBC isolates.[54] Since some strains of the MTBC will grow better or only on solid media, the CDC-recommended gold standard for the detection of *M. tuberculosis* is to inoculate at least one tube each of solid and liquid media.[54] However, whether this is a cost- and/or labor-effective approach in endemic areas is not yet clear. Antibiotics and other additives can be added to media (whether solid or liquid) to make them more selective and inhibit other bacteria that may have survived the decontamination process.

Identification Methods from Culture

Once growth is detected in the culture medium (whether it is solid or liquid), it is important to identify the isolate, as well as to perform drug susceptibility testing. In the past, either biochemical methods or chromatography were used for this purpose; however, they have been replaced with newer rapid molecular or antigen-based tests.

Some identification techniques will only differentiate *M. tuberculosis* (or members of the MTBC) from NTM. An example of this involves detecting the presence of a *M. tuberculosis* complex-specific antigen, MPT64.[55] If the antigen is present, the isolate is identified as *M. tuberculosis*, and if absent, it is presumed to be one of the NTMs. However, the test should be performed on a positive culture with sufficient bacterial load, as false negatives have been reported.[56,57] A number of commercial lateral flow assays are available, and are a quick, easy, and relatively inexpensive way of confirming that the isolate in culture is *M. tuberculosis*.

Other assays, usually molecular, are able to identify both *M. tuberculosis* as well as certain NTMs. Molecular assays for identification are usually based on reverse hybridization, although sequence-based assays also exist. Certain tests are also able to differentiate between members of the MTBC. This is of particular relevance in children when BCG disease is suspected. Examples of molecular kits able to speciate mycobacteria are the Accuprobe (Gen-Probe, San Diego, Calif.), Inno-LiPA Mycobacteria assay (Innogenetics, Ghent, Belgium), the GenoType MTBC assay and Genotype Mycobacteria CM/AS assays (Hain Lifesciences, Nehren, Germany), and the MicroSeq 500 system (Applied Biosystems, Calif.).[58–62]

Drug Susceptibility Testing (DST)

Multidrug-resistant tuberculosis (MDR-TB) is associated with longer, more expensive, and more toxic treatment courses, as well as with worse outcomes.[63] The more recent recognition of extensively drug-resistant tuberculosis (XDR-TB) has reemphasized the need for regimens based on drug-susceptibility testing results, and has highlighted the importance of expediting the availability of these results.[64,65]

DST of mycobacteria can be performed phenotypically and genotypically. The principle of phenotypic testing assesses whether the organism can survive and/or grow in the presence of the antibiotic. This is used to infer whether the patient infected with the strain is likely to respond to treatment. Genotypic methods involve detecting the presence of genes or mutations known to be associated with resistance; again, the inference is that a strain with the mutation will not respond to

treatment with the drug. Phenotypic susceptibility testing is often regarded as the gold standard; however, it is time-consuming since it relies on growth of the organism. Molecular methods are much faster, and, for certain antibiotics, there is excellent correlation between the presence of a specific mutation/s and phenotypic resistance.

DST can also be direct or indirect. "Direct" testing refers to testing drug susceptibility directly on the clinical specimen. Typically this involves an acid-fast smear-positive specimen's being inoculated onto antibiotic-containing and antibiotic-free medium after decontamination. "Indirect" testing implies that the DST is performed once the organism has been isolated in culture.

Phenotypic DST

The three standard methods of phenotypic DST are the absolute concentration method, the resistant ratio method, and the proportion method. All three have been described in numerous reviews.[66–72] Most commonly used in routine laboratories is the proportion method, which assumes that if more than 1% of the organisms in a given population are resistant to a drug, the strain will be resistant to that drug. Agar plates containing a defined concentration (called the critical concentration) of the drug are used. After inoculation of the isolate onto both antibiotic-containing and antibiotic-free media, the plates are incubated for up to three weeks. The number of colonies on both plates is counted and compared, and the proportion of resistant colonies (i.e., those growing on the antibiotic containing medium) is calculated.

When performed in liquid culture, the isolate is inoculated into a vial with the critical concentration of antibiotic, and into an antibiotic-free vial. There are numerous commercial non-radiometric culture systems that can be used to perform DST. Although the algorithms, critical concentrations, and inoculation procedures may differ across systems, they all follow the essential principle of comparing the growth in the antibiotic-containing vial to growth in the antibiotic-free vial to determine whether the isolate is susceptible. A major advantage of using liquid culture is the faster time to generate a result, but results can still take 10 to 14 days after the initial isolation of the organism. Although not widely implemented, direct DST can be performed with re-suspended sediments using the MGIT DST method, which avoids the need to have an isolate from the original culture and shortens the time to results.[73]

A key factor in performing the proportion method is the critical concentration, which is the lowest concentration of the agent that inhibits growth of wild-type (susceptible) strains.[71] The critical concentration varies for different culture media. Critical concentrations for many antibiotics were published by the WHO in 2008,[74] and updated in 2012.[75] Phenotypic DST results using current critical concentrations are very reliable for rifampicin and isoniazid, but less so for ethambutol and streptomycin.[76,77] The current critical concentrations for fluoroquinolones and injectable agents (amikacin, kanamycin, and capreomycin) also yield reliable results; however, the evidence for this may not be as strong as for rifampicin and isoniazid.[77–79] Critical concentrations have been suggested for testing pyrazinamide (PZA), but testing is difficult since the drug is more active at a low pH, which itself inhibits mycobacterial growth.[80] The reliability of the proposed critical concentrations and methodology for PZA has been questioned, based on studies correlating phenotypic DST to molecular methods.[81,82]

Genotypic DST

Drug resistance in *M. tuberculosis* is due to chromosomal mutations; acquisition of resistance genes through mobile genetic elements such as phages has not been described. Molecular assays in general are based either on detecting the presence of a specific mutation and/or detecting the presence or absence of a wild-type gene (or region of the gene). Molecular assays work best when resistance is associated with either a limited number of mutations, or mutations in limited regions of the genome. This is probably best exemplified by rifampicin resistance. The vast majority (>95%) of rifampicin-resistant isolates (based on phenotypic DST) have mutations in an 81bp region of the *rpoB* gene that encodes RNA polymerase B, the target of rifampicin.[83,84]

The more diverse the range of mutations responsible for resistance, the more technically challenging molecular DST becomes, although with the advent of next-generation sequencing technology this may become less of an issue. Most molecular assays use DNA probes corresponding to wild-type sequences or specific mutations and determine whether specific mutations or wild-type sequences are present in the isolate's DNA. It is likely that in the future sequence-based techniques will become more widely used.

Commercial reverse-hybridization assays are available for determining rifampicin and isoniazid resistance. The Inno-LiPA Rif TB assay (Innogenetics, Ghent, Belgium) detects resistance to rifampicin only, and the GenoType MTBDR*plus* assay tests for both rifampicin and isoniazid resistance. Both have excellent sensitivity when it comes to rifampicin resistance, ranging from 95–100% compared to phenotypic results. The sensitivity of the GenoType MTBDR*plus* system for isoniazid resistance is on the order of 73–90%, and is due to the greater variety of molecular resistance mechanisms for isoniazid compared to rifampicin's. Both assays are close to 100% specific.[74,85,86] Both systems can detect resistance directly from smear-positive clinical specimens, and while the performance may not be quite as good as when performed on cultured isolates, it is still excellent.[87] A more sensitive second version of the GenoType MTBDR*plus* assay is now available and allows its use with acid-fast smear-negative sputum specimens. The main drawback to the routine implementation of these methods for drug susceptibility testing (whether it be from culture or specimen), is expense. The Hain Genotype MTBDR*sl* line probe assay detects resistance to the fluoroquinolones, injectable agents (amikacin, kanamycin, and capreomycin), and ethambutol. The performance of this assay was recently reviewed.[88,89] In summary, the assay performs well for both the fluoroquinolones and injectable agents, but is less reliable for ethambutol. For the fluoroquinolones and injectable drugs, the specificity was higher than its sensitivity, and the assay is thus probably more suitable as a rule-in test than a rule-out test (i.e., more reliable to detect resistance than to detect susceptibility), and phenotypic testing should be performed in addition to the molecular assay. A new version of the MTBDR*sl* has been released recently, which has removed the probes for *embB* (ethambutol), and replaced them with probes for the *eis* gene (to detect additional kanamycin resistance). The use of the assay will vary, depending on the local prevalence of resistance to these agents, as well as on local distribution of specific resistance mutations. As with the GenoType MTBDR*plus*, this assay can be performed both on clinical specimens and cultured isolates.[88] This more sensitive version of the MTBDR*sl* assay will also allow the testing of smear-negative specimens.

The GeneXpert MTB/RIF assay (Cepheid, Sunnyvale, Calif.) is an automated, semi-nested real-time PCR assay that both detects the presence of *M. tuberculosis* in clinical specimens and uses molecular beacons to determine whether wild-type *rpo*B sequences are present in the amplicons. The assay is designed for use on clinical specimens, primarily sputum, although more evidence is accumulating to describe its use in extrapulmonary specimens. It combines automated DNA extraction with amplification and detection in a cartridge format, and can be used by technicians with even with minimal formal training in molecular techniques. As with other molecular assays for detection of rifampicin resistance, it has excellent sensitivity and specificity.[90] Furthermore, the next-generation GeneXpert assays are being designed to have sensitivity more equivalent to cultures' and will detect fluoroquinolone resistance.

CONCLUSION

Although laboratory techniques described more than 100 years ago are still in use, and a perfect, quick and sensitive point-of-care tuberculosis diagnostic test is not yet available, more effort is being made to improve microbiological confirmation in children, especially as rates of drug resistance increase. However, the paucibacillary nature of childhood tuberculosis remains a major limitation of new sampling methods and laboratory techniques. It is encouraging to see children included in reviews of current and potential future technologies[51,91] as well as collaborations between end-users and product developers regarding the targets and specifications that should be met for new diagnostic methods.[92]

REFERENCES

1. Pfyffer GE, Palicova F. Mycobacterium: general characteristics, laboratory detection, and staining procedures. In: Murray PR, Baron EJ, American Society for Microbiology, eds. *Manual of Clinical Microbiology*. 10th ed. Washington, DC: ASM Press; 2011:472–502.
2. List of Prokaryotic Names with Standing in Nomenclature (LPSN). Available from: http://www.bacterio.net.
3. Rue-Albrecht K, Magee DA, Killick KE, Nalpas NC, Gordon SV, MacHugh DE. Comparative functional genomics and the bovine macrophage

4. Parsons SD, Drewe JA, Gey van Pittius NC, Warren RM, van Helden PD. Novel cause of tuberculosis in meerkats, South Africa. *Emerg Infect Dis*. 2013;19(12):2004–2007.
5. Veyrier FJ, Dufort A, Behr MA. The rise and fall of the *Mycobacterium tuberculosis* genome. *Trends Microbiol*. 2011;19(4):156–161.
6. Galagan JE. Genomic insights into tuberculosis. *Nat Rev Genet*. 2014;15(5):307–320.
7. World Health Organization. *WHO policy on TB infection control in health-care facilities, congregate settings and households*, WHO/HTM/TB/2009.419. Geneva: World Health Organization; 2009. Available from: http://whqlibdoc.who.int/publications/2009/9789241598323_eng.pdf.
8. Schluger NW. The pathogenesis of tuberculosis: the first one hundred (and twenty-three) years. *Am J Resp Cell Molec Biol*. 2005;32(4):251–256.
9. Marais BJ. Tuberculosis in children. *J Paediatr Child Health*. 2014;50(10):759–767.
10. Hunter RL. Pathology of post primary tuberculosis of the lung: an illustrated critical review. *Tuberculosis*. 2011;91(6):497–509.
11. Marais BJ, Gie RP, Schaaf HS, et al. The natural history of childhood intra-thoracic tuberculosis: a critical review of literature from the pre-chemotherapy era. *IJTLD*. 2004;8(4):392–402.
12. Perez-Velez CM, Marais BJ. Tuberculosis in children. *N Engl J Med*. 2012;367(4):348–361.
13. Cruz AT, Starke JR. A current review of infection control for childhood tuberculosis. *Tuberculosis (Edinb)*. 2011;91(Suppl 1):S11–S15.
14. Behr MA, Waters WR. Is tuberculosis a lymphatic disease with a pulmonary portal? *Lancet Infect Dis*. 2014;14(3):250–255.
15. Horsburgh CR, Jr. Tuberculosis. *ERR*. 2014;23(131):36–39.
16. Ginsberg AM. Tuberculosis drug development: progress, challenges, and the road ahead. *Tuberculosis*. 2010;90(3):162–167.
17. Zhang Y, Yew WW, Barer MR. Targeting persisters for tuberculosis control. *Antimicrob Agents Chemother*. 2012;56(5):2223–2230.
18. Zhang Y. Persisters, persistent infections and the Yin-Yang model. *Emerg Microbes Infect*. 2014;3:e3.
19. Flynn JL, Chan J, Lin PL. Macrophages and control of granulomatous inflammation in tuberculosis. *Mucosal Immunol*. 2011;4(3):271–278.

response to strains of the genus. *Front Immunol*. 2014;5:536.

20. Lin PL, Rodgers M, Smith LK, et al. Quantitative comparison of active and latent tuberculosis in the cynomolgus macaque model. *Infect Immun.* 2009;77(10):4631–4642.

21. Toman K, Frieden T, Toman K, World Health Organization. *Toman's Tuberculosis. Case Detection, Treatment, and Monitoring: Questions and Answers.* Geneva: WHO; 2004.

22. Marais BJ, Gie RP, Schaaf HS, Beyers N, Donald PR, Starke JR. Childhood pulmonary tuberculosis: old wisdom and new challenges. *Am J Respir Crit Care Med.* 2006;173(10):1078–1090.

23. Marais BJ, Gie RP, Schaaf HS, et al. A proposed radiological classification of childhood intra-thoracic tuberculosis. *Pediatr Radiol.* 2004;34(11):886–894.

24. Whitelaw AC, Sturm WA. Chapter 18—Microbiological testing for *Mycobacterium tuberculosis.* In: Schaaf HS, Zumla AI, Grange JM, et al., eds. *Tuberculosis.* Edinburgh: W.B. Saunders; 2009:169–178.

25. Warren JR, Bhattacharya M, De Almeida KN, Trakas K, Peterson LR. A minimum 5.0 ml of sputum improves the sensitivity of acid-fast smear for *Mycobacterium tuberculosis. Am J Respir Crit Care Med.* 2000;161(5):1559–1562.

26. Graham SM, Ahmed T, Amanullah F, et al. Evaluation of tuberculosis diagnostics in children: 1. Proposed clinical case definitions for classification of intrathoracic tuberculosis disease. Consensus from an expert panel. *J Infect Dis.* 2012;205(Suppl 2):S199–S208.

27. Cuevas LE, Browning R, Bossuyt P, et al. Evaluation of tuberculosis diagnostics in children: 2. Methodological issues for conducting and reporting research evaluations of tuberculosis diagnostics for intrathoracic tuberculosis in children. Consensus from an expert panel. *J Infect Dis.* 2012;205(Suppl 2):S209–S15.

28. Newton SM, Brent AJ, Anderson S, Whittaker E, Kampmann B. Paediatric tuberculosis. *Lancet Infect Dis.* 2008;8(8):498–510.

29. Kim SJ, Lee SH, Kim IS, Kim HJ, Kim SK, Rieder HL. Risk of occupational tuberculosis in National Tuberculosis Programme laboratories in Korea. *IJTLD.* 2007;11(2):138–142.

30. World Health Organization. *Guidance for National Tuberculosis Programmes on the Management of Tuberculosis in Children.* 2nd ed. WHO/HTM/TB/2014.03, 2014. Available from: http://www.who.int/tb/publications/childtb_guidelines/en/.

31. World Health Organization. *Tuberculosis Laboratory Biosafety Manual.* WHO/HTM/TB/2012.11, 2012. Available from: http://www.who.int/tb/publications/2012/tb_biosafety/en/.

32. Francis J. Curry National Tuberculosis Center, California Department of Public Health. *Pediatric Tuberculosis: A Guide to the Gastric Aspirate (GA) Procedure,* 2014. Available from: http://www.currytbcenter.ucsf.edu/catalogue/epub/index.cfm?tableName=GAP.

33. Grant LR, Hammitt LL, Murdoch DR, O'Brien KL, Scott JA. Procedures for collection of induced sputum specimens from children. *Clin Infect Dis.* 2012;54(Suppl 2):S140–S145.

34. Kolwijck E, Mitchell M, Venter A, Friedrich SO, Dawson R, Diacon AH. Short-term storage does not affect the quantitative yield of *Mycobacterium tuberculosis* in sputum in early-bactericidal-activity studies. *J Clin Microbiol.* 2013;51(4):1094–1098.

35. Wright CA, Bamford C, Prince Y, et al. Mycobacterial transport medium for routine culture of fine needle aspiration biopsies. *Arch Dis Child.* 2010;95(1):48–50.

36. Kitai I, Demers AM. Chapter 9: *Pediatric Tuberculosis, Canadian Tuberculosis Standards.* 7th ed. Public Health Agency of Canada, Canadian Lung Association/Canadian Thoracic Society; 2013. Available from: http://www.respiratoryguidelines.ca/tb-standards-2013.

37. Parashar D, Kabra SK, Lodha R, et al. Does neutralization of gastric aspirates from children with suspected intrathoracic tuberculosis affect mycobacterial yields on MGIT culture? *J Clin Microbiol.* 2013;51(6):1753–1756.

38. American Society for Microbiology. *Clinical Microbiology Procedures Handbook.* 3rd ed. Washington, DC: American Society of Microbiology; 2010.

39. Whitelaw AC, Mentoor K, Zar HJ, Nicol MP. Standard mycobacterial decontamination protocols may be inappropriate for samples from paediatric patients. Oral Presentation. 41st Union World Conference on Lung Health, 11–15 November 2010, Berlin, Germany

40. McCarthy KD, Metchock B, Kanphukiew A, et al. Monitoring the performance of mycobacteriology laboratories: a proposal for standardized indicators. *Int J Tuberc Lung Dis.* 2008;12(9):1015–1020.

41. Association of Public Health Laboratories. *Mycobacteriology Tuberculosis: Assessing Your Laboratory,* 2009. Available from: http://www.aphl.org/aphlprograms/infectious/tuberculosis/Documents/Mycobacteria_TuberculosisAssessingYourLaboratory.pdf.

42. Global Laboratory Initiative STP. *Laboratory Diagnosis of Tuberculosis by Sputum Microscopy—The Handbook, 2013.* Available

from: http://www.stoptb.org/wg/gli/assets/documents/TBLabDiagnosisSputum%20Microscopy_Handbook.pdf.

43. Steingart KR, Ng V, Henry M, et al. Sputum processing methods to improve the sensitivity of smear microscopy for tuberculosis: a systematic review. *Lancet Infect Dis.* 2006;6(10):664–674.

44. Steingart KR, Henry M, Ng V, et al. Fluorescence versus conventional sputum smear microscopy for tuberculosis: a systematic review. *Lancet Infect Dis.* 2006;6(9):570–581.

45. Rodrigues C, Vadwai V. Tuberculosis: laboratory diagnosis. *Clin Lab Med.* 2012;32(2):111–127.

46. World Health Organization. *Fluorescent Light-Emitting Diode (LED) Microscopy for Diagnosis of Tuberculosis: Policy Statement.* WHO/HTM/TB/2011.8, 2011. Available from: http://apps.who.int/iris/bitstream/10665/44602/1/9789241501613_eng.pdf?ua=1&ua=1.

47. American Thoracic Society. Diagnostic standards and classification of tuberculosis in adults and children. *Am J Respir Crit Care Med.* 2000;161(4 Pt 1):1376–1395.

48. European Centre for Disease Prevention and Control. *ERLN-TB Expert Opinion on the Use of the Rapid Molecular Assays for the Diagnosis of Tuberculosis and Detection of Drug-Resistance.* Stockholm: ECDC; 2013. Available from: http://www.ecdc.europa.eu/en/publications/Publications/ERLN-TB-use-rapid-molecular-assays-diagnosis-tuberculosis-detection-drug-resistance.pdf.

49. Nicol MP, Zar HJ. New specimens and laboratory diagnostics for childhood pulmonary TB: progress and prospects. *Paediatr Respir Rev.* 2011;12(1):16–21.

50. Pai M, Minion J, Jamieson F, Wolfe J, Behr M. Chapter 3: Diagnosis of active tuberculosis and drug resistance. In: *Canadian Tuberculosis Standards.* 7th ed. Public Health Agency of Canada, Canadian Lung Association/Canadian Thoracic Society, 2013. Available from: http://www.respiratoryguidelines.ca/tb-standards-2013.

51. UNITAID. *Tuberculosis Diagnostics Technology and Market Landscape.* 3rd ed. 2014. Available from: http://www.unitaid.eu/images/marketdynamics/publications/UNITAID_TB_Diagnostics_Landscape_3rd-edition.pdf.

52. Joloba ML, Johnson JL, Feng PJ, et al. What is the most reliable solid culture medium for tuberculosis treatment trials? *Tuberculosis.* 2014;94(3):311–316.

53. World Health Organization. *Use of Liquid TB Culture and Drug Susceptibility Testing (DST) in Low and Medium Income Settings,* 2007. Available from: http://www.who.int/tb/laboratory/use_of_liquid_tb_culture_summary_report.pdf?ua=1.

54. Parsons LM, Somoskovi A, Gutierrez C, et al. Laboratory diagnosis of tuberculosis in resource-poor countries: challenges and opportunities. *Clin Microbiol Rev.* 2011;24(2):314–350.

55. Brent AJ, Mugo D, Musyimi R, et al. Performance of the MGIT TBc identification test and meta-analysis of MPT64 assays for identification of the *Mycobacterium tuberculosis* complex in liquid culture. *J Clin Microbiol.* 2011;49(12):4343–4346.

56. Vadwai V, Sadani M, Sable R, et al. Immunochromatographic assays for detection of *Mycobacterium tuberculosis*: what is the perfect time to test? *Diagn Microbiol Infect Dis.* 2012;74(3):282–287.

57. Global Laboratory Initiative Stop TB Partnership (STP). *Mycobacteriology Laboratory Manual.* 1st ed. 2014. Available from: http://www.stoptb.org/wg/gli/assets/documents/gli_mycobacteriology_lab_manual_web.pdf.

58. Hall L, Doerr KA, Wohlfiel SL, Roberts GD. Evaluation of the MicroSeq system for identification of mycobacteria by 16S ribosomal DNA sequencing and its integration into a routine clinical mycobacteriology laboratory. *J Clin Microbiol.* 2003;41(4):1447.

59. Somoskovi A, Song Q, Mester J, et al. Use of molecular methods to identify the *Mycobacterium tuberculosis* complex (MTBC) and other mycobacterial species and to detect rifampin resistance in MTBC isolates following growth detection with the BACTEC MGIT 960 system. *J Clin Microbiol.* 2003;41(7):2822–2826.

60. Lebrun L, Gonullu N, Boutros N, et al. Use of INNO-LIPA assay for rapid identification of mycobacteria. *Diagn Microbiol Infect Dis.* 2003;46(2):151–153.

61. Richter E, Weizenegger M, Fahr AM, Rusch-Gerdes S. Usefulness of the GenoType MTBC assay for differentiating species of the *Mycobacterium tuberculosis* complex in cultures obtained from clinical specimens. *J Clin Microbiol.* 2004;42(9):4303–4306.

62. Makinen J, Marjamaki M, Marttila H, Soini H. Evaluation of a novel strip test, GenoType Mycobacterium CM/AS, for species identification of mycobacterial cultures. *Clin Microbiol Infect.* 2006;12(5):481–483.

63. Ettehad D, Schaaf HS, Seddon JA, Cooke GS, Ford N. Treatment outcomes for children with multidrug-resistant tuberculosis: a systematic review and meta-analysis. *Lancet Infect Dis.* 2012;12(6):449–456.

64. Pillay M, Sturm AW. Evolution of the extensively drug-resistant F15/LAM4/KZN strain of *Mycobacterium tuberculosis* in KwaZulu-Natal, South Africa. *Clin Infect Dis.* 2007;45(11):1409–1414.

65. Centers for Disease Control. Emergence of *Mycobacterium tuberculosis* with extensive resistance to second-line drugs—worldwide, 2000–2004. *MMWR Morb Mortal Wkly Rep.* 2006;55(11):301–305.

66. Inderlied C, Nash K. Antimycobacterial agents: in vitro susceptibility testing and mechanisms of action and resistance. In: V. Lorian, editor. *Antibiotics in Laboratory Medicine.* 5th ed. Philadelphia, PA: Lippincott Williams & Wilkins; 2005:155–225.

67. Drobniewski F, Rusch-Gerdes S, Hoffner S, Subcommittee on Antimicrobial Susceptibility Testing of *Mycobacterium Tuberculosis* of the European Committee for Antimicrobial Susceptibility Testing [EUCAST] of the European Society of Clinical Microbiology and Infectious Diseases [ESCMID]. Antimicrobial susceptibility testing of *Mycobacterium tuberculosis* (EUCAST document E.DEF 8.1)—report of the Subcommittee on Antimicrobial Susceptibility Testing of *Mycobacterium tuberculosis* of the EUCAST of the ESCMID. *Clin Microbiol Infect.* 2007;13(12):1144–1156.

68. Woods GL, Lin S-YG, Desmond EP. Susceptibility test methods: mycobacteria, nocardia, and other actinomycetes. In: Murray PR, Baron EJ, American Society for Microbiology, eds. *Manual of Clinical Microbiology.* 10th ed. Washington, DC: ASM Press; 2011:472–502.

69. Kim SJ. Drug-susceptibility testing in tuberculosis: methods and reliability of results. *Eur Respir J.* 2005;25(3):564–569.

70. European Centre for Disease Prevention and Control. *Mastering the Basics of TB Control: Development of a Handbook on TB Diagnostic Methods.* Stockholm: European Centre for Disease Prevention and Control; [updated 2011]. Available from: http://www.ecdc.europa.eu/en/publications/Publications/1105_TER_Basics_TB_control.pdf.

71. Clinical and Laboratory Standards Institute (CLSI). *Susceptibility Testing of Mycobacteria, Nocardiae and Other Aerobic Actinomycetes.* M24–A2. 2nd ed. 2011.

72. Francis J. Curry National Tuberculosis Center, California Department of Public Health. *Drug-Resistant Tuberculosis: A Survival Guide for Clinicians.* 2nd ed. 2008. Available from: http://www.currytbcenter.ucsf.edu/products/drug-resistant-tuberculosis-survival-guide-clinicians-2nd-edition.

73. Siddiqi S, Ahmed A, Asif S, et al. Direct drug susceptibility testing of *Mycobacterium tuberculosis* for rapid detection of multidrug resistance using the Bactec MGIT 960 system: a multicenter study. *J Clin Microbiol.* 2012;50(2):435–440.

74. World Health Organization. *Policy Guidance on Drug-Susceptibility Testing (DST) of Second-Line Antituberculosis Drugs.* WHO/HTM/TB/2008.392, 2008. Available from: http://www.who.int/tb/publications/2008/whohtmtb_2008_392/en/.

75. World Health Organization. *Updated Critical Concentrations for First-Line and Second-Line DST.* May, 2012. Available from: http://www.stoptb.org/wg/gli/assets/documents/Updated%20critical%20concentration%20table_1st%20and%202nd%20line%20drugs.pdf.

76. Angra PK, Taylor TH, Iademarco MF, Metchock B, Astles JR, Ridderhof JC. Performance of tuberculosis drug susceptibility testing in U.S. laboratories from 1994 to 2008. *J Clin Microbiol.* 2012;50(4):1233–1239.

77. Horne DJ, Pinto LM, Arentz M, et al. Diagnostic accuracy and reproducibility of WHO-endorsed phenotypic drug susceptibility testing methods for first-line and second-line antituberculosis drugs. *J Clin Microbiol.* 2013;51(2):393–401.

78. Kruuner A, Yates MD, Drobniewski FA. Evaluation of MGIT 960-based antimicrobial testing and determination of critical concentrations of first- and second-line antimicrobial drugs with drug-resistant clinical strains of *Mycobacterium tuberculosis.* *J Clin Microbiol.* 2006;44(3):811–818.

79. Updated guidelines for the use of nucleic acid amplification tests in the diagnosis of tuberculosis. *MMWR Morb Mortal Wkly Rep.* 2009;58(1):7–10.

80. Chang KC, Yew WW, Zhang Y. Pyrazinamide susceptibility testing in *Mycobacterium tuberculosis*: a systematic review with meta-analyses. *Antimicrob Agents Chemother.* 2011;55(10):4499–4505.

81. Dormandy J, Somoskovi A, Kreiswirth BN, Driscoll JR, Ashkin D, Salfinger M. Discrepant results between pyrazinamide susceptibility testing by the reference BACTEC 460TB method and pncA DNA sequencing in patients infected with multidrug-resistant W-Beijing

Mycobacterium tuberculosis strains. *Chest.* 2007;131(2):497–501.

82. Werngren J, Sturegard E, Jureen P, Angeby K, Hoffner S, Schon T. Reevaluation of the critical concentration for drug susceptibility testing of *Mycobacterium tuberculosis* against pyrazinamide using wild-type MIC distributions and pncA gene sequencing. *Antimicrob Agents Chemother.* 2012;56(3):1253–1257.

83. Gillespie SH. Evolution of drug resistance in *Mycobacterium tuberculosis*: clinical and molecular perspective. *Antimicrob Agents Chemother.* 2002;46(2):267–274.

84. Ramaswamy S, Musser JM. Molecular genetic basis of antimicrobial agent resistance in *Mycobacterium tuberculosis*: 1998 update. *Tuber Lung Dis.* 1998;79(1):3–29.

85. Makinen J, Marttila HJ, Marjamaki M, Viljanen MK, Soini H. Comparison of two commercially available DNA line probe assays for detection of multidrug-resistant *Mycobacterium tuberculosis*. *J Clin Microbiol.* 2006;44(2):350–352.

86. Hillemann D, Weizenegger M, Kubica T, Richter E, Niemann S. Use of the genotype MTBDR assay for rapid detection of rifampin and isoniazid resistance in *Mycobacterium tuberculosis* complex isolates. *J Clin Microbiol.* 2005;43(8):3699–3703.

87. Hillemann D, Rusch-Gerdes S, Richter E. Application of the GenoType MTBDR assay directly on sputum specimens. *IJTLD.* 2006;10(9):1057–1059.

88. World Health Organization. *The Use of Molecular Line Probe Assay for the Detection of Resistance to Second-Line Anti-Tuberculosis Drugs: Expert Group Meeting Report*, February, 2013. WHO/HTM/TB/2013.01, 2013. Available from: http://apps.who.int/iris/bitstream/10665/78099/1/WHO_HTM_TB_2013.01.eng.pdf?ua=1.

89. Theron G, Peter J, Richardson M, et al. The diagnostic accuracy of the GenoType° MTBDR*sl* assay for the detection of resistance to second-line anti-tuberculosis drugs. *Cochrane Database Syst Rev.* 2014;10:CD010705.

90. World Health Organization. *Automated Real-Time Nucleic Acid Amplification Technology for Rapid and Simultaneous Detection of Tuberculosis and Rifampicin Resistance: Xpert MTB/RIF Assay for the Diagnosis of Pulmonary and Extrapulmonary TB in Adults and Children. Policy Update.* WHO/HTM/TB/2013.16, 2013. Available from: http://www.who.int/tb/laboratory/xpert_policyupdate/en/.

91. Polly Clayden SC, Daniels C, Frick M, et al.; Benzacar A, ed. *2014 Pipeline Report. HIV, Hepatitis C Virus (HCV), and Tuberculosis (TB) Drugs, Diagnostics, Vaccines, Preventive Technologies, Research Toward a Cure, and Immune-Based and Gene Therapies in Development.* HIV i-Base/Treatment Action Group: 2014. Available from: http://www.pipelinereport.org/download.

92. World Health Organization. *High-Priority Target Product Profiles for New Tuberculosis Diagnostics: Report of a Consensus Meeting.* WHO/HTM/TB/2014.18, 2014. Available from: http://www.who.int/tb/publications/tpp_report/en/.

93. Zar HJ, Hanslo D, Apolles P, Swingler G, Hussey G. Induced sputum versus gastric lavage for microbiological confirmation of pulmonary tuberculosis in infants and young children: a prospective study. *Lancet.* 2005;365(9454):130–134.

94. Arlaud K, Gorincour G, Bouvenot J, Dutau H, Dubus JC. Could CT scan avoid unnecessary flexible bronchoscopy in children with active pulmonary tuberculosis? A retrospective study. *Arch Dis Child.* 2010;95(2):125–129.

95. Kiwanuka J, Graham SM, Coulter JB, et al. Diagnosis of pulmonary tuberculosis in children in an HIV-endemic area, Malawi. *Ann Trop Paediatr.* 2001;21(1):5–14.

96. Thakur A, Coulter JB, Zutshi K, et al. Laryngeal swabs for diagnosing tuberculosis. *Ann Trop Paediatr.* 1999;19(4):333–336.

97. Achkar JM, Lawn SD, Moosa MY, Wright CA, Kasprowicz VO. Adjunctive tests for diagnosis of tuberculosis: serology, ELISPOT for site-specific lymphocytes, urinary lipoarabinomannan, string test, and fine needle aspiration. *J Infect Dis.* 2011;204(Suppl 4):S1130–S1141.

98. Wright CA, Warren RM, Marais BJ. Fine needle aspiration biopsy: an undervalued diagnostic modality in paediatric mycobacterial disease. *IJTLD.* 2009;13(12):1467–1475.

99. Donald PR, Schaaf HS, Gie RP, Beyers N, Sirgel FA, Venter A. Stool microscopy and culture to assist the diagnosis of pulmonary tuberculosis in childhood. *J Trop Pediatr.* 1996;42(5):311–312.

100. Walters E, Gie RP, Hesseling AC, Friedrich SO, Diacon AH. Rapid diagnosis of pediatric intrathoracic tuberculosis from stool samples using the Xpert MTB/RIF assay: a pilot study. *Pediatr Infect Dis J.* 2012;31(12):1316.

101. Van Rie A. The challenge of diagnosing TB in people with HIV. Is stool the new tool? *IJTLD.* 2013;17(8):995.

102. Nicol MP, Spiers K, Workman L, et al. Xpert MTB/RIF testing of stool samples for the diagnosis of pulmonary tuberculosis in children. *Clin Infect Dis.* 2013;57(3):e18–e21.

103. Peter J, Green C, Hoelscher M, Mwaba P, Zumla A, Dheda K. Urine for the diagnosis of tuberculosis: current approaches, clinical applicability, and new developments. *Curr Opin Pulm Med.* 2010;16(3):262–270.

104. Green C, Huggett JF, Talbot E, Mwaba P, Reither K, Zumla AI. Rapid diagnosis of tuberculosis through the detection of mycobacterial DNA in urine by nucleic acid amplification methods. *Lancet Infect Dis.* 2009;9(8):505–511.

105. Gray KD, Cunningham CK, Clifton DC, et al. Prevalence of mycobacteremia among HIV-infected infants and children in northern Tanzania. *Pediat Infect Dis J.* 2013;32(7):754–756.

106. Rose PC, Schaaf HS, Marais BJ, Gie RP, Stefan DC. Value of bone marrow biopsy in children with suspected disseminated mycobacterial disease. *IJTLD.* 2011;15(2):200–204, i.

107. Starke JR, Cruz AT. Tuberculosis. In: Remington JS, Klein JO, Wilson CB, Nizet V, Maldonado YA, eds. *Infectious Diseases of the Fetus and Newborn Infant.* 7th ed. Philadelphia: W.B. Saunders Company; 2011:577–600.

3

IMMUNOLOGY OF TUBERCULOSIS IN CHILDREN

Beate Kampmann and Elizabeth Whittaker

HIGHLIGHTS OF THIS CHAPTER

- The identification of inherited defects in the interferon-gamma (IFNγ) receptors, IFNγ genes, and associated signaling pathways has provided key mechanistic insights into the important role of IFNγ in the defense against *M. tuberculosis* in humans.
- Key lessons about immune control of mycobacteria can be learned from children presenting with congenital or acquired T-cell deficiencies, such as severe combined immunodeficiency (SCID) or HIV infection.
- A partial explanation for the increased rate of progression from tuberculosis infection to disease in young children may be that they have deficient macrophage phagocytosis and recruitment, with consequences for the initiation of an antigen-specific immune response.
- There is strong evidence that regulatory T cells are involved in the immune response against *M. tuberculosis*, although whether this is protective or pathogenic remains a topic of debate.
- The key concept for human immunity to tuberculosis is *balance* between beneficial and destructive immune responses; both genetic and environmental factors probably determine the array of responses in any individual.

THE IMMUNE responses induced by *Mycobacterium tuberculosis* are complex, both in adults and in children. Although much progress has been made in dissecting the essential elements needed to contain the mycobacteria, the "holy grail" of understanding the correlates of protection against the development of tuberculosis disease is, unfortunately, still not within our reach. Our current knowledge of immunity in the human host is primarily derived from observations of adults and children presenting with "extreme phenotypes" of disease manifestations, and from experimental data obtained from observational research studies.

This chapter aims to provide current insights into the fundamental immune mechanisms required for control of mycobacteria. First, we illustrate key mechanisms through examples of clinical presentations of patients with extreme phenotypes of mycobacterial infections. Second, we summarize results from research studies in childhood tuberculosis, which tell us more about additional cell populations and mechanisms that are also likely to play an important role.

WHAT DO DISSEMINATED MYCOBACTERIAL INFECTIONS TELL US ABOUT THE IMMUNE RESPONSES NEEDED TO CONTAIN MYCOBACTERIA, INCLUDING *M. TUBERCULOSIS*?

In the early 1990s, several investigators reported patients and case series of individuals with unusual manifestations of disseminated mycobacterial infections.[1-3] These dramatic clinical presentations, which appeared to cluster in families, were primarily attributable to nontuberculous mycobacteria, but also included disseminated BCG infections and some cases of *M. tuberculosis*.[4] The subsequent identification of inherited defects in the interferon-gamma (IFNγ) receptors, IFNγ genes, and associated signaling pathways provided key mechanistic insights into the important role of IFNγ in humans, which had earlier been demonstrated in the mouse model.[5] Through the identification of significant mutations within the IFNγ/IFNγ receptor (IFNγR) pathways, it became clear that both the cytokine and its receptors play a central role in containment of mycobacteria.

A hallmark of the clinical presentation in patients with complete IFNγR deficiency is impaired granuloma formation, reflecting the importance of IFNγ for containment of mycobacteria within granulomata. The term "Mendelian susceptibility to mycobacterial disease" (MSMD) evolved, as more and more defects also involving the interleukin-12 (IL12) receptor, IL12 genes, and signaling pathways were described. To date, more than ten inherited defects have been described[6] (Figure 3.1).

Depending on the location of the defect, treatment with regular subcutaneous injections of IFNγ[7] in conjunction with combination therapy of antimycobacterial medication represent a treatment option for some of the milder defects

associated with the IL12 pathway, while other individuals with defects in IFNγ/IFGR have undergone successful bone marrow transplantation.[8] Investigation of the IFNγ/IL12 pathway has become part of the intense workup of patients who present with unusually severe, or atypical, widely disseminated forms of mycobacterial disease, especially in the context of familial cases or consanguinity.

The prevalence of MSMD in tuberculosis endemic settings might be underestimated, since sophisticated immunological investigations are rarely available. However, large genetic cohorts from a variety of settings have not reproducibly revealed polymorphisms that could explain susceptibility to *M. tuberculosis* at a population level. It is therefore likely that such mutations cannot be maintained in populations exposed to high pressure of infectious diseases, as affected patients simply do not survive beyond early childhood.

WHAT HAVE WE LEARNED ABOUT MYCOBACTERIAL IMMUNITY FROM CHILDREN WITH IMPAIRED B AND T-CELL FUNCTION?

Key lessons about immune control of mycobacteria can be learned from children presenting with congenital or acquired T-cell deficiencies, such as SCID or HIV infection. SCID is a group of inherited disorders that cause severe abnormalities of the immune system by affecting numbers and functions of T- and B-lymphocytes. A diagnosis of SCID is often first considered if an infant vaccinated with BCG at birth presents with multisystem disease and dissemination of BCG within the first three to six months of life, and BCG can be grown from various organs. This is a serious and often fatal condition, unless antimycobacterial treatment and bone marrow transplantation can be provided swiftly.

In 1995, Casanova et al.[9] reviewed 121 published cases of disseminated BCG infections. They found 61 cases of definitive immunodeficiency disease: 45 cases were SCID, 11 cases were chronic granulomatous disease (CGD), 4 cases were acquired immunodeficiency syndrome and 1 case had complete DiGeorge syndrome (CDGS). Norouzi et al.[10] reported that, out of 158 patients with disseminated BCG infection (BCGosis), 120 patients had immunodeficiency disease. These results indicate that immunogenetic factors affecting T-cell function are

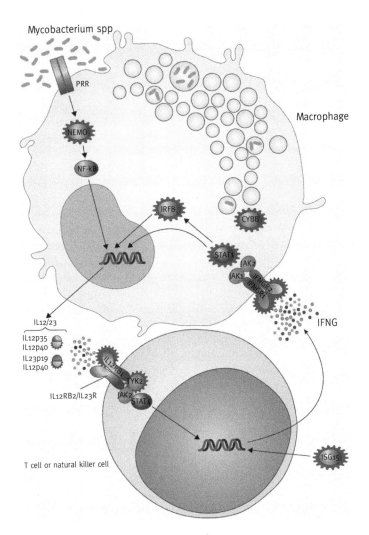

FIGURE 3.1   The identified defects in the IFNγ/IL12 pathway.

Figure courtesy of Dr. Begona Santiago, with additional permission from *Lancet Respiratory Medicine.*

critical for containment of mycobacteria, be they BCG, NTM, or *M. tuberculosis.*

HIV is the preeminent risk factor for the development of tuberculosis disease, and the HIV epidemic is well recognized as the key contributor to the resurgence in tuberculosis incidence in many settings. One in eight incident cases of tuberculosis occurs in persons living with HIV infection, with a quarter of all tuberculosis-related deaths occurring in persons living with HIV infection, while around a fifth of HIV-related deaths occur in incident tuberculosis cases.[11]

T-cell immunity is well recognized as essential for protection against tuberculosis infection and disease, and CD4+ T-cell depletion, the hallmark

of HIV infection, is a contributing factor to tuberculosis susceptibility. Immune reconstitution with antiretroviral drugs leads to normalization of CD4+ numbers, but despite this, higher susceptibility to tuberculosis remains a key feature of HIV infection.[12] Restoration of CD4+ numbers is not associated with significant increases in production of IFNγ in response to mycobacteria, as shown previously by Kampmann et al.[13]

Although we understand the role that CD4 T cells play in protecting against bacterial replication, we have not yet fully defined either their capacity to mediate protection or the mechanisms by which they mediate immunity. MTB-specific CD4+ T cells primarily produce Th1 cytokines, which include

IFNγ, IL-2 and TNFα, and it was thought that the ability of T cells to produce several cytokines at once would be an indicator for the increased potential to protect an individual from tuberculosis. Various CD4+ T-cell cytokine-producing effector subtypes have been described, ranging from early activated cells making only IL-2, to cells making IFN-γ, to multifunctional cells expressing IL-2, IFNγ, and tumor-necrosis factor (TNF). These polyfunctional cells are seen at high frequency in tuberculosis patients, in people living in high incidence areas, and in BCG-vaccinated infants.[14-16] However, recent studies do not support a role for these cells in protection against tuberculosis disease in response to either BCG or the novel anti-tuberculosis vaccine candidate MVA85A, as recently tested in a large phase IIb vaccine trial.[17,18]

Murine studies using a variety of knockout models have demonstrated that CD4 T cells are essential for protection against M. tuberculosis, and that CD8 T cells play a lesser role. Although CD8 knockout mice survive and control infection, they do so with a higher bacillary burden, suggesting a role for CD8 T cells in bacterial control.[19] Mycobacterial-specific CD8 T cells, in addition to secreting IFNγ and TNFα alongside CD4 T cells, have direct cytotoxic effects, expressing perforins and granulysins that can kill mycobacteria.[20,21]

M. tuberculosis residing within the phagosome ensures presentation of antigens via the major histocompatibility complex (MHC) Class II antigen processing pathways to CD4 T cells. Naïve CD4 T cells then differentiate into MTB-specific Th1 cells producing IFNγ, IL2, and TNFα, promoted by the local cytokine milieu, including IL12, IL18, and IL23.[22,23] IL12 and IL23 promote clonal expansion of these Th1 lymphocytes and further production of cytokines. IFNγ is a potent activator of macrophages, and TNFα facilitates mononuclear cell recruitment and activation as described below. Thus, CD4 T cells play an essential part in the cell-mediated response to mycobacteria, characterized by granuloma formation and containment of M. tuberculosis. The part of CD4 T cells in the generation of granulomas, and the depletion of such cells with HIV disease progression, may explain the increased risk of disseminated and extrapulmonary tuberculosis (EPTB) also seen in HIV-infected patients.[24]

It is now well recognized that activated CD4 T cells are the main target of HIV. Cell entry occurs via interactions with CD4 and the chemokine co-receptors, CCR5 and CXCR4. In turn, M. tuberculosis enhances HIV replication by transcriptional activation of long terminal repeats in HIV.[25] Furthermore, patients with tuberculosis have increased expression of HIV co-receptors CXCR4 and CCR5 on CD4 T cells, allowing more rapid infection of CD4 T cells by HIV.[26] South African studies in the pre-antiretroviral era have shown that the incidence of tuberculosis doubled in patients in the year following initial HIV infection, with increasing incidence as CD4 T-cell counts fell, reaching a peak of 25.7/100 person-years in patients with CD4 T-cell counts of fewer than 50 cells per μL.[27,28] This clinical recognition of the vital role played by CD4 T cells is validated by extensive experimental evidence over the last 20 years.

Further work in TB-HIV co-infected individuals to characterize functional defects in CD4 T cells has increased our understanding of these cells in the immune response to M. tuberculosis. Interestingly, investigation of the impact of HIV on cytokine responses showed no correlation between IFNγ production and total CD4 T-cell count in tuberculosis infected or uninfected HIV-infected patients: although IFNγ responses to purified protein derivative (PPD) were lower in HIV-infected individuals, responses to the M. tuberculosis-specific antigens ESAT 6 and CFP10 were preserved.[29] HIV preferentially infects and depletes MTB-specific T cells, most likely due to their activated, CD27-expressing, IL2-producing state.[30]

The consequences of an acquired T-cell defect for response to mycobacteria can also be appreciated in perinatally HIV-infected children, who are inadvertently vaccinated with BCG at birth. Data from South Africa show that the incidence of BCGosis in these children can be as high as 999/100.000.[31] For this reason, BCG vaccination is not recommended in hosts known to be immunocompromised, such as HIV-infected children.

However, with over half a million cases of tuberculosis per year worldwide in children alone, we must not forget that tuberculosis is a frequent and often serious infection in many non-HIV-infected children, also.[32] Extensive epidemiological evidence and data from household contact studies show that younger children are more susceptible to developing tuberculosis disease and more likely to present with disseminated forms of tuberculosis than their older peers.[33] It is highly probable that both epidemiological and immunological factors interact.

Figure 3.2 summarizes the relationship between dissemination of M. tuberculosis and age in

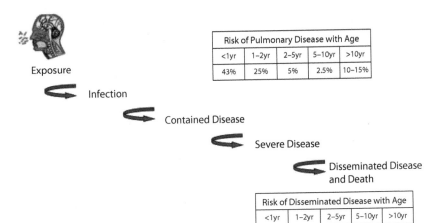

Risk of Pulmonary Disease with Age				
<1yr	1–2yr	2–5yr	5–10yr	>10yr
43%	25%	5%	2.5%	10–15%

Exposure

Infection

Contained Disease

Severe Disease

Disseminated Disease and Death

Risk of Disseminated Disease with Age				
<1yr	1–2yr	2–5yr	5–10yr	>10yr
20%	5%	2.5%	1<%	<1%

Marais AJRCCM 2006

FIGURE 3.2   The pathway from TB exposure to disease and the impact of age. In adults, following tuberculosis infection, 90% contain the mycobacteria within a granuloma. 10% of these individuals will develop late reactivation of disease in their lifetime. Primary progression of disease is less common in adults, but in the absence of intervention, almost 50% of very young children, and in particular infants under 1 year of age, will develop progressive pulmonary disease. 20% of those will develop a disseminated form of disease such as tuberculous meningitis or miliary tuberculosis. This risk decreases with age, as shown in the table Adapted from[35].

immunocompetent individuals in the absence of intervention. As a consequence, it is recommended that children under the age of five years should receive treatment if significantly exposed to a smear-positive tuberculosis case.[34,35]

WHY ARE YOUNGER CHILDREN MORE SUSCEPTIBLE TO TUBERCULOSIS THAN OLDER CHILDREN, EVEN IN THE ABSENCE OF HIV INFECTION?

Although it is assumed that differences in the immune response between adults and children are responsible for the differences in their susceptibility to infection and development of severe disease, only a limited number of studies have assessed the impact of age on crucial aspects of the immune response to *M. tuberculosis*.

The fate of *M. tuberculosis* within the macrophage in the granuloma has four possible outcomes: MTB infection can cause primary tuberculosis disease, can become dormant in a granuloma, can be eliminated, or can reactivate later to cause disease. Factors associated with innate as well as acquired immune responses will determine the ultimate outcome, as well as the mycobacteria themselves. A dynamic

balance between bacterial persistence and host defense develops, and, in young children, this balance tips in the favor of the mycobacteria more frequently than in adults.

There is good evidence that innate and acquired immune functions undergo changes after birth, and rather than describing the infant response as "immature," it is more helpful to think of these as differently regulated.[36] The immunological factors influencing this are not yet fully elucidated, but the following differences are likely to play a role. The maturation of toll-like receptors (TLR) over the first year of life, which has been documented by several research groups,[37,38] might affect the initial immune response to *M. tuberculosis*, since the organism is recognized via TLRs. Antigen-presenting cells, such as macrophages and dendritic cells (DCs), play a vital role in the initial response to mycobacteria. After engulfing *M. tuberculosis*, these phagocytic cells undergo activation and maturation with the resulting synthesis of inflammatory cytokines and chemokines, in particular IL1, IL12, and TNFα, which elicit a specific immune response. Multiple cell types, in particular CD4+ and gammadelta (γδ) T cells, are recruited to the disease site. Mature DCs then migrate to the lymph node where they present MHC-peptide complexes to T cells and, through co-stimulatory molecules and cytokines, including

IL12p70, trigger the expansion and differentiation of naïve T cells.

Young children demonstrate deficient macrophage phagocytosis and recruitment, with consequences for the initiation of an antigen-specific response. In addition, infants have fewer circulating DCs than adults, and their functional capacity is weaker. In particular, the ability of DCs to present antigen to naïve T cells appears to be reduced until the second year of life,[39] and the production of IL12p70 is impaired compared to adult levels until 12 years of age. Together, these may contribute to younger children's susceptibility to infection and disease. Other aspects of the initial innate response to mycobacteria are altered in neonates and early infancy, such as collectin levels and the complement pathway.[40,41] Neonatal CD4+ T cells exhibit reduced capacity to express Th1-effector function, partly attributed to hypermethylation of the proximal promoter of the IFNγ gene.[42] This results in a highly restricted pattern of IFNγ response to a variety of stimuli.

However, studies of immune responses to the BCG vaccine at birth or at slightly later time points have shown that infants of all ages respond well to this antigen challenge with a live attenuated bacterium and are capable of producing good levels of cytokines, indicative of strong immunogenicity.[43-45] It is possible that the response to a specific stimulus such as a live vaccine matures more rapidly than responses to a non-specific stimulus such as phytohemagglutin (PHA) or lipopolysaccharide (LPS), which are reagents often used as controls in immunoassays but which do not elicit an antigen-specific response. Nevertheless, despite robust responses, BCG vaccine does not protect all infants from dissemination of M. tuberculosis, and why it works for some children and not for others is still not sufficiently explained through immune mechanisms.[46]

To date, no conclusive deficits in immune mechanisms have been defined to explain why infants and toddlers are more prone to developing tuberculosis disease after infection, other than substantial T-cell defects, as seen in HIV-infected individuals, for whom tuberculosis is 24 times more common than in non-HIV-infected individuals[47]; congenital immunodeficiencies like those described above; and the mutations in key receptors and signaling pathways, also described in this chapter.

A summary of the key components of innate and adaptive immune mechanisms in the response to M. tuberculosis is illustrated in Figure 3.3.

DO NEUTROPHILS CONTRIBUTE TO THE CONTROL OF M. TUBERCULOSIS?

Neutrophils are less well studied than other components of the host response to tuberculosis infection, although they are the most commonly infected phagocyte in human tuberculosis disease.[48] Recently, a neutrophil-driven, IFN-inducible transcript signature in human whole blood was identified that correlated with the clinical severity of tuberculosis, raising the possibility that neutrophils may directly contribute to disease pathogenesis.[49] Neutrophils are recruited early to the site of mycobacterial infection, peaking at 24 hours. Following their arrival, neutrophils directly interact with, and internalize, mycobacteria. Although neutrophils contain antimycobacterial peptides, it is unclear whether neutrophils can directly kill the internalized mycobacteria, and it has been hypothesized that they traffic mycobacteria to distal sites in a "Trojan horse" fashion. Macrophages phagocytose apoptotic neutrophils and may deploy these neutrophil peptides. The peptides described include the α defensins human neutrophil peptides (HNPs) human cathelicidin LL-37 and lipocalin 2, the latter of which is iron-dependent. As shown by Martineau et al.,[50] neutrophils were required for mycobacterial growth inhibition in whole blood in vitro, and the peptides were found either to directly kill mycobacteria or to restrict mycobacterial growth in broth. Neutrophils appear to be important in early disease, but excessive numbers of neutrophils in later stages are associated with poor granuloma formation. IFNγ-deficient mice are reported to have increased levels of IL17, a cytokine linked to neutrophil recruitment, in association with enhanced numbers of neutrophils and poor control of bacterial growth, which can be reversed by exogenous IFNγ.[51] In adult patients with tuberculosis, high numbers of neutrophils in peripheral blood at the time of diagnosis have been associated with poor prognosis and slow sputum-culture conversion.[52,53] Whether neutrophils are responsible for disease severity or are simply accumulating in response to tissue inflammation and causing further tissue damage is as yet unclear, and further research is required. The occurrence of BCG vaccine complications in children diagnosed with chronic granulomatous disease (CGD) further confirms a role of neutrophils in containment of mycobacteria.[54]

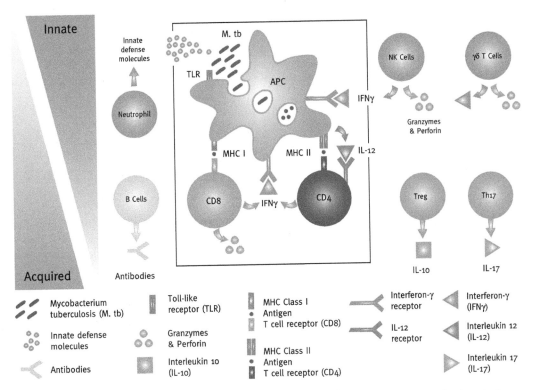

FIGURE 3.3 This figure illustrates the key components of innate and adaptive immune mechanisms in the response to *Mycobacterium tuberculosis*.

Illustration © Hugh Gifford, 2010.

CGD is caused by a defect in the burst of oxygen consumption that normally accompanies phagocytosis in myeloid cells (i.e., neutrophils, eosinophils, monocytes, and macrophages). As a result of the failure to mount a respiratory burst in their phagocytes due to a defect in nicotinamide adenine dinucleotide phosphate (NADPH) oxidase NOX2, the majority of CGD patients suffer from severe recurrent infections and also from dysregulated Th-17-lymphocyte-controled inflammation. Neutrophils are the cells primarily affected.

There are numerous case reports of BCG complications in patients with CGD, and retrospective studies estimate that between 6% and 57% of CGD patients will develop BCG complications if vaccinated. In the majority of CGD patients, BCG disease will present as a local or regional complication such as swelling, fistula formation, or lymphadenitis. Medical treatment often leads to an apparent full clinical recovery; however, recurrence is often observed. Although disseminated BCG disease is less commonly seen in CGD than SCID or MSMD

(15% vs. 67% or 33%, respectively), it has substantial mortality. IFNγ treatment has been used with some success in this cohort.[55] Furthermore, in the last 15 years, increasing numbers of tuberculosis cases have been described in patients with CGD, most commonly from regions with high endemicity for tuberculosis, such as Iran, China, and Argentina. In Hong Kong, it is estimated that patients with CGD are 140 times more likely to contract tuberculosis than those unaffected.[54] According to some authors, tuberculosis is more severe in CGD patients than in immunocompetent patients,[56,57] and treatment failure and recurrence are observed in the former group more frequently.

ARE THERE ADDITIONAL PLAYERS IN THE IMMUNE RESPONSE TO TUBERCULOSIS?

Although CD4+ T cells and IFNγ are important components of an effective antimycobacterial immune response, they do not fully explain observed differences in host susceptibility to tuberculosis. More recently, the role of non-conventional T cells, such as gammadelta (γδ) T cells and natural killer (NK) cells, has been investigated in the immunoprotective response to mycobacteria.

It has been noted that patients with tuberculosis infections have large expansions of the peripheral γδ T-cell subset, sometimes comprising up to 80% of all T cells.[58] HIV infection results in rapid and specific depletion of the peripheral Vδ2 T-cell population with consequences for the host's ability to resist intercurrent infections such as tuberculosis.[59] Interestingly, γδ T-cell levels and activity are high among patients who have natural control of HIV without the use of antiretroviral therapy.[60] Initial studies demonstrated that M. tuberculosis selectively expands human γδ T cells from healthy donors in vitro, and γδ T cells were found to proliferate rapidly and display effector T-cell functions such as IFNγ production and granulysin release in response to lipid antigens of M. tuberculosis.[61] In adults, the percentage and absolute number of γδ T cells were unchanged during tuberculosis disease.[58,62] However, in children, although the frequency of γδ T cells did not differ between those with and without tuberculosis infection, the proliferative capacity was much greater in those with infection. γδ T cells from children with tuberculosis infection produce more IFNγ and granulysin than did those from children with tuberculosis disease.[61]

As the search for a protective vaccine continues, γδ T cells have been investigated further. BCG vaccine elicits both expansion and IFNγ responses by γδ T cells; however, as with CD4 T cells, the relationship between γδ T cells and protection is uncertain.[63,64] In infants immunized with BCG at birth, the frequency of IFNγ-producing γδ T cells after immunization did not correlate with protection against tuberculosis.[17]

NK cells are a further source of IFNγ following vaccination with BCG and infection with M. tuberculosis and, in addition, produce IFNγ, perforin, and granzyme-A when stimulated with BCG in vitro.[21,64] NK cells are CD3−CD56+ lymphocytes, constituting approximately 10% of peripheral blood lymphocytes. The vast majority are cytotoxic and produce granulysin to lyse cells, and the remaining 5–10% are IFNγ-producing. Like γδ T cells, they link the innate and adaptive immune systems. They are an important source of early IFNγ, which is critical for activating macrophages and may directly present mycobacterial antigens to T cells promoting expansion of an effector Th1 response. In vitro, NK cells directly lyse M. tuberculosis-infected monocytes and enhance CD8 T-cell effector functions.[65] Recent evidence shows that activated NK cells reduce the expansion of regulatory T cells by direct lysis of M. tuberculosis-specific regulatory T cells, favoring Th1 responses.[66] In adults with tuberculosis disease, however, NK activity was decreased, and regulatory T-cell numbers increased.[65] In children, although serum granulysin levels have been identified to be reduced in tuberculosis disease, and return to normal following treatment, the source of the granulysin was not identified. Further studies into the role of NK cells in the pediatric immune response to mycobacteria are warranted.[67]

There is strong evidence that regulatory T cells are involved in the immune response against M. tuberculosis, although whether this is protective or pathogenic remains a topic of debate. Regulatory T cells with the CD4+CD25+FOXP3+ phenotype actively suppress Th1 T cells. Adults with tuberculosis infection and disease, particularly patients with extrapulmonary tuberculosis, have greater numbers of regulatory T cells than do healthy controls.[68] Raised numbers of regulatory T cells persist, even in patients with "cured" extrapulmonary tuberculosis.[69] Additionally, regulatory T cells have been shown to suppress IFNγ production in patients with tuberculosis.[70,71] Semple et al.[21,72] recently reported a greater increase in regulatory T cells in patients with tuberculosis disease compared to infection, particularly in bronchoalveolar lavage (BAL) samples; that regulatory T cells mediated suppression of T-helper cell proliferation in a dose-dependent manner; and that mycobacterial growth restriction in infected alveolar macrophages was affected by the addition of regulatory T cells. Their role as part of an effective mycobacterial vaccine response has been investigated in several animal and human models. In a murine model, despite the inactivation of regulatory T cells' leading to increased numbers of antigen-specific IFNγ+ CD4 T cells, this was not associated with increased protection from virulent tuberculosis infection.[73] In a human study of the vaccine candidate MVA85A, regulatory T cells were induced and higher levels were associated with the individuals who had preexisting immune responses to mycobacterial antigens.[74]

While regulatory T cells may dampen immune responses to infection with M. tuberculosis, they are probably required, similarly, to dampen potentially pathogenic proinflammatory responses and limit damage to infected tissue. Thus, a balance between the proinflammatory responses of monocytes/macrophages and effector T cells and the suppression of inflammation by regulatory T cells may be essential for maintenance of the granuloma and containment of the organisms. More "potent" regulatory T cells may therefore play a role in the development of tuberculosis disease. More data from pediatric populations are required.

WHAT CAN WE LEARN FROM THE ASSOCIATION OF SOME ANTI-TNF AGENTS WITH THE OCCURRENCE OF TUBERCULOSIS?

As mentioned above, TNFα is a key cytokine involved in the response to mycobacteria and is probably responsible for some of the clinical manifestations of tuberculosis disease, including weight loss, night sweats, and tissue destruction. Yet, TNFα plays a central part in the effective host response against the organism by recruiting and activating monocytes and promoting granuloma formation and containment of the disease. In 2001, a paper in the *New England Journal of Medicine* described 70 reported cases of tuberculosis in patients started on a then-new monoclonal antibody treatment for rheumatoid arthritis, Infliximab.[75] Infliximab is a humanized monoclonal antibody against TNFα and was approved in 1998 by the U.S. Food and Drug Administration (FDA) for patients who did not have a response to other anti-inflammatory agents. The clinical pattern of disease and the interval between the initiation of Infliximab and onset of disease was evaluated in these patients. The median interval from the start of treatment with Infliximab until the development of tuberculosis was 12 weeks. More than half of the patients had EPTB, and approximately one quarter had disseminated tuberculosis. The incidence of tuberculosis disease in this cohort was 24.4/100,000, compared to a similar study, which found one case of tuberculosis in 10,782 geographically dispersed patients with rheumatoid arthritis, who were followed prospectively for approximately 18 months. Interestingly, only 9 cases of tuberculosis were reported in equivalent numbers treated with another monoclonal antibody against TNF,

Etanercept. Etanercept binds only trimeric soluble TNF, while Infliximab binds both monomeric and trimeric soluble TNF, which may explain the difference in causing susceptibility to tuberculosis. The pattern of tuberculosis observed after anti-TNFα treatment may be due to the failure of granulomas to contain the organism, but the underlying mechanism is unclear. One mechanism by which TNFα is thought to mediate a successful host response to mycobacteria is the orderly induction of macrophage apoptosis after bacillary infection, which is a prominent feature of tuberculosis-associated granulomas.[76]

Infection with mycobacteria or treatment with specific mycobacterial molecules has been shown to induce TNFα secretion by macrophages.[77] *In vitro* studies have demonstrated that TNFα increases the ability of macrophages to phagocytose and kill mycobacteria and stimulates macrophage apoptosis, depriving the bacilli of their niche cells; this leads to increased killing and presentation of mycobacterial antigens by dendritic cells.[78] TNFα coordinates the inflammatory response through the induction of IL1 and IL6 and by recruitment of immune and inflammatory cells through the induction of chemokine release and upregulation of adhesion molecules.[79,80] TNFα produced in a local infection site recruits macrophages, NK cells, and γδ T cells, and promotes their activation. TNFα additionally activates CD8+ T cells, which, as described, directly kill intracellular bacteria. Thus, TNFα elicits a pro-inflammatory response, and absence of this cytokine is associated with severe tuberculosis progression. Yet excessive TNFα promotes immunopathology by interfering with cell-death processes and induction of a hyper-inflammatory milieu. As with so many factors in the immune response to tuberculosis, balance is the key. Given the high likelihood of reactivation of tuberculosis in patients receiving anti-TNF agents, it is recommended that all patients starting biologics be screened for tuberculosis infection beforehand.[81]

WHAT ABOUT DISSEMINATED BCG OR TUBERCULOSIS IN CHILDREN WITHOUT A SPECIFIC UNDERLYING IMMUNE DEFECT?

Infection, even disseminated infection, caused by BCG has occasionally been reported in individuals without identified defects in any particular immune pathway. The incidence of BCGosis is approximately 1:10,000–1:1,000,000.[82] It can be assumed that children with subtler complications of BCG vaccination, such as large ipsilateral lymphadenopathy or developing a continuously discharging BCG vaccine site, have some form of immune dysregulation. However, despite extensive immunological investigations, most of these children do not carry any known mutation beyond the already known MSMD abnormalities.

TUBERCULOSIS AND MALNUTRITION—CHICKEN OR EGG?

In highly endemic settings, malnutrition and tuberculosis are frequently seen to go hand in hand, and malnutrition appears to be an important risk factor for tuberculosis. Nutrition, immune function, and infection interact in complex and dynamic patterns. Protein-energy malnutrition compromises cell-mediated immunity (CMI), which is key to the defense against *M. tuberculosis*, and therefore increases susceptibility to or severity of infections.[83] However, most of the time, it is not clear which comes first: does the presence of malnutrition facilitate the occurrence of tuberculosis disease by lowering the threshold for infection to become active, or by changing the nature of innate immune responses that might have protected an exposed child from becoming infected? In malnourished individuals, the likelihood of tuberculosis infection's progressing to disease is increased. However, there is no evidence for a direct relationship between malnutrition and the risk of initial infection.

It is likely that the production of significant amounts of TNFα during tuberculosis disease leads to cachexia and weight loss, further disabling the underlying immune response and in turn contributing to malnutrition. Conversely, infection can also lead to nutritional stress and weight loss, thereby worsening nutritional status and immunological function. Therefore, understanding the temporal relationship between the onset of malnutrition and the development of the infectious disease is crucial to correctly assessing any possible cause and effect relationship, and much work is still required to tease out the precise mechanisms involved in the context of tuberculosis.

WHAT ELSE COULD CONTRIBUTE TO THE HIGHER SUSCEPTIBILITY IN YOUNGER CHILDREN?

In addition to the outlined contribution of immunological mechanisms to the containment of *M. tuberculosis*, it is also likely that environmental factors play a role: very young infants are much more likely to live in close proximity to a tuberculosis-infected parent or household contact. They will often be cared for more intensely than older children; for example, if they are breastfed by a coughing mother or carried close to her body, as is the case in many high-incidence countries.

In addition to the immune responses, it is important to remember that differences in exposure-intensity and also the virulence of the infecting strain might play a role, and there is some evidence that *M. tuberculosis* strains of certain lineages carry a higher risk of causing disseminated disease.[84] These studies are not conclusive at present, and very little work has been carried out that relates epidemiological and bacteriological parameters to detailed immunological findings.

Our ability to study immune responses, even in young children, using small blood samples, has significantly increased over the last ten years, and new, even more sophisticated tools are constantly evolving. In conjunction with epidemiological and microbiological parameters, further studies of age-related susceptibility are clearly warranted, as these will greatly enhance our understanding of the correlates of risk and protection, which is essential in order to finally develop better vaccines and equally improve diagnostics and therapeutics. Much can be learned about immunity to tuberculosis for all age groups through detailed studies of the disease in children.

WHAT CAN THE CLINICIAN DO IF PRESENTED WITH UNUSUALLY SEVERE MANIFESTATIONS OF TUBERCULOSIS?

While it is likely that a young child presenting with typical signs and symptoms and a known tuberculosis contact, or living in a highly endemic setting, simply has developed tuberculosis rather than suffering from a rare immunodeficiency, it is important not to overlook patients with unusual presentations, where any of the conditions described above could play a role. In order to exclude such known immune defects, it is therefore worth considering a range of investigations, which should include those listed in Table 3.1.

If there is sufficient clinical suspicion for immunodeficiency in a child with presumed or proven tuberculosis, the evaluation of immunological function should involve the analysis of lymphocyte subsets, the detection of immunoglobulins, complement factors C3, C4, and CH50 to exclude significant T-, B-cell and complement defects; and the analysis of NADPH oxidase activity in neutrophils to exclude CGD. The detection of functional defects in the type I-cytokine pathway is possible by incubating whole blood with positive stimuli to activate macrophages and T cells, including negative

Table 3.1 Suggested investigations in children presenting with unusual manifestations of *M. tuberculosis* and other mycobacterial infections

	INVESTIGATION	EXPLANATION
All disorders	Full blood count and blood film	Basic measure of presence and morphology of white blood cell populations, including lymphocyte count
Neutrophil disorders	Nitroblue tetrazolium (NBT)	Semi-quantitative method for evaluating neutrophil oxidative burst dysfunction
	Dihydrorhodamine (DHR)	Flow cytometry based assay—more commonly used diagnostic screening test for CGD
	Molecular genotyping	Confirmatory tests for CGD—4 genes associated with CGD and *CYBB* gene
Severe combined immunodeficiency	Lymphocyte subsets (basic)	Measurement of T (CD4 and CD8), B, NK, and double negative (CD4–CD8–) T cell populations
	Lymphocyte subsets (incl. memory markers)	Presence of naïve and different memory T cell populations (CD4 and CD8)
	Immunoglobulin level	Quantification of levels of IgG, IgA, IgM, and IgE
	Complement pathway	Measurement of C3/C4, THC levels
	Vaccine responses	Antibody responses to common vaccine antigens—tetanus, HiB, measles—to probe B cell memory
	T cell receptor excision circles (TRECS)	Recent thymic emigrants—evaluating thymic function in patients with cellular or combined primary immunodeficiencies
	T cell receptor gene rearrangement—V beta repertoire	The marked diversity of somatic TCR-gene rearrangements is important for normal immune functions
Mendelian susceptibility to mycobacterial disease (MSMD)	IFNγ/IL12 pathway defects	Stimulation of whole blood or PBMC with LPS +/– IL12 to induce production of IFNγ

controls. The readout of such an assay is the production of IFNγ and IL-12 in order to analyze the interactions between macrophages and T cells, which could be affected by known genetic polymorphisms. The expression of the IL12- or IFNγ receptors can also be demonstrated by flow cytometry. If such assays reveal normal results, it is unlikely that a defect in the IFNγ/IL12 pathway will be found by gene sequencing. However, if the results are abnormal, gene sequencing can be applied to identify the known mutations. Whole exome sequencing might also be able to detect novel mutations. It is advisable to examine the blood samples of parents and siblings when conducting these in-depth investigations for MSMD.

REFERENCES

1. Levin M, Newport MJ, Kalabalikis P, et al. Familial disseminated atypical mycobacterial infection in childhood: a human mycobacterial susceptibility gene? *Lancet.* 1995;345:29–83.
2. Newport MJ, Huxley CM, Huston S, et al. A mutation in the interferon-gamma-receptor gene and susceptibility to mycobacterial infection. *N Engl J Med.* 1996;335:2941–1949.
3. Jouanguy E, Altare F, Lamhamedi S, et al. Interferon-γ—receptor deficiency in an infant with fatal Bacille Calmette–Guérin infection. *N Engl J Med.* 1996;335:2956–1962.
4. Boisson-Dupuis S, Baghdadi El J, Parvaneh N, et al. IL-12Rβ1 deficiency in two of fifty children with severe tuberculosis from Iran, Morocco, and Turkey. *PLoS ONE.* 2011;6:e18524.
5. Blackwell JM, Barton CH, White JK, et al. Genetic regulation of leishmanial and mycobacterial infections: the LSH/ITY/BCG gene story continues. *Immunol Lett.* 1994;43:29–107.
6. Bustamante J, Boisson-Dupuis S, Abel L, Casanova J-L. Mendelian susceptibility to mycobacterial disease: genetic, immunological, and clinical features of inborn errors of IFN-γ immunity. *Semin Immunol.* 2014;26:254–470.
7. Dorman SE, Picard C, Lammas D, et al. Clinical features of dominant and recessive interferon gamma receptor 1 deficiencies. *Lancet.* 2004;364:2113–2121.
8. Chantrain CF, Bruwier A, Brichard B, et al. Successful hematopoietic stem cell transplantation in a child with active disseminated *Mycobacterium fortuitum* infection and interferon-gamma receptor 1 deficiency. *Bone Marrow Transpl.* 2006;38:25–76.
9. Casanova J-L, Jouanguy E, Lamhamedi S, Blanche S, Fischer A. Immunological conditions of children with BCG disseminated infection. *Lancet.* 1995;346:281.
10. Norouzi S, Aghamohammadi A, Mamishi S, Rosenzweig SD, Rezaei N. Bacillus Calmette-Guérin (BCG) complications associated with primary immunodeficiency diseases. *J Infect.* 2012;64:243–554.
11. UNAIDS. *UNAIDS Report on the Global AIDS Epidemic.* 2014.
12. Rekha B, Swaminathan S. Childhood tuberculosis—global epidemiology and the impact of HIV. *Paediatr Respir Rev.* 2007;8:29–106.
13. Kampmann B, Tena-Coki GN, Nicol MP, Levin M, Eley B. Reconstitution of antimycobacterial immune responses in HIV-infected children receiving HAART. *AIDS.* 2006;20:2011–1018.
14. Caccamo N, Guggino G, Joosten SA, et al. Multifunctional CD4(+) T cells correlate with active *Mycobacterium tuberculosis* infection. *Eur J Immunol.* 2010;40:2211–2220.
15. Scriba TJ, Kalsdorf B, Abrahams D-A, et al. Distinct, specific IL-17- and IL-22-producing CD4+ T cell subsets contribute to the human anti-mycobacterial immune response. *J Immunol.* 2008;180:2962–1970.
16. Soares AP, Scriba TJ, Joseph S, et al. Bacillus Calmette-Guérin vaccination of human newborns induces T cells with complex cytokine and phenotypic profiles. *J Immunol.* 2008;180:2569–3577.
17. Kagina BMN, Abel B, Scriba TJ, et al. Specific T cell frequency and cytokine expression profile do not correlate with protection against tuberculosis after bacillus Calmette-Guérin vaccination of newborns. *Am J Respir Crit Care Med.* 2010;182:2073–1079.
18. Tameris M, McShane H, Mcclain JB, et al. Lessons learnt from the first efficacy trial of a new infant tuberculosis vaccine since BCG. *Tuberculosis (Edinb).* 2013. doi:10.1016/j.tube.2013.01.003
19. Mogues T. The relative importance of T cell subsets in immunity and immunopathology of airborne *Mycobacterium tuberculosis* infection in mice. *J Exp Med.* 2001;193:271–280.
20. Tena-Coki NG, Scriba TJ, Peteni N, et al. CD4 and CD8 T-cell responses to mycobacterial antigens in African children. *Am J Respir Crit Care Med.* 2010;182:220–129.
21. Semple PL, Watkins M, Davids V, et al. Induction of granulysin and perforin cytolytic mediator expression in 10-week-old infants vaccinated with BCG at birth. *Clin Dev Immunol.* 2011;2011:238463.

22. Kaufmann SH. How can immunology contribute to the control of tuberculosis? *Nat Rev Immunol.* 2001;1:20–30.

23. Khader SA, Bell GK, Pearl JE, et al. IL-23 and IL-17 in the establishment of protective pulmonary CD4+ T cell responses after vaccination and during *Mycobacterium tuberculosis* challenge. *Nat Immunol.* 2007;8:269–377.

24. Gilks CF, Brindle RJ, Otieno LS, et al. Extrapulmonary and disseminated tuberculosis in HIV-1-seropositive patients presenting to the acute medical services in Nairobi. *AIDS.* 1990;4:281–985.

25. Zhang Y, Nakata K, Weiden M, Rom WN. *Mycobacterium tuberculosis* enhances human immunodeficiency virus-1 replication by transcriptional activation at the long terminal repeat. *J Clin Invest.* 1995;95:2324–2331.

26. Juffermans NP, Speelman P, Verbon A, et al. Patients with active tuberculosis have increased expression of HIV coreceptors CXCR4 and CCR5 on CD4+ T cells. *Clin Infect Dis.* 2001;32:250–652.

27. Sonnenberg P, Glynn JR, Fielding K, Murray J, Godfrey-Faussett P, Shearer S. How soon after infection with HIV does the risk of tuberculosis start to increase? A retrospective cohort study in South African gold miners. *J Infect Dis.* 2005;191:250–158.

28. Holmes CB, Wood R, Badri M, et al. CD4 Decline and incidence of opportunistic infections in Cape Town, South Africa. *JAIDS.* 2006;42:264–469.

29. Rangaka MX, Wilkinson KA, Seldon R, et al. Effect of HIV-1 infection on T-cell-based and skin test detection of tuberculosis infection. *Am J Respir Crit Care Med.* 2007;175:214–520.

30. Geldmacher C, Ngwenyama N, Schuetz A, et al. Preferential infection and depletion of *Mycobacterium tuberculosis*-specific CD4 T cells after HIV-1 infection. *J Exp Med.* 2010;207:2869–2881.

31. Hesseling AC, Marais BJ, Gie RP, et al. The risk of disseminated Bacille Calmette-Guerin (BCG) disease in HIV-infected children. *Vaccine.* 2007;25:24–18.

32. WHO Publication. *Global Tuberculosis Control, 2011.* World Health Organisation, 2011; WHO/HTM/TB/2011.16:2–258.

33. Newton SM, Brent AJ, Anderson S, Whittaker E, Kampmann B. Paediatric tuberculosis. *Lancet Infect Dis.* 2008;8:298–510.

34. Graham SM. Treatment of paediatric TB: revised WHO guidelines. *Paediatr Respir Rev.* 2011;12:22–26.

35. Marais BJ. Childhood tuberculosis: epidemiology and natural history of disease. *Indian J Pediatr.* 2011. doi:10.1007/s12098-010-0353-1

36. Jones C, Whittaker E, Bamford A, Kampmann B. Immunology and pathogenesis of childhood TB. *Paediatr Respir Rev.* 2011;12:2–8.

37. Burl S, Townend J, Njie-Jobe J, et al. Age-dependent maturation of Toll-like receptor-mediated cytokine responses in Gambian infants. *PLoS ONE.* 2011;6: e18185.

38. Shey MS, Nemes E, Whatney W, et al. Maturation of innate responses to mycobacteria over the first nine months of life. *J Immunol.* 2014;192:2833–4843.

39. Smith S, Jacobs RF, Wilson CB. Immunobiology of childhood tuberculosis: a window on the ontogeny of cellular immunity. *J Pediatr.* 1997;131:26–26.

40. Cosar H, Ozkinay F, Onay H, et al. Low levels of mannose-binding lectin confers protection against tuberculosis in Turkish children. *Eur J Clin Microbiol Infect Dis.* 2008;27:2165–1169.

41. Davis CA, Vallota EH, Forristal J. Serum complement levels in infancy: age related changes. *Pediatr Res.* 1979;13:2043–1046.

42. White GP, Watt PM, Holt BJ, Holt PG. Differential patterns of methylation of the IFN-gamma promoter at CpG and non-CpG sites underlie differences in IFN-gamma gene expression between human neonatal and adult CD45RO- T cells. *J Immunol.* 2002;168:2820–2827.

43. Vekemans J, Amedei A, Ota MO, et al. Neonatal bacillus Calmette-Guérin vaccination induces adult-like IFN-gamma production by CD4+ T lymphocytes. *Eur J Immunol.* 2001;31:2531–1535.

44. Kampmann B, Tena GN, Mzazi S, Eley B, Young DB, Levin M. Novel human in vitro system for evaluating antimycobacterial vaccines. *Infect Immun.* 2004;72:2401–6407.

45. Hanekom WA. The immune response to BCG vaccination of newborns. *Ann N Y Acad Sci.* 2005;1062:29–78.

46. Lalor MK, Ben-Smith A, Gorak-Stolinska P, et al. Population differences in immune responses to Bacille Calmette-Guérin vaccination in infancy. *J Infect Dis.* 2009. doi:10.1086/597069

47. Hesseling AC, Cotton MF, Jennings T, et al. High incidence of tuberculosis among HIV-infected infants: evidence from a South African population-based study highlights the need for improved tuberculosis control strategies. *Clin Infect Dis.* 2009;48:208–114.

48. Eum S-Y, Kong J-H, Hong M-S, et al. Neutrophils are the predominant infected phagocytic cells in the airways of patients with active pulmonary TB. *Chest.* 2010;137:222–128.

49. Berry MPR, Graham CM, Mcnab FW, et al. An interferon-inducible neutrophil-driven blood transcriptional signature in human tuberculosis. *Nature.* 2010;466:273–977.

50. Martineau AR, Newton SM, Wilkinson KA, et al. Neutrophil-mediated innate immune resistance to mycobacteria. *J Clin Invest.* 2007;117:2988–1994.

51. Cruz A, Khader SA, Torrado E, et al. Cutting edge: IFN-gamma regulates the induction and expansion of IL-17-producing CD4 T cells during mycobacterial infection. *J Immunol.* 2006;177:2416–1420.

52. Martineau AR, Timms PM, Bothamley GH, et al. High-dose vitamin D(3) during intensive-phase antimicrobial treatment of pulmonary tuberculosis: a double-blind randomised controlled trial. *Lancet.* 2011;377:242–250.

53. Lowe DM, Bandara AK, Packe GE, et al. Neutrophilia independently predicts death in tuberculosis. *Eur Respir J.* 2013;42:2752–1757.

54. Deffert C, Cachat J, Krause K-H. Phagocyte NADPH oxidase, chronic granulomatous disease and mycobacterial infections. *Cell Microbiol.* 2014;16:2168–1178.

55. Marciano BE, Wesley R, De Carlo ES, et al. Long-term interferon-γ therapy for patients with chronic granulomatous disease. *Clin Infect Dis.* 2004;39:292–699.

56. Köker MY, Camcıoğlu Y, van Leeuwen K, et al. Clinical, functional, and genetic characterization of chronic granulomatous disease in 89 Turkish patients. *J Allerg Clin Immunol.* 2013;132:2156–1163.e5.

57. Fattahi F, Badalzadeh M, Sedighipour L, et al. Inheritance pattern and clinical aspects of 93 Iranian patients with chronic granulomatous disease. *J Clin Immunol.* 2011;31:292–801.

58. Barnes PF, Grisso CL, Abrams JS, Band H, Rea TH, Modlin RL. Gamma delta T lymphocytes in human tuberculosis. *J Infect Dis.* 1992;165:206–512.

59. Hinz T, Wesch D, Friese K, Reckziegel A, Arden B, Kabelitz D. T cell receptor gamma delta repertoire in HIV-1-infected individuals. *Eur J Immunol.* 1994;24:2044–3049.

60. Riedel DJ, Sajadi MM, Armstrong CL, et al. Natural viral suppressors of HIV-1 have a unique capacity to maintain gammadelta T cells. *AIDS.* 2009;23:2955–1964.

61. Dieli F, Sireci G, Caccamo N, et al. Selective depression of interferon-gamma and granulysin production with increase of proliferative response by Vgamma9/Vdelta2 T cells in children with tuberculosis. *J Infect Dis.* 2002;186:2835–1839.

62. Carvalho ACC, Matteelli A, Airò P, et al. Gammadelta T lymphocytes in the peripheral blood of patients with tuberculosis with and without HIV co-infection. *Thorax.* 2002;57:257–360.

63. Mazzola TN, Da Silva MTN, Moreno YMF, et al. Robust gammadelta+ T cell expansion in infants immunized at birth with BCG vaccine. *Vaccine.* 2007;25:2313–6320.

64. Zufferey C, Germano S, Dutta B, Ritz N, Curtis N. The contribution of non-conventional T cells and NK cells in the mycobacterial-specific IFNγ response in Bacille Calmette-Guérin (BCG)-immunized infants. *PLoS ONE.* 2013;8: e77334.

65. Vankayalapati R, Barnes PF. Innate and adaptive immune responses to human *Mycobacterium tuberculosis* infection. *Tuberculosis (Edinb).* 2009;89(Suppl 1): S77–S80.

66. Roy S, Barnes PF, Garg A, Wu S, Cosman D, Vankayalapati R. NK cells lyse T regulatory cells that expand in response to an intracellular pathogen. *J Immunol.* 2008;180:2729–1736.

67. Di Liberto D, Buccheri S, Caccamo N, et al. Decreased serum granulysin levels in childhood tuberculosis which reverse after therapy. *Tuberculosis (Edinb).* 2007;87:222–328.

68. Hougardy J-M, Verscheure V, Locht C, Mascart F. In vitro expansion of CD4+CD25highFOXP3+CD127low/- regulatory T cells from peripheral blood lymphocytes of healthy *Mycobacterium tuberculosis*-infected humans. *Microb Infect.* 2007;9:2325–1332.

69. de Almeida AS, Fiske CT, Sterling TR, Kalams SA. Increased frequency of regulatory T cells and T lymphocyte activation in persons with previously treated extrapulmonary tuberculosis. *Clin Vaccine Immunol.* 2012;19:25–52.

70. Hougardy J-M, Place S, Hildebrand M, et al. Regulatory T cells depress immune responses to protective antigens in active tuberculosis. *Am J Respir Crit Care Med.* 2007;176:209–416.

71. Chen X, Zhou B, Li M, et al. CD4(+) CD25(+)FoxP3(+) regulatory T cells suppress *Mycobacterium tuberculosis* immunity in patients with active disease. *Clin Immunol.* 2007;123:20–59.

72. Semple PL, Binder AB, Davids M, Maredza A, Van Zyl-Smit RN, Dheda K. Regulatory T-cells attenuate mycobacterial stasis in alveolar and blood-derived macrophages from patients

with TB. *Am J Respir Crit Care Med.* 2013. doi:10.1164/rccm.201210-1934OC

73. Quinn KM, Rich FJ, Goldsack LM, et al. Accelerating the secondary immune response by inactivating CD4+CD25+ T regulatory cells prior to BCG vaccination does not enhance protection against tuberculosis. *Eur J Immunol.* 2008;38:295–705.

74. de Cassan SC, Pathan AA, Sander CR, et al. Investigating the induction of vaccine-induced Th17 and regulatory T cells in healthy, *Mycobacterium bovis* BCG-immunized adults vaccinated with a new tuberculosis vaccine, MVA85A. *Clin Vaccine Immunol.* 2010;17:2066–1073.

75. Keane J, Gershon S, Wise RP, et al. Tuberculosis associated with Infliximab, a tumor necrosis factor α–neutralizing agent. *N Engl J Med.* 2001;345:2098–1104.

76. Lügering A, Schmidt M, Lügering N, Pauels HG, Domschke W, Kucharzik T. Infliximab induces apoptosis in monocytes from patients with chronic active Crohn's disease by using a caspase-dependent pathway. *Gastroenterology.* 2001;121:2145–1157.

77. Roach TI, Barton CH, Chatterjee D, Blackwell JM. Macrophage activation: lipoarabinomannan from avirulent and virulent strains of *Mycobacterium tuberculosis* differentially induces the early genes c-fos, KC, JE, and tumor necrosis factor-alpha. *J Immunol.* 1993;150:2886–1896.

78. Keane J, Balcewicz-Sablinska MK, Remold HG, et al. Infection by *Mycobacterium tuberculosis* promotes human alveolar macrophage apoptosis. *Infect Immun.* 1997;65:298–304.

79. Ramírez GML, Rom WN, Ciotoli C, et al. *Mycobacterium tuberculosis* alters expression of adhesion molecules on monocytic cells. *Infect Immun.* 1994;62:2515–2520.

80. Roach DR, Bean AGD, Demangel C, France MP, Briscoe H, Britton WJ. TNF regulates chemokine induction essential for cell recruitment, granuloma formation, and clearance of mycobacterial infection. *J Immunol.* 2002;168:2620–4627.

81. Solovic I, Sester M, Gomez-Reino JJ, et al. The risk of tuberculosis related to tumour necrosis factor antagonist therapies: a TBNET consensus statement. *Eur Respir J.* 2010:2185–206.

82. Ying W, Sun J, Liu D, et al. Clinical characteristics and immunogenetics of BCGosis/BCGitis in Chinese children: a 6-year follow-up study. *PLoS ONE.* 2014;9: e94485.

83. Jones KDJ, Berkley JA. Severe acute malnutrition and infection. *Paediatr Int Child Health.* 2014;34(Suppl 1): S1–S29.

84. Nicol MP, Wilkinson RJ. The clinical consequences of strain diversity in *Mycobacterium tuberculosis.* *Trans R Soc Trop Med Hyg.* 2008;102:255–965.

4

NATURAL HISTORY OF CHILDHOOD TUBERCULOSIS

Ben J. Marais

HIGHLIGHTS OF THIS CHAPTER

- There is a predictable time table of events after tuberculosis infection in children that can be represented by five discernible phases.
- The most important determinants of the expression of infection by *M. tuberculosis* are the child's age and immune status.
- Children less than a year of age with untreated tuberculosis infection have a 40–50% chance of developing disease, with frequent progression to meningitis and other forms of disseminated tuberculosis.
- Adolescence present the second high-risk period, with frequent and rapid progression to adult type disease following documented primary infection.
- Children infected between five and ten years of age experience the least risk of disease progression (which is why this age range is sometimes referred to as "the favored age"), although they do contribute to the disease burden seen in endemic areas, given the frequency with which primary infection occurs during this period.

FOLLOWING EARLY autopsy studies that identified the underlying pathology in patients dying from tuberculosis, and the discovery of *Mycobacterium tuberculosis* as the causative agent by Robert Koch in 1882, major advances in the diagnosis and treatment of tuberculosis occurred in the twentieth century. Detection of infection became possible with refinement of the tuberculin skin test (TST) by von Pirque and Mantoux, and chest radiography became widely available after the First World War, increasing the capacity to detect and monitor the development of lung disease following *M. tuberculosis* infection. The most important diagnostic advance was the ability to perform direct sputum-smear microscopy, but this had limited benefit for children who are often unable to expectorate and usually have paucibacillary disease.

The period from 1920 to 1950 represented a golden opportunity for natural history of disease descriptions, as it was possible to identify *M. tuberculosis* infection (using the TST), describe various forms of lung involvement (using chest radiography), and identify *M. tuberculosis* in clinical specimens (using microscopy and culture) without any chemotherapeutic interference. The first antituberculosis drugs (para-amino salicylic acid and streptomycin) were only introduced during the Second World War, with more effective drugs becoming available in the 1950s; combination therapy with isoniazid[1,2] and rifampicin (discovered in 1959)[3] enabled most tuberculosis cases to be cured. During this time, many high-quality observational studies were conducted with meticulous long-term follow-up, providing detailed descriptions of disease presentation and progression.

NATURAL HISTORY STUDIES

Table 4.1 provides a summary of studies that reported on large numbers of children (more than 1,000) with untreated primary *M. tuberculosis* infection who were followed for a prolonged period of time (maximum of at least 10 years).[4-13] The table also includes a few studies that failed to meet these criteria, but provided unique insight: (1) a Norwegian study by Tobias Gedde-Dahl that was interrupted by the Second World War after eight years of follow-up[9]; (2) observations by Arvid Wallgren based on a lifetime of personal experience as the childhood tuberculosis expert in all of Scandanavia[6,7]; and (3) a classic report by Edith Lincoln that followed 964 children with radiological signs suggestive of primary *M. tuberculosis* infection to the age of 25 years.[12] Gedde-Dahl's study provided the only description of an active community surveillance program, while Arvid Wallgren and Edith Lincoln were the most highly regarded childhood tuberculosis experts on either side of the Atlantic. Table 4.2 provides a summary of the key findings and major limitations of studies listed in Table 4.1; studies are reported in chronological order to illustrate the progression in knowledge.

PIONEERS FROM THE PRE-CHEMOTHERAPY ERA

Arvid Johan Wallgren (1889–1973) trained and started working as a pediatrician in Gothenburg, Sweden, before moving to the Karolinska Institute in Stockholm, where he spent most of his professional life (Figure 4.1). His engaging manner and broad interests in all aspects of child health and social development made him an outstanding teacher and influential child health advocate. He helped ensure that children's best interests were considered during the reconstruction of Europe after the Second World War and that the World Health Organization included a strong focus on maternal and child health. His contribution to a better understanding of childhood tuberculosis benefitted from his meticulous attention to detail and careful recording of observations when taking clinical care of patients. In particular, a prospective study of 100 children who developed primary *M. tuberculosis* infection following documented tuberculosis exposure assisted description of the various clinical phases observed, which became known as the influential 'time table of primary tuberculosis'.

Edith Maas Lincoln (1899–1971) graduated from Johns Hopkins Medical School (Baltimore, Maryland) in 1916 and led the Children's Chest Clinic at Bellevue Hospital, New York City, from 1922 on (Figure 4.2). The novel chest radiograph observations described by Escherich in Austria required a pediatrician with clinical acumen and persistence to establish the long-term consequences of these findings. Edith Lincoln took on the challenge, and she embarked on a study to enroll 1,000 children with radiographic evidence of primary tuberculosis and follow them until age 25. Other studies conducted at Bellevue Hospital included studies of adolescents with adult-type cavitary disease, and very young children (<2 years of age) with a positive TST and normal chest radiograph. The last child was enrolled into the observational study in 1947. *Tuberculosis in Children*, published in 1963, reported on the long-term outcomes of 2,500 children with various tuberculosis disease manifestations, including 964 children with radiological evidence of primary *M. tuberculosis* infection.[12] It was a seminal publication in the field. Lincoln also pioneered the use of new antituberculosis drugs in children, for both the treatment and the prevention of tuberculosis in high-risk cases.

PRIMARY PULMONARY INFECTION

Pulmonary infection occurs when an inhaled infectious droplet, containing only a few bacilli, settles

Table 4.1. Description of original studies documenting the natural history of tuberculosis in children*

INDIVIDUAL STUDY REFERENCE	TIME FRAME	STUDY TYPE	STUDY POPULATION	DATA COLLECTION METHODS
1) Wallgren A—1935, 1938, 1948 Children's Hospital, Gothenburg and the Karolinska Medical Institute, Stockholm, Sweden. Primary pulmonary tuberculosis in childhood.[5] Relation of childhood infection to the disease in adults.[6] The time-table of tuberculosis.[7]	1930–1950 Follow-up period not specified	—Prospective descriptive, hospital-based —Personal experience	100 newly infected children All children with TB seen on referral	—Children observed after household exposure —Meticulous documentation of signs/symptoms following infection —In addition, Wallgren drew from vast personal experience
2) Brailey M—1940 Johns Hopkins (Harriet Lane Clinic), Baltimore, Maryland. Prognosis in white and colored tuberculous children according to initial chest X-ray findings.[8]	1928–1937 Follow-up period of 1–10 yrs	Retrospective descriptive, outpatient-based	285 families with 1383 children <15 yrs 40% white 60% black	—All children from tuberculous households —TST (Old tuberculin at 0.1 or 1mg) —Annual CXR if TST positive
3) Gedde-Dahl T—1951 Kinn District, Bergen, Norway. Tuberculous infection in the light of tuberculin matriculation/conversion.[9]	1937–1944 Follow-up period of 1–8 yrs	Prospective TST survey, community-based	6739 people 3138 children <15 yrs	—Annual community-based TST survey (Von Pirquet) —Documented TST conversion —Annual CXR if TST positive
4) Bentley FJ, Grzbowski S, Benjamin B—1954 High Wood Hospital for Children, Brentwood, Essex, UK. Tuberculosis in childhood and adolescence.[10]	1942–1952 Follow-up period of 5–10 yrs	—Retrospective descriptive, hospital-based —Literature review	1) Sanatorium patients 1049 children <16 yrs 2) Death Investigation: 100 consecutive TB deaths notified in children	—Successive referrals admitted over a 10-year period —Observation and CXR in hospital —Review CXR 5–10 years after hospital discharge

(continued)

Table 4.1. Continued

INDIVIDUAL STUDY REFERENCE	TIME FRAME	STUDY TYPE	STUDY POPULATION	DATA COLLECTION METHODS
5) Davies PDB—1961 Brompton Hospital, London. The natural history of tuberculosis in children.[11]	1930–1954 Follow-up period of 2–25 yrs	Retrospective descriptive, outpatient-based	2377 children <15 yrs	—All asymptomatic household contacts —Different TSTs compared —Annual CXR —70% follow-up achieved
6) Lincoln EM, Sewell EM—1963 Bellevue Hospital, New York. Tuberculosis in children.[12]	1930–1960 Follow-up period of 10–25 yrs	Prospective descriptive, hospital-based	Sanatorium patients 954 <15 yrs 50% white 25% black 25% Puerto Rican	—Children referred with evidence of recent (uncalcified) TB —Observation and CXR in hospital —Hospitalized for extended periods with careful documentation of disease progression —Annual CXR after discharge —90% follow-up achieved
7) Miller FJW, Seal RME, Taylor MD—1963 Royal Victoria Infirmary, Newcastle upon Tyne, and Children's Sanatorium at Stannington, Northumberland, UK Tuberculosis in children.[13]	1) 1941–1951 2) 1951–1961 Follow-up period of 1–10 yrs	—Retrospective descriptive, outpatient-based —Literature review	1) Children <7 yrs from 1000 families with an adult source case 2) 1500 children <5 yrs in household contact with an adult source case	1) 1000 family study —Household contacts <7 yrs —Annual CXR+TST (until positive) —99 TST converted 2) Household contact study —Household contacts <5 yrs —Annual CXR+TST (until positive) —72 TST converted

TST—tuberculin skin test; CXR—chest radiograph; TB—tuberculosis.
Adapted from Marais BJ, Gie RP, Schaaf HS, et al. The natural history of childhood intra-thoracic tuberculosis—a critical review of the pre-chemotherapy literature. Int J Tuberc Lung Dis. 2004;8:392–402.

Table 4.2 Summary of key findings and major limitations of natural history studies*

CITATION	AGE GROUPS	UNIQUE FEATURE	KEY FINDINGS	MAJOR LIMITATIONS
Wallgren	2 groups <3, 3–14 yrs	—Meticulous observation —Detailed description of symptoms and signs following primary infection	—Age at primary infection and time since primary infection were major determinants of risk for disease development following infection. It also influenced the type of disease manifestation. —Host immunity was influenced by age and considered to be of crucial importance. —Documented the timetable of disease.	—Study methodology was not specified. —Observations were illustrated with case studies. —Guidelines provided were dogmatic.
Brailey	5 groups <1, 1–2, 2–4, 5–9, 10–14 yrs	—Relevant age groups —Racial differences	—In all children <2 yrs and in black children <5 yrs, segmental lung lesions were predominant. —Black children suffered increased morbidity and mortality.	—Public health entry point selected the poor. —Type of segmental lesion not specified. —Socio-economic differences not evaluated.
Gedde-Dahl	3 groups <5, 5–9, 10–14 yrs	—TST conversion in the community	—Enlarged nodes were visible on CXR in the vast majority of recently infected children. —All CXR changes apart from cavitation and calcification seen within 1 year after infection	—Preschool children were poorly and selectively represented. —Isolated community.
Bentley et al.	4 groups <1, 1–4, 5–9, 10–15 yrs	—First dedicated childhood TB study in UK	—Described the slow rate at which adenopathy undergoes radiological regression. —Suggested a focus on high-risk groups: (<2 yrs and >10 yrs of age).	—Excessive pre-selection occurred due to the referral system and long waiting periods. —Disease progression was not well documented.

Table 4.2 Continued

CITATION	AGE GROUPS	UNIQUE FEATURE	KEY FINDINGS	MAJOR LIMITATIONS
Davies	4 groups <1, 1–4, 5–9, 10–14 yrs	—UK study with longest follow-up period	—Progression of disease was documented even after calcification became visible. —Risk of cavitating disease was dependent on age at primary infection (>10 yrs).	—Selected only asymptomatic children at study entry, to ensure clinical unity. —Majority of children were already infected at study entry.
Lincoln et al.	4 groups <1, 1–4, 5–9, 10–14 yrs	Detailed description of disease progression	—Meticulously documented disease progression, together with the signs, symptoms and outcome associated with each specific disease entity.	—Study inclusion was selective (symptomatic children with CXR evidence of recent infection). —Limited racial sub-analysis.
Miller et al.	5 groups <1, 1–2, 2–4, 5–9, 10–14 yrs	Relevant age groups Comprehensive literature review	—Informative illustrations of lymph drainage and TB lung pathology. —Re-emphasized high-risk groups following primary infection (<2 yrs and adolescents). —Cavitating disease may follow primary infection, re-infection, or reactivation.	—Cavitation with visible calcification was accepted as proof of re-activation. —Validity of studies quoted were not evaluated.

TST—tuberculin skin test; CXR—chest radiograph; UK—United Kingdom; TB—tuberculosis.

Adapted from Marais BJ, Gie RP, Schaaf HS, et al. The natural history of childhood intra-thoracic tuberculosis—a critical review of the pre-chemotherapy literature. *Int J Tuberc Lung Dis.* 2004;8:392–402.

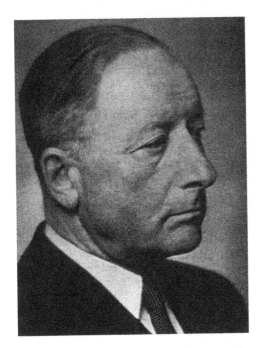

FIGURE 4.1   Arvid Johan Wallgren (1889–1973).

in a terminal airway. This triggers a localized pneumonic process with parenchymal inflammation known as the "primary focus." From the primary or Ghon focus, named after Anton Ghon, bacilli drain

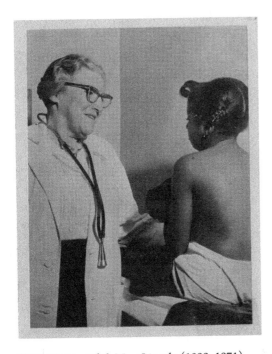

FIGURE 4.2   Edith Maas Lincoln (1899–1971).

via local lymphatics to the regional lymph nodes. Ranke first described the primary lung complex in 1917,[14] which includes the primary parenchymal focus, often with overlying pleural reaction and associated tuberculous lymphangitis, together with involvement of the regional lymph nodes. From the regional lymph nodes, bacilli may enter the systemic circulation via the lymphatic duct, resulting in occult hematogenous dissemination before immune responses are able to contain its spread. After occult dissemination, bacilli may survive in target organs for prolonged periods of time, with the risk of future disease development depending on the dynamic balance between local host-immunity and pathogen-related factors (Figure 4.3).[15]

Wallgren summarized the sequence of pathology following primary pulmonary infection in the classic timetable of primary tuberculosis in childhood; later confirmed and expanded by other investigators (Figure 4.4).[4] The timetable described the most commonly observed clinical patterns and did not represent dogmatic rules regarding the course of disease in children infected with *M. tuberculosis*. An important observation was the fact that, in children, the vast majority of disease manifestations occurred within the first 6–12 months after primary infection.

Timetable of Primary Tuberculosis in Childhood

- **Phase 1** occurs 3–8 weeks after primary infection.[5,7] The end of the initial asymptomatic incubation period is heralded clinically by hypersensitivity reactions such as initial fever, erythema nodosum, a positive TST, and visible elements of the primary complex on chest radiograph.[5,7]
- **Phase 2** follows 1–3 months after primary infection.[7] This period follows the occult hematogenous spread that occurs during incubation, and represents the period of highest risk for the development of tuberculous meningitis and miliary tuberculosis in young children.[5,7] However, tuberculous meningitis or miliary disease may occur after any time interval if there is local disease progression with hematogenous dissemination, often serving as the final terminal pathway in children with advanced disease.[9,10,12,13]
- **Phase 3** occurs 3–9 months after primary infection.[7] It is associated with pleural effusion in older children and with lymph node, airway

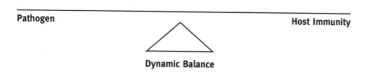

Pathogen   Host Immunity

Dynamic Balance

Pathogen	Host Immunity
Infecting dose (limited)	Innate Immunity
Virulence	Acquired immunity
Persistence	Local defences
(Preferential growth in the lung apices)	(Pronounced lymphadenopathy ‹5yrs)
	(Excessive tissue necrosis ›10yrs)

FIGURE 4.3   Factors influencing the dynamic pathogen–host interaction.*
Virulence and persistence may be related to the specific *M. tuberculosis* strain, but also to the metabolic state of the organism and the nature of the host immune response.

*Adapted from Marais BJ, Donald PR, Gie RP, Schaaf HS, Beyers N. Diversity of disease manifestations in childhood pulmonary tuberculosis. *Ann Trop Paed.* 2005;25:79–86.

disease, or parenchymal disease in children less than five years of age.[9,10,12,13]

- **Phase 4** lasts until the primary complex is calcified, which usually occurs one to three years after primary infection. This is the period of osteoarticular tuberculosis in children under five years of age[7,13] and adult-type disease in adolescents, although adult-type cavitary lung disease may manifest earlier in adolescents with rapid disease progression.[6–13] As a general rule, the risk of disease progression is greatly reduced by the time calcification appears within the primary complex,[8–13] although adult-type disease may occur with delayed clinical onset following reactivation of the initial infection.[11,13]
- **Phase 5** develops more than three years after primary infection. This represents the late manifestations of tuberculosis, including renal tuberculosis and pulmonary reactivation disease.[10,13]

PATHOLOGY-BASED DISEASE CLASSIFICATION AND "WINDOW OF RISK"

A pathology-based disease classification was developed to combine the findings from various studies (Table 4.3). This is illustrated by Figure 4.5, which provides a pictorial description of the diverse pulmonary disease manifestations observed in children.[16] The prognosis of primary infection was usually favorable, but the risk of disease progression was highly dependent on the age at the time of primary infection.[5–13] (Table 4.4) As illustrated by the timetable of primary tuberculosis in children, time since infection was another critical factor, with more than 90% of all disease manifestations observed within the first year. The 12 months following primary infection were commonly referred to as the "window of risk."

Primary Pulmonary Infection

Primary pulmonary infection was identified after active contact tracing or presentation after documented tuberculosis exposure. Primary pulmonary infection was associated with TST conversion and nonspecific, self-limiting, viral-like, respiratory symptoms.[5–7,10,13] Enlarged lymph nodes on the chest radiograph was the most typical finding, with or without a visible parenchymal focus.[9–13] Following primary infection, 50–70% of children showed radiological signs of infection, irrespective of symptoms.[9,11,13] Good quality antero-posterior and lateral views were required for optimal visualization of enlarged regional lymph nodes. The primary (Ghon) focus had no predilection for any specific part of the lung[9,11,12]: a focus in the apex of the lung affected the ipsilateral paratracheal nodes[10,12]; a focus in other parts of the right lung caused right-sided hilar adenopathy; and a focus in the left lung usually caused bilateral hilar adenopathy.[10,12] Paratracheal

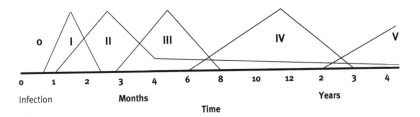

FIGURE 4.4 Schematic timeline of primary tuberculosis*
Phases of disease—adapted from the timetable of tuberculosis described by Wallgren[3]

0	Incubation
I	Hypersensitivity with development of tuberculin positivity
II	Dissemination with miliary tuberculosis and/or tuberculous meningitis
III	Segmental lesions in children <5 years and pleural effusion in those ≥5 years
IV	Osteoarticular tuberculosis in children <5 years and adult-type disease in those ≥10 years
V	Late manifestations, including renal disease and pulmonary reactivation

Different "phases" are not equally common and are highly age-dependent. While hypersensitivity is a nearly universal phenomenon following primary infection, the late manifestations are extremely rare. Table 4.4 provides an indication of how common the most important of these disease manifestations are in specific age groups, and Table 4.5 gives a more detailed, age-specific breakdown.

Adapted from Marais BJ, Gie RP, Schaaf HS, et al. The natural history of childhood intra-thoracic tuberculosis—a critical review of the pre-chemotherapy literature. *Int J Tuberc Lung Dis.* 2004;8:392–402.

node involvement reflected a focus in the lung apex, secondary spread from hilar glands, or hematogenous spread.[10] Paratracheal nodes were more frequently observed in children under two years of age and were associated with increased hematogenous spread, even with correction for age.[10]

During the first three to four months, the lymph nodes were vaguely defined, cloudy, and homogeneous on chest radiography, indicating a phase of "full activity."[10] Over the following months, the radiological signs of "activity" regressed, the shadow became denser, and the border better defined.[10] With serial radiographs, 40% of lesions cleared within six months, a further 30% within one year, but the remaining 30% persisted up to four years.[10,13] Calcification developed in 20–50% of infected children with visible lymph node involvement,[10,11,13] although this was reduced following the provision of chemotherapy. Calcification usually occurred between 12 and 24 months, but was sometimes delayed up to four years after primary infection.[10,13] Calcification in young children tended to be more extensive and developed earlier (within 6–12 months) than in older children.[10,11] In general, calcification was an indication of clinical quiescence, but not a guarantee thereof.[11-13] The disappearance of calcification was rare and attributed to either resorption or bronchial escape of a

pneumolyth.[13] The prognosis of pulmonary infection was usually favorable, with the associated risk mainly dependent on the child's age at the time of primary infection,[5-13] and the time since its inception. Neither the presence of a visible parenchymal lesion nor the size of regional hilar lymph nodes influenced the prognosis, apart from an increase in segmental lesions that were mostly seen in very young children.[10]

Pulmonary Disease

Host immunity was considered to be the major determinant of risk for disease development following infection. Infants with immature immune systems were at highest risk,[5,13] with pulmonary disease developing in 30–40% and tuberculous meningitis (TBM) or miliary disease in a further 10–20%.[8,10,12,13] The risk decreased considerably in the second year of life, but stayed high with 10–20% of infected children developing pulmonary disease and a further 2–5% TBM or miliary disease.[12,13] The risk decreased further in the 2–5-year age group, before reaching its lowest level at 5–10 years of age.[8,10,12,13] Intrathoracic lymph node disease was the dominant disease manifestation in children under 5 years.[10-13] Disease progression was least common in children aged 5–10 years,[10-13] although they were

Table 4.3   Disease classification used as template*

Pulmonary Infection	Tuberculosis infection uncomplicated by clinical symptoms (other than self-limiting, viral-like illness) or radiological abnormalities (other than the primary complex). The primary complex includes the Ghon focus with associated tuberculous lymphangitis and affected regional lymph nodes. Pulmonary infection without progression to disease implies successful containment of the organism.
Pulmonary Disease	Tuberculosis infection complicated by marked clinical symptoms or additional radiological abnormalities apart from the primary complex. Pulmonary disease includes a diverse spectrum of pathology, described as separate disease entities.
Separate Disease Entities: Ghon Focus with/without cavitation	Progressive parenchymal caseation surrounding the Ghon focus represents poor organism containment. The caseated area may discharge into a bronchus, resulting in the formation of a cavity with possible endobronchial spread.
Lymph Node Disease	Regional lymph node enlargement forms part of the primary complex, but the presence of marked clinical symptoms differentiates lymph node disease from pulmonary infection.
Bronchial Disease	With pulmonary infection, affected regional lymph nodes attach to the bronchus, but rarely progress to clinical or radiological disease. If disease progression follows this "lympho-bronchial involvement," the affected bronchus may become partially or totally obstructed as a result of nodal compression, inflammatory edema, polyps, granulomatous tissue, or caseous material extruded from ulcerated lymph nodes. Parenchymal disease may result from aspiration of caseous material. Variation in the degree of airway obstruction, dose, and virulence of the bacilli aspirated and the immune status of the host determines the degree of pathology.
—with airway obstruction	Airway obstruction occurs due to enlarged matted nodes encircling and compressing an airway, together with associated inflammation or additional processes described above.
—with collapse/ hyperinflation	Complete airway obstruction leads to resorption of distal air and collapse, while partial airway obstruction may cause a ball-valve effect with hyperinflation of the segment or lobe supplied.
—with allergic consolidation	Nodal perforation into an airway with endobronchial aspiration of allergic products causes an acute hypersensitivity response (epituberculosis) with dense consolidation.
—with bronchopneumonic consolidation	Nodal perforation into an airway with endobronchial aspiration of live bacilli causes local areas of caseation surrounding the airways, resulting in patchy consolidation.
—with caseating consolidation	Nodal airway obstruction with perforation and endobronchial aspiration of live bacilli causes extensive parenchymal caseation, resulting in dense, expansile consolidation of the affected segment or lobe.
Pleural Disease —with effusion	Pleural involvement occurs after direct spread of caseous material from a sub-pleural parenchymal or lymph node focus, or from hematogenous spread. Variation in the dose and virulence of bacilli that enter the pleural space, together with the immune status of the host, determines the degree of pathology.

Table 4.3   Continued

—with empyema	The presence of caseous material in the pleural space triggers a hypersensitivity inflammatory response with the accumulation of serous straw-colored fluid, containing few tuberculosis bacilli.
Adult-Type Disease	Active caseation in the pleural space causes thick, loculated pus, containing many tuberculosis bacilli.
Hematogenous Spread	Excessive local containment may cause parenchymal destruction and resultant cavity formation. Tubercle bacilli flourish in these cavities from whence they disseminate to other parts of the lung via endobronchial spread. Endobronchial spread occurs directly from these infected cavities and is not dependent on lympho-bronchial breakthrough, as in bronchial disease.
—with miliary disease	Tuberculosis bacilli may enter the bloodstream via pulmonary lymphatic drainage, from affected regional lymph nodes, or directly from the parenchymal focus. Hematogenous spread is a condition of infinite gradation, depending on the frequency, dose, and virulence of the bacilli released, as well as host immunity. During occult spread, bacilli are seeded into susceptible organs, while the child remains asymptomatic. Following invasion of the bloodstream, tuberculosis bacilli lodge in small capillaries, where they may progress to form tubercles, visible on chest radiograph as typical even-sized, miliary lesions (<2 mm) or atypical lesions of differing size.

More than one disease entity may coexist, or develop during the course of disease.

*Adapted from Marais BJ, Gie RP, Schaaf HS, et al. The natural history of childhood intra-thoracic tuberculosis—a critical review of the pre-chemotherapy literature. *Int J Tuberc Lung Dis.* 2004;8:392–402.

not infrequently seen in clinical practice, since older children are more frequently infected in the community than the very young. Adult-type disease was only seen among children older than 8 years, becoming the dominant disease manifestation after 10 years of age.[10–13] Primary infection during adolescence was associated with a high risk (10–20%) of developing adult-type disease.[4–13] The dominant type of disease that followed primary infection in relevant age groups is also summarized in Table 4.4.

Ghon Focus With/Without Cavitation

A Ghon focus with radiologically visible cavitation was rare. It occurred predominantly in black children under the age of two.[8,10,12,13] Clinical symptoms of Ghon focus cavitation included weight loss, fatigue, fever, and chronic cough.[12,13] In those with cavitation, the disease progressed to death within one year in the majority of cases.[12,13] Healing was rare, and even those who survived the initial illness ultimately died from tuberculosis or associated complications.[8] Cavitation following primary infection occurred frequently during adolescence,[6,9–13] but in

this age group, parenchymal breakdown probably reflected excessive tissue destruction rather than poor disease containment, as is the case in the very young whose T-cell responses are immature.[15]

Lymph Node Disease

Enlarged regional lymph nodes on chest radiograph were the most common sign of disease. In many instances, this was essentially only a marker of recent infection, not being associated with symptoms and showing spontaneous resolution. Respiratory symptoms were apparent when enlarged lymph nodes caused bronchial irritation or obstruction, while excessive nodal caseation caused persistent fever and weight loss.[13] The subcarinal nodes were most commonly involved and pericardial effusion developed rarely following nodal erosion with caseous discharge into the pericardial space.[13]

Bronchial Disease

Different degrees of airway obstruction and/or parenchymal involvement were observed with

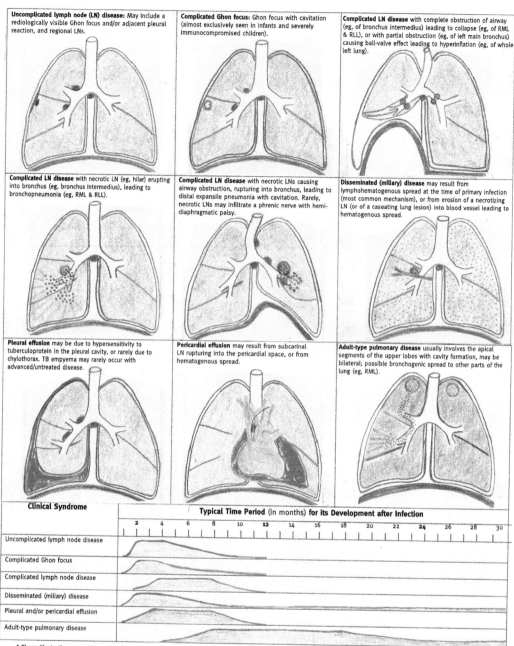

FIGURE 4.5   Pictorial description of different pulmonary disease manifestations.

bronchial disease. Bronchial disease occurred predominantly in children under five years of age, being more frequent in younger children, boys,[10–13] and black children.[4] The most frequently affected lobes were the right upper lobe (anterior segment), the right middle lobe, and the left upper lobe.[10–13] The lobes most frequently affected in combination were the right middle and lower lobes, indicating bronchus intermedius involvement.[10,13] Rebound enlargement of segmental lesions did occur after cessation of high-dose steroid treatment and was attributed to immune

Table 4.4   Age-specific risk for disease progression following primary infection*

AGE AT PRIMARY INFECTION	RISK OF DISEASE FOLLOWING PRIMARY INFECTION IMMUNE-COMPETENT CHILDREN (DOMINANT DISEASE ENTITY INDICATED IN BRACKETS)
<1 year	No disease 50% Pulmonary disease [Ghon focus, lymph node, or bronchial] 30–40% TBM or miliary disease 10–20%
1–2 years	No disease 70–80% Pulmonary disease [Ghon focus, lymph node, or bronchial] 10–20% TBM or miliary disease 2–5%
2–5 years	No disease 95% Pulmonary disease [lymph node or bronchial] 5% TBM or miliary disease 0.5%
5–10 years	No disease 98% Pulmonary disease [lymph node, bronchial, effusion, or adult-type] 2% TBM or miliary disease <0.5%
>10 years	No disease 80–90% Pulmonary disease [effusion or adult-type] 10–20% TBM or miliary disease <0.5%

TBM—tuberculous meningitis.

*Adapted from Marais BJ, Gie RP, Schaaf HS, et al. The natural history of childhood intra-thoracic tuberculosis—a critical review of the pre-chemotherapy literature. *Int J Tuberc Lung Dis.* 2004;8:392–402.

reconstitution.[13] Bronchoscopy revealed a spectrum of pathology from no visible involvement, to obstruction from external nodal compression, endobronchial nodal breakthrough with caseous drainage, and granulation tissue with polyps and fistula formation.[10,12] A very rare sequel was the expectoration of a pneumolyth, which occurred after perforation of a calcified lymph node into an airway.[12,13] The prognosis of bronchial disease and associated segmental or lobar involvement depended on the type and duration of involvement.[10,12,13]

AIRWAY OBSTRUCTION

Symptoms varied according to the degree of airway irritation and obstruction. Infants frequently developed a persistent cough, sometimes mimicking pertussis.[12,13] With disease progression, the cough became more prominent, often brassy or bi-tonal with associated large airway wheeze or stridor.[5,12,13] Imminent total airway obstruction was viewed as an indication for surgery.[13]

COLLAPSE/HYPERINFLATION

Collapse and hyperinflation were mostly a radiological diagnosis, with minimal clinical symptoms unless large lung segments collapsed, or hyperinflation caused symptoms related to mediastinal shift or pressure on surrounding structures.[10,12]

ALLERGIC INFLAMMATION (EPITUBERCULOSIS)

The onset of symptoms could be dramatic, with a high fever, acute respiratory symptoms, and signs of consolidation, or it could occur subclinically.[12] Chest radiography revealed a densely consolidated segment or lobe with minimal volume change.[12,13] Consolidation resolved completely within months, or quicker with steroid therapy, and left no permanent sequelae.[12]

BRONCHOPNEUMONIC CONSOLIDATION

Bronchopneumonic consolidation was rare. Symptoms were not well described, but depended on the extent of involvement. On chest radiography, patchy infiltration usually involved more than one lobe of a single lung.[10] Bilateral patchy infiltration was a sign of severe disease that could have resulted from hematogenous dissemination with local progression of initial miliary lesions.[10]

CASEATING CONSOLIDATION

Children with caseating consolidation were ill, with high undulating fever, chronic cough, and even hemoptysis.[12] Chest radiography demonstrated dense lobar consolidation, often with volume increase (expansile), with or without areas of parenchymal breakdown. *M. tuberculosis* cultures were positive in more than 80% of cases.[10,12,13] Bacterial infection often complicated the picture, making it difficult to establish the primary pathogen, although it was mostly considered to be *M. tuberculosis*.[10,13] Bronchoscopy showed total airway obstruction. Reestablishment of airway patency with surgical lymph node enucleation, together with penicillin, gave dramatic symptomatic relief.[12,13] Following resolution of the consolidation, non-collapsing parenchymal bullae appeared with extensive fibrotic scarring in the surrounding lung tissue.[10,12] Without intervention the prognosis was poor, with frequent hematogenous spread mostly terminating in tuberculous meningitis (TBM).[10,12]

The result of bronchopneumonic or caseating consolidation was a contracted, fibrotic area.[10–13] Contracted segments were often impossible to visualize on follow-up chest radiographs.[10,12] Bronchiectasis was a common sequel to peribronchial caseation.[10–13] Bronchial damage ranged from saccular bronchiectasis to bronchial stenosis.[12,13] Most children with bronchiectasis remained asymptomatic on long-term follow-up.[10–13] Apical lesions hardly ever caused complications, but large bronchiectatic lesions in the lower lobes predisposed to suppurative lung disease on long-term follow-up.[10–13] A few case reports of the "middle lobe syndrome" (recurrent bacterial pneumonia in individuals with previous tuberculous damage of the right middle lobe) were quoted, but this was uncommon.[13] Surgery was only indicated when a bronchiectatic lobe caused chronic symptomatic disease.[10,12,13] Very rarely, massive fibrosis and contraction of a whole lung (chronic fibroid lung) following resolution of the underlying tuberculosis caused mediastinal shift and scoliosis.[10,12]

Pleural Disease

EFFUSION

Localized pleurisy overlying a peripheral Ghon focus was common and was considered to be part of the primary complex.[12] Limited adhesions sometimes developed between the visceral and parietal pleura, but this did not cause symptoms or lung-function abnormality.[8] Effusions were rare in children under five years of age and most common in adolescent children,[10,11,13] usually signifying recent primary infection. Pleural effusion had a characteristic clinical course, starting with pleuritic pain localized to one side of the chest, accompanied by a high fever in the absence of acute illness, ill-defined loss of vigor, and a dry cough.[10,12,13] The sizes of the effusions were highly variable, ranging from small effusions that only obliterated the costophrenic angle, to massive fluid collections with mediastinal shift to the opposite side.[10,12] In most cases, a third to a half of the lung was obliterated with a visible meniscus sign,[10] making it impossible to evaluate lesions in the underlying lung.[10,12] Some localized interlobular effusions required radiological differentiation from segmental lung lesions.[13] A unilateral effusion, ipsilateral to the parenchymal focus, indicated direct pleural spread of bacilli or antigens from a sub-pleural focus. Bilateral effusions indicated hematogenous spread or bilateral primary foci, and were uncommon.[10–13] Pleural fluid was typically straw-colored with high protein content and lymphocyte predominance,[12,13] with the number of polymorphonuclear cells depending on the acuteness of onset.[13] Direct microscopy was negative, but culture yields were as high as 70% with immediate inoculation.[12] In general, the TST was highly reactive.[10,12]

In children, the prognosis of effusion was generally good. The high fever showed gradual resolution over 3–4 weeks,[6,8] while the fluid collection resolved more often over 3–6 months.[10,13] Obliteration of the costophrenic angle and slight pleural thickening remained permanently.[10,12,13] The main complication described was future adult-type disease, which was not a complication of the effusion per se, but reflected the risk associated with primary infection at an older age.[10,13] Rarely, extensive pleural fibrosis caused contraction of the affected hemi-thorax with scoliosis.[8,10] Bilateral effusions were associated with increased risk of hematogenous spread and future adult-type disease.[10–13]

EMPYEMA

The presence of caseating empyema was indicated by a persistent, high, swinging fever and a loculated pleural collection on chest radiograph.[13] Aspiration was difficult due to thick pus, but if successful, bacilli could be visualized on microscopy.[13] Caseating empyema was rare and the prognosis was variable, with either slow disease progression or slow resolution with the ultimate result of pleural calcification and fibrosis.[13]

Adult-Type Disease

Adult-type disease resulted following primary infection, endogenous reactivation or exogenous reinfection.[13] All these processes operated in the same community at the same time.[12] Adult-type disease was most common after recent primary infection in children over ten years of age.[6,8–13] The interval from primary infection to adult-type disease was widely variable (3 months to 20 years), mostly dependent on the age at primary infection.[10–12] The shortest time intervals and highest risk followed primary infection during adolescence, especially in girls of peri-menarchal age.[9–13] Disease started off with minimal symptoms such as cough, loss of appetite, and fatigue.[12] With disease progression, typical tuberculosis symptoms of chronic cough, chest pain, lethargy, anorexia, and weight loss became evident.[9,10,12,13] Children with advanced disease became anemic, and developed an oscillating fever and, rarely, hemoptysis.[12] A frequent complaint, even in the absence of fever, was excessive night sweats.[12] On chest radiograph, an initial rounded homogeneous shadow 2–3 cm in diameter situated in the vicinity of the clavicle was typical. Parenchymal breakdown and cavity formation of the lesion often occurred with alarming speed.[12,13] Cavities did not contain a fluid level and were characteristically surrounded by a rim of inflammation.[13] The sputa from these children were acid-fast bacilli smear-positive and transmitted infection to others. Bilateral disease was not uncommon, mainly involving the apical segments of the upper lobes; lower lobe involvement was far less frequent.[13] Previous radiographic appearances were non-predictive and highly variable, ranging from no visible abnormality detected to a densely calcified primary complex.[10] A correlation existed between the lesions that represented primary infection in the older age group, such as pleural effusion, and adult-type disease.[10–13] Without treatment, the prognosis of adult-type disease was poor, and 50–60% died within 5–10 years.[9–13]

Hematogenous Spread

During incubation and occult hematogenous spread, bacilli seeded to susceptible organs, especially the spleen, bone, kidney, and cerebral cortex,[5,12,13] and possibly to the apices of the lungs (Simon foci).[17] The age at the time of infection and the time since infection were the major determinants of risk for metastatic disease development. Infection of children under two years of age carried a significant risk of serious disease, even if the radiograph was considered normal initially.[10,13] TBM was present in over 30% of children who presented with tuberculosis before two years of age.[10,13] The risk of TBM after three years of age was greatly reduced, but it often remained the final terminal pathway in those with advanced disease.[12,13]

MILIARY DISEASE

Infants were most vulnerable to developing miliary disease.[4,12,13] Children appeared unwell, with prolonged fever, lethargy, anorexia, and weight loss,[10,12,13] but the severity of disease was easily underestimated. In the absence of TBM, children had no localizing signs, mostly presenting with only slight tachypnea and palpable hepatosplenomegaly.[10,12] Radiological mottling followed 7–21 days after febrile onset, starting as barely visible nodules that slowly progressed to large, poorly defined patches.[12] Early miliary lesions were often difficult to visualize, with 30–40% of autopsy-proven miliary lesions missed on initial chest radiograph.[10] Bone marrow biopsy and ophthalmoscopy were useful diagnostic aids,[10] although the reported presence of choroidal tubercles varied from less than 15% to more than 50%.[10,12,13] The majority of children were TST positive, but up to 20% were initially TST negative. Among TST negative children who were able to access treatment, all experienced TST conversion within 1–4 months of treatment initiation.[12] Without treatment, the prognosis of miliary disease was poor, with persistent fever, increased irritability, and weight loss, and usually

Table 4.5 Different clinical syndromes associated with tuberculosis in children*

PATHOLOGICAL CLASSIFICATION	DISEASE PHASE (TIME PERIOD)	CLINICAL SYNDROMES	RISK GROUPS	PATHOGENESIS	IMAGING MANIFESTATIONS
Primary MTB infection	**Incubation** (0–6 weeks)	Asymptomatic	All ages	No adaptive immunity TST(–); IGRA(–)	None
	Infection (1–3 months)	Self-limiting symptoms (mild, viral-like)		Adaptive immunity IGRA(+); TST(+) No test to register reinfection	Transient hilar or mediastinal lymphadenopathy (50–70% of cases), rarely visible transient Ghon focus
		Hypersensitivity reactions (fever; erythema nodosum; phlyctenular conjunctivitis)			
Early disease progression >90% of disease occurs within 12 months of primary infection	**Very early** (2–6 months)	Uncomplicated LN disease	<10 years	Inadequate innate and/or adaptive immunity; TST(+); IGRA(+). May be negative with immune compromise or extensive disease, cannot be used as "rule-out" tests	Hilar or mediastinal lymphadenopathy without airway or parenchymal involvement
		Progressive Ghon focus	<1 year		Ghon focus with visible cavitation
		Disseminated disease: —Miliary disease —TB meningitis	<3 years		—Discrete lung nodules (1–2 mm); hepato- splenomegaly —Hydrocephalus; basal enhancement; brain infarcts or tuberculomas

	Disease	Timeline	Immunity	Imaging/features
Early (4–12 months)	Complicated LN disease —Airway compression —Expansile caseating pneumonia —Infiltration of adjacent anatomical structures (esophagus, phrenic nerve, pericardium)	<5 years		—Hyperinflation or atelectasis/collapse —Expansile consolidation of a segment or lobe —Tracheo-/broncho-esophageal fistula; Pericardial effusion; Hemidiaphragmatic palsy
	Pleural disease —Exudative effusion (rarely, empyema; or chylothorax)	>3 years		Effusion usually unilateral; some pleural thickening and loculations
	Lymphadenitis —Most common extra-thoracic manifestation; usually cervical	1–10 years		Usually not needed, matting and edema of adjacent soft tissue
Late (1–3 years)	Adult-type pulmonary disease —Difficult to differentiate primary infection; reactivation and reinfection disease	>10 years	"Over-aggressive" innate and/or adaptive immunity	Apical cavities; may be bilateral; minimal or no LN enlargement (Previously referred to as "post-primary TB")
Late disease progression Generally rare, apart from adult-type disease in adolescents	Osteoarticular disease: —Spondylitis/arthritis/osteomyelitis	~5 years	Inadequate local control; usually local manifestations only, but can disseminate from any active focus	Periarticular osteopenia, subchondral cystic erosions, joint space narrowing
Very late (>3 years)	Urinary tract (renal, ureter, bladder) disease	>5 years		Renal calcifications; hydronephrosis, calyceal dilation and/or ureter stricture

*Adapted from Simon G. Die Tuberkulose der Lungenspitzen. *Beiträge klin Tuberk.* 1927;67:467–476; based on detailed disease descriptions by Arvid Wallgren and Edith Lincoln.
Age ranges, risk groups, and timelines specified provide general guidance only; HIV-infected children are particularly vulnerable and may present with atypical features.
TST—tuberculin skin test; TB—tuberculosis; IGRA—interferon-γ release assay; LN—lymph node.

terminating in TBM.[6,8,9] The majority died within six months, but chronic forms were occasionally seen where children eventually died from toxemia, malnutrition, or amyloidosis.[12] Typical even-sized miliary mottling pointed to an acute invasion of the bloodstream. Protracted release of bacilli from a chronic focus such as a matted lymph node mass or, rarely, a skeletal lesion, also occured.[12] The symptoms of protracted seeding were similar to the symptoms of acute invasion, but were initially more intermittent, presumably corresponding to periods of bacilli or toxic product release; eventual progression occurred with either acute or chronic deterioration.[12]

SUMMARY

Recent primary infection posed the greatest risk of disease progression, with more than 90% of disease occurring within one year of infection (Table 4.5). Children under 2–3 years of age experienced the greatest risk of disease progression and represented the first high-risk period, with frequent progression to miliary disease or TBM, often without significant preceding symptoms. Children infected between 5 and 10 years of age experienced the least risk of disease progression (which is why this age range is sometimes referred to as "the favored age"), although they do contribute to the disease burden seen in endemic areas, given the frequency with which primary infection occurs during this period. In older children (>3 years of age), persistent, non-remitting symptoms preceded progression to serious disease, providing a window of opportunity for clinical diagnosis. Adolescence represented the second high-risk period, with frequent and rapid progression to adult-type disease following documented primary infection.

The natural history disease descriptions provided by the pre-chemotherapy literature do not include the influence of HIV infection. However, disease descriptions in HIV-infected children of all ages suggest that those with significant immune compromise are at high risk of disease progression and illustrate poor disease containment, similar to what was seen in young (<2–3 years of age) children with immature T-cell responses.[18–21]

A number of challenges emerge regarding the diagnosis and optimal management of *M. tuberculosis* infection in children. The first challenge is to identify any untreated infection (recent or past, primary or reinfection) with a high degree of sensitivity and specificity, especially in very young or immune-compromised children at high risk of disease progression. Current markers of *M. tuberculosis* infection have inadequate sensitivity to rule out infection with certainty in those at high risk of disease progression, while no marker of reinfection currently exists. The second challenge is to identify disease progression as early as possible, in order to prevent the morbidity and mortality caused by tuberculosis. The non-specificity of early symptoms and signs, together with the high rate of spontaneous resolution of early radiographic signs in those with asymptomatic infection, complicates clinical diagnosis and case definitions for research purposes.[22,23] The third challenge is the need for accurate disease classification, since the highly variable disease phenotype described reflects differences in pathology.[24,25] Knowledge gained by exploring these phenotypical differences and the distinct age-relatedness of disease patterns observed may offer unique mechanistic insight into the ontogeny of immune responses in children and the underlying disease processes across the age spectrum.[26]

REFERENCES

1. Robitzek EH, Selikoff IJ. Hydrazine derivatives of isonicotinic acid (Rimifon, Marsalid) in the treatment of active progressive caseous-pneumonic tuberculosis. *Am Rev Tuberc.* 1952;65:402–428.
2. Domagk G, Klee P. Die Behandelung der Tuberkulose mit Neoteben (Isonikotinsäuerhydrazid). *Deutsch Med Wschr.* 1952;77:578–581.
3. Sensi P, Margilith P, Timbal MT. Rifamycin, a new antibiotic. Preliminary report. *Farmaco Ed Sci.* 1959;14:146–147.
4. Marais BJ, Gie RP, Schaaf HS, et al. The natural history of childhood intra-thoracic tuberculosis—a critical review of the pre-chemotherapy literature. *Int J Tuberc Lung Dis.* 2004;8:392–402.
5. Wallgren A. Primary pulmonary tuberculosis in childhood. *Am J Dis Child.* 1935;49:1105–1136.
6. Wallgren A. Pulmonary tuberculosis—relation of childhood infection to disease in adults. *Lancet.* 1938;1:5973–5976.
7. Wallgren A. The time-table of tuberculosis. *Tubercle.* 1948;29:245–251.

8. Brailey M. Prognosis in white and colored tuberculous children according to initial chest X-ray findings. *Am J Public Health.* 1943;33:343–352.

9. Gedde-Dahl T. Tuberculous infection in the light of tuberculin matriculation. *Am J Hygiene.* 1952;56:139–214.

10. Bentley FJ, Grzybowski S, Benjamin B. Tuberculosis in childhood and adolescence. London: National Association for the Prevention of Tuberculosis. Waterlow & Sons, Ltd.; 1954:1–213 and 238–253.

11. Davies PDB. The natural history of tuberculosis in children. *Tubercle.* 1961;42(Suppl):1–40.

12. Lincoln EM, Sewell EM. *Tuberculosis in Children.* New York: McGraw-Hill Book Company; 1963:1–315.

13. Miller FJW, Seal RME, Taylor MD. *Tuberculosis in Children.* London: J. and A. Churchill, Ltd.; 1963:163–275 and 466–587.

14. Ranke KE. Primare, sekundare and tertiare tuberculose des menschen. *Münch med Wchschr.* 1917;64:305–308.

15. Marais BJ, Donald PR, Gie RP, Schaaf HS, Beyers N. Diversity of disease manifestations in childhood pulmonary tuberculosis. *Ann Trop Paed.* 2005;25:79–86.

16. Perez-Velez CM, Marais BJ. Tuberculosis in children. *N Engl J Med.* 2012;367:348–361.

17. Simon G. Die Tuberkulose der Lungenspitzen. *Beitrage klin Tuberk.* 1927;67:467–476.

18. Jeena PM, Pillay P, Pillay T, et al. Impact of HIV-1 co-infection on presentation and hospital-related mortality in children with culture proven pulmonary tuberculosis in Durban, South Africa. *Int J Tuberc Lung Dis.* 2002;6:672–678.

19. Chan SP, Birnbaum J, Rao M, et al. Clinical manifestations and outcome of tuberculosis in children with acquired immune deficiency syndrome. *Pediatr Infect Dis J.* 1996;15:443–447.

20. Mukadi YD, Wiktor SZ, et al. Impact of HIV infection on the development, clinical presentation and outcome of tuberculosis among children in Abidjan, Cote d'Ivoire. *AIDS.* 1997;11:1151–1158.

21. Marais BJ, Cotton M, Graham S, Beyers N. Diagnosis and management challenges of childhood TB in the era of HIV. *J Infect Dis.* 2007;196(Suppl 1):S76–S85.

22. Marais BJ, Gie RP, Schaaf HS, Donald PR, Beyers N, Starke J. Childhood pulmonary tuberculosis—old wisdom and new challenges. *Am J Resp Crit Care Med.* 2006;173:1078–1090.

23. Graham SM, Ahmed T, Amanullah F, et al. Evaluation of TB diagnostics in children: proposed clinical case definitions for classification of intrathoracic tuberculosis disease. Consensus from an expert panel. *J Infect Dis.* 2012;205:199–208.

24. Marais BJ, Gie RP, Schaaf HS, et al. A proposed radiologic classification of childhood intra-thoracic tuberculosis. *Pediatr Rad.* 2004;33:886–894.

25. Cuevas LE, Ahmed T, Amanullah F, et al. Evaluation of TB diagnostics in children: methodological issues for conducting and reporting research evaluations of TB diagnostics for intrathoracic tuberculosis in children. Consensus from an expert panel. *J Infect Dis.* 2012;205:S209–S215.

26. Donald PR, Marais BJ, Barry CE 3rd. The influence of age on the epidemiology and pathology of tuberculosis. *Lancet.* 2010;375:1852–1854.

5

GLOBAL EPIDEMIOLOGY OF PEDIATRIC TUBERCULOSIS

Charalambos Sismanidis, Philippe Glaziou, Malgosia Grzemska,
Katherine Floyd, and Mario Raviglione

HIGHLIGHTS OF THIS CHAPTER

- Accurate estimation of the incidence, prevalence, and mortality of tuberculosis in children is hampered by the difficulty in confirming the diagnosis microbiologically, especially where the only available test is microscopy.
- The lack of child-appropriate tools to confirm diagnosis of tuberculosis disease, standard case-definitions, and the incomplete recording and reporting of children who are diagnosed with tuberculosis and put on treatment continue to pose significant shortcomings to the robust estimation of burden due to tuberculosis in children.
- The WHO estimated that in 2014 there were 1 million cases of tuberculosis disease in children aged 0-14 and 136,000 deaths caused by tuberculosis, 55,000 of whom in HIV-infected children. Researchers estimate 53 million children in the world with untreated tuberculosis infection.
- Availability and robustness of estimates of disease burden caused by TB in children have greatly benefited the last few years from, improved data reporting, collaborative efforts between burden estimation groups, and availability of funding for analytical work and generation of new data.

INTRODUCTION

Tuberculosis is likely to have affected humans for most of their history[1,2] and remains a major cause of morbidity and mortality worldwide, despite the discovery of effective and affordable chemotherapy more than 60 years ago. In 2014, there were an estimated 9.6 million incident cases of tuberculosis and 1.5 million deaths from the disease (1.1 among HIV-uninfected and 0.4 million among HIV-infected people).[3] Tuberculosis and the human immunodeficiency virus (HIV) are the top causes of death from an infectious agent.[4,5] Tuberculosis is a leading killer among people in the most economically productive age groups and those living with HIV.[6]

Every year, the World Health Organization (WHO) publishes estimates of tuberculosis incidence, prevalence, and mortality at global, regional, and country levels, along with an analysis of progress towards achievement of global international targets for tuberculosis (UN Millennium Development Goal 6c's target of halting and reversing tuberculosis incidence, and other international targets of halving its prevalence and mortality by 50% compared with 1990 levels).[3,3A] Increased global attention to maternal and child health has created a demand for, and interest in, tuberculosis disease burden estimates disaggregated by age and sex. Tuberculosis disease burden estimates for children (throughout this chapter, a "child" is defined as aged less than 15 years) were published for the first time by WHO in 2012.[7]

Overburdened health systems traditionally gave low priority to the largely noninfectious tuberculosis cases among children. As a result, currently much is left to be desired in terms of availability of child-appropriate diagnostic and treatment tools, as well as robust and nationally representative surveillance and survey data. As a direct result of the global focus on maternal and child health, clearly articulated actions have been defined for all stakeholders involved to address historical shortcomings in the identification and reporting of childhood tuberculosis, including: (a) strengthening surveillance through better recording and reporting and engagement with the private sector, especially pediatricians; (b) incorporating tuberculosis screening in existing maternal and child health services, especially in tuberculosis-endemic settings; and (c) addressing knowledge and research gaps in epidemiology, basic and operational research, and the development of new tools such as diagnostics, drugs, vaccines.[8]

This chapter describes our current understanding of the global burden of pediatric tuberculosis disease; the reasons why it remains difficult to estimate disease burden in children; the data sources available to inform disease burden estimation in children; the progress made in recent years through the collaboration of key partners with the development of complementary methods to produce burden estimates; and the next steps planned to improve those estimates.

TUBERCULOSIS EPIDEMIOLOGY

Tuberculosis is contagious and airborne.[9] Susceptible individuals acquire *Mycobacterium tuberculosis* infection through inhalation of bacteria contained in droplet nuclei dispersed in the environment by individuals with tuberculosis of the lungs or the airways. When coughing, sneezing, or speaking, such individuals aerosolize droplet nuclei that are then passed to others. Other routes of transmission are very uncommon and of no epidemiological significance. The probability of contact with a person who has an infectious form of tuberculosis, the intimacy and duration of that contact, the degree of infectiousness of the case, the virulence of the bacterial strain, and the shared environment in which the contact takes place are all important determinants of the likelihood of transmission. About one third of the world's population is estimated to be latently infected with *M. tuberculosis*.[10] Of those infected, only a small proportion (fewer than 15%) will ultimately become sick with tuberculosis,[11,12] but very young children, people with weakened immune systems, people living with HIV; and patients with renal insufficiency, silicosis, diabetes, and other morbidities, have a much greater risk of falling ill from tuberculosis. We know from historical data that, if left untreated, smear-positive, infectious tuberculosis among HIV-uninfected individuals has a 10-year case fatality variously reported between 53% and 86%, with a weighted mean of 70%,[13] compared with about 3% of HIV-uninfected tuberculosis patients who receive adequate treatment.[14] Tuberculosis is a disease of poverty that thrives where social and economic determinants of ill health prevail. It affects mostly young adults in their most productive years living in the developing world.[10]

GLOBAL MONITORING OF THE BURDEN OF CHILDHOOD TUBERCULOSIS

Existing Challenges to Estimating Disease Burden in Children

There are important challenges that currently prevent the accurate measurement of the number of tuberculosis cases and deaths among children. First of all, there is no point-of-care, easy-to-use, and accurate diagnostic test for confirming tuberculosis disease in children. Most children have pauci-bacillary pulmonary tuberculosis that is harder to diagnose with available laboratory tests (such as sputum-smear microscopy and culture). Children are often not able to expectorate sputum, which means that obtaining a specimen requires induced special techniques such as gastric lavage, nebulization, or bronchoalveolar lavage. These procedures usually require a hospital setting, overnight hospitalization, an appropriate infection-control environment and trained personnel. Therefore, diagnosis is usually made using a combination of clinical criteria and a nonspecific test for tuberculosis infection such as the tuberculin skin test (TST) or interferon-gamma release assay (IGRA). There are several diagnostic clinical algorithms that have been proposed, but none has been thoroughly validated and universally applied, making comparisons over time and space difficult. Furthermore, the definitive diagnosis of extrapulmonary tuberculosis requires specialized services that are usually available only in referral tertiary hospitals, and thus often not accessible to those most in need. Besides the known diagnostic challenges, children diagnosed with tuberculosis are not always reported to national surveillance systems because of the lack of linkages among individual pediatricians and pediatric hospitals, and national tuberculosis programs. In addition, data from national surveys that include children are limited. Many countries lack vital registration (VR) systems in which deaths from tuberculosis are reported and disaggregated by age.

Tuberculosis Incidence

Tuberculosis incidence has never been measured at the national level because this would require long-term studies among large cohorts of people (hundreds of thousands) at high cost and with challenging logistics. However, health information systems in many countries are not yet capable of providing a direct measure of tuberculosis incidence, as an unknown number of cases are either treated but not reported, or go undiagnosed. The major reasons why cases are missing from official notification data include laboratory errors,[15] lack of notification of cases by public[16] and private providers,[17] the failure of people accessing health services to be identified as potential tuberculosis cases,[18] and lack of access to health services.[19] The best approach to estimating tuberculosis incidence is from routine surveillance systems in which case

reports disaggregated by age and sex are more or less complete, such that notifications can be considered a close proxy of incidence. This is possible in settings with universal health care coverage,[20,21] and where operational research has been used to quantify the small fraction of cases that are treated but not reported to surveillance systems.[22] Recent efforts to improve our understanding of the gap between tuberculosis surveillance systems and the true incidence level are very promising and include the design and implementation of nationwide inventory surveys to measure underreporting of childhood tuberculosis, primarily from the private but also the public sector, in high-priority countries in Asia.[23,24]

Tuberculosis Mortality

Tuberculosis mortality among HIV-negative people can be directly measured using age-disaggregated data from national VR systems, provided that these systems have high coverage and the causes of death are accurately coded according to the latest revision of the *International Classification of Diseases* (ICD-10).[25] Sample VR systems covering representative areas of the country (e.g., China) provide an interim solution. The parts of the world where there are major gaps in the availability of VR data are the African region and parts of the Southeast Asia region; in the latter, Indonesia is currently building a sample VR system.

TB mortality among HIV-infected children is hard to measure directly, even when national VR systems with standard coding of causes of death are in place, because deaths among HIV-infected people are coded as HIV deaths, and contributory causes (such as tuberculosis) are generally not reliably recorded. This will need to be corrected in future iterations of the ICD to permit a proper assessment of tuberculosis mortality. In the interim, indirect estimation of tuberculosis mortality among HIV-infected children is the only option, using data on contributory causes of AIDS death from well-monitored cohorts of HIV-infected people on care and autopsy studies.

Tuberculosis Prevalence

There is currently no global data source available that monitors the prevalence of tuberculosis disease in children. Bacteriologically confirmed disease prevalence among adults (aged 15 or older) is measured in nationwide population-based surveys in countries with a high burden of tuberculosis.[26,27] Since 2002, 22 countries have successfully measured the prevalence of tuberculosis disease through such surveys, including ten in Africa,[28,29,30,31,3] while an additional ten countries (three in Africa) have planned to implement a survey by 2015.

Review of historical data from national surveys of pulmonary tuberculosis targeting children found that, while the group including some of, or the entire, 0–14 age category made up between 20–30% of the total sample size of the survey, it only included between 1–4% of the total number of acid-fast bacilli smear-positive and 2–7% of bacteriologically confirmed tuberculosis cases found by the survey (Table 5.1). Furthermore, in the context of the current design of national prevalence surveys to estimate pulmonary tuberculosis:

- The inclusion of children in a survey would not lead to a precise estimate of tuberculosis prevalence among children, since only a few bacteriologically confirmed cases would be found. Even existing surveys are not able to provide precise estimates for different age groups.
- There are ethical considerations associated with mass screening of all children, most of whom are healthy. While evidence exists that chest radiograph screening is safe for adults, similar evidence does not exist for children. Furthermore, there is no simple and reliable tool that could be used to restrict the number of children screened by radiography.
- Among adults, "over-reading" of radiographs is encouraged to minimize the number of cases that are missed. Among children, use of tests for tuberculosis infection and over-reading of radiographs would lead to unnecessary efforts to obtain specimens, which among young children requires invasive and uncomfortable procedures.
- Referral hospitals are needed for the follow-up and diagnostic confirmation of tuberculosis in children. These are often not available in the rural areas that account for a large share of the clusters included in national prevalence surveys.
- Inclusion of children would approximately double the sample size and associated costs. The additional logistical complications of including children could also jeopardize the survey as a whole.

Taking all of the above into consideration, as well as the performance of existing screening and diagnosis tools, the inclusion of children in the current design of national prevalence surveys that estimate pulmonary tuberculosis is not currently recommended, but instead attention is focused on strengthening surveillance systems so they can provide reliable and complete data on new tuberculosis cases and tuberculosis-related deaths among children. Those adult cases that are found as part of prevalence surveys of pulmonary tuberculosis provide an opportunity for household-contact investigation and identification of children with tuberculosis disease and/or those under than 5 years eligible for isoniazid treatment of tuberculosis infection.

Drug-Resistant Tuberculosis

Estimates of the incidence and mortality of multidrug-resistant tuberculosis (MDR-TB) are derived from periodic surveys or from routine drug-susceptibility testing (DST) if the coverage of patient testing is sufficiently representative.[3] The global surveillance of resistance to the two most important first-line anti-TB drugs—isoniazid and rifampicin—has been coordinated by WHO since 1994.[32, 32A] Due to the lack of consistently reported age-disaggregated results from these surveys, WHO does not currently publish global estimates of drug resistance among children. Research groups have attempted to address this gap, estimating the global incidence of MDR-TB cases among children for 2013 at 32,000 (95% confidence interval [CI] 26,000–39,000).[33]

Burden of Tuberculosis Infection

Nationally representative TST surveys were traditionally used to measure the prevalence of tuberculosis infection and determine the annual risk of infection (which under a number of assumptions was also translated into an estimate of incidence of tuberculosis disease). However, well-documented shortcomings with the conduct, analysis, and interpretation of such data, as well as evidence that contradicted the underlying assumptions, discontinued the conduct of such surveys.[34,35,36] In the absence of an accurate diagnostic test for infection, and due to the lack of recent nationally representative data, WHO does not currently publish global estimates of the burden of tuberculosis infection. However, a mathematical

Table 5.1 Evidence from past national tuberculosis prevalence surveys that included children: numbers and rates per 100,000 of acid-fast smear-positive and bacteriologically-confirmed cases among the age group including some of or the entire 0–14 childhood age category

NATIONAL SURVEYS[1]	AGE GROUP INCLUDING CHILDREN (COLUMN B)	TOTAL NUMBER OF SURVEY PARTICIPANTS— ALL AGES (%[3])	NUMBER OF S+[4] CASES N (%[5])	S+[4] RATE PER 100,000	NUMBER OF B+[6] CASES N (%[5])	B+[6] RATE PER 100,000
China 1990[a]	0–14	401,997 (28)	30 (2)	7	51 (2)	13
China 2000[2,b]	0–14	89,295 (24)	6 (1)	7	11 (2)	12
Cambodia 2002[2,c]	10–14	4,591 (21)	3 (4)	65	4 (1)	87
Philippines 1997[d]	10–19	4,989 (31)	6 (9)	120	18 (10)	361
Philippines 2007[e]	10–19	6,728 (29)	1 (2)	15	11 (7)	163
Republic of Korea 1990[f]	5–19	16,468 (34)	2 (3)	12	5 (4)	30
Republic of Korea 1995[g]	5–19	19,005 (29)	1 (2)	5	2 (1)	11

[1] Pulmonary tuberculosis with chest radiograph screening; [2] Additional symptoms screening; [3] Percentage calculated as the number of participants in the age group including children (column B) over total number of survey participants (all ages); [4] Smear-positive tuberculosis; [5] Percentage calculated as the number of cases in the age group including children (column B) over total number of survey cases (all ages); [6] Bacteriologically-confirmed tuberculosis cases (smear and/or culture positive).

[a] Ministry of Public Health—China (1990). Nationwide random survey for the epidemiology of tuberculosis in 1990. Beijing, China.
[b] Ministry of Public Health—China (2000). Nationwide random survey for the epidemiology of tuberculosis in 2000. Beijing, China.
[c] Ministry of Health—Cambodia (2005). Report of the national tuberculosis prevalence survey, 2002.
[d] Tropical Disease Foundation Inc and Department of Health (1997). Final report of the national tuberculosis prevalence survey 1997. Navotas City, Philippines.
[e] Tropical Disease Foundation Inc and Department of Health (2008). Final report of the nationwide tuberculosis prevalence survey 2007. Navotas City, Philippines.
[f] Ministry of Health & Social Affairs and the Korean National Tuberculosis Association (1990). Report on the 6th Tuberculosis Prevalence Survey in Korea, 1990 Seoul, Republic of Korea.
[g] Ministry of Health & Social Affairs and the Korean National Tuberculosis Association (1996). Report on the 7th tuberculosis prevalence survey in Korea, 1995. Seoul, Republic of Korea.

modelling exercise has attempted to address this gap and estimated that in 2010 there were about 53 million (95% CI 41–69 million) children with mostly untreated tuberculosis infection in just the 22 highest-burden countries in the world.[37]

INCIDENCE

Age-Disaggregated Tuberculosis Case Notifications

Routine recording and reporting of the numbers of tuberculosis cases diagnosed and treated by national tuberculosis programs (NTPs) and monitoring of treatment outcomes was one of the five components of the global tuberculosis strategy (directly observed therapy short course [DOTS]) launched by WHO in the mid-1990s,[38] and remained a core element of its successors, the *Stop TB Strategy*[39,39A] and the *End TB Strategy*.[40] With the standard definitions of cases and treatment outcomes recommended by WHO and associated recording and reporting framework as a foundation, global monitoring of trends in case notifications and treatment outcomes has been possible since 1995.

Age and sex disaggregation of acid-fast smear-positive tuberculosis case notifications has been requested from countries since the establishment of the data collection system in 1995, but few countries had actually been reporting these data to WHO. In 2006, the data collection system was revised to additionally monitor age-disaggregated notifications for smear-negative and extrapulmonary tuberculosis. The revision also included a further disaggregation of the 0–14 age group category to differentiate the very young (0–4) from the older children (5–14). While reporting of age-disaggregated data was limited in the early years of the data collection system, coverage kept improving until, for 2012 case notifications, it reached 99%, 83%, and 83% out of total acid-fast smear-positive, smear-negative, and extrapulmonary tuberculosis case notifications notified, respectively, that were age- and sex-disaggregated (Figure 5.1). Finally, in 2013, another revision of the recording and reporting system was necessary to allow the capture of cases diagnosed using WHO-approved rapid diagnostic tests (such as Xpert MTB/RIF).[41] This current revision of the system requests the reporting of all new and relapse case notifications by age and sex (but not separately by case type). The countries that reported age-disaggregated data in 2013 can be seen in Figure 5.2.

While there are some nationwide surveys that have quantified the amount of under-reporting of cases diagnosed in the health sector outside the network of the NTPs,[42,43,22] none have produced precise enough age-disaggregated results. Small-scale, conveniently sampled studies in some settings indicate that *under-reporting of childhood tuberculosis is very high*,[44] but extrapolation to nationally representative, regional, and global settings is not yet possible. This shortcoming is currently being addressed through the plans for implementation of national-scale surveys in high-priority countries in Asia to measure under-reporting of tuberculosis in children.[24]

Complementary Methods of Estimation

The first estimation approach to quantify tuberculosis incidence in children, published by WHO in 2012, was based on case notifications corrected for the estimated gap from true incidence due to under-reporting and under-diagnosis with well-described strengths and limitations.[7] Since then, alternative approaches to indirectly estimating incidence and improving our understanding of disease burden in children were commissioned to research groups that were presented and reviewed during a global consultation in 2013 on methods to estimate childhood tuberculosis burden. By early 2014, both these approaches[37,33] and an additional independent approach[45] were published. Comparing results between approaches shows large discordance that ultimately highlights the weaknesses of the underlying data and the urgent need for strengthening surveillance and improving the direct measurement of tuberculosis disease in children.

To estimate TB incidence in children for 2014, an ensemble statistical approach was used to combine results from the original WHO approach and the two commissioned approaches from the research groups.[3] The third method has been refined with additional data review efforts to inform parameters critical to the estimation process.[46] The fourth method is currently excluded due to the lack of information on the uncertainty of the estimate.[45]

Childhood tuberculosis incidence in 2014 was estimated to be 1,000,000 (range, 900,000–1,100,000),

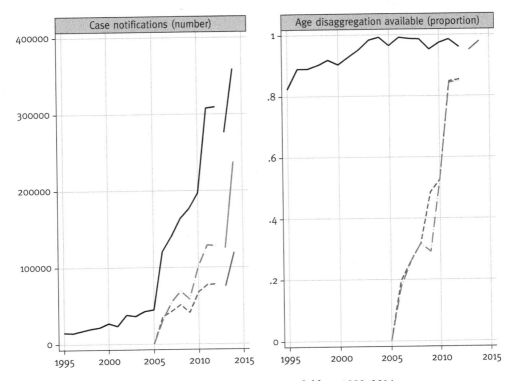

FIGURE 5.1 Global progress in reporting of TB cases among children, 1995–2014.
Left panel: Number of notifications of cases reported to WHO among the 0-14 (solid), 0–4 (dash) and 5–14 (longdash-dot) age groups.
Right panel: Proportion of case notifications reported to WHO that are age-disaggregated among new smear-positive (solid), new smear-negative and smear not done (dash), new extra-pulmonary (longdash-dot) before 2013, and new and relapse (solid) after 2013.

Before 2013 childhood case notifications included smear-positive, smear-negative, smear not done and extrapulmonary TB for all new patients. After 2013 (shown as a gap in the graph) childhood case notifications include all new and relapse cases irrespective of case type.

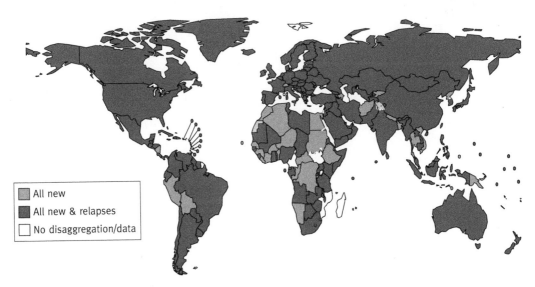

FIGURE 5.2 Reporting of new and relapse TB case notifications disaggregated by age, 2014.

equivalent to about 10% of the total 9.6 million incident (all ages) cases in the world.[3]

Next Steps to Improve Estimation and Ongoing Analytical Work

The key future efforts that will contribute most to the improvement of the estimation of tuberculosis incidence among children are: first, the promotion of case-based electronic recording and reporting systems that will facilitate the compilation and analysis of age-disaggregated data at national and sub-national levels; second, the implementation of nationwide inventory surveys in high-priority countries to measure under-reporting of childhood tuberculosis; and third, intensified household-contact-tracing activities of index adult tuberculosis cases, as well as the integration of tuberculosis activities in maternal, newborn, and child health services, to identify childhood cases that would otherwise go undiagnosed.

Finally, the currently ongoing analytical work, coordinated by WHO and conducted by collaborating research groups, aims to produce robust estimates of incidence for regions and countries, as well as disaggregate global tuberculosis incidence by HIV-status and multi-drug-resistance status, by the end of 2016.

MORTALITY

Mortality data reported to WHO from VR systems that were disaggregated by age were available for 113 countries for 2014 (Figure 5.3). These data were used to calculate tuberculosis death rates per 100,000 population for children and adults, after adjustment for incomplete coverage and ill-defined causes, and impute data for countries without VR.[3] The total number of deaths from tuberculosis among HIV-uninfected children was estimated to be 81,000 (range, 69,000–93,000), equivalent to about 7% of the total number of 1,100,000 tuberculosis-related deaths among HIV-uninfected people in 2014.[3] An alternative independent approach produced a lower estimate of about 60,000 deaths.[45] There were an additional 55,000 (range, 50,000–60,000) TB deaths among HIV-positive children, equivalent to 14% of the total number of HIV-positive TB deaths. The total number of TB deaths among children (136,000, range 115,000–157,000) corresponds to a case fatality rate of 13.6%.

To improve estimates of tuberculosis mortality among children, the next steps are: first, to collect age-specific data from sample vital registration systems and mortality surveys in high-burden countries, including China, India, and Indonesia; and second, to advocate the further development of,

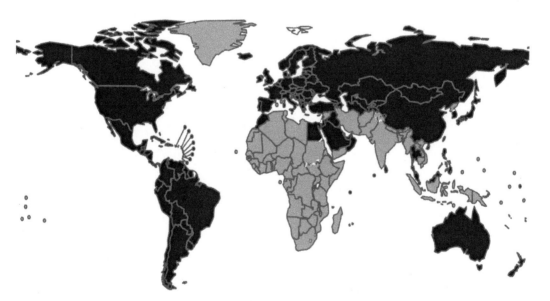

FIGURE 5.3   Countries (in black) for which tuberculosis mortality is estimated using age-disaggregated measurements from vital registration systems, 2014.

and continued investment in, robust and accurate VR systems. Current analytical work aims to produce robust estimates of tuberculosis mortality for regions and countries, by the end of 2016.

EPIDEMIOLOGICAL STRATEGIES TO DECREASE TUBERCULOSIS BURDEN AMONG CHILDREN

WHO currently recommends the active screening for tuberculosis disease of all children, especially those living with HIV or in the households of adults diagnosed with tuberculosis disease.[47,48,49] The main purposes of contact screening and management are: first, the early identification of all child contacts of an index case with undiagnosed tuberculosis disease to improve treatment outcomes and prevent further transmission of infection; and second, to identify all child contacts recently infected who do not have tuberculosis disease and are eligible for provision of chemotherapy to prevent the onset of disease. Among asymptomatic children in close contact with a tuberculosis case, those recommended by WHO for treatment are all children under the age of five years and all HIV-infected children.

CONCLUSIONS

The lack of child-appropriate tools to confirm diagnosis of tuberculosis disease, standard case-definitions, and the incomplete recording and reporting of children who are diagnosed with tuberculosis and put on treatment continue to pose significant shortcomings to the robust estimation of burden due to tuberculosis in children. Despite that, remarkable progress has been made since the first official set of WHO estimates for childhood tuberculosis was published in 2012. Since then, global interest in improving these estimates has been ignited, with countries around the world improving their recording and reporting practices for age-disaggregated data, multiple collaborating research groups working with WHO to improve our understanding of tuberculosis disease burden in children, and for the first time ever, a number of high-priority countries in Asia are planning to implement national scale studies to measure the level of tuberculosis under-reporting in children.

WHO estimates that in 2014 there were 1,000,000 (range, 900,000–1,100,000) new tuberculosis cases and 136,000 (range, 115,000/157,000) deaths in children. Independent research groups estimate there are 32,000 (95% CI 26,000–39,000) children with MDR-TB and an astounding 53 million (95% confidence interval 41,000,000–69,000,000) children with tuberculosis infection in the 22 high-burden countries, the future pool of tuberculosis cases of tomorrow. The sheer magnitude of tuberculosis infection and tuberculosis morbidity and mortality places childhood tuberculosis high as a global public health priority and demands our continued attention and commitment.

REFERENCES

1. Holloway KL, Henneberg RJ, de Barros Lopes M, Henneberg M. Evolution of human tuberculosis: a systematic review and meta-analysis of paleopathological evidence. *Homo: internationale Zeitschrift fur die vergleichende Forschung am Menschen.* 2011;62:402–458.
2. Comas I, Coscolla M, Luo T, et al. Out-of-Africa migration and Neolithic coexpansion of *Mycobacterium tuberculosis* with modern humans. *Nature Genetics.* 2013;45:1176–1182.
3. WHO. *Global TB Report 2015.* Geneva: WHO; 2015.
3A. Squire SB, Obasi A, Nhlema-Simwaka B. The Global Plan to Stop TB: a unique opportunity to address poverty and the Millennium Development Goals. *Lancet.* 2006;367:955–957.
4. Lozano R, Naghavi M, Foreman K, et al. Global and regional mortality from 235 causes of death for 20 age groups in 1990 and 2010: a systematic analysis for the Global Burden of Disease Study 2010. *Lancet.* 2012;380:2095–2128.
5. Ortblad KF, Lozano R, Murray CJ. The burden of HIV: insights from the Global Burden of Disease Study 2010. *AIDS.* 2013;27:2003–2017.
6. Lopez AD, Mathers CD, Ezzati M, Jamison DT, Murray CJ. Global and regional burden of disease and risk factors, 2001: systematic analysis of population health data. *Lancet.* 2006;367:1747–1757.
7. WHO. *Global TB Report 2012.* Geneva: WHO; 2012.
8. WHO. *Roadmap for Childhood Tuberculosis.* Geneva: WHO; 2013.
9. Riley RL. The contagiosity of tuberculosis. *Schweiz Med Wochenschr.* 1983;113:75–79.
10. WHO. Tuberculosis. Fact sheet No 104. http://www.who.int/mediacentre/factsheets/fs104/en/, accessed 21 November 2015.
11. Vynnycky E, Fine PE. Lifetime risks, incubation period, and serial interval of tuberculosis. *Am J Epidemiol.* 2000;152:247–263.

12. Borgdorff MW, Sebek M, Geskus RB, Kremer K, Kalisvaart N, van Soolingen D. The incubation period distribution of tuberculosis estimated with a molecular epidemiological approach. *Int J Epidemiol.* 2011;40:964–970.

13. Tiemersma EW, van der Werf MJ, Borgdorff MW, Williams BG, Nagelkerke NJ. Natural history of tuberculosis: duration and fatality of untreated pulmonary tuberculosis in HIV negative patients: a systematic review. *PLoS One.* 2011;6:e17601.

14. Straetemans M, Glaziou P, Bierrenbach AL, Sismanidis C, van der Werf MJ. Assessing tuberculosis case fatality ratio: a meta-analysis. *PLoS ONE.* 2011;6:e20755.

15. Botha E, den Boon S, Lawrence KA, et al. From suspect to patient: tuberculosis diagnosis and treatment initiation in health facilities in South Africa. *Int J Tuberc Lung Dis.* 2008;12:936–941.

16. Dye C, Scheele S, Dolin P, Pathania V, Raviglione MC. Consensus statement. Global burden of tuberculosis: estimated incidence, prevalence, and mortality by country. WHO Global Surveillance and Monitoring Project. *JAMA.* 1999;282:677–686.

17. Uplekar M, Pathania V, Raviglione M. Private practitioners and public health: weak links in tuberculosis control. *Lancet.* 2001;358:912–916.

18. Meintjes G, Schoeman H, Morroni C, Wilson D, Maartens G. Patient and provider delay in tuberculosis suspects from communities with a high HIV prevalence in South Africa: a cross-sectional study. *BMC Infect Dis.* 2008;8:72.

19. Veron LJ, Blanc LJ, Suchi M, Raviglione MC. DOTS expansion: will we reach the 2005 targets? International Journal of Tuberculosis and Lung Diseases, 2004, 8:139–146. 376.

20. Moreno-Serra R, Smith PC. Does progress towards universal health coverage improve population health? *Lancet.* 2012;380:917–923.

21. O'Neill K, Takane M, Sheffel A, Abou-Zahr C, Boerma T. 2013. Monitoring service delivery for universal health coverage: the Service Availability and Readiness Assessment. *Bull World Health Organ.* 1994;91:923–931.

22. Van Hest N, Story A, Grant AD, Antoine D, Crofts JP, Watson JM. Record-linkage and capture-recapture analysis to estimate the incidence and completeness of reporting of tuberculosis in England 1999–2002. *Epidemiol Infect.* 2008;136:1606–1616.

23. WHO. *Assessing Tuberculosis Under-Reporting Through Inventory Studies.* Geneva: WHO; 2012.

24. WHO. *Protocol Development Workshop for Inventory Studies to Measure TB Under-Reporting.*

Geneva: WHO; 2014. Available at http://www.who.int/tb/advisory_bodies/impact_measurement_taskforce/meetings/sep14indonesia_inventorystudyworkshop/en/.

25. Korenromp EL, ALB, Williams BG, Dye C. The measurement and estimation of tuberculosis mortality. *Int J Tuberc Lung Dis.* 2009;13:283–303.

26. Glaziou P, van der Werf MJ, Onozaki I, et al. Tuberculosis prevalence surveys: rationale and cost. *Int J Tuberc Lung Dis.* 2008;12:1003–1008.

27. WHO. *Tuberculosis Prevalence Surveys: A Handbook.* Geneva: WHO; 2011.

28. Hong YP, Kim SJ, Lew WJ, Lee EK, Han YC. The seventh nationwide tuberculosis prevalence survey in Korea, 1995. *Int J Tuberc Lung Dis.* 1998;2:27–36.

29. Tupasi TE, Radhakrishna S, Rivera AB, et al. The 1997 Nationwide Tuberculosis Prevalence Survey in the Philippines. *Int J Tuberc Lung Dis.* 1999;3:471–477.

30. Dye C, Fengzeng Z, Scheele S, Williams B. Evaluating the impact of tuberculosis control: number of deaths prevented by short-course chemotherapy in China. *Int J Epidemiol.* 2000;29:558–564.

31. Soemantri S, Senewe FP, Tjandrarini DH, et al. Three-fold reduction in the prevalence of tuberculosis over 25 years in Indonesia. *Int J Tuberc Lung Dis.* 2007;11:398–404.

32. Pablos-Méndez A, Raviglione MC, Laszlo A, et al., for the WHO/IUATLD Working Group on Anti-tuberculosis Drug Resistance Surveillance. Global surveillance for antituberculosis-drug resistance: 1994–1997. *N Engl J Med.* 1998;338:1641–1649.

32A. Zignol M, van Gemert W, Falzon D, et al. Surveillance of anti-tuberculosis drug resistance in the world: an updated analysis, 2007–2010. *Bull World Health Organ.* 2012;90:111–119D.

33. Jenkins HE, Tolman AW, Yuen CM, et al. Incidence of multidrug-resistant tuberculosis disease in children: systematic review and global estimate. *Lancet.* 2014;383:1572–1579.

34. Dye C. Breaking a law: tuberculosis disobeys Styblo's rule. *Bull World Health Organ.* 2008;86:4.

35. Van Leth F, Van der Werf MJ, Borgdorff MW. Prevalence of tuberculous infection and incidence of tuberculosis: a re-assessment of the Styblo rule. *Bull World Health Organ.* 2008;86:20–26.

36. WHO. *TB Impact Measurement Policy and Recommendations for How to Assess the Epidemiological Burden of TB and the Impact of TB Control.* (Stop TB policy paper; no. 2).

Geneva: WHO; 2009 (WHO/HTM/TB/2009.416). Available at http://whqlibdoc.who.int/publications/2009/9789241598828_eng.pdf?ua=1.

37. Dodd PJ, Gardiner E, Coghlan R, Seddon JA. Burden of childhood tuberculosis in 22 high-burden countries: a mathematical modelling study. *Lancet Global Health*. 2014;2:453–459.

38. WHO. *WHO Tuberculosis Programme: Framework for Effective Tuberculosis Control*. Geneva: WHO; 1994 (WHO/TB/94.179).

39. Raviglione MC, Uplekar MW. WHO's new Stop TB Strategy. *Lancet*. 2006;367:952–955.

39A. Raviglione M, Marais B, Floyd K, et al. Scaling up interventions to achieve global tuberculosis control: progress and new developments. *Lancet*. 2012;379:1902–1913.

40. WHO. *WHO Factsheet: The End TB Strategy*. Geneva: WHO; 2014. Available at http://www.who.int/tb/post2015_TBstrategy.pdf?ua=1.

41. WHO. *Definitions and Reporting Framework for Tuberculosis—2013 Revision*. Geneva: WHO; 2013 (WHO/HTM/TB/2013.2). Available at http://www.who.int/tb/publications/definitions/en/.

42. Bassili A, et al. Estimating tuberculosis case detection rate in resource-limited countries: a capture–recapture study in Egypt. *Int J Tub Lung Dis*. 2010;14:727–732.

43. Van Hest NA, et al. Completeness of notification of tuberculosis in the Netherlands: how reliable is record-linkage and capture-recapture analysis? *Epidemiol Infect*. 2007;135:1021–1029.

44. Lestari T, Probandari A, Hurtig AK, Utarini A. High caseload of childhood tuberculosis in hospitals on Java Island, Indonesia: a cross sectional study. *BMC Public Health*. 2011;11:784.

45. Murray CJL, et al. Global, regional, and national incidence and mortality for HIV, tuberculosis, and malaria during 1990–2013: a systematic analysis for the Global Burden of Disease Study 2013. *Lancet*. 2014;384:1005–1070.

46. Sismanidis C, Glaziou P, Law I, Floyd K. The burden of tuberculosis disease in children. *Lancet*. 2014;384:9951.

47. WHO. Guidelines for intensified tuberculosis case-finding and isoniazid preventive therapy for people living with HIV in resource-constrained settings. 2011. Geneva: WHO; 2011. Available at http://whqlibdoc.who.int/publications/2011/9789241500708_eng.pdf?ua=1.

48. WHO. *Recommendations for Investigating Contacts of Persons with Infectious Tuberculosis in Low- and Middle-Income Countries*. Geneva: WHO; 2012. Available at http://apps.who.int/iris/bitstream/10665/77741/1/9789241504492_eng.pdf.

49. WHO. *Guidance for National Tuberculosis Programmes on the Management of Tuberculosis in Children*. 2nd ed. Geneva: WHO; 2014. Available at http://apps.who.int/iris/bitstream/10665/112360/1/9789241548748_eng.pdf?ua=1.

6

DIAGNOSIS OF TUBERCULOSIS INFECTION IN CHILDREN

Anna M. Mandalakas and Andrew DiNardo

HIGHLIGHTS OF THIS CHAPTER

- The sensitivity for confirming tuberculosis infection with disease is comparable among all the IGRAs and the TST. None of the tests can differentiate between tuberculosis infection and disease.
- A negative result from the TST or IGRA does not exclude tuberculosis disease. Clinically significant tuberculosis exposure, symptoms, physical examination, and chest radiography remain the cornerstones of diagnosis in children.
- Among children with high risk of tuberculosis infection and progression to disease, or who may already have tuberculosis disease, combined use of a TST and IGRA can maximize sensitivity. Children falling into this category include young, malnourished, HIV-infected, and immune-compromised children (including those about to start immune-suppressive therapy).
- For children five years of age or older who have not received the BCG, either the TST or IGRA is acceptable.
- For BCG-vaccinated children five years of age or older, IGRAs are preferable. If a TST is completed and negative, no other testing is required. If a positive TST result is obtained, an IGRA may help determine if the TST result was caused by tuberculosis infection or the previous BCG vaccination.

IN 2010, 15.3 million children in the world shared a household with an individual with infectious tuberculosis, resulting in 7.6 million children becoming infected with *Mycobacterium tuberculosis*.[1] Modeling estimates further suggest that cumulative exposure has resulted in a prevalence of over 50 million infected children in the 22 high tuberculosis burden countries in 2010, most of whom have gone undetected and untreated. Most children with *M. tuberculosis* infection develop a latent tuberculosis infection characterized by a positive tuberculin skin test or interferon-γ release assay result but no symptoms or radiographic abnormalities.[2] Following infection with *M. tuberculosis*, the five-year risk of developing tuberculosis disease is 33% in children under 5 years of age and 20% for those ages 5–14 years.[3] The risk is greatest in the year following infection and highest among young, malnourished, and immune-compromised children; up to 50% of children infected during the first year of life develop disease in the absence of effective treatment.[4] Treatment of tuberculosis infection decreases subsequent tuberculosis morbidity and mortality among adult contacts[5,6] and markedly reduces risk in child contacts.[7,8] Nevertheless, in 2010, over 650,000 children developed tuberculosis,[1] and 74,000 HIV-uninfected children died of tuberculosis,[9] suggesting a need for improvements in detection and treatment of the reservoir of infected children.

The World Health Organization (WHO) has a goal to eliminate tuberculosis by 2050, an achievement that will depend on many activities, including detection and treatment of tuberculosis infection to reduce the potential disease burden originating from the large reservoir of infected individuals. Targeted treatment of tuberculosis infection has been a tuberculosis control strategy for over a decade,[10] but it remains hampered by poor detection and implementation. The WHO released recommendations to guide the investigation of tuberculosis contacts in middle and high burden settings in 2012[11] and for the provision of treatment of tuberculosis infection in 2015.[12]

The course of tuberculosis infection is influenced largely by the child's immune response to the organism.[2,13–15] Although children classically have been thought to progress from no infection, to infection, to disease in a linear, unidirectional fashion, a growing body of evidence suggests that a more complex, dynamic bidirectional continuum of responses exists, leading to a spectrum of tuberculosis infection and disease states[16] (Figure 6.1). It is further hypothesized that the phase of the host response may be associated with the magnitude of the mycobacterial load harbored by the host. Improved understanding of this dynamic interplay is vital as new tests of infection, vaccines, and treatment of tuberculosis disease and infection are developed.

EPIDEMIOLOGY AND TEST PERFORMANCE

As there is no reference standard test for infection with *M. tuberculosis*, clinicians and public health

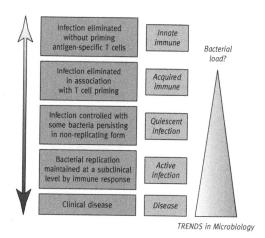

FIGURE 6.1   A spectrum of responses to *M. tuberculosis* infection.[16]

practitioners must consider risk factors for transmission and infection when developing guidelines for control activities and interpreting available tests to guide clinical decision-making. Transmission of *M. tuberculosis* is generally person-to-person and occurs via inhalation of mucous droplets that become airborne when an individual with pulmonary or laryngeal tuberculosis coughs, sneezes, speaks, laughs, or sings. After drying, the droplet nuclei can remain suspended in the air for hours. Only small droplets (<1–5 μm in diameter) can reach alveoli. Droplet nuclei also can be produced by aerosol treatments, sputum induction, aerosolization during bronchoscopy, and through manipulation of lesions or processing of tissue or secretions in the hospital or laboratory. Transmission rarely occurs by direct contact with infected body fluids or fomites.

Many factors are associated with the risk for acquiring tuberculosis infection, including the extent of contact with the infectious case, the burden of organisms in the sputum, and the frequency of cough in the index case.[17] Adults with acid-fast sputum-smear-positive pulmonary tuberculosis are more likely to transmit infection; risk of infection to contacts increases as the sputum smear grade (density of organisms seen) of the case increases. In addition, the risk for transmission is directly correlated with the degree of contact with a contagious case. Most transmission to young children occurs in their homes.[18] A child's risk of infection is directly correlated with tuberculosis in the primary caregiver, sleep proximity and exposure to the index case, infectiousness of the index case, and having multiple cases of tuberculosis in the home.[19] Markers of close contact such as urban living and overcrowding also correlate with risk of infection in all age groups.[20] An increased risk for infection has been demonstrated in institutional settings, including nursing homes, schools, correctional institutions, homeless shelters, orphanages, and refugee camps.[21–23] The quality and amount of air circulation in the environment is another important factor; generally, low air quality in homes compared with commercial buildings is a part of the reason why transmission tends to be greater in the home. The general risk for acquiring infection increases with age from infancy to early adulthood, probably because of increasing contacts with infectious persons.

The sensitivity and specificity of available methods to detect tuberculosis infection are inherent properties of the tests. However, the positive and negative predictive values depend on the population in which the test is used. Therefore, all tests are more accurate and the positive predictive value is much higher when used in a population with established risk factors (i.e., high pre-test probability) for tuberculosis infection. Additionally, treatment of tuberculosis infection is most effective in children with a high risk of progression to tuberculosis disease. This target population of children with either a high risk of infection or progression to disease can be identified by asking the child's caretaker a collection of screening questions tailored to provide specificity for the clinical setting[11,19,24] (Table 6.1). The performance of a test can be further improved by using population specific guidelines for test interpretation as have been developed for the tuberculin skin test.

AVAILABLE TESTS FOR TUBERCULOSIS INFECTION

There is no accepted reference standard measure of infection by *M. tuberculosis*. There are three commonly used immune-based tests of infection that all measure the cell-mediated immune response in which interferon-gamma (IFN-ϒ) plays a major role[25] (Figure 6.2). The tuberculin skin test has well-recognized limitations, including limited positive predictive value in BCG-vaccinated populations. The identification of genes in the *M. tuberculosis* genome that are absent from *Mycobacterium bovis*-BCG[26] and most nontuberculous mycobacteria[27] supported the development of more specific interferon-γ release assays (IGRAs) that quantify the *in vitro* production of IFN-ϒ by T cells after stimulation with *M. tuberculosis*-specific antigens.[25]

The Tuberculin Skin Test

The TST remains the most widely employed test for the diagnosis of tuberculosis infection in children. Infection with *M. tuberculosis* produces a delayed-type hypersensitivity reaction to specific antigenic components of the bacilli that are contained in extracts of culture filtrates called "tuberculins." A batch of purified protein derivative (PPD) called PPD-S, produced by Siebert and Glenn in 1939, historically had served as the standard reference material worldwide. All PPD lots were bioassayed to demonstrate equal potency to PPD-S. The standard test dose of a commercially available preparation is now defined as the dose of that product that is expected to be biologically equivalent to 5 tuberculin units (TU) of PPD-S or 2 TU of PPD-RT (Research Tuberculin) 23. PPD-S is the most commonly used preparation of PPD, but PPD-RT 23 is used in many parts of the world. A small amount of Tween 80 is added to the diluent of PPD to reduce adsorption by glass and plastic. To minimize adsorption and subsequent loss of potency, tuberculin should never be transferred between containers and should be delivered as soon as possible after transfer to the syringe. Tuberculin should be stored refrigerated and in the dark, which limits its utility in areas where electricity is lacking or is only available intermittently. In response to the antigens, previously sensitized T cells release lymphokines that induce local vasodilation, edema, fibrin deposition, and recruitment of other inflammatory cells (Figure 6.2). The reaction to tuberculin typically begins 5 to 6 hours after injection and reaches maximal induration at 48–72 hours. In some individuals, the reaction may peak after 72 hours, and the largest reaction size is considered the result. The typical reaction consists of centralized induration with surrounding erythema and swelling (Figure 6.3). Vesiculation and necrosis rarely occur,[28–30] but when they do, repeat tuberculin testing should be avoided. Topical application of corticosteroids may reduce the degree of vesiculation, while local injection of corticosteroid may reduce the amount of necrosis that develops.

Variability of the results of the TST may be reduced by careful attention to details of administration and reading. A 1–2 cm, 27-gauge needle and tuberculin syringe are employed to inject

Table 6.1　Tuberculosis screening questions

TUBERCULOSIS LOW-BURDEN SETTING[24]	TUBERCULOSIS HIGH-BURDEN SETTING[19]
Has a family member or contact had tuberculosis disease?	Is the index case the child's mother?
	Is the index case the child's primary caretaker?
Has a family member had a (recently converted) positive tuberculin skin test result?	Does the index case sleep in the same bed as the child?
Was your child born in a high-risk country (countries other than the U.S., Canada, Australia, New Zealand, or Western and Northern Europe)?	Does the index case sleep in the same room as the child?
	Does the index case live in the same household as the child?
Has your child traveled (had contact with resident population) to a high-risk country for more than 1 week?	Does the index case see the child every day?
	Is the index case coughing?
	Does the index case have reported pulmonary tuberculosis?
	Does the index case have smear-positive sputum?
	Is there more than one index case in the child's household?

0.1 mL of 5-TU PPD or 2-TU RT-23 intradermally (Mantoux method) into the volar or dorsal aspect of the forearm. If done correctly, a discrete, pale wheal 6–10 mm in diameter is produced. If the first test is administered improperly, another test dose may be employed at once in a site several centimeters from the original site. The TST should be interpreted 48–72 hours following injection. The diameter of induration (not erythema) should be measured transversely to the long axis of the forearm and

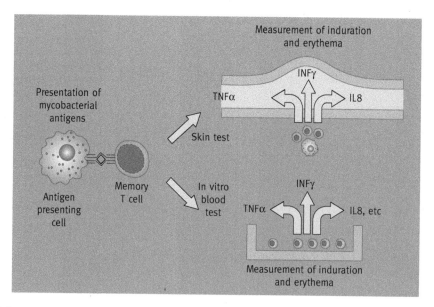

FIGURE 6.2　Basic principles of immunological tests for tuberculosis infection.[25]

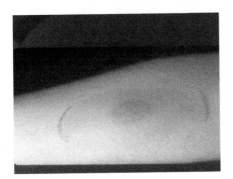

FIGURE 6.3 Typical tuberculin skin test response, with the ballpoint pen method used to demarcate the area of induration in the longitudinal axis (usually done in the transverse axis).

recorded in millimeters, even if the result is 0 mm. Use of the ballpoint pen method developed by Sokal minimizes interobserver variability.[31] The technique is completed by lightly drawing the pen across the arm until the pen meets resistance. At this point, a line is drawn to better define the two borders of the transverse axis of reaction. A ruler is then used to measure the distance between the two lines (Figure 6.3). An impartial, trained health professional should interpret all skin tests.

A number of factors can diminish reactivity to the TST, resulting in a false-negative reaction (Table 6.2) and decreased TST sensitivity. The administration of live-attenuated virus vaccines results in immune system suppression that appears more than 48 hours after vaccination and can cause a false-negative TST result. Tuberculin skin testing may be performed on either the same day as vaccination with live virus, or four to six weeks later. Studies have demonstrated that up to 10% of immunocompetent children with reactive anergy tests and culture-confirmed pulmonary tuberculosis have false-negative reactions to tuberculin testing.[32,33] In many of these children, TST conversion occurs after several months of treatment, suggesting that the infection was recently acquired or resulted in suppression of the immune response. The rate of false-negative TST results is higher in children with serious or life-threatening forms of tuberculosis, such as meningitis or disseminated disease. Therefore, a negative TST result *never* excludes tuberculosis disease. Among U.S. children diagnosed with tuberculosis, 89% have a positive TST; however, children who were diagnosed with

Table 6.2 Causes of Diminished Tuberculin Reactivity Associated with False-Negative TST

Factors Related to the Person Being Tested

Infections

Viral (measles, mumps, chickenpox, HIV)

Bacterial (typhoid fever, brucellosis, typhus, leprosy, pertussis, overwhelming tuberculosis, tuberculosis pleurisy)

Fungal (blastomycosis)

Live virus vaccinations (measles, mumps, polio, varicella)

Metabolic derangements (chronic renal failure)

Low protein states (severe protein depletion, afibrinogenemia)

Diseases affecting lymphoid organs (Hodgkin's disease, lymphoma, chronic leukemia, sarcoidosis)

Drugs (corticosteroids and other immunosuppressive agents)

Age (newborns, elderly patients with "waned" sensitivity)

Stress (surgery, burns, mental illness, graft-versus-host reactions)

Factors Related to the Tuberculin Used: Improper storage (exposure to light and heat), improper dilutions

Chemical denaturation

Contamination

Adsorption (partially controlled by adding Tween 80)

Factors Related to the Method of Administration: Injection of too little antigen

Subcutaneous injection

Delayed administration after drawing into syringe injection too close to other skin tests

Factors Related to Reading the Test and Recording Results: Inexperienced reader

Conscious or unconscious bias

Error in recording

disseminated or meningeal tuberculosis were less likely to have a positive TST result (57.6% and 54.6%, respectively) than those with pulmonary tuberculosis (90.6%).[33] This important finding emphasizes that a negative TST does not exclude any form of tuberculosis disease.

Many factors have been associated with false-positive tuberculin reactions and decreased tuberculin test positive predictive value. Because some antigens in PPD are shared with nontuberculous mycobacteria (NTM), false-positive reactions can occur in children who have been infected with NTMs. Exposure to NTMs varies geographically and generally results in smaller, transient indurations than those caused by infection with M. tuberculosis, but there is no reliable method of distinguishing TST reactivity secondary to NTM infection from TST reactivity secondary to tuberculosis infection.

Previous immunization with a BCG vaccine causes some TST reactivity in a significant portion of patients. The degree of BCG cross-reactivity is dependent on several factors, including the strain of BCG employed, age and nutritional status at vaccination, frequency of skin testing, and years since vaccination.[34-37] In most studies of children who received a BCG vaccine during the newborn period, only 50% reacted to tuberculin testing at 12 months, and 80–90% lost reactivity within two to three years. BCG vaccination of older children or adults results in greater initial and more persistent TST reactivity. While some evidence suggests that individuals lose TST reactivity within ten years of vaccination unless they also have become infected with M. tuberculosis,[38] new evidence suggests that neonatal BCG and BCG given more than ten years prior to testing can be associated with positive TST reactions that are generally less than 15 mm in size.[39] Guidelines in the United States recommend that the TST be interpreted the same for patients who have and who have not received a BCG vaccination.[24] Although these guidelines will lead to some children with false-positive TST results being treated, they are the most commonly followed and cited guidelines in settings that routinely use TST.

For persons living in tuberculosis high-burden settings, the WHO recommends systematic TST screening and treatment of M. tuberculosis in two specific populations: children younger than five years of age who are household contacts of tuberculosis cases,[11] and people living with HIV.[40] However, with limited access to TST, a positive TST is not required to initiate treatment in these situations. WHO guidelines recommend that a TST be considered positive when greater than or equal to 10 mm in HIV-uninfected children and greater than or equal to 5 mm in HIV-infected children.[41] Recognizing that the decision to test is a decision to treat, national tuberculosis programs must consider their local epidemiology and resources when deciding if a given at-risk population should be targeted for systematic testing with subsequent treatment for M. tuberculosis infection. National guidelines vary considerably and reflect cost constraints and the economic reality of using a lower (more sensitive but less specific) definition of positive. The use of the TST in tuberculosis high-burden settings remains infrequent due to the limited availability of PPD, limited allocation of resources to support testing, and limited treatment for M. tuberculosis infection despite existing guidelines recommending it. Where available, the TST is generally used in children being evaluated for tuberculosis disease or recent close contact with an infectious tuberculosis patient, and as part of a comprehensive package of HIV care. In these children, with a high risk of infection or disease, the most commonly used interpretation considers the TST to be positive when greater than or equal to 10 mm in HIV-uninfected children and greater than or equal to 5 mm in HIV-infected children.

The likelihood that positive TST or IGRA results represent true infection with M. tuberculosis (positive predictive value) increases as the prevalence of tuberculosis infection increases within the population. Testing populations or individuals without a known or likely exposure to M. tuberculosis can result in many false-positive reactions. In contrast, the high prevalence of tuberculosis infection in close contacts of individuals with infectious tuberculosis or persons who have lived in high-burden countries means that TSTs and IGRAs have much higher positive-predictive values in these target populations—most of the positive results are true positives.

Varying the interpretation of the TST based on a child's individual risk factors for tuberculosis infection minimizes false-positive and false-negative readings. Hence, many guidelines recommend that interpretation of TST reactions be based on risk for infection. (Table 6.3) lists the suggested interpretation of the TST in the United States where the burden of disease is low and the population is mainly not immunized with a BCG vaccine. For children

Table 6.3 Interpretation of the Tuberculin Skin Test

Induration ≥5 mm

Children in close contact with known or suspected contagious case of tuberculosis disease

Children suspected to have tuberculosis disease:

- Findings on chest radiograph consistent with active or previous tuberculosis
- Clinical evidence of tuberculosis disease

Children receiving immunosuppressive therapy or with immunosuppressive conditions, including HIV infection

Induration ≥10 mm

Children at increased risk for disseminated disease:

- Those younger than 4 years of age
- Those with other medical conditions, including Hodgkin's disease, lymphoma, diabetes mellitus, chronic renal failure, or malnutrition

Children with increased exposure to tuberculosis disease:

- Those born, or whose parents were born, in high-prevalence regions of the world

Those frequently exposed to adults who are HIV-infected, homeless, users of illicit drugs, residents of nursing homes, incarcerated or institutionalized, or migrant farm workers

Those who travel to high-prevalence regions of the world

Induration ≥15 mm

Children 4 years of age or older without any risk factors

with the greatest risk for infection or developing tuberculosis disease after infection, or those with suspected tuberculosis disease, an induration greater than or equal to 5 mm is considered positive. For children with an increased risk for infection or progression to disseminated disease, an induration greater than or equal to 10 mm is considered positive. Children with low risk must have an induration greater than or equal to 15 mm to be considered positive.

The annual risk of tuberculous infection (ARTI) is an epidemiological index derived from TST surveys among children to measure the extent of transmission of M. tuberculosis in a community. The measurement estimates the probability of acquiring new infection or reinfection over a period of one year. ARTI trends are a critical indicator for tuberculosis control in a community. Although the Styblo rule served as the basis of the estimate for decades,[42] new techniques are now favored to estimate the ARTI.[43,44] It is also well recognized that the operating characteristics of the TST result in a tradeoff between sensitivity and specificity that varies according to the prevalence of M. tuberculosis infection and other mycobacteria, including BCG, in the population. Although recent discussion has focused on the potential use of IGRAs to estimate the ARTI,[7] current evidence is conflicting regarding the potential gain in specificity and ultimate impact of replacing the TST with IGRAs.[43,45]

Interferon-Gamma Release Assays

The identification of genes in the M. tuberculosis genome that are absent from M. bovis BCG[26] and most NTMs[27] has supported the development of more specific, and possibly more sensitive, tests for detection of tuberculosis infection.[25] M. bovis BCG has 16-gene deletions including the region of difference 1 (RD-1) that encodes for early secretory antigen target-6 (ESAT-6) and culture filtrate protein 10 (CFP-10).[27,46] ESAT-6 and CFP-10 are strong targets of the cellular immune response in patients with tuberculosis infection and disease in whom sensitized memory and effector T cells produce IFN-γ in response to M. tuberculosis antigens, forming the biological basis for both the TST and IGRAs.[47,48] Research over the past two decades has resulted in the development of two commercially available IGRAs.[25,49,50] The latest generation, Quantiferon TB Gold In-tube assay (QFT) (Qiagen, USA), is an enzyme-linked immunosorbent assay (ELISA)–based whole-blood assay measuring the amount of IFN-γ produced in response to three M. tuberculosis antigens (ESAT-6, CFP-10, TB 7.7). In contrast, the enzyme-linked immunospot (ELISPOT)–based T.SPOT.TB (T-Spot) (Oxford Immunotec, UK) uses quantified peripheral mononuclear cells to detect the number of INF-γ-producing T cells after exposure to two M. tuberculosis antigens (ESAT-6, CFP-10). Manufacturer guidelines regarding test interpretation primarily are based on results for adults, despite existing data suggesting that test outcomes are age-dependent.[51]

It is important to understand the origin of indeterminate (Quantiferon) and invalid (T-Spot) results when interpreting IGRA results. In both IGRAs, immune cells are stimulated with (1) negative controls, (2) *M. tuberculosis*-specific stimuli (a combination of ESAT-6, CFP-10, and/or TB 7.7), and (3) a nonspecific positive control stimulant, such as phytohemagglutinin (PHA). Results are then interpreted based on the immune cells responding to the *M. tuberculosis*-specific stimulus compared to the negative controls. For example, a positive T-Spot response is one in which the *M. tuberculosis*-specific response has eight spots more than the negative stimulus. A lack of positive response to the PHA positive control is interpreted as an indeterminate or invalid result. Similarly, a positive response to the negative stimuli is considered an invalid result (Figure 6.4).

REVERSION, CONVERSION, AND BOOSTING

The TST and the IGRAs are based on the dynamic host immune response. Therefore, a dynamic test response should be expected. Conversion is defined as the change to a positive test result following a previous negative test result. True conversion represents the development of new or enhanced hypersensitivity due to new infection with *M. tuberculosis* or NTM, including BCG vaccination. Reversion is defined as the change to a negative test result following a previous positive test result. Among some children who are infected with *M. tuberculosis*, the ability to react to the TST may wane over time, resulting in a false-negative TST. However, the placement of the TST may stimulate the immune system, causing a positive or boosted reaction to subsequent TSTs. Completing a second TST after an initial negative TST reaction is called "two-step testing" and is used only when serial skin testing may be employed, such as for health care workers. The second TST may produce a larger reading due to the immune response's being "boosted" by the first TST. Boosting is maximal if the second TST is placed between one and five weeks after the initial test. The second boosted response should be used for decision-making or future comparison. When employing two-step testing, TST conversion is defined as a reaction to the second TST of more than 10 mm and an increase of at least 6 mm compared to the first TST. Individuals

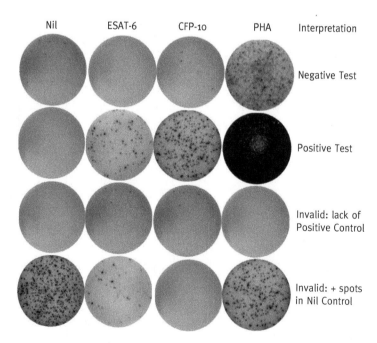

FIGURE 6.4   A T-spot positive result is defined as the number of CFP-10 or ESAT-6 minus Nil spots or greater than 8. Either a lack of positive control (row 3) or a positive Nil control (row 4) are considered invalid results.

showing TST conversion after the second test should be considered to be previously infected with a mycobacterium—*M. tuberculosis* or an NTM—or may have been BCG-vaccinated, whereas individuals with a negative reaction to the second TST should be considered uninfected.

Despite the T-Spot and the Quantiferon having continuous results, they are reported as either positive or negative. This creates some confusion, as repeat testing of health-care workers in tuberculosis low-burden settings has high rates of low-level conversions (a positive test that was previously negative) and reversions (a negative test that was previously positive). Most of these conversions and reversions are related to borderline positive results near the manufacturer-recommended cut-point, deemed the so-called "wobble" zone. Unlike the TST, in which results are interpreted based on an individual's risk of exposure, disease progression, and immune compromise (Table 6.3), the IGRAs do not have population-specific cutoffs. These findings have called into question: (1) the precise nature of the test; and (2) the need for population-specific cutoffs based on an individual's risk. While further studies are needed to clarify these issues, especially in children, many experts have recommended that IGRA's interpretation be based on an individual's risk for exposure, disease progression, and immune compromise, similar to TSTs.[46,47]

The introduction of IGRAs has resulted in new data regarding TST and IGRA testing for *M. tuberculosis*. TST reversion was previously thought to occur in fewer than 10% of healthy people and to be associated with older age, initially small TST responses, and an initial boosted response.[52] Nevertheless, new data indicate that conversions and reversions are common for all tests. Among South African children with recent tuberculosis exposure and an 87% BCG-vaccination rate, conversion and reversion were common for all tests of infection: TST (11% conversion, 15% reversion), Quantiferon (9% conversion, 8% reversion), and T-SPOT (11% conversion, 11% reversion).[53] Additionally, in this study, TST conversion was more common in HIV-infected children who had completed frequent tuberculin skin testing. The interpretation of serial testing in previously BCG-vaccinated children in tuberculosis high-burden settings is complicated by the inability to differentiate between increases in the test response resulting from conversion secondary to recent infection, and boosting resulting from previous exposure to mycobacteria, including BCG vaccination.

Internationally adopted children joining families in the United States are a unique group, as they are born in tuberculosis high-burden settings but have little to no risk of tuberculosis exposure after joining their adoptive families. Among these children, TST conversion was more common in younger children, suggesting that BCG-vaccination was associated with TST conversion.[37] Additionally, adult evidence suggests that recent TST may be associated with boosting of IGRA when the initial response is near the cut-point for positive.[54] Additional studies are needed, particularly in BCG-vaccinated children living in TB high-burden settings where there is a lack of data on repeat testing.

COMPARISON OF TEST PERFORMANCE

In the absence of a gold standard for infection, many studies have assessed the utility of IGRAs for the detection of tuberculosis infection, utilizing children with bacteriologically confirmed and clinically diagnosed tuberculosis disease (who are infected with *M. tuberculosis*). Systematic review of pediatric studies estimated the specificity of commercially approved IGRAs for detecting tuberculosis infection in tuberculosis diseased children at 91% for the ELISA-based tests and 94% for the ELISPOT-based test, compared with 88% for the TST (positive defined as 10 mm).[55] Estimates of test sensitivity were similar for the three tests: 83% (QFT assays), 84% (T-Spot), and 84% (TST), respectively. Similarly, a second pediatric systematic review found the performance of the TST and QFT assays to be no different for the detection of tuberculosis infection in children with tuberculosis disease.[56] Although a qualitative review of four pediatric studies concluded that the QFT assays were more specific for detection of tuberculosis infection in children than was the TST,[56] a larger pooled analysis was unable to demonstrate a statistically significant difference between these tests.[55] Like the TST, IGRAs cannot differentiate between tuberculosis infection and disease.

The lack of a gold standard for detection of tuberculosis infection complicates studies of diagnostic accuracy,[57] many of which have employed surrogate measures of infection to serve as the reference standard for tuberculosis infection.[55] The association between IGRA positivity and tuberculosis exposure is well described in low-burden countries.[58–60] Results from high-burden countries are conflicting, and demonstrate both advantages of the T-Spot[61] and no difference in T-Spot performance compared to TST and QFT.[62] Although the majority of these studies have used simple dichotomous measures of exposure, a few key studies have illustrated that exposure may be quantified to support direct comparison of tests of infection.[19,59,61,62] Pooled analysis of studies employing a measure of tuberculosis exposure demonstrates that positive IGRA results are more strongly correlated with tuberculosis exposure than the TST results.[55]

There is limited and conflicting evidence regarding IGRA use in young, malnourished, immune-compromised, or impoverished children, the groups most likely to develop tuberculosis disease following infection. Studies have demonstrated a variable association between indeterminate IGRA results and young age, with some studies showing an association[63-68] and others showing no association.[28,29,62,69] A seminal study of European immigrant children found that indeterminate IGRA results were more frequent among young children, but notably demonstrated that indeterminate results occurred at clinically insignificant rates of 1.8% and 1.6% for the QFT and T-Spot, respectively.[68] Most studies have reported rates less than 10%.[55] Emerging evidence further demonstrates that a number of factors related to poverty (malnourishment,[28,29,70] micronutrient deficiency,[71] and helminth infection[72,73]) may lead to diminished IGRA sensitivity. More evidence is needed to guide the interpretation of IGRAs in the vulnerable groups of children at high risk of tuberculosis progression following infection.

Limited data are available regarding IGRA performance in immune-compromised and HIV-infected children, in whom the performance of the TST is impaired.[74-76] Two studies suggest that test failures described as indeterminate or invalid results are common among pediatric oncology patients.[77,78] Two studies have shown a noncommercial IFN-γ ELISPOT assay to have higher sensitivity for detecting tuberculosis infection compared with the TST in HIV-infected children.[74,79] A comparison of the QFT-gold assay and the TST for the detection of tuberculosis infection in 36 young, HIV-infected children with culture-confirmed tuberculosis disease found comparable sensitivity in children with CD4+ count >200 cells/ml; unfortunately, indeterminate QFT-gold results were reported in 25% of children tested.[80] A study of 23 HIV-infected children demonstrated high levels of discordant and indeterminate IGRA results and suggested that the T-Spot may have improved sensitivity for the detection of tuberculosis infection in this group of children.[51] In a head-to-head comparison among 130 HIV-infected and 120 HIV-uninfected children, the TST and IGRAs performed similarly for the detection of tuberculosis infection in well-nourished HIV-uninfected children, but test performance was differentially affected by chronic malnutrition, HIV infection, and age.[29] In a study of over 1,300 children, IGRAs correlated better with tuberculosis exposure than the TST ($p = 0.0011$).[28] Indeterminate QFT results were more frequent in HIV-infected (4.7%) than HIV-uninfected children (1.9%), while T-Spot invalid results were rare (0.2%) and were not affected by HIV-infection. Conversion, reversion, and operational measures were not associated with HIV status. Among HIV-infected children, test sensitivities declined as malnutrition worsened. As a conclusion from the available evidence, clinicians should take age and nutritional and HIV status into consideration when interpreting IGRAs.

The purpose of the TST and IGRAs is to determine whether the person is infected with *M. tuberculosis* and guide subsequent evaluation and treatment. In general, the decision to test is a decision to treat for either tuberculosis disease or infection. If resources are available such that a test result could change the treatment, then attributes of the child and the purpose of the testing should inform the choice of which diagnostic test to use. In the absence of treatment for tuberculosis infection, ~40% of children younger than two years of age will progress to tuberculosis disease within one year of infection. Hence, in this population, testing strategies should optimize sensitivity and guide the provision of treatment. In BCG-vaccinated or NTM-exposed children, use of the TST will result in a considerable proportion of false-positive results and poor allocation of resources. Hence, in low-risk BCG-vaccinated children, high specificity is desired, making the IGRAs preferable. When sensitivity must be maximized, a positive result with either the TST or IGRA should be considered evidence of tuberculosis infection. Although it may compromise the specificity of the testing strategy, both an IGRA and a TST should be performed in a child with a high suspicion of tuberculosis disease or a child with a high risk rapid progression to disease. Both the TST and the IGRAs have limitations, but use of the tests in targeted populations with increased risk of tuberculosis infection or disease maximizes the impact of testing.

COMBINED USE AND PRACTICAL CONSIDERATIONS

IGRAs offer several pragmatic advantages over the TST (Table 6.4). Use of M. tuberculosis–specific antigens leads to improved specificity, which decreases the probability of false-positive responses, particularly in young, BCG-vaccinated children. Use of internal positive controls allows for the assessment of anergy, which can be useful in immune-compromised and young children. Additionally, IGRAs do not require a second visit to measure the response and thus eliminate the chance of a missed reading. Hence, IGRAs may be particularly useful in settings where it may be difficult for patients to return, such as emergency departments and testing of migrants and homeless individuals. Although the direct cost of the IGRA assays is greater than that of the TST, evidence in adults suggests that IGRAs may be cost-effective in certain populations and settings by decreasing the number of false-positive results and subsequent evaluation and treatment of patients.[81–84]

Treatment of tuberculosis infection substantially decreases rates of progression to disease, morbidity, and mortality among close contacts of infectious cases.[5] Nevertheless, in many tuberculosis high-burden settings, limited resources are allocated to support the effective delivery of treatment of infected individuals. As a result, risk factors such as age and recent tuberculosis exposure are used as indications for recommending treatment. Accurate identification of children with M. tuberculosis infection could potentially narrow the group of children for whom treatment is recommended. One cost-effectiveness analysis, set in South Africa, has compared the cost-effectiveness of five tuberculosis infection screening strategies in child household tuberculosis contacts identified through contact tracing.[85] Simulating WHO guidelines, the study included a unique no-testing strategy in which treatment was offered to child contacts based on their age. The model also included two dual testing methods to assess strategies maximizing test sensitivity (IGRA after negative TST) and specificity (IGRA after positive TST). Assessment of both strategies is important because young children might benefit from confirmatory IGRA testing to maximize specificity in the presence of BCG vaccination and from confirmatory IGRA testing to maximize sensitivity in recently exposed child contacts. These models employed 2011 estimates of IGRA performance and suggested that provision of treatment to recent contacts of tuberculosis cases without testing for infection is the most cost-effective strategy in children under three years of age in high-burden settings and probably the preferred strategy in older children due to cost considerations.[85] Due to the lack of definitive pediatric data and concerns regarding cost-effectiveness, the WHO has recommended against the use of IGRAs in children living in low- and middle-income countries.[86]

IGRAs are commonly used in children living in upper-income, low-burden countries and have influenced clinical decision-making.[79] National guidelines continue to change, vary dramatically among countries, and often lag behind the rapidly emerging evidence. Pragmatic approaches to the use of IGRAs and TST have emerged through clinical practice and are emerging in formal guidelines.[87] Child characteristics and test purpose should guide the selection and combined use of tests (Figure 6.5). Only children who have risk of tuberculosis exposure, underlying health conditions that require immune suppression, or suspected tuberculosis disease should be tested for tuberculosis infection in tuberculosis low-burden settings. When high specificity is desired, the IGRAs are the preferred test. When high sensitivity is desired, a positive result with either an IGRA or a TST should be considered indicative of tuberculosis infection. When caring for a child in whom there is a high clinical suspicion of disease, high risk of infection, or high risk of disease progression, test sensitivity can be optimized by performing both a TST and IGRA[87] (Figure 6.5). Although this approach decreases test specificity and may result in overtreatment, the benefits of avoiding disease progression generally outweigh the risk of overtreatment, particularly since children tolerate treatment of tuberculosis infection with few side-effects.

FUTURE TESTS OF INFECTION, AND PERSPECTIVE

The current diagnostic tests for tuberculosis infection, the TST and IGRAs, are indirect measures of host cell-mediated immunity. The TST requires a

Table 6.4 Comparison of the tuberculin skin test (TST) and interferon-gamma release assays (IGRAs)

CONSIDERATION	TST	IGRA	IDEAL TEST
Sampling	Intradermal injection	Blood draw	
Patient visits required	Two	One	One
BCG cross-reactivity	Yes	No	No
NTM cross-reactivity	Yes	Infrequent*	No
Boosting associated with repeat testing	Yes	No	No
Boosting associated with prior TST	Yes	Possible	No
Population-specific interpretation	Yes	No	Not needed
Internal controls for anergy	No	Yes	Not needed
Subject to human variability	Yes	No	No
Subject to laboratory error	No	Yes	No
Location of trained staff	Peripheral health services	Centralized lab services	Peripheral health services
Requires trained clinical staff	Yes	No	No
Requires trained lab staff	No	Yes	No
Relies on host immune function	Yes	Yes	No
Distinguishes infection from disease	No	No	Yes
Predicts disease progression	No	No	Yes
Distinguishes remote and recent infection	No	No	Yes
Performs similarly regardless of HIV status	No	Possible	Yes
Monitors treatment efficacy	No	No	Yes

* IGRA positivity results from infection with the following organisms thereby decreasing test specificity: *Mycobacterium marinum, Mycobacterium kansasii, Mycobacterium szulgai,* and *Mycobacterium flavescens.*

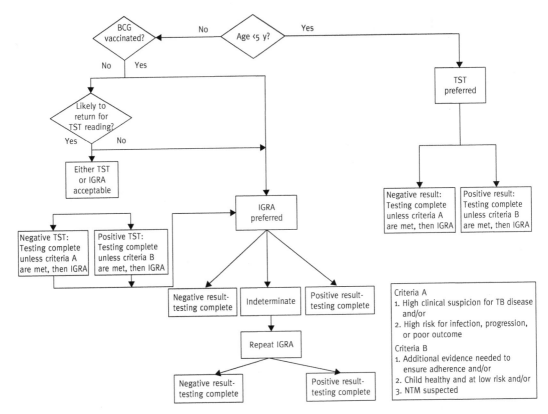

FIGURE 6.5   Am algorithm for the use of TSTs and IGRAs in children with risk of tuberculosis infection in low-burden settings.[87]

trained clinician and multiple patient visits, while having cross-reactivity with the BCG vaccine and some common NTMs and only a 60–90% sensitivity.[55,88] The IGRAs avoid a second patient visit and cross-reactivity with BCG and most NTMs, have similar diagnostic accuracy to that of the TST, but are more expensive and require a trained laboratory staff. Considering the burden of tuberculosis in HIV-infected and immunocompromised individuals, the ideal test of infection would not depend on host immune function. An ideal test would be economical and require minimally trained staff, being either point of care or near point of care. Furthermore, clinicians would benefit from a test that accurately differentiated between infection and disease, especially in high-burden settings. A test that identifies those at high risk for disease progression would permit improved targeted treatment of tuberculosis infection. Developing technologies are attempting to fulfill these stringent criteria while recognizing the new paradigm that sees tuberculosis states as a continuum of host–pathogen interactions.

While still relying on host response, polyfunctional flow cytometry measurement of CD4 cells producing TNF, IL-2, and INF-γ after TB-specific stimulation with ESAT-6 and CFP-10 was able to differentiate infection and disease with a sensitivity of 67% and specificity of 92%.[89] Flow cytometry with accompanying intracellular staining is unlikely to be scalable to a point of care test, considering the tedium of peripheral blood mononuclear cell isolation, limited availability of multi-parameter flow cytometry, and excessive cost. A more realistic application of this research would be the development of a multi-parameter in-tube ELISA assay.

Relying on host immune response, RNA transcription signatures, also known as transcriptomics or gene micro-array studies, are another promising technology. Current micro-array capacity, which is able of detecting the expression regulation of the entire functional genome (>40,000 genes), is being applied to distinguishing among tuberculosis infection, disease, and healthy controls. Current methods are challenged to differentiate other causes of granulomatous lung diseases that have similar transcriptional signatures.[90] In a three-country study of childhood tuberculosis, a 51-transcript signature had 82% sensitivity and 83% specificity in detecting culture-confirmed disease.[91] Considerable work is still required for this technology to be scaled up and rolled out in resource-limited settings.

The diagnostic yield of serological tests detecting antibodies against *M. tuberculosis*[92] and the organism's antigens[93] have thus far been suboptimal, with the WHO formally recommending against their use. Despite the poor results thus far, scientific advances in numerous technologies offer the promise of meeting some of the stringent criteria for an ideal test. For example, matrix-assisted laser desorption/ionization time-of-flight mass spectrometry (MALDI TOF MS) is advancing the field of proteomics to screen plasma, serum, cerebrospinal fluid, sputum,[94] and urine for potential biomarkers of tuberculosis infection.[95] Combined with chemical, mechanical, and/or nanopore trap enrichment processes, proof of concept papers are holding out the promise of femtomolar (10^{-15} mole per liter) detection of *M. tuberculosis* peptides using MALDI-MS.[96]

Another application of mass spectroscopy includes detection of volatile organic compounds (VOCs). Evolving from historical reports of Hippocrates burning human sputum to diagnose tuberculosis via its unique odor, the anecdotal reports of dogs detecting cancers[97] and *C. difficile* infection,[98] and the African giant pouch rat's ability to sniff out tuberculosis,[99,100] significant investments have been made to develop "e-noses." Using gas chromatography, ion mobility, or proton-transfer variations of mass spectroscopy, potential point-of-care e-noses detect exhaled VOCs at the parts per billion limit of detection. Similarly, progress is being made in the detection of VOCs from the aroma of urine and stool samples.[101,102]

Despite over 100 years of tuberculosis infection diagnosis relying on the TST, there is optimism in the scientific advances in flow cytometry, ELISA, transcription micro-arrays, proteomics, peptidomics, and e-nose detection. Lessons may be applicable from the use of nucleic acid amplification tests for the diagnosis of tuberculosis disease. While available for over a decade, the ubiquity of this method occurred when Gene Xpert MTB/RIF converted the laborious process of PCR into an automated platform requiring less than five minutes of hands-on time, analogous to a single-serve coffeemaker.

To meet the WHO's 2050 goal of eliminating tuberculosis, there will need to be economical and scalable scientific advances in detecting tuberculosis infection. Considering the lack of a comparator gold standard, future studies will require robust, longitudinal clinical correlation. In addition, young and HIV-infected children must be included in future studies, as they carry the highest burden of disease progression. Once developed, the impact of any new diagnostic test will depend on a broad rollout to support a sustainable market price in low-income, high-burden countries. While awaiting these advances, a focus on strengthening current health infrastructure able to implement current diagnostics while retaining and providing effective preventative therapy is needed to reduce the infectious reservoir of future cases.

REFERENCES

1. Dodd PJ, et al. Burden of childhood tuberculosis in 22 high-burden countries: a mathematical modelling study. *Lancet Glob Health.* 2014;2(8):e453–e459.
2. Smith S, Jacobs RF, Wilson CB. Immunobiology of childhood tuberculosis: a window on the ontogeny of cellular immunity. *J Pediatr.* 1997;131(1 Pt 1):16–26.
3. Sloot R, et al. Risk of Tuberculosis after Recent Exposure. A 10-Year Follow-up Study of Contacts in Amsterdam. *Am J Respir Crit Care Med.* 2014;190(9):1044–1052.
4. Marais BJ, et al. The natural history of childhood intra-thoracic tuberculosis: a critical review of literature from the pre-chemotherapy era. *Int J Tuberc Lung Dis.* 2004;8(4):392–402.
5. Smieja M, et al. Isoniazid for preventing tuberculosis in non-HIV infected persons. *Cochrane Database of Systematic Reviews.* 1999; Art. No.: CD001363(1).
6. Woldehana and J. Volmink, Treatment of latent tuberculosis infection in HIV infected persons 2004, *Cochrane Database of Sytematic Reviews,* (1):CD000171.
7. Hsu KH, Isoniazid in the prevention and treatment of tuberculosis. A 20-year study of the effectiveness in children. *Jama.* 1974;229(5):528–533.
8. Ayieko J, et al. Efficacy of isoniazid prophylactic therapy in prevention of tuberculosis in children: a meta-analysis. *BMC Infect Dis.* 2014;14:91.
9. Getahun H, et al. Prevention, diagnosis, and treatment of tuberculosis in children and

mothers: evidence for action for maternal, neonatal, and child health services. *J Infect Dis.* 2012;205 Suppl 2:S216–S227.

10. Targeted tuberculin testing and treatment of latent tuberculosis infection. American Thoracic Society. *MMWR Recomm Rep.* 2000;49(RR-6):1–51.

11. WHO, *Recommendations for Investigating Contacts of Persons with Infectious Tuberculosis in Low- and Middle-Income Countries.* World Health Organization; Geneva, 2012.

12. WHO, *Guidelines on the management of latent tuberculosis infection.* World Health Organization; Geneva, 2015.

13. Schluger NW, Rom WN. The host immune response to tuberculosis. *Am J Respir Crit Care Med.* 1998;157(3 Pt 1):679–91.

14. Barnes P. Immunology of tuberculosis. *Semin Pediatr Infect Dis.* 1993;4:232.

15. Barnes PF, et al. Gamma delta T lymphocytes in human tuberculosis. *J Infect Dis.* 1992;165(3):506–512.

16. Young DB, Gideon HP, Wilkinson RJ. Eliminating latent tuberculosis. *Trends Microbiol.* 2009;17(5):183–188.

17. Comstock G. Epidemiology of tuberculosis. In: Riechman LB, Hershfield E, eds. *Tuberculosis: A Comprehensive International Approach.* New York: Marcel Dekker; 2000:129–148.

18. Beyers N, et al. A prospective evaluation of children under the age of 5 years living in the same household as adults with recently diagnosed pulmonary tuberculosis. *Int J Tuberc Lung Dis.* 1997;1(1):38–43.

19. Mandalakas A, et al. Well Quantified Tuberculosis Exposure is a Reliable Surrogate Measure of Tuberculosis Infection in children. *Int J Tuberc Lung Dis.* 2012;16:1033–1039.

20. Wood R, et al. Tuberculosis transmission to young children in a South African community: modeling household and community infection risks. *Clin Infect Dis.* 2010;51(4):401–408.

21. Sutter RW, Haefliger E. Tuberculosis morbidity and infection in Vietnamese in Southeast Asian refugee camps. *Am Rev Respir Dis.* 1990;141(6):1483–1486.

22. Mandalakas AM, et al. Predictors of Mycobacterium tuberculosis infection in international adoptees. *Pediatrics.* 2007;120(3):e610–e616.

23. Saiman L, et al. Prevalence of infectious diseases among internationally adopted children. *Pediatrics.* 2001;108(3):608–612.

24. AAP. *Tuberculosis, in Red Book, 2009 report of the Committee on Infectious Diseases,* Pickering LK. et al. Editors. 2012, American Academy of Pediatrics: Elk Grove Village, IL, USA.

25. Anderson, P. and e. al., Specific immune-base diagnosis of TB. *Lancet.* 2000;356:1099–1104.

26. Mahairas GG, et al. Molecular analysis of genetic differences between Mycobacterium bovis BCG and virulent M. bovis. *J Bacteriol.* 1996;178(5):1274–1282.

27. Harboe M, et al. Evidence for occurrence of the ESAT-6 protein in Mycobacterium tuberculosis and virulent Mycobacterium bovis and for its absence in Mycobacterium bovis BCG. *Infect Immun.* 1996;64(1):16–22.

28. Mandalakas AM, et al. Optimizing the Detection of Recent Tuberculosis Infection in Children in a High TB-HIV Burden Setting. *Am J Respir Crit Care Med.* 2015; 191:820-830.

29. Mandalakas AM, et al. Detecting Tuberculosis Infection in HIV-Infected Children: A Study of Diagnostic Accuracy, Confounding and Interaction. *Pediatr Infect Dis J.* 2012;32:e111–e113.

30. Felten MK, van der Merwe CA, Random variation in tuberculin sensitivity in schoolchildren. Serial skin testing before and after preventive treatment for tuberculosis. *Am Rev Respir Dis.* 1989;140(4):1001–1006.

31. Sokol JE, Measurement of delayed skin test reponses. *N Engl J Med.* 1975;293:501–502.

32. Lincoln E, Gilbert L, Morales S. Chronic pulmonary tuberculosis in individuals with known previous primary tuberculosis. *Chest.* 1960;38:473.

33. Steiner P, et al. Persistently negative tuberculin reactions: their presence among children with culture positive for Mycobacterium tuberculosis (tuberculin-negative tuberculosis). *Am J Dis Child.* 1980;134(8):747–750.

34. Karalliedde S, Katugaha LP, Uragoda CG. Tuberculin response of Sri Lankan children after BCG vaccination at birth. *Tubercle.* 1987;68(1):33–38.

35. Menzies R, Vissandjee B, Amyot D. Factors associated with tuberculin reactivity among the foreign-born in Montreal. *Am Rev Respir Dis.* 1992;146(3):752–756.

36. Menzies, R. and B. Vissandjee, Effect of bacille Calmette-Guerin vaccination on tuberculin reactivity. *Am Rev Respir Dis.* 1992;145(3):621–625.

37. Mandalakas AM, et al. Interpretation of repeat tuberculin skin testing in international

adoptees: conversions or boosting. *Pediatr Infect Dis J.* 2008;27(10):913–919.

38. Farhat M, et al. False-positive tuberculin skin tests: what is the absolute effect of BCG and non-tuberculous mycobacteria? *Int J Tuberc Lung Dis.* 2006;10(11):1192–1204.

39. Chuke SO, et al. Tuberculin Skin Tests versus Interferon-Gamma Release Assays in Tuberculosis Screening among Immigrant Visa Applicants. *Tuberc Res Treat.* 2014;2014:217969.

40. WHO, *Guidelines for intensified tuberculosis case finding and isoniazid preventive therapy for people living with HIV in resource constrained settings.* 2011, World Health Organization: Geneva, Switzerland.

41. WHO, *Guidance for national tuberculosis programmes on the management of tuberculosis in children.* World Health Organization: Geneva, 2015.

42. Styblo K, The relationship between the risk of tuberculous infection and the risk of developing infectious tuberculosis. *Bull IUAT.* 1985;60:117–119.

43. Shanaube K, et al. Annual risk of tuberculous infection using different methods in communities with a high prevalence of TB and HIV in Zambia and South Africa. *PLoS One.* 2009;4(11):e7749.

44. van Leth F, M.J. van der Werf, Borgdorff MW. Prevalence of tuberculous infection and incidence of tuberculosis: a re-assessment of the Styblo rule. *Bull World Health Organ.* 2008;86(1):20–26.

45. Diez N, et al. Use of interferon-gamma release assays to calculate the annual risk of tuberculosis infection. *Pediatr Infect Dis J.* 2015;34(2):219–221.

46. Colangeli R, et al. MTSA-10, the product of the Rv3874 gene of Mycobacterium tuberculosis, elicits tuberculosis-specific, delayed-type hypersensitivity in guinea pigs. *Infect Immun.* 2000;68(2):990–993.

47. Lein AD, et al. Cellular immune responses to ESAT-6 discriminate between patients with pulmonary disease due to Mycobacterium avium complex and those with pulmonary disease due to Mycobacterium tuberculosis. *Clin Diagn Lab Immunol.* 1999;6(4):606–609.

48. Arend SM, et al. Detection of active tuberculosis infection by T cell responses to early-secreted antigenic target 6-kDa protein and culture filtrate protein 10. *J Infect Dis.* 2000;181(5):1850–1854.

49. Lalvani A, Spotting latent infection: the path to better tuberculosis control. *Thorax.* 2003;58(11):916–918.

50. Wood, P.R., Jones SL. BOVIGAM: an in vitro cellular diagnostic test for bovine tuberculosis. *Tuberculosis (Edinb).* 2001;81(1–2):147–155.

51. Mandalakas AM, et al. High level of discordant IGRA results in HIV-infected adults and children. *Int J Tuberc Lung Dis.* 2008;12(4):417–423.

52. Menzies D, Interpretation of repeated tuberculin tests. Boosting, conversion, and reversion. *Am J Respir Crit Care Med.* 1999;159(1):15–21.

53. Mandalakas AM, et al. Optimizing the Detection of Recent Tuberculosis Infection in Children in a high TB-HIV Burden Setting. *Am J Respir Crit Care Med.* 2015;e-Pub ahead of print.

54. van Zyl-Smit RN, et al. Within-subject variability of interferon-g assay results for tuberculosis and boosting effect of tuberculin skin testing: a systematic review. *PLoS One.* 2009;4(12):e8517.

55. Mandalakas AM, et al. Interferon-gamma release assays and childhood tuberculosis: systematic review and meta-analysis. *Int J Tuberc Lung Dis.* 2011;15(8):1018–1032.

56. Machingaidze S, et al. The utility of an interferon gamma release assay for diagnosis of latent tuberculosis infection and disease in children: a systematic review and meta-analysis. *Pediatr Infect Dis J.* 2011;30(8):694–700.

57. Bossuyt PM, et al. Towards complete and accurate reporting of studies of diagnostic accuracy: the STARD initiative. *Bmj.* 2003;326(7379):41–44.

58. Arend SM, et al. Comparison of two interferon-gamma assays and tuberculin skin test for tracing tuberculosis contacts. *Am J Respir Crit Care Med.* 2007;175(6):618–627.

59. Ewer K, et al. Comparison of T-cell-based assay with tuberculin skin test for diagnosis of Mycobacterium tuberculosis infection in a school tuberculosis outbreak. *Lancet.* 2003;361(9364):1168–1173.

60. Soysal A, et al. Effect of BCG vaccination on risk of Mycobacterium tuberculosis infection in children with household tuberculosis contact: a prospective community-based study. *Lancet.* 2005;366(9495):1443–1451.

61. Hesseling AC, et al. Highly discordant T cell responses in individuals with recent exposure to household tuberculosis. *Thorax.* 2009;64(10):840–846.

62. Tieu HV, et al. Comparing interferon-gamma release assays to tuberculin skin test in Thai children with tuberculosis exposure. *PLoS One.* 2014;9(8):e105003.

63. Connell TG, et al. A three-way comparison of tuberculin skin testing, QuantiFERON-TB gold and T-SPOT.TB in children. *PLoS One.* 2008;3(7):e2624.

64. Critselis E, et al. The effect of age on whole blood interferon-gamma release assay response among

children investigated for latent tuberculosis infection. *J Pediatr.* 2012;161(4):632–638.

65. Bergamini BM, et al. Performance of commercial blood tests for the diagnosis of latent tuberculosis infection in children and adolescents. *Pediatrics.* 2009;123(3):e419–e424.

66. Kasambira TS, et al. QuantiFERON-TB Gold In-Tube for the detection of Mycobacterium tuberculosis infection in children with household tuberculosis contact. *Int J Tuberc Lung Dis.* 2011;15(5):628–634.

67. Blandinieres A, et al. QuantiFERON to diagnose infection by Mycobacterium tuberculosis: performance in infants and older children. *J Infect.* 2013;67(5):391–398.

68. Basu Roy R, et al. Identifying predictors of interferon-gamma release assay results in pediatric latent tuberculosis: a protective role of bacillus Calmette-Guerin?: a pTB-NET collaborative study. *Am J Respir Crit Care Med.* 2012;186(4):378–384.

69. Pavic I, et al. Interferon-gamma release assay for the diagnosis of latent tuberculosis in children younger than 5 years of age. *Pediatr Infect Dis J.* 2011;30(10):866–870.

70. Jenum S, et al. Influence of Age and Nutirional Status on the Performance of the Tuiberculin Skin Test and QuantiFERON-TB Gold In-Tube in Young Children Evaluated for Tuberculosis in Southern India. *Ped Infectious Dis J.* 2014; 33: e260-e269.

71. Mukherjee A, et al. Effect of micronutrient deficiency on QuantiFERON-TB Gold In-Tube test and tuberculin skin test in diagnosis of childhood intrathoracic tuberculosis. *Eur J Clin Nutr.* 2014;68(1):38–42.

72. Riazi S, et al. Rapid diagnosis of Mycobacterium tuberculosis infection in children using interferon-gamma release assays (IGRAs). *Allergy Asthma Proc.* 2012;33(3):217–226.

73. van Soelen N, et al. Effect of Ascaris Lumbricoides specific IgE on tuberculin skin test responses in children in a high-burden setting: a cross-sectional community-based study. *BMC Infect Dis.* 2012;12(1):211.

74. Davies MA, et al. Detection of tuberculosis in HIV-infected children using an enzyme-linked immunospot assay. *Aids.* 2009;23(8):961–969.

75. Marais BJ, et al. Diagnostic and management challenges for childhood tuberculosis in the era of HIV. *J Infect Dis.* 2007;196 Suppl 1:S76–S85.

76. Kumar A, Upadhyay S, Kumari G. Clinical Presentation, treatment outcome and survival among the HIV infected children with culture confirmed tuberculosis. *Curr HIV Res.* 2007;5(5):499–504.

77. Carvalho A, Schumacher R, Bigoni S. *NEED TO UPDATE REFERENCE.* 2013.

78. Stefan DC DA, Detjen AK, Schaaf HS, Marais BJ, Kriel B, Loebenberg L, Walzl G, Hesseling AC, Interferon-gamma release assays for the detection of Mycobacterium tuberculosis infection in children with cancer. *Int J Tuber Lung Dis.* 2010;14(6):689–694.

79. Ling DI, Crepeau CA, Dufrense M, et al. Evaluation of the Impact of Interferon-Gamma Release Assays on Management of Childhood Tuberculosis. *Pediatr Infect Dis J.* 2012;31:1258–1262.

80. Stavri H, et al. Comparison of tuberculin skin test with whole-blood interferon gamma release assay and ELISA, in HIV positive children and adolescents with TB. *Roum Arch Microbiol Immunol.* 2009;68:14–19.

81. Diel R, et al. Cost-optimisation of screening for latent tuberculosis in close contacts. *Eur Respir J.* 2006;28(1):35–44.

82. Diel R, Nienhaus A, Loddenkemper R. Cost-effectiveness of Interferon-{gamma} Release Assay Screening for Latent Tuberculosis Infection Treatment in Germany. *Chest.* 2007;131(5):1424–1434.

83. Diel R, P. Wrighton-Smith, Zellweger JP. Cost-effectiveness of IGRA testing for the treatment of latent tuberculosis in Switzerland. *Eur Respir J.* 2007;30:321–332.

84. Deuffic-Burban S, et al. Cost-effectiveness of QuantiFERON-TB test vs. tuberculin skin test in the diagnosis of latent tuberculosis infection. *Int J Tuberc Lung Dis.* 2010;14(4):471–481.

85. Mandalakas AM, et al. Modelling the cost-effectiveness of strategies to prevent tuberculosis in child contacts in a high-burden setting. *Thorax.* 2012;68:247–252.

86. WHO, Use of tuberculosis interferon-gamma release assays (IGRAs) in low- and middle income countries; policy statement. *2011;*World health Organization: Geneva.

87. Starke JR, D. Committee On Infectious, and D. Committee On Infectious, Interferon-gamma Release Assays for Diagnosis of Tuberculosis Infection and Disease in Children. *Pediatrics.* 2014;134(6):e1763–e1773.

88. Pai M, Zwerling A, Menzies D. Systematic review: T-cell-based assays for the diagnosis of latent tuberculosis infection: an update. *Ann Intern Med.* 2008;149(3):177–184.

89. Harari A, et al. Dominant TNF-alpha+ Mycobacterium tuberculosis-specific CD4+ T cell responses discriminate between latent infection and active disease. *Nat Med.* 2011;17(3):372–376.

90. Blankley S, et al. The application of transcriptional blood signatures to enhance our understanding of the host response to infection: the example of tuberculosis. *Philos Trans R Soc Lond B Biol Sci.* 2014;369(1645):20130427.

91. Anderson ST, et al. Diagnosis of childhood tuberculosis and host RNA expression in Africa. *N Engl J Med.* 2014;370(18):1712–1723.

92. Steingart KR, et al. Commercial serological tests for the diagnosis of active pulmonary and extrapulmonary tuberculosis: an updated systematic review and meta-analysis. *PLoS Med.* 2011;8(8):e1001062.

93. Flores LL, et al. Systematic review and meta-analysis of antigen detection tests for the diagnosis of tuberculosis. *Clin Vaccine Immunol.* 2011;18(10):1616–1627.

94. O'Sullivan DM, et al. Detection of Mycobacterium tuberculosis in sputum by gas chromatography-mass spectrometry of methyl mycocerosates released by thermochemolysis. *PLoS One.* 2012;7(3):e32836.

95. Cunningham R, Ma D, Li L. Mass Spectrometry-based Proteomics and Peptidomics for Systems Biology and Biomarker Discovery. *Front Biol (Beijing).* 2012;7(4):313–335.

96. Wu HJ, et al. Antibody-free detection of Mycobacterium tuberculosis antigen using customized nanotraps. *Anal Chem.* 2014;86(4):1988–1996.

97. de Boer NK, et al. The scent of colorectal cancer: detection by volatile organic compound analysis. *Clin Gastroenterol Hepatol.* 2014;12(7):1085–1089.

98. Bomers MK, et al. A detection dog to identify patients with Clostridium difficile infection during a hospital outbreak. *J Infect.* 2014;69(5):456–461.

99. Weetjens BJ, et al. African pouched rats for the detection of pulmonary tuberculosis in sputum samples. *Int J Tuberc Lung Dis.* 2009;13(6):737–743.

100. Mgode GF, et al. Diagnosis of tuberculosis by trained African giant pouched rats and confounding impact of pathogens and microflora of the respiratory tract. *J Clin Microbiol.* 2012;50(2):274–280.

101. Banday KM, et al. Use of urine volatile organic compounds to discriminate tuberculosis patients from healthy subjects. *Anal Chem.* 2011;83(14):5526–5534.

102. Purkhart R, et al. Chronic intestinal Mycobacteria infection: discrimination via VOC analysis in exhaled breath and headspace of feces using differential ion mobility spectrometry. *J Breath Res.* 2011;5(2):027103.

7

MICROBIOLOGICAL DIAGNOSIS OF PULMONARY TUBERCULOSIS IN CHILDREN

Mark P. Nicol and Heather J. Zar

HIGHLIGHTS OF THIS CHAPTER

- Diagnosis of childhood pulmonary tuberculosis (PTB) remains challenging, especially in young or immunosuppressed children.
- Clinical symptoms and signs, including clinical scoring systems, are unreliable for diagnosis in children.
- Interpretation of chest radiographs is subject to wide inter- and intra-observer variability.
- Microbiological confirmation in children has become increasingly important for diagnosis, case notification, to better define the true pediatric burden of disease, and to enable optimal drug therapy in the context of drug resistance.
- The efficacy of microbiological diagnostic testing depends on the quality of the sample, sample volume, and number of samples taken.
- Induced sputum (IS) provides a feasible and effective specimen that can be used in children of all ages for microbiological diagnosis.
- Children have paucibacillary disease, so acid-fast smear is seldom a useful investigation. Microbiological confirmation rests on PCR-based (polymerase chain reaction) detection (Xpert MTB/RIF [Xpert]) and culture.
- Xpert enables rapid microbiological confirmation and detection of rifampicin resistance; Xpert on induced sputum or gastric lavage detects approximately two thirds of children with culture-confirmed PTB.
- At least two specimens for Xpert and culture should be taken in children to improve diagnostic sensitivity.
- Training of health-care workers is needed to improve appropriate specimen collection. *Widespread implementation of IS collection is needed.*
- A rapid, highly sensitive point-of-care diagnostic test is still needed for pediatric PTB.

THE DIFFICULTY OF ESTABLISHING A DIAGNOSIS OF PTB IN CHILDREN

Accurate diagnosis of pulmonary tuberculosis (PTB) in children is important, as timely, effective treatment is key to preventing progression to severe disease and chronic morbidity or death. Infants or children with immunosuppression, such as those with malnutrition or HIV infection, are at particular risk of developing severe, disseminated disease. HIV-infected children who commence antiretroviral therapy (ART) are also at risk of developing an immune reconstitution syndrome if they have untreated tuberculosis. The rise in incidence of multidrug-resistant tuberculosis (MDR-TB) and extensively drug-resistant tuberculosis (XDR-TB) underscores the importance of microbiological confirmation and drug susceptibility testing (DST) for effective treatment. Definitive diagnosis is also important given the issues of pill burden and adherence to therapy.[1]

However, PTB in children may be difficult to definitively diagnose, due to its nonspecific clinical and radiological signs, paucibacillary disease, and lack of capacity for microbiological diagnosis.[2] Structured diagnostic scoring systems based on clinical and radiological findings and tuberculin skin testing (TST) show high variability in case yield, and poor agreement.[3] Radiological changes may be nonspecific, and interpretation is further complicated by wide inter- and intra-observer variation in the interpretation of the presence of mediastinal lymphadenopathy, one of the major radiological features of PTB.[4] Interferon-gamma release assays (IGRAs) offer little advantage over TST, with limited additional value to the current diagnostic workup of children suspected to have tuberculosis disease.[5] While clinical diagnosis has relied on chronic symptoms such as prolonged coughing or failure to thrive, recent studies have shown that tuberculosis in children may also cause *acute* pneumonia (rather than chronic disease), with culture-confirmed disease occurring in 8–15% of children with acute pneumonia living in tuberculosis-endemic areas.[6] Diagnostic uncertainty is compounded in HIV-infected children in whom chronic lung disease, anergy, and nonspecific clinical and radiological signs make definitive diagnosis even more challenging.

Microbiological confirmation of PTB in children has not been part of routine care in most high-burden settings, due to the unavailability of facilities, the perceived difficulty in obtaining samples, the poor performance of acid-fast smear microscopy, and the perception that microbiological yield is low. However, several studies have confirmed the feasibility and usefulness of microbiological confirmation in young children with suspected PTB.[6-14] The evidence indicates that adequate specimens can be obtained and a confirmed microbiological diagnosis made, even when done in primary care settings by nurses. Although microbiological confirmation, if done optimally, is typically obtained in approximately 50% of children with clinically diagnosed disease, microbiological diagnosis increases the number of children treated for PTB and allows rapid initiation of appropriate therapy.[7]

As pediatric disease is frequently paucibacillary, the yield of direct acid-fast smear microscopy is very low. Therefore new PCR-based methods (e.g., Xpert MTB/RIF [Xpert]) and mycobacterial culture are required for establishing a confirmed diagnosis. To optimize microbiological testing, good-quality samples must be obtained with meticulous attention to sample collection technique. Studies have also shown that, in children, multiple specimens are needed for optimal sensitivity, either from culture or from PCR.[6-14] Furthermore, specimen collection from several anatomical sites such as expectorated or induced sputum, nasopharyngeal aspirate, gastric lavage, and fine needle aspirate (FNA) of palpable nodes may increase the yield of microbiological diagnosis.

SAMPLE COLLECTION FOR MICROBIOLOGICAL DIAGNOSIS

Sputum

In older children, expectorated sputum may provide a good specimen. However, for young children or those who cannot spontaneously produce sputum, sputum induction can be used to obtain an induced sputum (IS) specimen. IS has been used successfully in several studies to obtain a lower respiratory tract specimen for Xpert and culture. Sputum induction has a number of advantages over gastric lavage (GL), as it can be done as an outpatient procedure, is relatively easy to perform, and the yield is higher. In two large studies of infants hospitalized in a tertiary care facility in South Africa (median ages 9 and 13 months), samples were successfully obtained from 95% of children.[8,9] In the first study, one IS sample yielded more positive cultures (10% of samples) than three sequential GL samples (6% of samples); while in the second study, the cumulative yield from three IS samples (87%) was greater than that of three GL samples (65%); a single IS sample was equivalent to three GL samples. The yield was similar in HIV-infected and uninfected children.

Sputum induction has also been used in children with milder illness. Among children with mild illness admitted to a case-verification ward as part of an infant tuberculosis vaccine trial, the yields of a single IS and GL sample were equivalent; however, positive cultures (from two GL and two IS samples) were obtained in only 10% of children admitted.[10] A study in a primary care clinic investigated 270 children (median age 38 months) with suspected PTB with two IS specimens taken on sequential days.[7] In 11% of cases, a microbiological diagnosis was made; IS culture identified an additional 22% of cases above those diagnosed by clinical judgement. Furthermore, using a Likert scale, most IS procedures (91%) were rated as very easy or easy to perform by the health care worker performing the test. Combined data involving thousands of sputum induction procedures has found IS to be feasible, safe, and effective, even in infants, in primary care settings, and in HIV-infected and uninfected children.[11]

More recently, IS has been shown to be a useful specimen for microbiological diagnosis using Xpert. Pediatric studies from South Africa, Tanzania, and Uganda have reported sensitivities of 60–70% for Xpert in comparison with culture as a gold standard, with an increased yield when a second specimen is obtained and tested.[12–14]

To obtain an adequate IS sample, pretreatment with an inhaled bronchodilator and nebulization with hypertonic (3–5%) saline is performed and secretions obtained by suctioning or by expectoration in older children (Box 7.1). Precautions must be taken to prevent nosocomial transmission of the organism during sputum induction. The procedure should take place in a well-ventilated room equipped with ultraviolet lighting or in the open air, and sufficient time should be allowed between procedures. Staff should use appropriate protective masks (N95 or FFP3).

Nasopharyngeal Aspirate

Nasopharyngeal aspiration (NPA), achieved by passing a cannula through a nostril into the nasopharynx, is an attractive diagnostic procedure as it is minimally invasive and easy to perform. However, the culture yield from NPAs is lower than that from IS or from GL. A recent study[15] found that Xpert done on NPAs was useful, with a similar sensitivity (relative to culture of the same specimen) on two NPAs or two IS; however, IS provided a much higher yield of culture-positive cases.

Gastric Lavage

For years, collection of three consecutive early-morning GL aspirate samples was the standard of care for obtaining a microbiological diagnosis. However specimens must be taken on three sequential days for optimal yield, and the procedure is unpleasant, relatively invasive, and usually requires hospitalization. Although GL can be done in an outpatient setting, children need to fast and return to the health facility two to three times to enable collection of sequential specimens. Furthermore, in ill hospitalized children, the yield from culture from a single IS is equivalent to that of three GL[9]; in children with mild illness, the yield from culture for GL and IS has been reported to be similar. GL is a suitable specimen for Xpert; a Zambian study reported that Xpert on GL detected 69% of culture-confirmed cases.[16] Gastric lavage samples should be collected into a tube containing 100 mg of sodium carbonate (sufficient for 5–10 ml of aspirate) and processed in the laboratory as soon as possible.

Stool

Since young children swallow sputum, stool may contain *M. tuberculosis*. Stool has proved to be a poor specimen for culture, with very low culture yields of 1–2%. Xpert on stool has been reported to be promising, particularly in HIV-infected children, in two small studies,[17,18] but IS provided a higher yield. Further refinement of the processing and testing protocols for stool Xpert are needed.

Urine

Urine can be relatively easily collected and repeat specimens obtained. However, the yield for culture, Xpert, and antigen detection (lipoarabinomannan) has been

Box 7.1. Method for Obtaining an Induced Sputum Specimen

- Pretreat with two puffs of a short-acting bronchodilator via a spacer 5 minutes before the saline nebulization (give 1 puff every 10 secs).
- Fill the nebulizer chamber with 2–5 ml of 5% sterile hypertonic saline solution.
- Place nebulizer mask over the child's mouth and ensure that it fits tightly. An older child should be asked to tightly occlude his/her mouth around this.
- Use a jet nebulizer or oxygen at a flow rate of 5–8 l/min for nebulization. Continue nebulization until the hypertonic solution has emptied or until the child starts to cough.
- An older child should be instructed to expectorate whenever he/she coughs. If there is no spontaneous coughing, then ask the child to cough (if possible) after nebulization is complete.
- Infants and young children who cannot expectorate should be suctioned, using a size 7 or 8 French catheter after completing the nebulization. Children should be suctioned through the nasopharynx. The distance from the tip of nose to tragus of the ear should be measured, and children should be suctioned to this depth or until a cough is elicited.
- During suctioning, the child should be tightly swaddled and positioned on his/her side, lying with the head turned away from the operator (to avoid aspiration if the child vomits and to prevent droplet spray into the operator's face).
- Place the sample in a specimen container and send this to the laboratory; keep specimen in a refrigerator until transported to laboratory.

very low, even in HIV-infected children, making it currently unsuitable as a routine diagnostic specimen.[19]

String Test

The string test consists of a string inside a gel capsule that is swallowed by the child. The string unravels as it descends into the stomach; the capsule is left in the stomach for four hours, allowing it to dissolve while the string becomes coated with gastric secretions, which are retrieved. The string test is not suitable for young children (<4 years of age), but was well tolerated in a small study of older children (median age 8 years).[20] However, no child had a positive TB culture result in this small study.

Ear Swab

An ear swab (or, ideally, an aspirate of pus) provides a useful sample for culture that can be easily obtained, but is limited to situations where a child with suspected PTB has a discharging ear.

Fine Needle Aspirate

FNA for Xpert and culture is a useful adjunct to testing of respiratory specimens when an enlarged

peripheral lymph node is present and when staff have been appropriately trained in the procedure.[21] The procedure should be done using topical anesthesia and sedation in young children. At least two needle passes should be made using a 23 or 25 gauge needle. Cytological smears (for Papanicolaou and Ziehl-Neelsen [ZN] staining) should be prepared and the needle and syringe rinsed with mycobacterial culture medium or saline for subsequent culture and Xpert testing. The sensitivity and specificity of Xpert on FNA (compared to a combined reference standard of cytology plus culture) in children with tuberculous lymphadenopathy has been reported to be 80% and 94%, respectively.[21]

Bronchoalveolar Lavage Fluid

Broncho-alveolar lavage (BAL) is a resource-intensive and invasive procedure that has a lower yield for mycobacterial culture compared to GL. In adults, BAL does not provide a substantial additional culture yield over sputum or IS, while in children, comparative studies of GL vs. BAL have reported GL to be superior.[22,23] A pilot study of culture and Xpert testing of BAL samples from children with complicated intrathoracic tuberculosis showed that while culture had the higher yield, Xpert identified additional culture-negative cases.[24]

MICROBIOLOGICAL TESTS TO DIAGNOSE TUBERCULOSIS

The principles of microbiological testing for tuberculosis in children are the same as those for adults, and rely on the specific detection of whole *M. tuberculosis* bacilli (through acid-fast smear microscopy or bacterial culture) or bacterial components (such as DNA or cell wall molecules). However, as highlighted above, the primary challenge in achieving microbiological confirmation is the presence of very small numbers of *M. tuberculosis* bacilli in low-volume, difficult-to-collect samples. As a result, it is recommended to use the *most sensitive test or combination of tests on the most appropriate samples* in order to maximize diagnostic yield. Given that for most national tuberculosis control programs the number of specimens from adults far outnumbers those from children, use of the best available tests for all pediatric samples typically has minimal impact on laboratory costs for the program, and is warranted by the high morbidity and mortality associated with tuberculosis in young children.

Smear Microscopy

Smear microscopy, the oldest microbiological test for tuberculosis, is still in use; it relies on the visualization of bacilli stained with acid-fast dyes, which are retained within the waxy mycobacterial cell wall after decolorization with acid alcohol. The most efficient and sensitive microscopy procedures include fluorescent stains (such as auramine O) rather than the traditional ZN stain, but neither is entirely specific for *M. tuberculosis*. As a result, false-positive smears may occur, most frequently due to nontuberculous mycobacteria (NTM); however, in endemic settings, specificity is typically 95% or higher.[25] The sensitivity of smear microscopy is further improved by concentrating specimens using centrifugation.[26] Given the need for high sensitivity in children, optimized microscopy using a fluorescent stain on a concentrated sample is advised. Even so, the sensitivity of smear microscopy remains low in children, with an average of 22% of gastric lavage or aspirate and 29% of expectorated/induced sputum samples from culture-confirmed PTB cases being detected by microscopy in a recent review.[25] Smear microscopy

is more sensitive in older children, who are more likely to present with adult-type cavitary disease.

Mycobacterial Culture

Mycobacterial culture requires the growth of viable bacilli on solid or in liquid growth medium. Culture is challenging since *M. tuberculosis* grows very slowly, typically dividing only once every 24 hours, and since most respiratory samples are contaminated with other, faster growing, commensal bacteria and fungi. Respiratory (and other nonsterile) samples are therefore decontaminated using a strong solution of sodium hydroxide (NaOH, typically 1–1.5% final concentration) that kills most bacteria and fungi other than *M. tuberculosis*. Importantly, NaOH is also toxic for *M. tuberculosis*, so the balance between adequate decontamination and reduced mycobacterial viability needs to be carefully monitored in each laboratory. There is some evidence that decontamination with lower concentrations of NaOH than are typically used for adult specimens may improve the yield of culture from pediatric samples.[27] If feasible, laboratories should separately monitor contamination rates from pediatric and adult samples to determine whether less stringent decontamination protocols may be suitable for samples from children.

Following decontamination, samples are centrifuged and the pellet is inoculated into liquid or onto solid medium. Automated liquid culture systems, such as Mycobacterial Growth Indicator Tube (BACTEC MGIT, Becton Dickinson Microbiology Systems, Cockeysville, Maryland), offer optimal sensitivity, improved reproducibility, and reduced time to detection, but at a relatively higher cost than solid media (such as Lowenstein Jensen, or "LJ" slopes). Non-commercial liquid culture systems, such as the Microscopic Observation Drug Susceptibility (MODS) assay, which has been shown to perform better than LJ culture in children,[28] may offer some of the advantages of automated liquid culture at reduced cost, but are technically more demanding. Again, the principle should be to use the most sensitive available culture test. Since smear microscopy lacks sensitivity, all pediatric samples should be subjected to culture, where available.

A particular problem for pediatric tuberculosis is the risk of cross-contamination by *M. tuberculosis* between samples in the laboratory, which results in false-positive culture results. This is most likely to happen when samples with a high bacillary load, such as those from adult smear-positive cases, are processed in liquid media in the same laboratory batch as pediatric samples. Ideally, laboratories should process pediatric samples separately or at the beginning of each sample batch to reduce the risk of cross-contamination. Clinicians should be alert to this possibility and carefully review positive culture results where the clinical scenario does not support the diagnosis or where unexpectedly high rates of culture-positivity are noted.

A variety of extrapulmonary samples may be suitable for diagnosis of tuberculosis in children. These are comprehensively reviewed in chapters 2 and 10. Given the paucibacillary nature of most extrapulmonary tuberculosis, the largest possible volume of specimen should be collected and concentrated to maximize sensitivity.

It is important to note that a substantial proportion of children who are clinically diagnosed with tuberculosis have negative cultures, despite attempts to obtain and test suitable specimens.[2] In the absence of a highly accurate reference standard test, it is difficult to quantify how many of these children actually have tuberculosis disease; however, a negative culture cannot be used to rule out tuberculosis, but should be interpreted in the context of the clinical scenario.

Nucleic Acid Amplification Assays

In 2013, the World Health Organization endorsed the use of an automated, integrated nucleic acid amplification test, Xpert, for the diagnosis of TB in children (Box 7.2).[29] The recommendations support the use of Xpert as the initial diagnostic test in children suspected of having MDR-TB or HIV-associated tuberculosis and, subject to resource constraints, in all children suspected of having tuberculosis disease. DNA amplification tests for M. tuberculosis (also known as polymerase chain reaction [PCR] tests) are not new; however, the specific advantages of this test include relatively good sensitivity for smear-negative tuberculosis, simultaneous detection of rifampicin resistance, and a high degree of automation, which substantially reduces operator dependence and improves test reliability. Xpert is based on the real-time PCR amplification and detection of a fragment of the rpoB gene of M. tuberculosis. The assay starts with addition of a sample reagent to the sample that effectively sterilizes and liquefies sputum within 15 minutes. A fixed volume of the liquefied sputum is then added to a test cartridge where DNA extraction, PCR amplification, detection, and result reporting are accomplished in an automated manner. The assay includes a positive control, which controls for both DNA extraction and amplification.

Laboratory studies have demonstrated that Xpert reliably detects 130 bacilli per milliliter of sputum[30]—the "limit of detection"—that is less than that of liquid culture (10–100 bacilli/ml) but considerably better than that of unconcentrated smear microscopy (10,000 bacilli/ml). A recent systematic review of the accuracy of Xpert for the diagnosis of tuberculosis in children[25] demonstrated a pooled sensitivity of 66% for both expectorated/induced sputum as well as for GL or aspirate, when compared with culture, but with substantial variation between studies. Sensitivity was higher in children aged 5–15 years (83%) vs. younger children (57%), and in HIV-infected children (75%) vs. HIV-uninfected children (57%). However, only small numbers of HIV-infected children have been studied. Several researchers have investigated the incremental benefit of testing a second specimen with Xpert, and demonstrated an increment of between 8% and 17% for a second IS sample. There may be a further small increment from testing a third sample; however, this is unlikely to be practical

---

Box 7.2. WHO Recommendation (2013) for the Use of Xpert MTB/RIF for Diagnosis of Tuberculosis in Children

---

Xpert should be used rather than conventional microscopy, culture, and drug-susceptibility testing as:

- the initial diagnostic test in children suspected of having MDR-TB or HIV-associated tuberculosis (strong recommendation, very low-quality evidence).
- the initial diagnostic test in all children suspected of having tuberculosis (conditional recommendation acknowledging resource implications, very low-quality evidence).

in many situations. The incremental yield from a second specimen on nasopharyngeal samples is even larger, at 37%.[15] Importantly, the meta-analysis found that Xpert was only able to identify the presence of *M. tuberculosis* in 4–15% of samples from children clinically diagnosed with tuberculosis who had negative mycobacterial cultures. Specificity was excellent, ranging from 93–100%, suggesting that a positive test may be taken as a firm indication of the presence of tuberculosis disease; however, recent data from adults indicate that Xpert may remain positive for prolonged periods during and after treatment.[31] A positive Xpert result from a child recently treated for tuberculosis should therefore be interpreted with caution.

Xpert consistently detects a very high proportion (90–99%) of children with acid-fast smear-positive TB.[25] Clinicians should therefore consider using Xpert as a replacement for (rather than in addition to) smear microscopy. Splitting of small-volume samples to allow smear microscopy to be done together with Xpert may compromise sensitivity, although this has never been specifically studied.

There are few data on the use of Xpert for the diagnosis of extrapulmonary tuberculosis in children. Studies of tuberculous meningitis in children have been too small to adequately estimate test accuracy. However, pooled results of studies from adults and children show sensitivity of 80% when compared with culture.[25] Studies of peripheral lymph node aspirate or tissue in children also show good sensitivity (ranging from 77–100%). Xpert should not be used for testing clear fluids such as pleural or peritoneal fluid, as sensitivity for this is poor. There are currently insufficient data to make firm recommendations on other specimen types. WHO recommendations for Xpert testing of extrapulmonary samples are shown in Box 7.3.

In summary, Xpert is suitable for testing a range of specimen types, including expectorated and induced sputum, gastric lavage or aspirate, nasopharyngeal aspirates, cerebrospinal fluid (CSF) and peripheral lymph node aspirates or tissue. Xpert is useful as a rule-in test for tuberculosis in children, since, when positive, it supports rapid initiation of appropriate therapy. Sensitivity is suboptimal, particularly in younger children. Testing of additional specimens improves sensitivity; however, a negative Xpert test can never be used to rule out tuberculosis in a child. Although WHO recommends use of

Xpert "rather than" conventional microscopy and culture, given the precious nature of pediatric specimens and the limited sensitivity of Xpert, it may be argued that, where available, culture should be done in parallel with Xpert, either by splitting the specimen prior to processing or by testing multiple specimens.

Next-generation "fast-follower" nucleic acid amplification assays are increasingly being developed and undergoing evaluation. The utility of these assays for the diagnosis of tuberculosis in children will in large part be determined by assay sensitivity as well as their suitability for testing the range of specimen types from children with suspected tuberculosis. New tests need to be specifically evaluated in pediatric populations before use, since test performance may vary between adults and children.

Urinary Lipoarabinomannan

An alternative to nucleic acid detection is the rapid detection of mycobacterial cell wall components. Specifically, detection of mycobacterial lipoarabinomannan (LAM) in urine has shown potential as a diagnostic test for tuberculosis in adults with advanced HIV-infection.[32] Only one study in children has been reported to date, which showed disappointing specificity (48%) and sensitivity (61%).[19] Test accuracy was not better in children with HIV-infection. At present, this test should not be used in children, irrespective of their HIV-status.

MICROBIOLOGICAL TESTS FOR DRUG RESISTANCE

Microbiological testing not only provides confirmation of tuberculosis disease, but also is crucial for identifying the presence of drug resistance so that appropriate therapy can be given. Initial drug susceptibility testing aims to identify patients with MDR-TB, defined as disease caused by a strain of *M. tuberculosis* resistant to both rifampicin and isoniazid. Since resistance to rifampicin alone (without associated resistance to isoniazid) is relatively uncommon, testing for rifampicin resistance is a useful screen for MDR-TB. Once MDR-TB is identified it is important to test for susceptibility to second-line tuberculosis drugs, particularly fluoroquinolones and

> ### Box 7.3. WHO Recommendation (2013) for the Use of Xpert MTB/RIF for Testing of Extrapulmonary Samples (Adults and Children)
>
> - Xpert MTB/RIF should be used in preference to conventional microscopy and culture as the initial diagnostic test for CSF specimens from patients suspected of having tuberculous meningitis (strong recommendation given the urgency for rapid diagnosis, very low-quality evidence).
> - Xpert MTB/RIF may be used as a replacement test for usual practice (including conventional microscopy, culture, or histopathology) for testing specific non-respiratory specimens (lymph nodes and other tissues) from patients suspected of having extrapulmonary tuberculosis (conditional recommendation, very low-quality evidence).

injectables; resistance to both of these classes defines XDR-TB. Microbiological testing for drug-resistant tuberculosis in children is similar to that done for adult disease, with several particular considerations, described below.

Most drug resistance in *M. tuberculosis* results from specific chromosomal mutations (typically deletions or single base-pair changes in the DNA sequence of the bacterium, called single nucleotide polymorphisms [SNPs]). For some antibiotics, such as rifampicin, the mutations giving rise to drug resistance are well described, while for other drugs the relationship between genotype (the DNA mutation) and phenotype (drug resistance) are poorly understood. Laboratory assays for resistance are either phenotypic (compare the ability of the bacterium to grow in the presence vs. absence of antibiotic) or genotypic (screen for the presence of chromosomal mutations).

Phenotypic testing methods such as agar proportion or liquid-based automated methods (e.g., MGIT) are generally regarded as the reference standard methods for determining drug resistance; however, such methods are slow, labor intensive, require pure culture of *M. tuberculosis,* and pose substantial biohazard risks. These tests are reviewed in detail in Chapter 2. In contrast, genotypic testing is rapid, amenable to direct testing of specimens, and safer. However, reliable genotypic testing is not always possible, since not all resistance-conferring mutations are well defined, and since many different mutations may be responsible for resistance to one antibiotic.

Given the rapid progression, risk of dissemination, and high morbidity associated with tuberculosis in young children, there is a strong argument that drug susceptibility testing (specifically screening for

MDR-TB) should be done for all microbiologically confirmed cases of tuberculosis in children. Indeed, this is one of the most compelling reasons for the doing microbiological testing for all children with presumptive tuberculosis disease.

Commonly used genotypic tests for MDR-TB include Xpert[33] (which screens only for rifampicin resistance) and line probe assays (LPA) such as Genotype MTBDR*plus* (Hain Lifesciences, Hehren, Germany), which screens for both rifampicin and isoniazid resistance.[34] The Xpert assay includes five different fluorescent probes that target the rifampicin-resistance determining region of the *rpoB* gene. Binding of these probes to the sensitive (or "wild type") sequence can be measured by detecting fluorescent signal from each of the probes. Absence of fluorescence from one or two of these probes indicates that there is a mutation in this DNA region and that rifampicin resistance is present. LPAs target the same region to detect rifampicin resistance, but include additional targets for isoniazid resistance (*inhA* [mutations in this region give rise to low-level resistance] and *katG* [mutations give rise to high-level resistance]). LPAs use conventional or "end-point" PCR to amplify the relevant target sequences from DNA extracted from *M. tuberculosis,* followed by hybridization of the amplified DNA to a strip which contains probes for both the wild-type (sensitive) as well as the most common mutant (resistant) sequences. The banding pattern on the strip is then visually interpreted to determine resistance. LPA testing can be done on a cultured isolate of *M. tuberculosis* or directly from a specimen (usually restricted to smear-positive specimens, where *M. tuberculosis* is known to be present). The major advantages of Xpert over LPA are ease of use and reduced operator dependence. LPAs are relatively complex to perform, requiring highly trained staff and very strict adherence to laboratory protocol to avoid amplicon contamination (in which amplified DNA from one sample contaminates another sample, giving rise to incorrect results).

In many settings, genotypic methods are now used as the first-line method for screening for MDR-TB. Since any method may give incorrect results, although this is uncommon (the specificity of Xpert and LPA for rifampicin resistance is estimated as 98%[25] and 99%,[34] respectively), and given the clinical implications of diagnosing MDR-TB, resistance to rifampicin should be confirmed using a second method wherever possible. Expert advice should be sought for cases where discordant results are obtained from the different methods. In such cases, direct DNA sequencing of the relevant target gene and further detailed susceptibility testing may be necessary to resolve the discordance.

As Xpert tests for only rifampicin (and not isoniazid) resistance, the question arises as to the need for further testing for isoniazid resistance when an Xpert-positive, rifampicin-susceptible result is obtained. Since many children with tuberculosis are treated with a three-drug initial regimen, knowledge of isoniazid resistance is important to assess the need for a fourth drug. Where resources permit, it would therefore be appropriate to perform mycobacterial culture and isoniazid susceptibility testing for all such cases. In cases that are acid-fast smear-positive, direct line probe assay testing for isoniazid resistance on the sample may be a feasible and rapid alternative.

If first-line testing identifies the presence of MDR-TB (or rifampicin-resistant *M. tuberculosis*) then second-line drug susceptibility testing should be done. Rapid genotypic testing for resistance to fluoroquinolones and injectables is possible using LPA (e.g., Genotype MTBDR*sl*), custom microarrays, real-time PCR, or DNA sequencing. The MTBDR*sl* assay has been studied in detail; however, other genotypic methods have not been widely validated for clinical use. As a general rule, genotypic tests such as the MTBDR*sl* are highly specific (i.e., can be used as rule in tests for XDR-TB) but lack sensitivity (will miss approximately one quarter of XDR cases).[35] Confirmatory phenotypic testing should always be done.

REFERENCES

1. Connell TG, Zar HJ, Nicol MP. Advances in the diagnosis of pulmonary tuberculosis in HIV-infected and HIV-uninfected children. *J Infect Dis*. 2011 Nov 15;204(Suppl 4):S1151–S1158. PubMed PMID: 21996697. Pubmed Central PMCID: 3192545.
2. Perez-Velez CM, Marais BJ. Tuberculosis in children. *N Engl J Med*. 2012 Jul 26;367(4):348–361. PubMed PMID: 22830465.
3. Hatherill M, Hanslo M, Hawkridge T, et al. Structured approaches for the screening and diagnosis of childhood tuberculosis in a high prevalence region of South Africa. *Bull World Health Organ*. 2010;88(4):312–320. PubMed PMID: 20431796. Pubmed Central PMCID: 2855594.
4. Swingler GH, du Toit G, Andronikou S, van der Merwe L, Zar HJ. Diagnostic accuracy of chest radiography in detecting mediastinal lymphadenopathy in suspected pulmonary tuberculosis. *Arch Dis Child*. 2005;90(11):1153–1156. PubMed PMID: 16243870. Pubmed Central PMCID: 1720188.
5. Ling DI, Nicol MP, Pai M, Pienaar S, Dendukuri N, Zar HJ. Incremental value of T-SPOT.TB for diagnosis of active pulmonary tuberculosis in children in a high-burden setting: a multivariable analysis. *Thorax*. 2013;68(9):860–866. PubMed PMID: 23674550. Pubmed Central PMCID: 3862980.
6. Oliwa JN, Karumbi JM, Marais BJ, Madhi SA, Graham SM. Tuberculosis as a cause or comorbidity of childhood pneumonia in tuberculosis-endemic areas: a systematic review. *Lancet Respir Med*. 2015;3:235–243.
7. Moore HA, Apolles P, de Villiers PJ, Zar HJ. Sputum induction for microbiological diagnosis of childhood pulmonary tuberculosis in a community setting. *Int J Tuberc Lung Dis*. 2011;15(9):1185–1190, i. PubMed PMID: 21943843.
8. Zar HJ, Tannenbaum E, Apolles P, Roux P, Hanslo D, Hussey G. Sputum induction for the diagnosis of pulmonary tuberculosis in infants and young children in an urban setting in South Africa. *Arch Dis Child*. 2000;82(4):305–308. PubMed PMID: 10735837. Pubmed Central PMCID: 1718283.
9. Zar HJ, Hanslo D, Apolles P, Swingler G, Hussey G. Induced sputum versus gastric lavage for microbiological confirmation of pulmonary tuberculosis in infants and young

children: a prospective study. *Lancet*. 2005 Jan 8–14;365(9454):130–134. PubMed PMID: 15639294.

10. Hatherill M, Hawkridge T, Zar HJ, et al. Induced sputum or gastric lavage for community-based diagnosis of childhood pulmonary tuberculosis? *Arch Dis Child*. 2009;94(3):195–201. PubMed PMID: 18829621.

11. Planting NS, Visser GL, Nicol MP, Workman L, Isaacs W, Zar HJ. Safety and efficacy of induced sputum in young children hospitalised with suspected pulmonary tuberculosis. *Int J Tuberc Lung Dis*. 2014;18(1):8–12. PubMed PMID: 24365546.

12. Nicol MP, Workman L, Isaacs W, et al. Accuracy of the Xpert MTB/RIF test for the diagnosis of pulmonary tuberculosis in children admitted to hospital in Cape Town, South Africa: a descriptive study. *Lancet Infect Dis*. 2011;11(11):819–824. PubMed PMID: 21764384.

13. Rachow A, Clowes P, Saathoff E, et al. Increased and expedited case detection by Xpert MTB/RIF assay in childhood tuberculosis: a prospective cohort study. *Clin Infect Dis*. 2012 May;54(10):1388–1396. PubMed PMID: 22474220.

14. Sekadde MP, Wobudeya E, Joloba ML, et al. Evaluation of the Xpert MTB/RIF test for the diagnosis of childhood pulmonary tuberculosis in Uganda: a cross-sectional diagnostic study. *BMC Infect Dis*. 2013;13:133. PubMed PMID: 23497044. Pubmed Central PMCID: 3602671.

15. Zar HJ, Workman L, Isaacs W, et al. Rapid molecular diagnosis of pulmonary tuberculosis in children using nasopharyngeal specimens. *Clin Infect Dis*. 2012 Oct;55(8):1088–1095. PubMed PMID: 22752518. Pubmed Central PMCID: 3529610.

16. Bates M, O'Grady J, Maeurer M, et al. Assessment of the Xpert MTB/RIF assay for diagnosis of tuberculosis with gastric lavage aspirates in children in sub-Saharan Africa: a prospective descriptive study. *Lancet Infect Dis*. 2013;13(1):36–42. PubMed PMID: 23134697.

17. Nicol MP, Spiers K, Workman L, et al. Xpert MTB/RIF testing of stool samples for the diagnosis of pulmonary tuberculosis in children. *Clin Infect Dis*. 2013 Aug;57(3):e18–e21. PubMed PMID: 23580738. Pubmed Central PMCID: 3703104.

18. Walters E, Gie RP, Hesseling AC, Friedrich SO, Diacon AH, Gie RP. Rapid diagnosis of pediatric intrathoracic tuberculosis from stool samples using the Xpert MTB/RIF assay: a pilot study. *Pediatr Infect Dis J*. 2012;31(12):1316. PubMed PMID: 23188101.

19. Nicol MP, Allen V, Workman L, et al. Urine lipoarabinomannan testing for diagnosis of pulmonary tuberculosis in children: a prospective study. *Lancet Global Health*. 2014;2(5):e278–e284. PubMed PMID: 24818083. Pubmed Central PMCID: 4012567.

20. Chow F, Espiritu N, Gilman RH, et al. *La cuerda dulce*—a tolerability and acceptability study of a novel approach to specimen collection for diagnosis of paediatric pulmonary tuberculosis. *BMC Infect Dis*. 2006;6:67. PubMed PMID: 16595008. Pubmed Central PMCID: 1484483.

21. Coetzee L, Nicol MP, Jacobson R, et al. Rapid diagnosis of pediatric mycobacterial lymphadenitis using fine needle aspiration biopsy. *Pediatr Infect Dis J*. 2014;33(9):893–896. PubMed PMID: 25361020.

22. Bell DJ, Dacombe R, Graham SM, et al. Simple measures are as effective as invasive techniques in the diagnosis of pulmonary tuberculosis in Malawi. *Int J Tuberc Lung Dis*. 2009;13(1):99–104. PubMed PMID: 19105886. Pubmed Central PMCID: 2873674.

23. Abadco DL, Steiner P. Gastric lavage is better than bronchoalveolar lavage for isolation of Mycobacterium tuberculosis in childhood pulmonary tuberculosis. *Pediatr Infect Dis J*. 1992;11(9):735–738. PubMed PMID: 1448314.

24. Walters E, Goussard P, Bosch C, Hesseling AC, Gie RP. GeneXpert MTB/RIF on bronchoalveolar lavage samples in children with suspected complicated intrathoracic tuberculosis: a pilot study. *Pediatr Pulmonol*. 2014;49(11):1133–1137. PubMed PMID: 24339262.

25. Automated Real-Time Nucleic Acid Amplification Technology for Rapid and Simultaneous Detection of Tuberculosis and Rifampicin Resistance: Xpert MTB/RIF Assay for the Diagnosis of Pulmonary and Extrapulmonary TB in Adults and Children: Policy Update. WHO Guidelines Approved by the Guidelines Review Committee. Geneva; 2013.

26. Steingart KR, Ng V, Henry M, et al. Sputum processing methods to improve the sensitivity of smear microscopy for tuberculosis: a systematic review. *Lancet Infect Dis*. 2006;6(10):664–674. PubMed PMID: 17008175.

27. Whitelaw A, Mentoor K, Zar H, Nicol M. Standard Mycobacterial Decontamination Protocols May Be Inappropriate for Samples from

Paediatric Patients. Abstract FA-101237-13 2010. 41st Union World Conference on Lung Health, November 11–15. Berlin; 2010.

28. Tran ST, Renschler JP, Le HT, et al. Diagnostic accuracy of Microscopic Observation Drug Susceptibility (MODS) assay for pediatric tuberculosis in Hanoi, Vietnam. *PloS ONE*. 2013;8(9):e72100. PubMed PMID: 24023726. Pubmed Central PMCID: 3762843.

29. Automated Real-Time Nucleic Acid Amplification Technology for Rapid and Simultaneous Detection of Tuberculosis and Rifampicin Resistance: Xpert MTB/RIF System Policy Statement. WHO Guidelines Approved by the Guidelines Review Committee. Geneva; 2011.

30. Helb D, Jones M, Story E, et al. Rapid detection of Mycobacterium tuberculosis and rifampin resistance by use of on-demand, near-patient technology. *J Clin Microbiol*. 2010;48(1):229–237. PubMed PMID: 19864480. Pubmed Central PMCID: 2812290.

31. Friedrich SO, Rachow A, Saathoff E, et al. Assessment of the sensitivity and specificity of Xpert MTB/RIF assay as an early sputum biomarker of response to tuberculosis treatment. *Lancet Respir Med*. 2013 Aug;1(6):462–470. PubMed PMID: 24429244.

32. Lawn SD, Kerkhoff AD, Vogt M, Wood R. Diagnostic accuracy of a low-cost, urine antigen, point-of-care screening assay for HIV-associated pulmonary tuberculosis before antiretroviral therapy: a descriptive study. *Lancet Infect Dis*. 2012;12(3):201–209. PubMed PMID: 22015305. Pubmed Central PMCID: 3315025.

33. Boehme CC, Nabeta P, Hillemann D, et al. Rapid molecular detection of tuberculosis and rifampin resistance. *N Engl J Med*. 2010 Sep 9;363(11):1005–1015. PubMed PMID: 20825313. Pubmed Central PMCID: 2947799.

34. Ling DI, Zwerling AA, Pai M. GenoType MTBDR assays for the diagnosis of multidrug-resistant tuberculosis: a meta-analysis. *Eur Respir J*. 2008 Nov;32(5):1165–1174. PubMed PMID: 18614561.

35. Theron G, Peter J, Richardson M, et al. The diagnostic accuracy of the GenoType' MTBDR*sl* assay for the detection of resistance to second-line anti-tuberculosis drugs. *Cochrane Database Syst Rev*. 2014;10:CD010705. PubMed PMID: 25353401.

8

RADIOLOGY OF CHILDHOOD TUBERCULOSIS

Savvas Andronikou and Tracy Kilborn

HIGHLIGHTS OF THIS CHAPTER

- Imaging plays a crucial role in the diagnosis of tuberculosis in children when other tests are not diagnostic. It also detects complications and demonstrates extrapulmonary disease.
- The chest radiographic appearance of tuberculosis in children is dominated by the enlargement of the intrathoracic lymph nodes and their effect on adjacent structures.
- Modalities such as CT, MRI, and ultrasound provide much more specific detail than plain radiography, better define the anatomical abnormalities caused by tuberculosis and can aid in establishing the correct diagnosis.
- Radiographic features that are common and suggestive of tuberculous meningitis in children include basal enhancement, communicating or non-communicating hydrocephalus, evidence of stroke, and tuberculomas.
- It is critical that the clinician communicate with the radiologist that tuberculosis is a consideration so the optimal test and technique can be used and the studies be interpreted correctly.

RATIONALE FOR IMAGING IN SUSPECTED OR KNOWN TUBERCULOSIS IN CHILDREN

As long as the clinical and laboratory diagnosis of childhood tuberculosis remains elusive, clinicians will continue to look to diagnostic imaging to make the diagnosis. For imaging to remain relevant in the management of children with suspected tuberculosis, we need to change the way we use it, and we need to clarify what clinicians can expect from diagnostic imaging.

Chest radiography (CXR) is widely used because it is often the only method available for investigating patients with possible pulmonary tuberculosis (PTB) who have negative sputum smears. Chest radiographs for the diagnosis of childhood tuberculosis have been perceived to be "lack(ing in) specificity for PTB, . . . subjective and (is) neither standardized nor reproducible."[1] This perception stems largely from the poor inter-reader agreement and poor diagnostic accuracy demonstrated for diagnosing PTB.[2,3] Radiologists in practice continue to report radiographs in the detail that they are accustomed to provide for other pathologies and often report "possible" and "subtle" findings, a feature that distinguishes radiologists from other clinicians. However, it is this mismatch between what is required from imaging—a highly specific test for PTB; and what radiologists perceive is their duty—to be highly sensitive—that affects the clinical utility of radiographs. It is imperative that interpretation of radiographs be performed in the context where the sensitivity for PTB is dictated by the clinical suspicion and where radiographs are only reported positive for tuberculosis when the radiographic features of tuberculosis are obvious and incontestable.

Given the relatively poor specificity and sensitivity of chest radiographs in diagnosing childhood PTB, when facilities are available, the strategy should be to consider novel and affordable ways of using existing diagnostic modalities such as point-of-care ultrasound, dose-reduced CT scans, and fast MRI scanning. Even if these strategies succeed, we need to move beyond accepting that lymphadenopathy detection is adequate for diagnosing tuberculosis, and concentrate on imaging biomarkers, pathognomonic of the disease itself. Chest radiographs remain useful for detecting complications such as airway compression and for making alternative and additional diagnoses.

STRATEGIES FOR IMPROVED DIAGNOSTIC IMAGING FOR CHILDHOOD TUBERCULOSIS

Radiology Department vs. Point of Care

Considering the magnitude of the childhood tuberculosis burden in high tuberculosis incidence communities and the number of infected children potentially needing assessment, high-quality portable ultrasound machines for point-of-care sonography should become an integral part of the clinician's armamentarium at the community-clinic level. Physician-performed ultrasound at the clinic or bedside reduces the time to diagnosis, time to treatment, and referral to tertiary centers for advanced imaging and diagnosis. Point-of-care imaging, affordability, non-invasiveness, low-risk (no radiation dose), improved visualization of the mediastinum and no limit to the number of monitoring scans for response to treatment are important goals for imaging tuberculosis in children. Furthermore, because of its portability, ultrasound imaging is especially suitable for use in remote settings where there is no imaging, or only X-ray imaging, available.[4]

Clinician-Led Interpretation vs. Telereading

Many developing countries have limited radiology expertise within their borders, and this is a significant contributor to patient morbidity and mortality. For such countries, telereading (the electronic transfer of digital medical images from an area with no radiologist to a part of the world where expertise is available for interpretation) is being increasingly adopted to assist underserved areas. Simple telereading mechanisms include email and other free internet-based platforms that enable subspecialists to give expert opinions on diagnostic images.[4] There are many barriers to effective teleradiology, including lack of digital radiography for producing electronic images, poor radiographic quality, slow bandwidths, patient privacy issues, and even poor expertise of the telereaders in the diagnosis of diseases affecting the developing world. The alternative is that there must be task shifting of radiograph interpretation to clinicians (which is already a reality in developing countries) who must become proficient in interpreting radiographs and who benefit from continuous training courses.[5]

Looking for the Diagnosis Outside the Chest

The thoracic cage restricts ultrasound access to the internal structures, and it is for this reason that cross-sectional imaging with CT is so useful. However, an ultrasound diagnosis of *pulmonary* tuberculosis by identifying *abdominal* lymphadenopathy as a surrogate for mediastinal lymphadenopathy may present a simple additional diagnostic technique. One study showed abdominal lymphadenopathy in 19% and solid organ involvement in 23% of patients who presented with respiratory symptoms and had confirmed tuberculosis. Abdominal ultrasonographic features of tuberculosis had a sensitivity of 18% (95% CI 7.0–35.5%) with a specificity of 79% (95% CI 49.2–95.1%) when measured against chest radiographs for the presence of thoracic lymphadenopathy. Ultrasound also provided a 6% increase in the detection rate of tuberculous lymphadenopathy.[6]

A bedside ultrasound protocol for HIV/TB (focused assessment with sonography [FAS]) for HIV/TB has been developed to improve detection of extra-pulmonary tuberculosis in HIV-infected adults, and is now also being evaluated in young children who have a relatively high rate of extrapulmonary tuberculosis (EPTB).[4] Abdominal nodes; hepatic or splenic hypo-echoic lesions; as well as pericardial, pleural, or ascitic effusions, which are the main features of EPTB in high-prevalence settings, are easily recognizable following basic ultrasound training.[4] This concept also opens the door for other FAST and non-radiation-reliant whole-body imaging techniques such a fast whole body MRI using diffusion-weighted imaging (DWI) and short tau inversion recovery (STIR) (see below).

IMAGING APPEARANCES

Pulmonary Tuberculosis

Imaging findings of childhood PTB reflect the pathology. Initial infection usually involves one part of the lung parenchyma and may be small, peripheral, and seen as an airspace process accompanied by regional lymphadenopathy.[7] In young infants, hilar lymph nodes continue to enlarge, causing bronchial compression with air-trapping at first; but, with continued inflammation of the wall, perforation of the bronchus may occur, causing caseous material to enter the lumen, resulting in necrosis of the lung parenchyma with cavitation. This process is termed "lymphobronchial tuberculosis" or "epituberculosis" if there is a sudden onset of segmental or lobar opacification with minimal symptoms.[8,9] In children with untreated tuberculosis of the lower lobes, the disease can progress, resulting in scarring and bronchiectasis. Pleural effusion is a frequent association in older children but is rarely seen in children less than two years of age. Calcification can occur in the primary complex, especially in the lymph nodes when treatment is instituted early.[8] One of the major problems with radiographs for diagnosing childhood PTB is that many of the imaging features are common to other causes of pneumonia—lymphadenopathy may be the only distinguishing feature.[2,10] It should be the *goal* of those using imaging to make a diagnosis of PTB to *identify lymphadenopathy* or any surrogate marker of lymphadenopathy and any *complication* of the disease process. The sections that follow focus on the identification of lymphadenopathy and complications related to this disease process.

CHEST RADIOGRAPHS

The major role of imaging for diagnosis of PTB is the identification of lymphadenopathy. Du Toit and colleagues[2] showed only "fair" inter-observer and "moderate" intra-observer agreement among experienced pediatric pulmonologists in detecting lymphadenopathy on chest radiography in children with suspected PTB. This is lower than the agreement reported for other chest radiological features of pulmonary infection in children: unweighted kappas of 0.46–0.79 for consolidation/pneumonia and 0.78–0.83 for hyperinflation.[2] A more reproducible radiological sign is therefore needed that reflects lymphadenopathy.

Pediatric tuberculous lymphadenopathy on plain radiographs is seen as soft-tissue density masses in known locations. These are most obvious at the right paratracheal region and the hila. Problems identifying paratracheal lymphadenopathy arise because the thymus itself is a soft-tissue density mass in the mediastinum and is often indistinguishable from lymphadenopathy. However, the non-pathological thymus is known to be "soft" and does not cause displacement or compression of structures, and vessels can be seen through it[7,11,12] (see Figure 8.1).

Hilar lymphadenopathy causes obliteration of the normally "empty" V-on-the-side hilar points, formed by the divergent vessels on either side of the mediastinum (see Figure 8.2). A mass obliterating the hilar point and resulting in an outwardly convex appearance may represent tuberculous lymphadenopathy. The left hilum is usually hidden behind the heart if the patient is not rotated.[7] Considering this, however, it follows that an obvious left-sided hilar mass represents relatively large-volume lymphadenopathy (see Figures 8.3 and 8.4). On the occasion that the patient is rotated to the right, the right hilum is obscured, and the left becomes more visible. Sometimes extensive lymphadenopathy causes a confluent, outwardly lobulated contour to the mediastinal shadow (see Figure 8.5). In the study

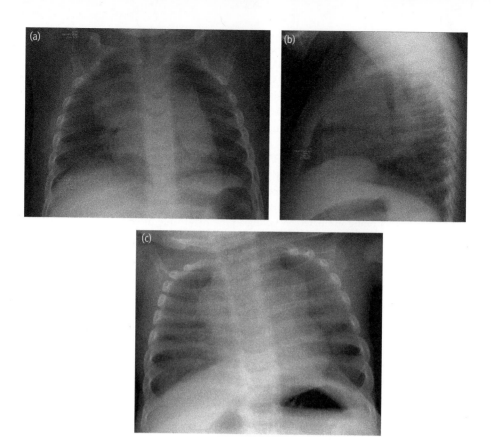

FIGURE 8.1   Mediastinal widening on frontal radiographs of infants with suspected tuberculosis—distinguishing the normal thymic shadow and identifying disease in: (*a, b*) an infant with tuberculosis, and (*c*) a normal infant. (*a*) There is mediastinal widening in this infant with proven tuberculosis, which may be due to a normal thymus or due to tuberculous lymphadenopathy. The indirect signs of airway compression at the bronchus intermedius are, however, in keeping with lymphadenopathy at the right hilum, and there is increased density behind the heart, representing left hilar nodes. (*b*) The lateral radiograph in this child confirms the normal thymic shadow in the anterior mediastinum but also demonstrates soft-tissue density behind the bronchus intermedius, supporting the diagnosis of tuberculous lymphadenopathy. (*c*) A different infant of the same age demonstrates mediastinal widening that represents a normal thymus.

by du Toit et al., there was greater agreement on the presence of lymphadenopathy (0.40) than on its absence (0.28).[2]

Lateral radiographs are useful for detecting lymphadenopathy posterior and inferior to the bronchus intermedius.[7] This retrocarinal, subcarinal, and superimposed hilar lymphadenopathy is represented as a lobulated density inferior and posterior to the bronchus intermedius. These soft-tissue densities complete the lower half of a "doughnut" formed superiorly by the right and left main pulmonary arteries and aortic arch[7] (see Figure 8.6).

Considering that tuberculous lymphadenopathy is known to involve the airways (lymphobronchial tuberculosis causing airway compression) in younger children, this finding may in itself represent a surrogate but more objective marker of tuberculous lymphadenopathy. Lymphobronchial tuberculosis usually affects the right main bronchus or bronchus intermedius, which is an area that is easily identified on plain radiographs. Airway compression is almost exclusive to children because their airways have a small caliber and they are compressible due to immature cartilage. Not only can demonstration of lymphobronchial tuberculosis assist in diagnosis, the finding is also relevant because prompt intervention to relieve the obstruction may salvage the affected lobe of lung segment[9] (see Figures 8.1, 8.2, 8.5).

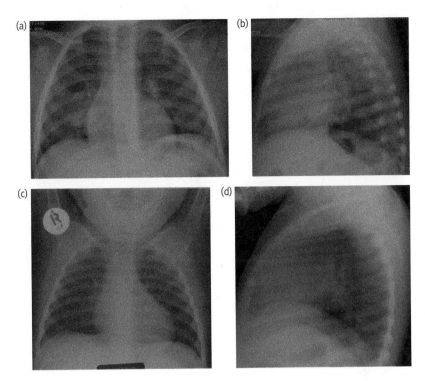

FIGURE 8.2   Frontal *(a)* and lateral *(b)* chest radiographs of an infant with tuberculosis, alongside *(c)* frontal and *(d)* lateral radiographs of a normal infant. *(a)* Oval lobulated soft-tissue density mass representing tuberculous lymphadenopathy partially obliterating the right hilum and preserving the right cardiac margin. There is associated narrowing of the bronchus intermedius, and the left main bronchus narrowing suggests the presence of subcarinal lymphadenopathy. *(b)* Oval soft-tissue density lymph node mass below and anterior to the hila, overlying the posterior cardiac shadow. *(c)* Normal right hilum is seen as an empty V-on-the-side, while the left hilum is hidden behind the heart on a non-rotated radiograph. *(d)* Normal lateral radiograph demonstrates densities in the shape of an upside-down horseshoe above the level of the bronchus intermedius. In particular, the region behind and below the bronchus intermedius shows no masses, and only diverging linear vessels are seen.

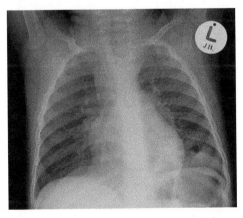

FIGURE 8.3   Large, left-sided tuberculous hilar lymph nodes projecting beyond the left cardiac margin seen as an outwardly convex dense mass. The lymphadenopathy causes moderate compression of the left main bronchus, and there is visible associated air-space disease in the left lower lobe.

Modification of plain radiography to demonstrate the airway, without resorting to CT, may improve its accuracy in diagnosing PTB and improve the inter-observer agreement. The frontal high-kilovolt (kV) radiograph has been used in the past to assess the effect of tuberculous adenopathy on the tracheobronchial tree and to detect endobronchial lesions. In one study, the specificity increased from 74.4% to 86.6% with the addition of the high-kV view, and sensitivity remained constant at 38.8%.[8] More recently, a very low-dose version of a chest radiograph using slit beam technology (Statscan—developed for whole-body imaging in trauma) has been studied and demonstrated that the trachea and left and right main bronchi were visualized better than with standard digital chest radiographic images. The authors recommended the use of this technology in developing countries with a high prevalence of PTB for detection

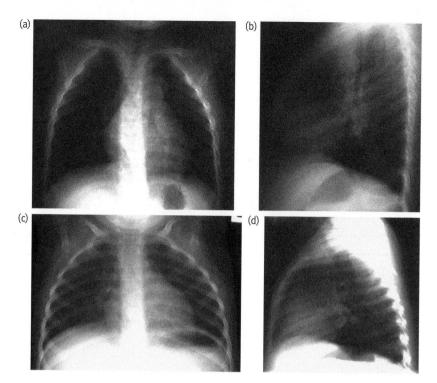

FIGURE 8.4   Frontal and lateral radiographs: at diagnosis of tuberculosis *(a, b)*, and after 6 months of anti-tuberculosis treatment *(c, d)*. *(a)* Left hilar tuberculous lymphadenopathy is not large enough to project beyond the cardiac margin on the frontal radiograph but is seen through the heart as an oval density occupying the left hilum. *(b)* Lobulated soft-tissue representing tuberculous lymphadenopathy is seen posterior and inferior to the bronchus intermedius on the lateral radiograph. *(c)* After 6 months of anti-tuberculosis treatment, the dense mass at the left hilum is no longer visible. *(d)* Post-anti-tuberculosis treatment, the lateral radiograph demonstrates normal diverging vessels posterior and inferior to the bronchus intermedius.

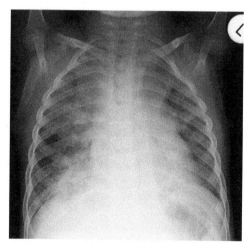

FIGURE 8.5   The frontal radiograph in a child diagnosed with tuberculosis: massive mediastinal and hilar lymphadenopathy resulting in mediastinal widening with a lobulated contour. There is significant airway compression and extensive bilateral air-space disease.

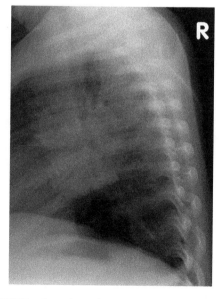

FIGURE 8.6   Tuberculous lymphadenopathy, seen as the "doughnut sign" on the lateral projection.

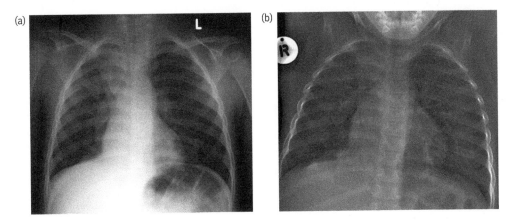

FIGURE 8.7   Hilar lymphadenopathy causing air-trapping. *(a)* Frontal chest radiograph shows filling in of the left hilar point, which suggests hilar lymphadenopathy. There is air-trapping of the left lung with shift of the mediastinum to the right. The left main bronchus is difficult to visualize. *(b)* Low-dose imaging using slit beam technology (LODOX) demonstrates the severe narrowing of the left main bronchus as an indirect marker of the left hilar lymphadenopathy. This is accounting for air-trapping on the left.

of mediastinal lymphadenopathy that can "distort the pliable pediatric tracheo-bronchial tree"[13] (see Figure 8.7).

Initial tuberculosis infection of the parenchyma is indistinguishable from other causes of pneumonia. Air-space disease can affect any part of the lung showing characteristic confluent density containing air bronchograms and obscuring cardiac, mediastinal, or diaphragmatic margins, depending on the location.[7] Alternatively, when disease is "contained" to the area of infection, a round or oval lesion representing a tuberculous granuloma is seen. This may

cavitate due to necrosis, or calcify[7] (see Figures 8.8, 8.9).

Much smaller, widely scattered multiple nodules are called "miliary nodules" and indicate hematogenous dissemination (including to other organs). These nodules are located in the interstitium and do not coalesce. The maintenance of multiple, discreet, sharply marginated nodules can be likened to stars in the night sky, whereas multifocal parenchymal disease can be likened to clouds in the daytime sky. Interstitial nodules are often best visualized at the costophrenic angles and the peripheral 1 cm

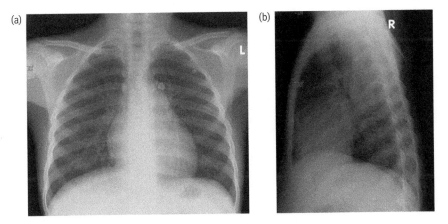

FIGURE 8.8   Obvious calcified tuberculous lymphadenopathy. *(a)* Frontal chest radiograph demonstrates calcified left mediastinal nodes and Ghon focus in the left upper lobe. *(b)* The lateral confirms the mediastinal location of the calcified lymph nodes.

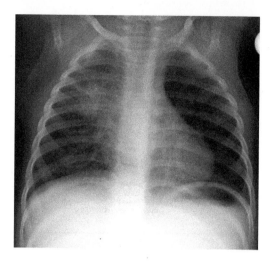

FIGURE 8.9   Frontal chest radiograph demonstrates a right hilar calcified lymph node mass in a child with proven tuberculosis.

of the lungs where few vessels are expected (see Figure 8.10).

PTB is one of the causes of necrotizing, cavitating pneumonia. Cavities are formed by liquefaction of caseous necrosis and subsequent fibrosis. In children, this can be caused by progressive primary infection or by bronchial obstruction with perforation and should not be classified as "reinfection" (see Figures 8.11, 8.12, 8.13). The walls of cavities contain a large population of rapidly multiplying bacilli and thus represent a risk for relapse and may harbor multidrug-resistant mutant strains. For this reason it is important to report all cavities and their characteristics, including the wall thickness

(cavities have thick walls ≥3 mm, while bullae or pneumatoceles have thin walls and little surrounding opacity).[7]

For the purposes of diagnosing childhood PTB, restricting the chest radiograph interpretation to the identification of, or absence of, only specific and repeatable signs of tuberculosis—i.e., indisputable lymph node masses, airway compression or displacement, and miliary nodules—may improve the utility of this modality. This is also the recommendation of du Toit and colleagues, who suggested the use of explicit criteria for reporting likely PTB.[2] Reporting the complications of PTB should be considered a separate activity where radiologists can add specific value thanks to their ability to identify subtle pathology. Pinto and colleagues developed a scoring system to aid the diagnosis of PTB, using features recorded with the Chest Radiograph Reading and Recording System (CRRS) for adults and "reliably ruled out active PTB in acid-fast smear-negative HIV-uninfected patients."[1] A similar recording system focusing on identification of lymphadenopathy has been developed and is recommended for use in children.[14]

CT OF THE CHEST

Even when CT is available, chest radiography is still widely used, because CT has a much higher radiation dose, much higher cost, and there is a need for intravenous contrast.[2] However, it is accepted that CT can demonstrate tuberculous lymphadenopathy far better than plain radiographs, and it is also an excellent modality for demonstrating the complications

(a)
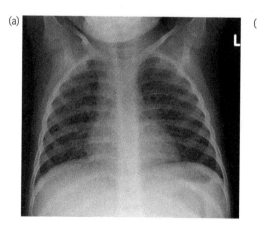

(b)
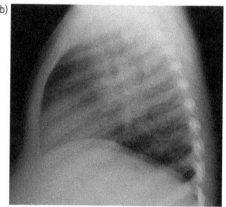

FIGURE 8.10   Miliary tuberculosis. Frontal (a) and lateral (b) chest radiographs demonstrate diffusely distributed, well-defined nodules in keeping with hematogenous dissemination of M. tuberculosis.

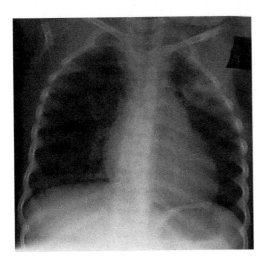

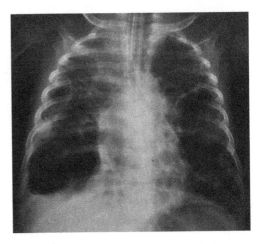

FIGURE 8.11 Example of childhood pulmonary tuberculosis causing cavitation: Frontal chest radiograph demonstrates a cavity within an oval nodule in the left upper lobe, much like that seen in adult pulmonary tuberculosis. There is no bronchial compression to account for this, and the findings probably represent uncontained primary infection, i.e., progressive primary disease.

FIGURE 8.13 Example of childhood pulmonary tuberculosis causing cavitation: Frontal chest radiograph demonstrates extensive bilateral cystic change involving the lung parenchyma in a young infant with progressive primary tuberculosis.

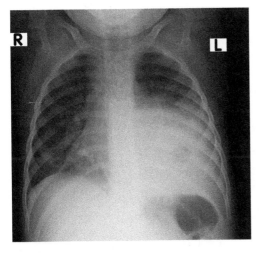

FIGURE 8.12 Example of childhood pulmonary tuberculosis causing cavitation: Frontal chest radiograph demonstrates a cavity within air-space consolidation of the lingula and left lower lobe. This is as a result of severe compression/obstruction of the left main bronchus. Other features of tuberculosis are the compression of bronchus intermedius, and compression with right middle lobe air-space disease (right cardiac margin obscured).

of PTB, including those resulting from lympho-bronchial tuberculosis and bronchiectasis.

Advanced multi-detector CT (MDCT) technology has markedly improved visualization and new iterative techniques of reconstruction have allowed significant dose-reduction. Ten years ago, using single-detector CT scanners, there was only moderate agreement among multiple readers for identifying tuberculous lymphadenopathy on pediatric contrast-enhanced CT scans. The readers had difficulty in distinguishing lymphadenopathy from normal thymus and were unable to distinguish "normal" from pathological nodes without being provided a predetermined size threshold for normality. Reliability was highest for the reported presence of lymphadenopathy in the right hilum and the sites around the carina.[15] Contrast-enhanced CT used to diagnose childhood PTB may demonstrate the characteristic rim-enhancement and low-density center of necrotic lymphadenopathy (see Figure 8.14). Matted lymphadenopathy, which loses its oval outline, may demonstrate rim enhancement and additional enhancing strands centrally within the mass, previously termed "ghost-like" because it was thought to have the appearance of multiple ghost-like figures.[7] CT studies found significant lymphadenopathy in up to 60% of PTB patients who had normal chest radiographs.[16]

The reported incidence of airway narrowing by tuberculous lymph nodes varies from 35% to 40%, with a higher prevalence in younger children (see

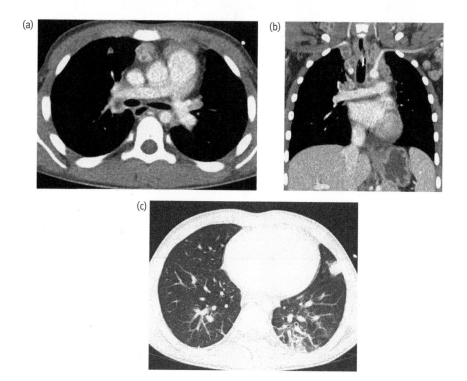

FIGURE 8.14   CT of pulmonary tuberculosis. *(a)* Axial contrast-enhanced CT at the level of the carinal bifurcation demonstrates ring-enhancing lymphadenopathy with low density centers at the right hilum and anterior mediastinum. *(b)* A coronal reformat demonstrates bilateral mediastinal rim-enhancing lymph nodes as well as the supraclavicular region on the right and the axilla on the left. *(c)* Axial CT on lung window demonstrates the associated Ghon focus in the lingula, as well as air-space disease in the left lower lobe.

Figure 8.15). CT of the chest is the imaging gold standard for demonstrating airway narrowing in children with PTB.[17] MDCT with three-dimensional volume rendering reconstruction has been shown to have a very good correlation with bronchoscopy in identifying airway compression due to tuberculous lymphadenopathy in children. It also provides information on the airway beyond severe obstructions,

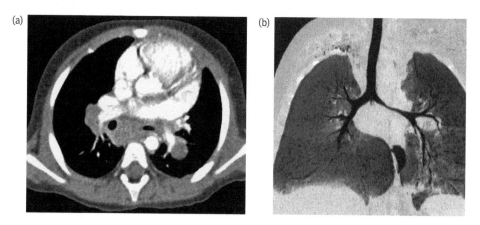

FIGURE 8.15   CT of complicated pulmonary tuberculosis. *(a)* Axial CT in the subcarinal region demonstrates bilateral hilar and subcarinal lymphadenopathy. There is compression of the left main bronchus. *(b)* Coronal thick-slab minimum intensity projection (MinIP) reconstruction, demonstrates the localized compression of the left main bronchus and patent right-sided airway.

an area invisible to the bronchoscope. CT with image post-processing also gives objective measurements of the degree and length of stenosis and can pinpoint the responsible lymphadenopathy for possible surgery[17] (see Figure 8.16).

Another post-processing reconstruction method for CT scans useful in detecting airway compression by tuberculous lymphadenopathy is the minimum intensity projection (MinIP). This provides an image highlighting only the airway within a slab

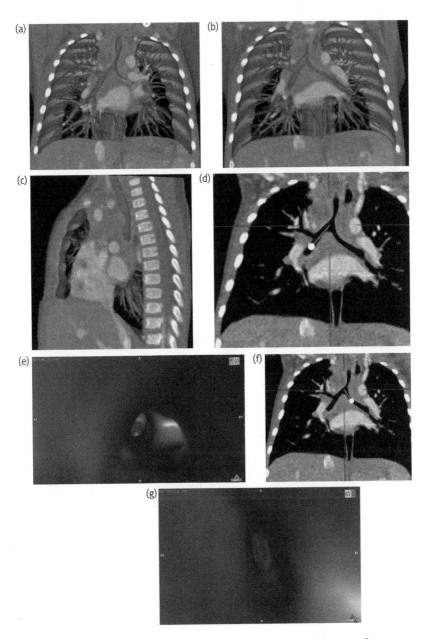

FIGURE 8.16   3-D volume–rendered reconstructions demonstrating the advantages of post-processing. (*a*) Anterior view with anterior chest wall removed demonstrates right tracheal compression as a result of right paratracheal lymphadenopathy. (*b*) Anterior view, dorsal to (*a*), demonstrates subcarinal lymphadenopathy compressing the left main bronchus against the normal blood vessels. (*c*) Midline lateral view demonstrates the anterior impression of the lymphadenopathy on the trachea. (*d*)–(*g*) Virtual bronchoscopy planning images and internal perspective views of the right main bronchus bifurcation (normal) and the left main bronchus (which shows narrowing).

of tissue. When coronal oblique reconstructions are created, the technique is most easily likened to a chest radiograph and easily identifies airway narrowing. These reconstructions can be produced by technologists without radiologist input based on predetermined criteria[18] (see Figure 8.15b).

Lucas and colleagues[9] showed that the bronchus intermedius is compressed most frequently (28% of all compressions), speculating that the narrow caliber (being a third-order bronchus), the length and vertical orientation, as well as its position between the two most commonly enlarged nodal groups (subcarinal and right hilar) in childhood PTB predispose to this finding. The left main bronchus, being longer and narrower than the right main bronchus, accounted for 24% of total airway compressions in their study. Airway compression was noted to be more frequent and more severe in infants who had relatively larger lymphadenopathy and smaller caliber airways which are more compressible.

CHEST ULTRASOUND: ROLE OF CHEST US AND FINDINGS

Mediastinal ultrasound (US) is currently being investigated as an alternative imaging test to diagnose childhood PTB. Windows for mediastinal US include the suprasternal notch and parasternal intercostal spaces, which allow detection of enlarged lymph nodes in the superior and anterior mediastinum. One pediatric imaging study demonstrated that mediastinal US detected lymphadenopathy in 67% of children with PTB who had a normal chest radiograph; the mediastinal US findings were confirmed on CT.[4]

A research group using mediastinal US in children with tuberculosis demonstrated lymphadenopathy in two-thirds of those with a normal chest radiograph and showed that US could be used to monitor response to treatment.[19,20] Another group developed and used a simplified technique for performing mediastinal sonography in children using a high-resolution, small-footprint sector transducer placed at the suprasternal notch. Using two views (coronal oblique and sagittal oblique), four zones were defined in relation to the blood vessels. Lymphadenopathy, which is relatively hypoechoic, is oval in all planes, and can displace structures, can be identified separately from normal, echo-free blood vessels, which often branch and become elongated structures in at least one plane (see Figures 8.17 and 8.18). The thymus can be identified as a homogeneous organ with well-defined

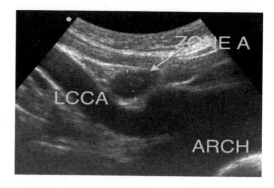

FIGURE 8.17 Sagittal ultrasound through the suprasternal notch demonstrates the normal vessels as long anechoic structures, while tuberculous lymphadenopathy is seen as single or multiple oval hypoechoic lesions.

LCCA = left common carotid artery; Zone A = indicates the lymphadenopathy anterior to the vessels.

margins that does not compress other structures in the anterior mediastinum[21] (see Figure 8.19).

MRI OF THE CHEST

The advantages of chest MRI are obvious—it does not involve ionizing radiation and provides high soft-tissue contrast without a need for intravenous contrast. The duration of the overall procedure as well as the sequences have been major stumbling blocks to its routine utilization, as has its high cost

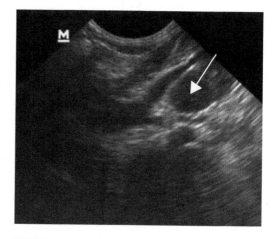

FIGURE 8.18 Coronal oblique ultrasound through the suprasternal notch performed by a pediatrician (non-radiologist) using low-cost portable ultrasound equipment at the bedside demonstrates the oval hypo-echoic lymph nodes as separate from the elongated anechoic vessels.

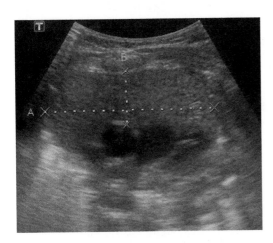

FIGURE 8.19 Coronal oblique ultrasound of the superior mediastinum through the suprasternal notch in a young child demonstrates the normal thymus as a homogenous rhomboidal structure anterior to the vessels and airway.

and unavailability. Recent technical advances in MR sequence speed, higher MRI signal, and improved resolution demand reinvestigation of this modality in identification of tuberculous lymphadenopathy (see Figure 8.20). The requirement of sedation or anesthesia, with its inherent risks for MRI studies in young children (under 6 year of age), calls for a rethinking of imaging strategies.

Limited sequences in the form of diffusion-weighted imaging (DWI; sensitive for lymphadenopathy) and Short Tau Inversion Recovery (STIR) (more characteristic of tuberculous lymphadenopathy) can be performed within 10-minute slots without sedation (unpublished research by chapter authors) (see Figure 8.21). Unlike lymphoma, in which lymphadenopathy demonstrates high signal on T2/STIR imaging, tuberculous lymph nodes may demonstrate characteristically low signal intensity. A T2 low-intensity pulmonary lesion on MRI might contain calcification, air, fibrous tissue, collagen tissue, and paramagnetic material. Tuberculosis-specific low T2/STIR signal intensity has been demonstrated in the parenchyma of older children with PTB who underwent MRI, with no calcification or air shown on CT. The reason for the shortening of the T2 signal is not clear, but it may be the result of the presence of paramagnetic free radicals in the enclosed macrophages.[22] Modified MRI may yet prove to be a specific biomarker for PTB.

Boiselle and Colleagues' Recommendations to Improve Access to MRI. [1] Create relationships to use MRI scanners outside of children's hospitals in order to increase available MRI capacity. [2] Use multichannel coils, parallel imaging, and new fast MRI sequences on 3T MRI scanners to improve image quality at decreased imaging times, without sedation.[23]

COMPLICATIONS AND PROGRESSION OF PTB

One of the major complications characteristic of childhood tuberculosis is lymphobronchial disease, with obstruction of airways by lymphadenopathy. This may result from external airway compression, erosion, ulceration, infiltration, intraluminal caseating material, or granulation tissue. The situation can become complicated further in a sequential process of air trapping, air-space consolidation, atelectasis, expansile pneumonia (bronchial filling by fluid or wet lung with bulging fissures) (see Figure 8.22), parenchymal necrosis (loss of vascular markings, lack of lung parenchymal enhancement) and eventual breakdown with cavity formation (see Figure 8.23). Erosion of tuberculous lymph nodes into the airways can also result in bronchial spread of the infection with resulting multifocal bronchopneumonic consolidation.[9,24] Even when radiographs are normal, air-space densities in the form of coalescing micronodules can be seen on CT when this occurs. These are different from miliary nodules, which remain discreet.[7]

Children with any of the above complications may benefit from surgical intervention by suction of an obstructing node to decompress a bronchus or by bronchoscopic removal of intraluminal content.[9] Maydel and colleagues[25] showed that patency of the airway and resolution of the parenchymal disease associated with obstruction can be achieved after surgical suction of offending lymphadenopathy. In these cases, CT scanning also allowed surgical planning and postsurgical follow-up.

Bronchiectasis and Cavitation. Cavities are formed by the necrosis and fibrosis that accompany lung destruction. Cavities predispose patients to relapse after treatment and are also considered responsible for harboring resistant strains of *M. tuberculosis*. It is therefore important to recognize cavities, as they may need surgical

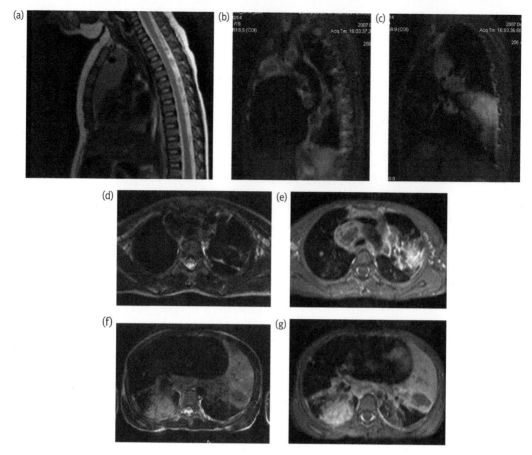

FIGURE 8.20   MR imaging of the chest in a normal infant (*a*) and in a child with pulmonary tuberculosis (*b-g*) to demonstrate the pathological features of tuberculosis. (*a*) Sagittal T2-weighted imaging of a normal infant chest demonstrates the position of the thymus in the anterior-superior mediastinum, anterior to the main branches of the aorta and deep to the venous structures. The thymus is seen as a single organ with a homogenous parenchyma of intermediate signal. (*b*) Parasagittal STIR image of the anterior mediastinum in a child with confirmed tuberculosis demonstrates multiple discreet nodular masses of low signal intensity replacing the thymus and separating vascular structures, representing characteristic tuberculous lymphadenopathy. (*c*) Parasagittal STIR image at the left hilum demonstrates an oval mass of lymphadenopathy surrounding the vascular structures and airways, which accounts for the plain radiographic "doughnut sign." The non-necrotic lung parenchymal consolidation shows a homogenous high signal. (*d*) Axial STIR imaging of the superior mediastinum demonstrates the low signal, right paratracheal tuberculous lymphadenopathy, in contrast to the high signal, reactive lymphadenopathy at the left axilla. (*e*) Axial T1 after IVI gadolinium demonstrates the typical rim-enhancement of tuberculous lymphadenopathy and partial enhancement of the consolidated parenchyma. (*f*) Axial STIR and (*g*) Corresponding T1 with gadolinium in the lower lobes demonstrates the high signal and enhancement of vital/non-necrotic lung at the right lower lobe with visible air bronchograms, in contrast to the necrotic air-space process in the lingula, with limited enhancement and non-enhancing true necrotic focus.

removal in certain difficult-to-treat cases of drug-resistant PTB. Cavities in children with PTB can form as part of the primary infection (progressive primary TB), can be due to reactivation or exogenous reinfection, may represent bronchial cavities/bronchiectasis, or may be distal to a proximal bronchial occlusion/erosion.[7] Air-filled oval areas with thick walls, often within an area of opacification/nodule, represent cavities and may contain air-fluid levels.

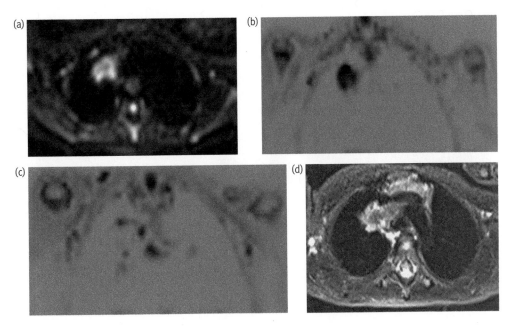

(a)

(b)

(c)

(d)

FIGURE 8.21   Rapid MRI protocol for diagnosing childhood tuberculosis performed in under 10 minutes without sedation or anesthesia incorporates DWI and STIR sequences. (a) Axial B500 image demonstrates the high signal lymphadenopathy at the right paratracheal region as well as "shotty" lymphadenopathy at the axillae. (b) Inverted coronal DWI reformat demonstrates the abnormal lymphadenopathy in the right paratracheal region and the smaller lymph nodes at the axillae as black structures against a suppressed background. (c) Coronal inverted DWI reformat at the level of the carina demonstrates additional regions of intrathoracic lymphadenopathy at the subcarinal region and both hila. (d) Axial STIR image of the paratracheal lymphadenopathy demonstrates that the center of the tuberculous lymphadenopathy has a characteristic low signal, while the periphery is of high signal, similar to that of the axillary reactive lymphadenopathy.

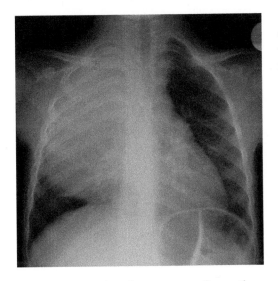

FIGURE 8.22   Tuberculosis as a cause of expansile pneumonia: This is an expansile pneumonia involving the right upper and middle lobes. The trachea and heart are displaced to the left, both by the expanded lung and by the presence of right-sided lymphadenopathy.

Bronchiectasis is difficult to identify with confidence on plain radiographs, but "ring shadows" and the "tram-track sign" are the main features. High resolution CT (HR-CT) is the imaging modality of choice in the diagnosis of bronchiectasis, demonstrating the "signet-ring sign" representing the dilated thick-walled bronchus ("ring") adjacent to the smaller blood vessel ("gem" of the ring). Traction bronchiectasis can complicate fibrosed and distorted lung.[7]

Lucas and colleagues[24] made an important observation that tuberculous lymphadenopathy can erode anything it comes into contact with. Reported examples of this are: broncho-esophageal fistula secondary to tuberculous glandular erosion into both the esophagus and bronchus[26] (see Figure 8.24); phrenic nerve palsy caused by tuberculous lymph gland infiltration of the phrenic nerve[27]; and chylous effusion caused by infiltration or compression of the thoracic duct by right paratracheal lymphadenopathy.[28]

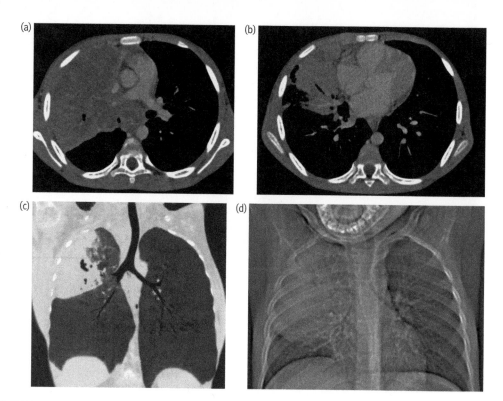

FIGURE 8.23 CT showing complications of lymphobronchial tuberculosis. *(a)* Axial contrast-enhanced CT of subcarinal and right hilar lymph node masses with faint strands of enhancement. There is compression of bronchus intermedius with the associated right-sided lung parenchymal necrosis and early cavitation. *(b)* Axial contrast-enhanced CT at a level more caudal to *(a)*, demonstrating an area of vital consolidated lung, where the parenchyma is enhancing, vessels are visible, and bronchi are patent (air-bronchograms). *(c)* Coronal thick slab MinIP reconstruction confirms the cutoff of the right upper lobe bronchus as well as the long segment narrowing of the bronchus intermedius. *(d)* The CT scanogram serves as the comparative 2-D correlate of the airway compression and expansile pneumonia.

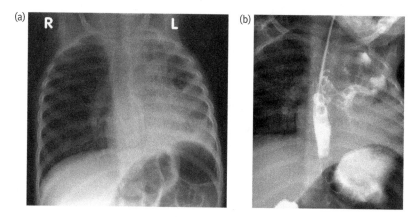

FIGURE 8.24 Tuberculosis causing a broncho-esophageal fistula. *(a)* Frontal chest radiograph demonstrates extensive air-space disease, a left upper lobe cavity, and pleural effusion in a patient diagnosed with tuberculosis. The lucency in the mediastinum (in addition to the normal tracheal lucency) is in keeping with an air-filled esophagus. *(b)* A contrast esophagogram using a tube placed in the esophagus demonstrates the broncho-esophageal fistula caused by tuberculous lymphadenopathy as well as the contrast filling of the left upper lobe cavity.

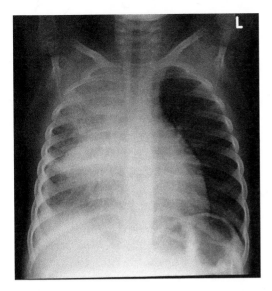

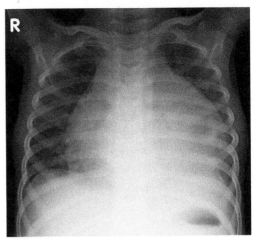

FIGURE 8.26   Tuberculous pericarditis: Tuberculous pericardial effusion causing globular cardiomegaly.

FIGURE 8.25   Tuberculosis with pleural effusion: Frontal radiograph demonstrates extensive right-sided air-space disease, bronchus intermedius compression, and a right pleural effusion.

Extensive cavitation can also be the result of uncontained primary infection, known as progressive primary disease. These patients are extremely ill, often require admission for ventilation, and have a high mortality rate[29] (see Figure 8.13).

Tuberculous pleurisy (see Figure 8.25) may also complicate, resulting in an empyema. This can progress to form a subcutaneous abscess or broncho-pleural fistula. Eventually, chronic pleural disease may results in a fibrothorax. Tuberculous pericarditis occurs in about 1% of childhood tuberculosis cases and often results from erosion of subcarinal lymph nodes into the pericardium[7] (see Figure 8.26).

An area of TB infection can result in vasculitis and thrombosis of pulmonary arteries and veins. Pseudoaneurysms of the pulmonary arteries occurring adjacent to tuberculous cavities are known as Rasmussen aneurysms. Hemoptysis resulting from these can be severe and life-threatening, requiring urgent angiographic arterial embolization while awaiting definitive therapy[7] (see Figure 8.27).

HIV/TB CO-INFECTION AND IMMUNE RECONSTITUTION INFLAMMATORY SYNDROME (IRIS)

HIV infection enhances the susceptibility to tuberculosis and hastens its progression with massive hematogenous dissemination after initial infection. Tuberculosis is a major cause of death in patients with HIV infection.

Chest radiography for tuberculosis in patients with HIV infection may be confusing because tuberculosis and HIV share some imaging features, and features of PTB may be more severe in patients with HIV infection. Chest radiographs in patients with tuberculosis and HIV co-infection may also be normal. There are multiple possible pathological conditions that may occur simultaneously (Kaposi sarcoma, lymphocytic interstitial pneumonitis, bacterial pneumonia).[30,31]

After initiation of anti-retroviral therapy, the child's immunity may be restored. This predisposes to the development of immune reconstitution

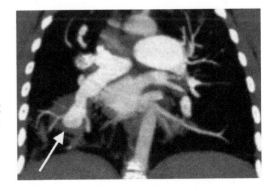

FIGURE 8.27   Rasmussen aneurysm: Contrast-enhanced CT (coronal reconstruction) demonstrates a right lower lobe, pulmonary artery aneurysm within a soft-tissue-density tuberculous lesion.

inflammatory syndrome (IRIS), which is a paradoxical deterioration as a result of the immune response to antigens of *M. tuberculosis*. The thoracic appearances of IRIS include lymphadenopathy not seen previously or worsening, new or worsening lung parenchymal disease, and/or effusion. IRIS usually occurs within three months of commencing antiretroviral treatment[32] (see Figure 8.28).

Classification as "Severe" or "Non-severe" Disease. A proposed classification system for evaluating patients or their radiographs with regard to PTB is based on the presence and extent of complications, and places imaging findings into the categories "severe" and "non-severe." This classification system may more accurately reflect the clinical disease spectrum in children, is relevant to clinical management, and may be valuable to inform research on diagnostic tools and treatment strategies in children. *Complications* refer to the presence of infiltration or compression of structures adjacent to the disease site. *Disseminated disease* is that from hematogenous spread; e.g., miliary tuberculosis; tuberculous meningitis; or renal, hepatic, or splenic tuberculous granulomata.

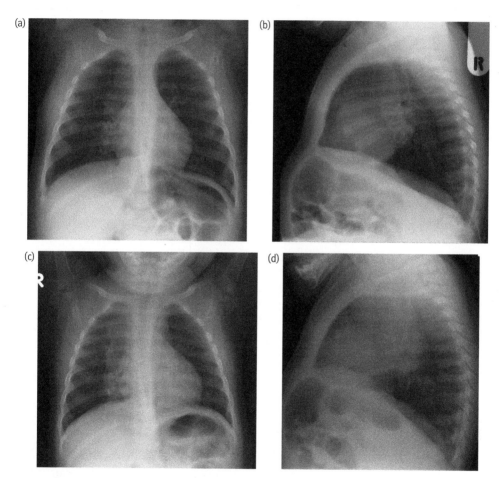

FIGURE 8.28   Pulmonary tuberculosis in a child with HIV infection, before and after the initiation of antiretroviral therapy (ART), demonstrating IRIS (immune reconstitution inflammatory syndrome).
(a) Right paratracheal and right hilar lymphadenopathy, with associated tracheal displacement to the left, and bronchus intermedius compression before initiation of ART. *(b)* Lateral radiograph before the initiation of ART, demonstrating hilar lymphadenopathy anterior and inferior to the bronchus intermedius. *(c)* Frontal radiograph in the same child as after initiation of ART, with progressive widening of the mediastinum and further compression of the bronchus intermedius, implying an increase in the volume of the lymphadenopathy. *(d)* Lateral radiograph post-ART, demonstrating a more obvious "doughnut sign" due to enlargement of the hilar lymph nodes.

Non-severe disease is limited (controlled), nondisseminated, and uncomplicated. Examples include: Ghon focus; non-expansile, non-bronchopneumonic, single-lobe alveolar disease; and effusion without or with lymphadenopathy that has not compressed or eroded any structures.

Severe disease is uncontrolled, as in disseminated disease or complicated thoracic disease, which includes expansile pneumonia, bronchopneumonia, multilobar alveolar disease, cavitation, nodal large-airway compression (lymphobronchial tuberculosis), empyema, and tuberculous pericarditis.[33]

CENTRAL NERVOUS SYSTEM TUBERCULOSIS

Blood-borne *M. tuberculosis* and, less commonly, direct spread of the organisms from the skull or middle ear, can cause tuberculosis of the CNS.[11] The result may be a focal lesion or a more diffuse process in the form of tuberculous meningitis (TBM).[11,12] Focal tuberculous lesions usually result in children's presenting with seizures, while meningitis can result in cranial nerve palsies, focal neurology, and a decreased level of consciousness.[12]

Imaging should be used for making an early diagnosis. CT serves the purposes of acute imaging because it is accessible and fast and therefore can be used to demonstrate complications that require urgent management, such as hydrocephalus, which is a treatable complication of TBM. CT can also contribute to assessing the patient's prognosis by identifying infarction and is useful for monitoring the response to treatment. MRI has restrictions in its accessibility and duration of the procedure and should therefore be reserved for the non-emergency setting. It has major advantages in demonstrating significant infarctions in TBM and also better demonstrates basal enhancement, which assists the clinician in making the diagnosis. MRI is also better than CT in differentiating focal tuberculous lesions from other lesions that may be considered in the differential diagnosis.[11,12]

Imaging of Focal Lesions

There are two types of focal tuberculous lesions that can be seen in the brain or spinal cord. Tuberculomas are the commonest of these (>95%), and they have characteristic appearances on both CT and MRI, usually being *smaller than* 2 cm with either ring or nodular enhancement and generating

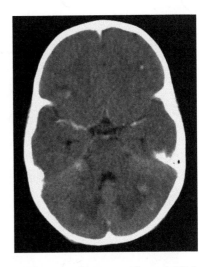

FIGURE 8.29   Axial contrast-enhanced CT showing multiple brain tuberculomas involving the cerebral and cerebellar hemispheres with ring-type and nodular enhancement and moderate surrounding edema.

moderate peri-lesional edema (see Figure 8.29). The density/signal intensity differentiate these from tuberculous abscesses or pyogenic abscesses. Tuberculomas demonstrate iso- or hyper-density centrally on CT (see Figure 8.30) and *characteristic*

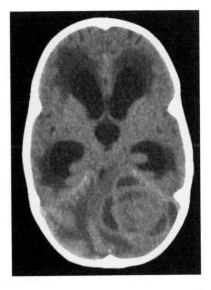

FIGURE 8.30   Axial contrast-enhanced CT of an unusually large left cerebellar tuberculoma demonstrates the typical isodense center with ring enhancement and moderate amounts of surrounding edema. The mass is compressing the fourth ventricle with consequent hydrocephalus.

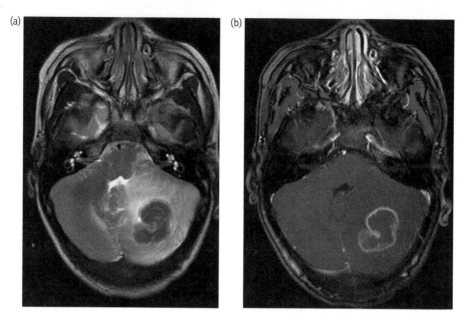

FIGURE 8.31   MRI of a large tuberculoma in the left cerebellar hemisphere. *(a)* Axial T2 demonstrates the typical low signal of caseous necrosis in a tuberculoma. There is also peripheral high signal, representing edema. *(b)* On axial T1, the lesion is isointense to cortex and demonstrates ring enhancement post-gadolinium, typical of a tuberculoma.

low signal on T2 and iso-intensity to cortex on T1 on MRI (see Figures 8.31 and 8.32). Tuberculomas are usually seen independently of meningitis (reported in less than 15% of children with TB meningitis).[11,12]

Tuberculous abscesses are less common lesions, are usually larger, and have features inseparable from those of pyogenic brain abscesses, such as low density on CT and low T1/high T2 signal on MRI.[12]

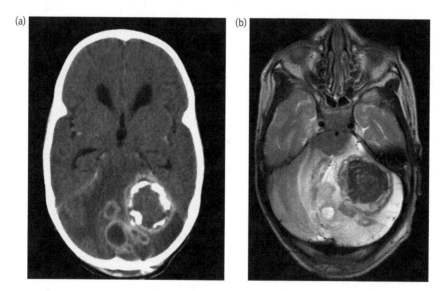

FIGURE 8.32   Follow-up imaging in a child with progressive disease. *(a)* Axial contrast-enhanced CT of the same child as in Figure 8.30, after two months of anti-tuberculosis treatment. The tuberculoma demonstrates an isodense center, rim enhancement, and peripheral calcification. New tuberculous abscesses have developed and demonstrate hypodense centers and rim-enhancement with surrounding edema. *(b)* Corresponding T2 MRI demonstrates the high signal intensity of the tuberculous abscesses, which are seen as satellites to the hypointense tuberculoma.

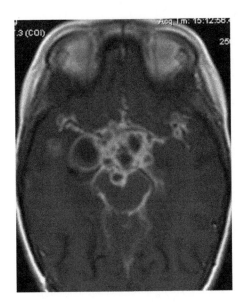

FIGURE 8.33   Post-contrast T1-weighted MRI of tuberculous abscesses resistant to treatment in the cisterns and parenchyma. The lesions have low signal centers on T1 and enhance avidly with gadolinium. This patient presented with blindness due to the inflammation and pressure on the optic chiasm.

Tuberculous brain abscesses may be difficult to treat medically and can cause complications such as seizures and blindness[34,35] (see Figure 8.33).

Intra-medullary spinal cord tuberculosis can demonstrate fusiform swelling of the cord containing focal tuberculous lesions that demonstrate features similar to those of brain tuberculomas.[36]

CT/MRI in Tuberculous Meningitis

The characteristic feature of TBM is abnormal basal enhancement involving the meninges or cisterns.[37] CT can demonstrate the abnormal basal enhancement in the vast majority of children with TBM (see Figure 8.34). Even non-contrast CT is useful because TBM typically demonstrates hyperdensity in the cisterns in about half of patients.[37] This "hyperdense cistern sign" is reported to be specific for TBM and probably represents both granulation tissue and exudate,[12] which enhances with contrast (see Figure 8.35). MRI is more sensitive than CT in detecting basal enhancement because the abnormal enhancement is not confused with blood vessels (which demonstrate flow voids) (see Figure 8.36). On CT, vessels and subtle enhancement of the edges of the cisterns are often indistinguishable.[12,38] In addition, MRI can demonstrate the miliary nodules deposited in the leptomeninges that account for some cases of TBM[39] (see Figure 8.37). There is a concordance between TBM and miliary tuberculosis in young children, suggesting a pathogenetic relationship. This is contrary to the perpetuated hypothesis that, in all cases of TBM, a preexisting caseous lesion (the Rich Focus) in the cortex ruptures into the meninges to cause meningitis.[40]

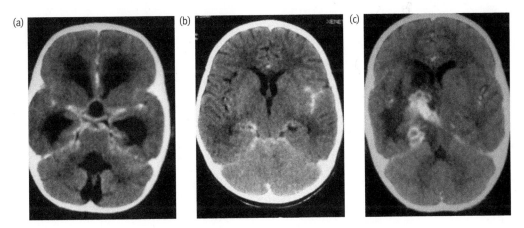

FIGURE 8.34   Axial contrast-enhanced CT of the brain in 3 different children with tuberculous meningitis. (a) Diffuse symmetrical meningeal enhancement outlining the suprasellar cistern and the accompanying hydrocephalus. (b) Asymmetrical localized enhancement in the left sylvian cistern, which is clearly different from the sylvian cistern on the right. (c) Nodular enhancement with meningeal-based tuberculomas anterior to the brainstem and along the tentorium.

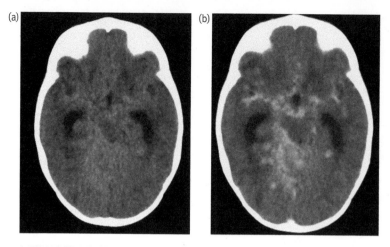

FIGURE 8.35   CT scanning in tuberculous meningitis, pre- and post-contrast. (*a*) Pre-contrast and (*b*) post-contrast CT demonstrating hyperdensity in the surrounding the brainstem and in the suprasellar cistern, which enhances post-contrast. In addition, there are multiple predominantly meningeal-based enhancing granulomas and hydrocephalus.

In addition to aiding in establishing a diagnosis of TBM, imaging is useful for demonstrating its complications. This is the true value of imaging, because these complications cannot be detected with laboratory testing, and it is these features of the disease that require urgent treatment and determine the prognosis.

Hydrocephalus is the most common complication of TBM; it is important to demonstrate it early

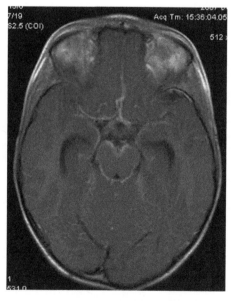

FIGURE 8.36   Post-contrast T1-weighted MRI showing abnormal meningeal enhancement of the suprasellar cistern outlining of the temporal lobe uncus bilaterally and surrounding the brainstem. The right middle cerebral artery is clearly distinguished from the adjacent frontal and temporal lobe meningeal enhancement by its flow void (i.e., signal free).

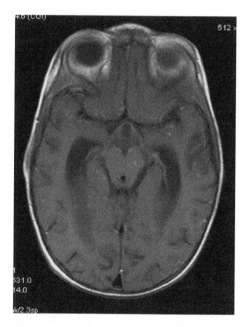

FIGURE 8.37   Post-contrast T1-weighted MRI in an HIV-infected child with tuberculous meningitis with scanty enhancement of the meninges at the cerebral peduncles; however, there are multiple enhancing miliary nodules with a pia-arachnoid meningeal distribution.

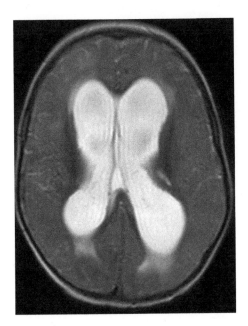

FIGURE 8.38   Axial T2-weighted MRI can demonstrate the ventriculomegaly and surrounding trans-ependymal fluid shift of hydrocephalus, and can be used for follow-up of patients without the radiation dose received during CT scanning.

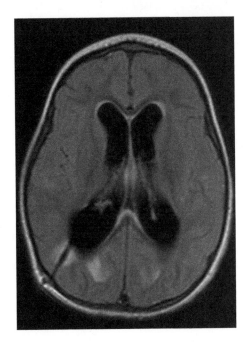

FIGURE 8.39   Fluid-attenuated inversion recovery (FLAIR) imaging is more useful than T2 for demonstrating trans-ependymal fluid shift, as it suppresses the intraventricular fluid and highlights the periventricular edema. In this child with tuberculous meningitis, the hydrocephalus was treated with ventricular drainage, and the drain is visualized entering the lateral ventricle from the right posterior.

(using CT or MRI) because it is treatable and has a poor outcome if treated late[41] (see Figures 8.34a and 8.38). Most hydrocephalus complicating TBM is "communicating" in nature and can be treated medically, without needing neurosurgical drainage.[41] Imaging must aim to identify the minority of patients who develop "non-communicating" hydrocephalus that requires surgical drainage to improve outcome[11,12] (see Figure 8.39). Standard CT and MRI are not reliable in differentiating the two types of hydrocephalus without intervention.[42] By injecting a small amount of air (5–10 ml) into the subarachnoid space after diagnostic lumbar puncture has been performed, non-communicating hydrocephalus can be distinguished when air fails to enter the ventricular system and remains trapped in the basal cisterns, as opposed to communicating hydrocephalus, which allows air in the ventricular system as well as the basal cisterns. The location of air can be evaluated after the procedure by radiography or CT (see Figures 8.40 and 8.41). To date, no other imaging study has been shown to be able to replace "air-encephalography" in differentiating the two entities.[41]

Another major complication of TBM is inflammatory pan-arteritis, which results in brain infarctions.

Prognosis is significantly affected by these infarctions in TBM, which usually involve the basal ganglia and internal capsules, often bilaterally,[11,12,43] and the brainstem.[44] Infarcts complicating TBM can lead to severe disability and death.[43] Even though CT is adequate to identify hydrocephalus in the emergency setting and can demonstrate early established infarcts (see Figure 8.42), MRI is the imaging modality of choice for demonstrating infarctions, especially those in the brainstem and pons. Diffusion-weighted imaging is used to show acute infarcts (see Figure 8.43).

The triad of basal enhancement, hydrocephalus, and infarction in the correct clinical setting is diagnostic of TBM.

Border-zone necrosis (BZN), present in approximately 50% of children with TBM, is found in advanced disease and indicates a poor prognosis. This phenomenon develops as a result of inflammation of the brain immediately underlying the tuberculous exudate and occurs by extension of disease along small proliferating vessels into the brain parenchyma,

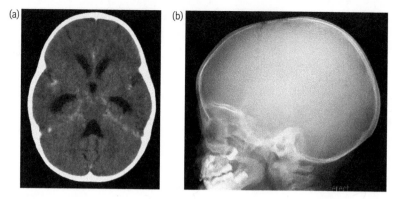

FIGURE 8.40 Non-communicating hydrocephalus. (a) Axial contrast-enhanced CT scan demonstrates moderate hydrocephalus as a result of tuberculous meningitis. (b) Lateral skull radiograph post-injection of 10 ml of air into the thecal sac after completing diagnostic lumbar puncture; i.e., air-encephalogram demonstrates that there is no air in the ventricular system. This finding is an indication for surgical ventricular drainage.

causing vasculitis and resulting in ischemic change. These infarcts are seen adjacent to severe meningeal/cisternal inflammation (most commonly seen in the Sylvian fissure, cerebral peduncles, midbrain, and pons) (see Figure 8.44). One MRI study in children with TBM demonstrated BZN as areas of restricted diffusion in 50% of patients, with the temporal lobe adjacent to the middle cerebral artery affected in 82% of these patients.[45]

Inflammation with exudate formation and granulation tissue in children with TBM is most prominent around the suprasellar cistern, which surrounds the pituitary gland and hypothalamus. It is thought that the vascular disease and associated destruction of the surrounding brain tissue in TBM may cause the syndrome of inappropriate anti-diuretic hormone secretion/diabetes insipidus in up to 71% of patients because of the proximity to the pituitary gland and hypothalamic-hypophyseal axis. Inflammation may result in leakage from the gland or brain edema with high intracranial pressure. The imaging correlate of the above is loss of the visualization of the posterior pituitary bright spot, which occurs in about half of children with TBM imaged with MRI (see Figure 8.45). An absent posterior pituitary bright spot has been reported to be associated with poor outcome at 6-month follow-up.[46]

Cranial nerve enhancement is seen in patients with and without cranial nerve palsies and can assist in identifying basal enhancement. Commonly, this affects the optic chiasm, and the occulomotor and trigeminal nerves (see Figure 8.46).

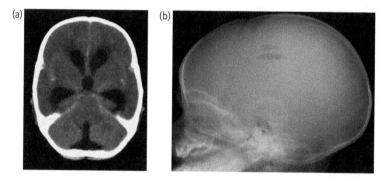

FIGURE 8.41 Communicating hydrocephalus. (a) Axial contrast-enhanced CT scan in this patient with tuberculous meningitis demonstrates more pronounced hydrocephalus than in the patient in Figure 8.40. (b) Lateral skull radiograph post-injection of 10 ml of air into the thecal sac after completing diagnostic lumbar puncture; i.e., air-encephalogram demonstrates air having gained access into the ventricular system after lumbar puncture. This warrants a trial of medical treatment.

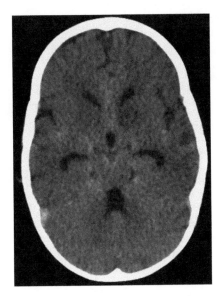

FIGURE 8.42   Axial contrast-enhanced CT scan demonstrates enhancement of the basal cisterns in keeping with tuberculous meningitis. Ill-defined low densities in the left caudate and lentiform nuclei represent infarction as a complication of the meningitis.

HIV/TUBERCULOSIS CO-INFECTION IN TBM

One of the major factors associated with poor outcome in TBM is HIV-coinfection.[41] The frequency of imaging abnormalities is similar in HIV-infected and HIV-uninfected adults with TBM.[47] In children, however, "intense" basal meningeal enhancement occurs less frequently in those who are HIV-infected (see Figure 8.47), and more often the enhancement is asymmetrical.[48] One study showed that HIV-infected children had more visible enhancing meningeal nodules on MR imaging than HIV-uninfected children with TBM, assisting in establishing the diagnosis.[48] Cerebral atrophy is more common in HIV-infected children,[47,48] and non-communicating hydrocephalus less common[48] (see Figure 8.48). Katrak et al.[49] have proposed that the decreased intensity of meningeal enhancement and obstructive hydrocephalus observed in HIV-infected patients (not on antiretroviral treatment) is due to the "immune suppression causing a reduced inflammatory response."

TB Arachnoiditis

Spinal arachnoiditis may not be as uncommon as previously thought, considering the involvement of the subarachnoid spaces in TBM. More cases of spinal arachnoiditis might be identified if the cord were imaged more often in patients with TBM. MRI with IV gadolinium demonstrates enhancement of the dura-arachnoid surrounding the cord. Tuberculous radiculomyelitis involves the thoracic

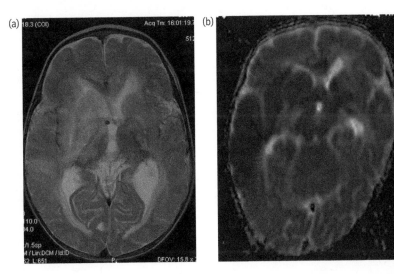

FIGURE 8.43   MRI scan demonstrating infarction. (a) Axial T2 demonstrates abnormal high signal involving the right caudate and both lentiform nuclei, right thalamus and possibly the left thalamus. (b) High DWI signal (not shown) and low apparent diffusion coefficient (ADC) signal represent restricted diffusion in keeping with an acute/subacute infarction. The ADC map demonstrates low signal in the right basal ganglia, as suspected on the T2-weighted study, but also indicates involvement of the left caudate, lentiform nuclei, as well as the right temporal operculum and insula.

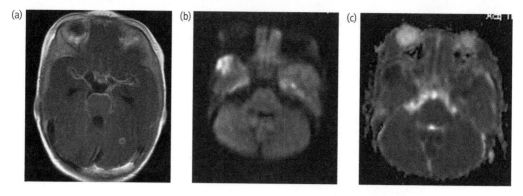

FIGURE 8.44 MRI demonstrating border-zone necrosis. *(a)* Post-contrast T1 image demonstrates the abnormal meningeal enhancement of the suprasellar cistern, middle cerebral artery cisterns, and surrounding the brainstem. *(b)* DWI and *(c)* Corresponding ADC map demonstrates restricted diffusion of the anterior temporal lobe adjacent to the abnormal meningeal disease, demonstrated on the T2-weighted sequence. This corresponds to border-zone necrosis of the parenchyma adjacent to the inflammation.

and cervical region most commonly.[11] Some reports indicate that CSF shows increased signal intensity on T1-weighted images and that there can be complete loss of the cord–CSF interface with an irregular cord outline. Imaging features of arachnoiditis include enhancing subarachnoid nodules, clumping of the cauda equina nerve roots, CSF loculations, and abnormal signal and enhancement of the cord[11,36] (see Figure 8.49).

ABDOMINAL TUBERCULOSIS

Abdominal tuberculosis is not as common in children as it is in adults.[11] Abdominal findings of tuberculosis in patients presenting with chest symptoms are becoming more evident as we search for

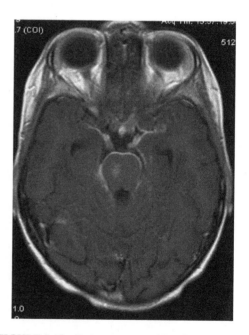

FIGURE 8.46 Post-contrast axial T1 showing abnormal enhancement of the meninges covering the optic chiasm and the occulomotor nerves, in addition to the typical enhancement around the brainstem. Abnormal enhancement within the brainstem may involve the nuclei.

FIGURE 8.45 Sagittal T1 (same patient as in Figure 8.54) demonstrates an absent posterior pituitary bright spot, which may relate to abnormal inflammation around the pituitary gland.

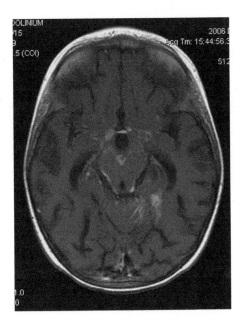

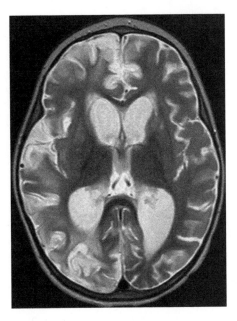

FIGURE 8.47　Post-contrast axial T1 in an HIV-infected child with tuberculous meningitis shows patchy enhancement of the basal cisterns and brainstem, as well as miliary nodular deposits. There is ventriculomegaly, but in the presence of increased surface markings, this may represent atrophy rather than hydrocephalus.

FIGURE 8.48　An HIV-infected child with tuberculous meningitis demonstrates ventriculomegaly with transependymal fluid shift in the presence of increased surface markings. This probably represents hydrocephalus in a patient with underlying atrophy. In addition, there is high signal in the caudate and lentiform nuclei, in keeping with bilateral infarctions.

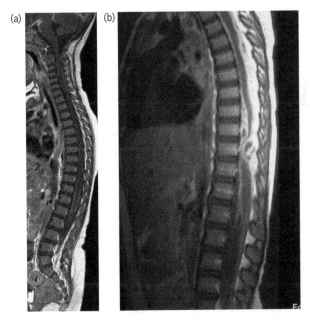

FIGURE 8.49　Post-contrast sagittal T1 of the spine in two children with tuberculous meningitis. (a) Demonstrating enhancement coating the cord, conus medullaris, and nerve roots of the cauda equine, in keeping with arachnoiditis. (b) Thick enhancement surrounding the cord, which is compressed and narrowed at the site of extra-medullary collections that show ring enhancement.

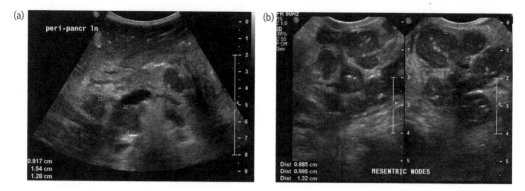

FIGURE 8.50 Ultrasound of intra-abdominal tuberculous lymphadenopathy. *(a)* Transverse image of the epigastric region, showing hypoechoic lymph nodes both deep and superficial to the pancreas. *(b)* Split screen of transverse ultrasound image in a different child demonstrates a conglomerate of abnormal hypoechoic mesenteric lymph nodes with typical echogenica hila.

diagnoses by imaging structures outside the chest. The incidence of extra-pulmonary tuberculosis may also be rising as a result of the HIV epidemic.

Ultrasound

Point-of-care sonography for tuberculosis can be performed by a physician at the patient's bedside. FASH (focused assessment with sonography for HIV/tuberculosis) is a predefined technique for demonstrating features of abdominal tuberculosis at the bedside. It is able to demonstrate typical US features that include lymphadenopathy (see Figure 8.50), hepatic or splenic hypoechoic lesions (see Figure 8.51), as well as associated pericardial, pleural, or ascitic effusions. FASH has become one of the most applied modalities in adult emergency rooms, and its value in children is especially promising, as it is non-invasive and well tolerated.[4,11]

CT Features

CT with contrast is a useful technique for demonstrating the features of abdominal tuberculosis. It can demonstrate lymphadenopathy, organ lesions (see Figure 8.52), conglomerate masses, and omental "cakes" (see Figure 8.53) separate from normal blood vessels. Characteristically, tuberculous lymphadenopathy is seen at the porta hepatis, para-aortic region, and the mesentery, causing fanning of the vessels and peripheralization of small bowel loops.

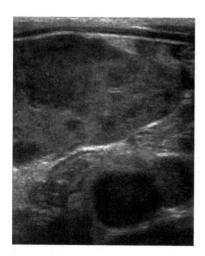

FIGURE 8.51 High-resolution ultrasound wimaging of the spleen demonstrates multiple, varying sized hypo-echoic lesions of the splenic parenchyma, in keeping with tuberculomas.

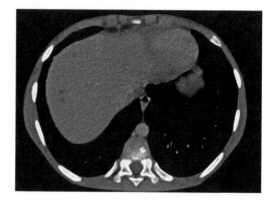

FIGURE 8.52 Axial contrast-enhanced CT in a child with pulmonary tuberculosis demonstrates multiple non-enhancing, low-density granulomata in the liver parenchyma.

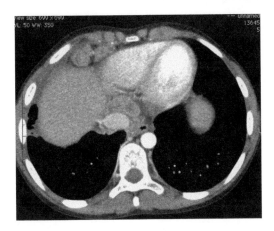

FIGURE 8.53   Axial contrast-enhanced CT of the abdomen demonstrates typical ring-enhancing porta-hepatis lymph nodes. In addition, soft-tissue masses are seen just deep to the anterior abdominal wall, representing tuberculous "omental cakes."

The typical appearance of this lymphadenopathy is ring-enhancement with low-density necrotic centers, although it may be calcified.[50] Organ tuberculomas are usually multifocal, non-enhancing oval lesions in the liver or spleen that may eventually calcify. Masses composed of bowel loops, omentum, and lymphadenopathy may develop, as may omental masses referred to as omental "cakes."[50]

MRI Features

Whole-body MRI can be performed using STIR/T2 imaging and DWI. Whole body DWIBS (diffusion-weighted whole-body imaging with background signal suppression) was primarily conceived to identify tumor. DWI identifies increased diffusion within pathological areas, including lymphadenopathy, lung parenchyma, organ lesions, and the musculoskeletal system. STIR/T2 sequences can confirm these pathological sites and also suggest the diagnosis of tuberculosis by demonstrating lesions that are of low signal (see Figure 8.54). DWIBS

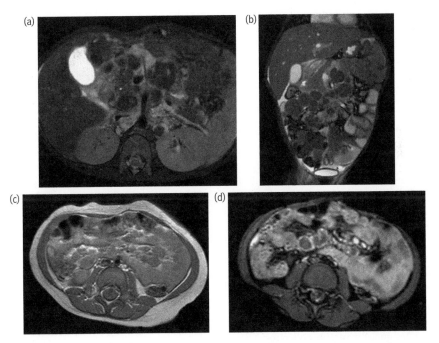

FIGURE 8.54   MRI in a child with abdominal tuberculosis. (a) Axial T2 with fat suppression showing multiple low signal/hypointense para-aortic lymph nodes that cause compression of the inferior vena cava. (b) Coronal T2 demonstrates low signal tuberculous lymphadenopathy interspersed within the mesentery and resulting peripheralization of the bowel. There are also multiple low-signal granulomata in the spleen. (c) Axial T1 without contrast and (d) Post-contrast with fat saturation, demonstrates rim enhancement of the mesenteric lymph nodes.

should not be interpreted in isolation as there are both false positive and false negative results, as it does not accurately identify the anatomical position of lesions.[51]

MR Enterography

MR enterography (MRE) is a modern MRI technique for assessing the bowel and can replace barium follow-through examinations without any radiation risk. It has been used extensively for the detection of Crohn's disease in children and is particularly useful for detecting additional findings such as disease outside the bowel and complications in the same sitting. Real-time assessment of peristalsis by cine MR is also possible. MRE has been reported to be useful for diseases other than Crohn's, including celiac disease, polyposis syndromes, and small bowel lymphoma. "MR enterography has the potential to be a useful test in the evaluation of abdominal tuberculosis."[52] Abnormal findings that may be relevant for tuberculosis include: wall thickness >3 mm, excess wall enhancement, diffusion restriction, DWI detection of lymph nodes, non-peristalsis on cine imaging, stricture, proximal bowel dilatation, submucosal edema (hyperintense bowel wall on T2), possible hypointensity on T2 in chronic fibrosis, and the presence of caseous necrosis.[52]

UROGENITAL TUBERCULOSIS

Tuberculosis of the renal tract results in papillary destruction and cavitation of the kidneys.[11] Bacilli can spread to the renal pelvis, ureter, and bladder, causing inflammation and eventually fibrosis. This in turn can cause strictures with obstruction at the calyceal infundibulum, the pelviureteric junction, and the vesicoureteric junction. When the entire collecting system is obstructed and the renal parenchyma is destroyed, the kidney may become nonfunctional.[53]

US findings include echogenic calyces and mixed or echo-free areas in the pyramids, indicating cavitation.[11] US can also show dilatation of the calyces and irregularity of the collecting system (see Figure 8.55). Increased echogenicity of the renal pelvis is a feature of fibrosis and scarring. The bladder may demonstrate urothelial thickening as well as focal echogenic granulomas. Ureters may be seen posterior to the bladder when there is a vesicoureteric junction stricture.[53]

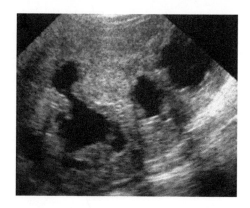

FIGURE 8.55 Longitudinal ultrasound of the kidney in a child with renal tuberculosis demonstrates cavitation associated with the calyces in the upper pole, as well as mild hydronephrosis.

Magnetic Resonance Imaging

MRI using heavily T2-weighted thick slab rapid acquisitions can show a dilated collecting system without having to rely on a functioning kidney. In addition, MRI will demonstrate features of renal tract tuberculosis traditionally described on an intravenous pyelogram: pericalyceal cavities (resembling papillary necrosis), which progress to resemble hydronephrosis (pseudohydronephrosis); and strictures at the infundibula, pelviureteric junctions, and ureterovesical junctions. Time-resolved gadolinium-enhanced images (with an IV diuretic) can also assist in detecting calyceal and ureteric stricturing as well as non-functioning of a kidney, indicating autonephrectomy.[53]

The ovaries can be involved in tuberculosis and may result in diagnostic confusion with diseases such as lymphoma and leukemia.[11]

MUSCULOSKELETAL TUBERCULOSIS

The most common form of musculoskeletal tuberculosis is spondylitis, which accounts for half of cases. Other forms of musculoskeletal tuberculosis are uncommon.

Tuberculous Spondylitis

Because the mechanism of infection is hematogenous, patients with tuberculous spondylitis often have a history of pulmonary or abdominal tuberculosis. Children may present refusing to walk due to pressure from an abscess or bony sequestra onto the spinal cord. Symptom duration is over weeks to months, in comparison to pyogenic spondylitis where symptoms are present over a few days or weeks only. The lower thoracic and upper lumbar levels are most commonly affected. Tuberculosis affects the vertebral bodies and exhibits disc destruction only late in the disease. The disease process usually begins in the anterior part of the vertebral body adjacent to either the superior or inferior end plates. The infection spreads to involve the adjoining disc spaces by (a) extension beneath the anterior or posterior longitudinal ligament, or (b) penetration of the subchondral bone plate. Involvement of the disc manifests as collapse of intervertebral disc space.[54]

Plain radiographs only identify vertebral disease after 50% destruction of the body has taken place. Tuberculous lesions are low-density areas of erosion that cause progressive vertebral collapse. The anterior wedging that results accounts for the characteristic kyphosis (see Figure 8.56). Erosion and scalloping of the anterior vertebral bodies occur due to subligamentous extension of disease.[54]

On CT, there are lytic vertebral lesions with foci of calcification within the surrounding conglomerate inflammatory soft-tissue mass that accompanies the destruction. One description refers to an "exploded" vertebral body. There are often accompanying psoas abscesses that may be calcified if the disease is long-standing.[54]

The imaging modality of choice is MRI because it demonstrates contiguous vertebral body destruction and consequent kyphosis better than other modalities and is useful in identifying multiple non-contiguous areas of disease. It also demonstrates the characteristic heterogeneous soft-tissue mass that returns intermediate signal on T1 and predominantly high signal on T2. In almost half of patients, the center of the mass has an intermediate signal on T2[55] (see Figure 8.57). Even though disc preservation between two destroyed end-plates is common in adults, in children the intervertebral discs are often involved at presentation, seen as a loss of the normal disc high signal on T2.[54,55]

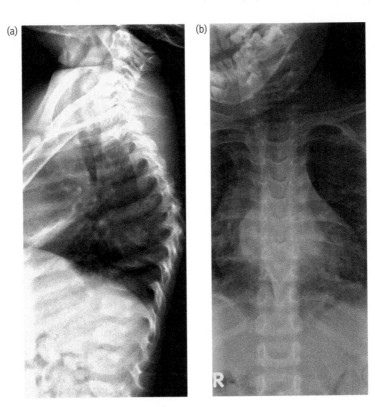

(a) (b)

FIGURE 8.56   Plain radiographs in tuberculous spondylitis. *(a)* Lateral showing mid-thoracic kyphosis as a result of the destruction of multiple vertebral bodies. Note also parenchymal lung disease in the middle lobe. *(b)* Frontal radiograph demonstrates a paraspinal soft-tissue mass corresponding to the area of the kyphosis seen on the lateral.

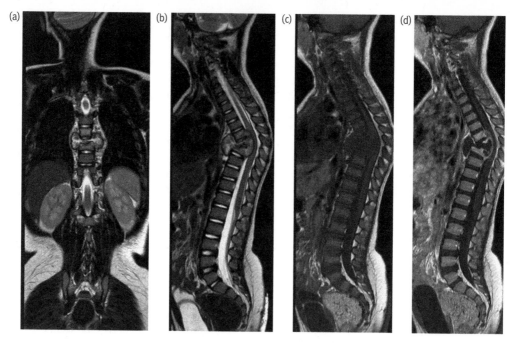

FIGURE 8.57   MRI of tuberculous spondylitis in the same child as in Figure 8.56. (*a*) Coronal T2 image demonstrates the circumferential soft-tissue mass that corresponds well to the frontal radiographs. (*b*) Sagittal T2 demonstrates kyphosis centered around the destroyed T6 and T7 vertebral bodies (identified by way of their intact posterior elements). Vertebral bodies of T5 and T8 are visible but have an abnormally high signal. An associated heterogeneous soft-tissue mass containing the destroyed bodies and discs of abnormal signal protrudes posteriorly into the spinal canal, compressing the spinal cord, and anteriorly under the anterior longitudinal ligament. A high signal collection, representing subligamentous spread, is seen anterior to and separate from the infective mass. (*c*) Pre-contrast sagittal T1 MRI and (*d*) Post-contrast sagittal T1 MRI, shows the mass to be of low signal and peripherally rim-enhancing. There is also enhancement of the T5 and T8 vertebral bodies.

Subligamentous spread of disease is typical of tuberculosis and is seen as a spindle-shaped mass or abscess extending over the anterior aspect of a number of vertebral bodies above and below the level of bone destruction.[54] The most significant complication that needs to be identified is compression of the cord by a soft-tissue mass extending posteriorly into the spinal canal, that can be compounded by the angulation of an associated kyphosis.[54] Involvement of the posterior vertebral elements is uncommon in tuberculosis but is important to recognize because it has surgical implications.[54]

Tuberculous Arthritis

Tuberculous arthritis is the second most common form of musculoskeletal tuberculosis and should be considered in any patient with features of chronic arthritis in an endemic tuberculosis area. This is characteristically a monoarthritis but less commonly can be multifocal. The larger weight-bearing joints, such as the hip, knee, or ankle, are more commonly involved, but wrist involvement is also reported.[54]

Plain radiographic features are indistinguishable from those in other arthritides and include joint effusion with tissue plane loss, osteopenia, soft-tissue swelling, marginal and peripheral erosions, and joint space narrowing (see Figure 8.58). Epiphyseal overgrowth can occur at the knee. Advanced disease can demonstrate bone sequestration, sinuses, and ankylosis of the joint. US can confirm a joint effusion and guide aspiration.

MRI is the imaging modality of choice because it can demonstrate the typical synovial low signal intensity on T2 and marked enhancement with IV gadolinium. MRI can also show arrow edema, periarticular bony erosion (loss of the normal cortical low signal), soft-tissue cold abscesses, myositis, teno-synovitis, or bursitis (see Figure 8.59). Fat-suppressed T2-weighted techniques are useful

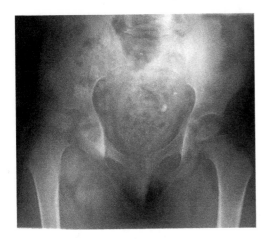

FIGURE 8.58 Radiograph of the pelvis in a child with confirmed tuberculous arthritis of the right hip, demonstrates lytic destruction of the acetabulum and subluxation of the proximal femur.

for showing sinus tracts. Tuberculosis can complicate by spreading across the physis in children.[54]

Bone Lesions Caused by Tuberculosis (X-ray, CT, MRI)

Bone infection by tuberculosis outside of the spine and large joints is less common, but when present, it usually involves the lower limbs. Lesions are most often metaphyseal, often precede joint involvement, and usually involve either end of the femur and tibia (see Figure 8.60). Lesions can demonstrate crossing

of the growth plate. Lesions of the diaphysis are rare. Spina ventosa or tuberculous dactylitis can present as a painless swelling presenting over months, affecting the hands more than the feet (proximal phalanx of the index or middle finger) (see Figure 8.61) and is a disease seen in children younger than six years of age.[54]

Early plain radiographic findings mainly show soft-tissue swelling. Delayed radiographic changes may be indistinguishable from chronic pyogenic osteomyelitis, tumors, or granulomatous lesions. There is a wide range of radiographic patterns, but cystic lesions are common in children (see Figure 8.62). These are focal, oval, osteolytic lesions eccentrically located in the bone, often causing cortical interruption without marginal sclerosis, and they may be multifocal. Alternatively, an infiltrative/permeative pattern of bone destruction with periosteal reaction can be seen, very similar to chronic osteomyelitis (see Figure 8.63). Localized erosions and lysis with cortical breakdown or a punched-out lesion is another type of pattern. Tuberculous dactylitis, also known as spina ventosa, demonstrates a typical expanding and fusiform abnormality with coarse trabecular pattern.[54]

MRI identifies soft-tissue swelling and intra-osseous involvement early on in the disease. These findings include marrow signal change as areas of low T1 or high T2 signal intensity (see Figure 8.64) with gadolinium enhancement. Necrotic regions have low T2W signal and do not enhance with gadolinium. MRI can also demonstrate soft-tissue fistulae, sinus tracts, and abscesses. Tuberculous lesions can

(a) 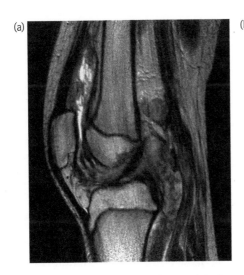 (b)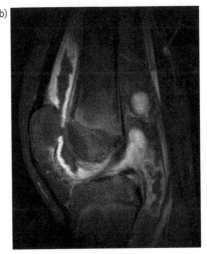

FIGURE 8.59 MRI of tuberculous synovitis of the knee in an adolescent. (a) Sagittal T2 MRI shows thickened low-signal synovium lining the suprapatellar bursa and popliteal fossa. (b) Corresponding sagittal post-contrast fat-saturated T1 with enhancement of the thickened synovium anterior and posteriorly.

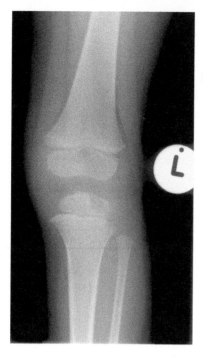

FIGURE 8.60   Tuberculosis of the long bones—a lytic (lucent) lesion in the proximal tibia, without sclerosis, involving mainly the epiphysis, but also crossing the physis to involve the lateral metaphysis.

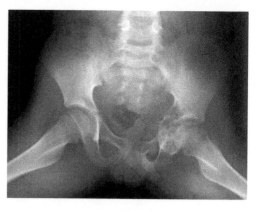

FIGURE 8.62   Cystic tuberculosis of the left acetabulum on plain radiograph: note the lack of sclerosis.

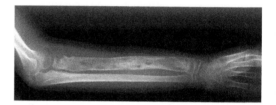

FIGURE 8.63   Plain radiograph of the radius in a child with confirmed bone tuberculosis demonstrates features indistinguishable from chronic osteomyelitis; namely, an infiltrative pattern of expansion, layered periosteal reaction sclerosis, and lucency involving the diaphysis and proximal metaphysis of the radius.

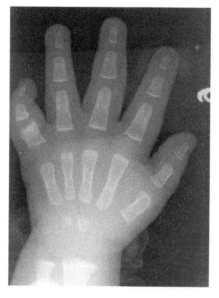

FIGURE 8.61   Tuberculous dactylitis involving the little finger demonstrates soft-tissue swelling with expansion and erosion of the proximal phalanx.

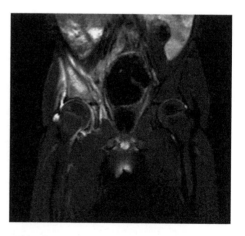

FIGURE 8.64   Coronal T2 with fat suppression of the pelvis in this child with confirmed tuberculosis of the bone. There is high signal of the marrow associated with expansion of the right ilium. Note the high signal of the surrounding soft-tissue and synovium.

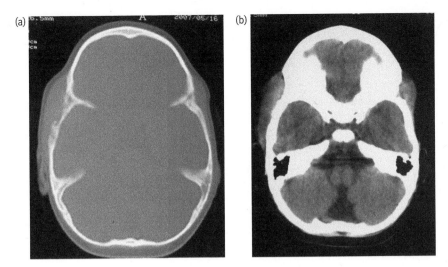

FIGURE 8.65   CT scan of calvarial tuberculosis. (*a*) Axial bone window with the bilateral erosion of the outer table of the squamous temporal bone, associated with soft-tissue thickening. (*b*) Axial soft-tissue window showing the soft-tissue component projecting outward as "Potts puffy tumor."

complicate pathological fracture, avascular necrosis, and growth disturbance.[54]

TB of the Skull and TB Osteomastoiditis

More than half of the cases of tuberculosis of the calvarium occur in children and adolescents. Clinically, there is a painless soft-tissue mass: Potts puffy tumor.[54] Tuberculosis is a cause of a lucent or lytic lesion of the skull (usually frontal or parietal) without sclerosis, involving inner and outer tables and associated with a soft-tissue mass (see Figure 8.65). When the lesion demonstrates a central "button" sequestrum, it may require surgical removal. On MRI, lesions have characteristic T2 low signal and are isointense to brain on T1 with a soft-tissue component intra- and extra-cranially (see Figure 8.66). Tuberculous osteomastoiditis causes chronic suppurative or acute otitis media/mastoiditis.[54] CT in tuberculous

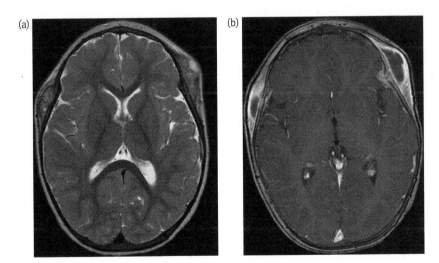

FIGURE 8.66   MRI of calvarial tuberculosis. (*a*) Axial T2 demonstrates bilateral extracranial soft-tissue masses with a heterogenous but predominantly low-signal center. Erosion of the outer table and involvement of the diploic space is well seen on the right. (*b*) Axial post-contrast T1 image with rim enhancement of the external soft-tissue masses and of the underlying bone. The internal soft-tissue component is now visible on the left.

osteomastoiditis demonstrates a soft-tissue density within the tympanic cavity with destruction of the middle ear structures.[54]

TUBERCULOSIS OF SOFT TISSUE

Tuberculosis can affect the soft tissue without or with bone or joint involvement (see Figure 8.67). Soft-tissue lesions take the form of cellulitis, fasciitis, bursitis, and tenosynovitis. Tuberculous bursitis is most common at the olecranon or prepatellar bursa. Cold abscesses usually involve the psoas muscles and are often associated with spondylitis.[54]

Plain radiographs demonstrate osteopenia in chronic bursitis due to hyperemia with or without features of arthritis or osteomyelitis. US demonstrates soft-tissue edema, joint effusion, and superficial collections with internal echoes indicating their complex nature. CT improves detection of deep collections, any related bone or joint disease, and calcification of psoas abscesses, which can be diagnostic. Collections typically show rim-enhancement and low-density necrotic centers. MRI is best suited to soft-tissue imaging and identifies collections as hyperintense on T2 with restricted diffusion and rim enhancement. Bursitis can distend the bursa overall or present with many small abscesses.[54]

CONCLUSION

Imaging plays a crucial role in primary diagnosis, when other tests are negative, for detecting

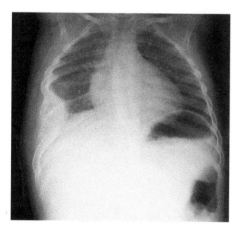

FIGURE 8.67　Chest radiograph demonstrates right-sided soft-tissue thickening (shown to be a tuberculous cold abscess on ultrasound). Also, expansion and erosion of the 5th, 6th, and 7th ribs.

complications and for demonstrating extrapulmonary disease, which on occasion requires planning for surgical intervention. Imaging also assists in narrowing down a differential diagnosis and in assessing response to treatment. New modalities are proving more specific for the diagnosis of tuberculosis, and these range from ultrasound, which can be performed at the point of care by non-radiologists, to advanced MRI technology, which can be used swiftly and without anesthesia or sedation. Radiologists and clinicians must be familiar with the imaging findings of childhood tuberculosis so that this diagnosis can be considered both in developing countries and developed countries where the disease persists.

REFERENCES

1. Pinto LM, Dheda K, Theron G, et al. Development of a simple reliable radiographic scoring system to aid the diagnosis of pulmonary tuberculosis. *PloS ONE.* 2013;8:e54235.
2. Du Toit G, Swingler G, Iloni K. Observer variation in detecting lymphadenopathy on chest radiography. *Int J Tuberc Lung Dis.* 2002;6:814–817.
3. Swingler GH, du Toit G, Andronikou S, van der Merwe L, Zar HJ. Diagnostic accuracy of chest radiography in detecting mediastinal lymphadenopathy in suspected pulmonary tuberculosis. *Arch Dis Child.* 2005;90:1153–1156.
4. Belard S, Andronikou S, Pillay T, Grobusch MP, Zar HJ. New imaging approaches for improving diagnosis of childhood tuberculosis. *SAMJ.* 2014;104:181–182.
5. Seddon JA, Padayachee T, Du Plessis AM, et al. Teaching chest X-ray reading for child tuberculosis suspects. *Int J Tuberc Lung Dis.* 2014;18:763–769.
6. Scheepers S, Andronikou S, Mapukata A, Donald P. Abdominal lymphadenopathy in children with tuberculosis presenting with respiratory symptoms. *Ultrasound.* 2011;19:134–139.
7. Andronikou S, Vanhoenacker FM, De Backer AI. Advances in imaging chest tuberculosis: blurring of differences between children and adults. *Clin Chest Med.* 2009;30:717–744, viii.
8. De Villiers RV, Andronikou S, Van de Westhuizen S. Specificity and sensitivity of chest radiographs in the diagnosis of paediatric pulmonary tuberculosis and the value of additional high-kilovolt radiographs. *Australas Radiol.* 2004;48:148–153.

9. Lucas S, Andronikou S, Goussard P, Gie R. CT features of lymphobronchial tuberculosis in children, including complications and associated abnormalities. *Pediatr Radiol.* 2012;42:923–931.

10. Graham SM. Chest radiography for diagnosis of tuberculosis in children: a problem of interpretation. *Int J Tuberc Lung Dis.* 2014;18:757.

11. Andronikou S, Wieselthaler N. Modern imaging of tuberculosis in children: thoracic, central nervous system and abdominal tuberculosis. *Pediatr Radiol.* 2004;34:861–875.

12. Andronikou S, Wieselthaler N. Imaging for tuberculosis in children. In: Schaaf HS, Zumla A, eds. *Tuberculosis: A Comprehensive Clinical Reference.* Philadelphia: Saunders Elsevier; 2009:261–295.

13. Daya RB, Kibel MA, Pitcher RD, Workman L, Douglas TS, Sanders V. A pilot study evaluating erect chest imaging in children, using the Lodox Statscan digital X-ray machine. *SAJR.* 2009;4:80–85.

14. Graham SM, Ahmed T, Amanullah F, et al. Evaluation of tuberculosis diagnostics in children: 1. Proposed clinical case definitions for classification of intrathoracic tuberculosis disease. Consensus from an expert panel. *J Infect Dis.* 2012;205(Suppl 2):S199–S208.

15. Andronikou S, Joseph E, Lucas S, et al. CT scanning for the detection of tuberculous mediastinal and hilar lymphadenopathy in children. *Pediatr Radiol.* 2004;34:232–236.

16. Delacourt C, Mani TM, Bonnerot V, et al. Computed tomography with normal chest radiograph in tuberculous infection. *Arch Dis Child.* 1993;69:430–432.

17. du Plessis J, Goussard P, Andronikou S, Gie R, George R. Comparing three-dimensional volume-rendered CT images with fibreoptic tracheobronchoscopy in the evaluation of airway compression caused by tuberculous lymphadenopathy in children. *Pediatr Radiol.* 2009;39:694–702.

18. Andronikou S, Irving B, Hlabangana LT, et al. Technical developments in postprocessing of paediatric airway imaging. *Pediatr Radiol.* 2013;43:269–284.

19. Bosch-Marcet J, Serres-Creixams X, Zuasnabar-Cotro A, Codina-Puig X, Catala-Puigbo M, Simon-Riazuelo JL. Comparison of ultrasound with plain radiography and CT for the detection of mediastinal lymphadenopathy in children with tuberculosis. *Pediatr Radiol.* 2004;34:895–900.

20. Bosch-Marcet J, Serres-Creixams X, Borras-Perez V, Coll-Sibina MT, Guitet-Julia M, Coll-Rosell E. Value of sonography for follow-up of mediastinal lymphadenopathy in children with tuberculosis. *JCU.* 2007;35:118–124.

21. Moseme T, Andronikou S. Through the eye of the suprasternal notch: point-of-care sonography for tuberculous mediastinal lymphadenopathy in children. *Pediatr Radiol.* 2014;44:681–684.

22. Peprah KO, Andronikou S, Goussard P. Characteristic magnetic resonance imaging low T2 signal intensity of necrotic lung parenchyma in children with pulmonary tuberculosis. *J Thorac Imaging.* 2012;27:171–174.

23. Boiselle PM, Biederer J, Gefter WB, Lee EY. Expert opinion: why is MRI still an under-utilized modality for evaluating thoracic disorders? *J Thorac Imaging.* 2013;28:137.

24. Lucas S, Andronikou S, Goussard P, Gie R. Tuberculous lymphadenopathy is not only obstructive but also inflammatory—it can erode anything it touches. Reply to Marchiori et al. *Pediatr Radiol.* 2013;43:254–255.

25. Maydell A, Goussard P, Andronikou S, Bezuidenhout F, Ackermann C, Gie R. Radiological changes post-lymph node enucleation for airway obstruction in children with pulmonary tuberculosis. *Eur J Cardiothorac Surg.* 2010;38:478–483.

26. Goussard P, Andronikou S. Tuberculous broncho-oesophageal fistula: images demonstrating the pathogenesis. *Pediatr Radiol.* 2010;40 Suppl 1:S78.

27. Goussard P, Gie RP, Kling S, Andronikou S, Janson JT, Roussouw GJ. Phrenic nerve palsy in children associated with confirmed intrathoracic tuberculosis: diagnosis and clinical course. *Pediatr Pulmonol.* 2009;44:345–350.

28. Grobbelaar M, Andronikou S, Goussard P, Theron S, Mapukata A, George R. Chylothorax as a complication of pulmonary tuberculosis in children. *Pediatr Radiol.* 2008;38:224–226.

29. Griffith-Richards SB, Goussard P, Andronikou S, et al. Cavitating pulmonary tuberculosis in children: correlating radiology with pathogenesis. *Pediatr Radiol.* 2007;37:798–804; quiz 848–799.

30. George R, Andronikou S, Theron S, et al. Pulmonary infections in HIV-positive children. *Pediatr Radiol.* 2009;39:545–554.

31. Theron S, Andronikou S, George R, et al. Non-infective pulmonary disease in HIV-positive children. *Pediatr Radiol.* 2009;39:555–564.

32. Kilborn T, Zampoli M. Immune reconstitution inflammatory syndrome after initiating highly

active antiretroviral therapy in HIV-infected children. *Pediatr Radiol.* 2009;39:569–574.

33. Wiseman CA, Gie RP, Starke JR, et al. A proposed comprehensive classification of tuberculosis disease severity in children. *Pediatr Infect Dis J.* 2012;31:347–352.

34. Andronikou S, Greyling PJ. Devastating yet treatable complication of tuberculous meningitis: the resistant TB abscess. *ChNS.* 2009;25:1105–1106; discussion 1107, 1109–1110.

35. Stefan DC, Andronikou S, Freeman N, Schoeman J. Recovery of vision after adjuvant thalidomide in a child with tuberculous meningitis and acute lymphoblastic leukemia. *J Child Neurol.* 2009;24:166–169.

36. Thwaites G, Fisher M, Hemingway C, Scott G, Solomon T, Innes J. British Infection Society guidelines for the diagnosis and treatment of tuberculosis of the central nervous system in adults and children. *J Infect.* 2009;59:167–187.

37. Andronikou S, Smith B, Hatherill M, Douis H, Wilmshurst J. Definitive neuroradiological diagnostic features of tuberculous meningitis in children. *Pediatr Radiol.* 2004;34:876–885.

38. Pienaar M, Andronikou S, van Toorn R. MRI to demonstrate diagnostic features and complications of TBM not seen with CT. *ChNS.* 2009;25:941–947.

39. Janse van Rensburg P, Andronikou S, van Toorn R, Pienaar M. Magnetic resonance imaging of miliary tuberculosis of the central nervous system in children with tuberculous meningitis. *Pediatr Radiol.* 2008;38:1306–1313.

40. van den Bos F, Terken M, Ypma L, et al. Tuberculous meningitis and miliary tuberculosis in young children. *Trop Med Int Health: TM & IH.* 2004;9:309–313.

41. van Well GT, Paes BF, Terwee CB, et al. Twenty years of pediatric tuberculous meningitis: a retrospective cohort study in the western cape of South Africa. *Pediatrics.* 2009;123:e1–e8.

42. Bruwer GE, Van der Westhuizen S, Lombard CJ, Schoeman JF. Can CT predict the level of CSF block in tuberculous hydrocephalus? *ChNS.* 2004;20:183–187.

43. Andronikou S, Wilmshurst J, Hatherill M, VanToorn R. Distribution of brain infarction in children with tuberculous meningitis and correlation with outcome score at 6 months. *Pediatr Radiol.* 2006;36:1289–1294.

44. van der Merwe DJ, Andronikou S, Van Toorn R, Pienaar M. Brainstem ischemic lesions on MRI in children with tuberculous meningitis: with diffusion weighted confirmation. *ChNS.* 2009;25:949–954.

45. Omar N, Andronikou S, van Toorn R, Pienaar M. Diffusion-weighted magnetic resonance imaging of borderzone necrosis in paediatric tuberculous meningitis. *J Med Imaging Radiat Oncol.* 2011;55:563–570.

46. Andronikou S, van Toorn R, Boerhout E. MR imaging of the posterior hypophysis in children with tuberculous meningitis. *Eur Radiol.* 2009;19:2249–2254.

47. Marais S, Pepper DJ, Marais BJ, Torok ME. HIV-associated tuberculous meningitis—diagnostic and therapeutic challenges. *Tuberculosis (Edinb).* 2010;90:367–374.

48. Dekker G, Andronikou S, van Toorn R, Scheepers S, Brandt A, Ackermann C. MRI findings in children with tuberculous meningitis: a comparison of HIV-infected and non-infected patients. *ChNS.* 2011;27:1943–1949.

49. Katrak SM, Shembalkar PK, Bijwe SR, Bhandarkar LD. The clinical, radiological and pathological profile of tuberculous meningitis in patients with and without human immunodeficiency virus infection. *J Neurol Sci.* 2000;181:118–126.

50. Andronikou S, Welman CJ, Kader E. The CT features of abdominal tuberculosis in children. *Pediatr Radiol.* 2002;32:75–81.

51. Murtz P, Krautmacher C, Traber F, Gieseke J, Schild HH, Willinek WA. Diffusion-weighted whole-body MR imaging with background body signal suppression: a feasibility study at 3.0 Tesla. *Eur Radiol.* 2007;17:3031–3037.

52. Chavhan GB, Babyn PS, Walters T. MR enterography in children: principles, technique, and clinical applications. *Indian J Radiol Imaging.* 2013;23:173–178.

53. Mapukata A, Andronikou S, Fasulakis S, McCulloch M, Grobbelaar M, Jee L. Modern imaging of renal tuberculosis in children. *Australas Radiol.* 2007;51:538–542.

54. Andronikou S, Bindapersad M, Govender N, et al. Musculoskeletal tuberculosis—imaging using low-end and advanced modalities for developing and developed countries. *Acta Radiol.* 2011;52:430–441.

55. Andronikou S, Jadwat S, Douis H. Patterns of disease on MRI in 53 children with tuberculous spondylitis and the role of gadolinium. *Pediatr Radiol.* 2002;32:798–805.

9

DIAGNOSIS OF INTRATHORACIC TUBERCULOSIS IN CHILDREN

Carlos M. Perez-Velez

HIGHLIGHTS OF THIS CHAPTER

- The majority of cases of intrathoracic tuberculosis are not bacteriologically confirmable with currently available microbiological tests. Until that is attainable, intrathoracic tuberculosis will continue to be a clinical diagnosis—especially if it is to be made at an earlier stage before significant complications occur.
- To optimize the accuracy of clinical diagnosis, and minimize both under- and over-diagnosis, a systematic diagnostic approach is necessary.
- The clinical presentation of intrathoracic tuberculosis in children is variable. Classifying a composite of clinical, radiological, laboratory, and endoscopic (when indicated) features into one of the intrathoracic clinical presentations that can be caused by tuberculosis will allow a more refined differential diagnosis and consequently guide the optimal specimen-collection strategy and diagnostic testing.
- The probability of tuberculosis increases with the number of findings supportive of it as the etiology, such as: recent exposure to a case; positive test of infection; biochemical markers of body fluids; suggestive histopathological findings; ruling out alternative diagnoses to the extent possible; and a satisfactory clinical and radiological response to tuberculosis treatment.

IN CHILDREN, pulmonary tuberculosis is frequently associated with intrathoracic lymphadenopathy, and sometimes with pleural or pericardial disease, so "intrathoracic tuberculosis" is the preferred term. Intrathoracic tuberculosis is the most common form of disease in children, occurring three to four times more frequently than extrathoracic manifestations. Although fewer than 30% of cases of intrathoracic tuberculosis in children can be confirmed microbiologically, with current tools, it is possible to clinically diagnose the majority of cases.[1] This chapter presents a systematic approach to the diagnosis of intrathoracic tuberculosis in children and reviews the most common presentations.

SPECTRUM OF INTRATHORACIC TUBERCULOSIS

Once infected with *Mycobacterium tuberculosis*, children are at higher risk than adults for progressing to both mild and severe forms of disease. The form the disease takes depends on the child's immune competence and an important determinant is age. Approximately 50% of young infants (<1 year old) who become infected with *M. tuberculosis* will progress to intrathoracic tuberculosis, and 10–20% develop meningitis or other forms of disseminated disease. In children 1–2 years of age, the risk of progressing to intrathoracic tuberculosis is 10–20% and to disseminated disease is 2–5%. These risks remain significant until after 5 years of age.[2]

Early diagnosis is therefore especially important for young children, and critical for infants. Because bacteriological confirmation in children is not attainable in the majority of cases, especially in the milder forms of disease, recognizing intrathoracic tuberculosis in its early stages requires understanding the

correlation between the bacterial load that is generally associated with the different outcomes in the spectrum of disease and the presence or absence of clinical and radiological abnormalities (Figure 9.1). Young children tend to have smaller bacterial burdens, and inflammation of intrathoracic lymph nodes is the dominant pathological process. As children get older and reach adolescence, they begin to present more often with adult-type disease with its larger bacterial burden.[3] The accurate diagnosis of children suspected of having intrathoracic tuberculosis requires recognition of the full clinical spectrum of intrathoracic presentations (Table 9.1).[4]

DIAGNOSTIC EVALUATION OF INTRATHORACIC TUBERCULOSIS: GENERAL CONCEPTS

Systematic Approach to the Diagnosis of Intrathoracic Tuberculosis in Children

Given that it is impossible to bacteriologically confirm tuberculosis in a very large proportion of

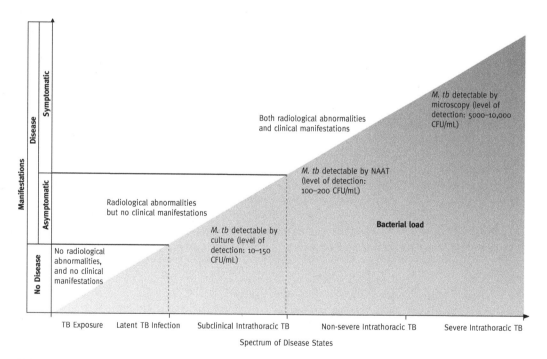

FIGURE 9.1   Spectrum of disease states after exposure to *M. tuberculosis* and correlations of manifestations with levels of bacterial detection.

Table 9.1. Classification of intrathoracic tuberculosis based on immunopathogenesis and containment of infection

TUBERCULOSIS CLASSIFICATION	IMMUNOPATHOGENESIS	IMMUNE-BASED TESTS (TST/IGRA)	POSSIBLE CHEST IMAGING ABNORMALITIES	CLINICAL FINDINGS (SYMPTOMS, PHYSICAL SIGNS)	MICROBIOLOGICAL STUDIES (MICROSCOPY, NAAT, CULTURE)
Exposure	*Innate immunity* (infection eliminated by innate immune response)	Negative	—None (i.e., normal chest imaging)	None	Negative
Infection	*Silent/quiescent infection* (infection contained by immune system, but some bacteria persisting in non-replicating state)	Positive	—Calcified non-enlarged regional lymph nodes —Calcified lung nodules —Pleural thickening (scarring) —None (i.e., normal chest imaging)	None	Negative
Subclinical intrathoracic tuberculosis	*Subclinical disease* (infection contained by immune system, but active bacterial replication without clinical manifestations)	Usually positive	—Uncomplicated hilar/mediastinal lymphadenopathies —Non-calcified lung nodules —Pleural effusion without severe underlying lung disease	None	Positive transiently
Non-severe intrathoracic tuberculosis	*Mild-to-moderate clinical disease* (infection only partially contained, active bacterial replication, limited disease with mild clinical manifestations)			Present	Positive cultures of respiratory specimens in ~10–30% of cases
Severe intrathoracic tuberculosis	*Severe clinical disease* (infection not contained, associated with bacterial replication and with clinical manifestations)	Usually positive (but may be initially negative in immuno-compromised patients, especially with overwhelming disease)	—Mediastinal/hilar lymphadenopathies with airway compression or expansile pneumonia —Bronchopneumonia —Multilobar pneumonia —Lung/parenchymal cavities —Pleural empyema or an effusion with severe underlying lung disease —Pericardial effusion —Diffuse micronodules (miliary tuberculosis)	Present	Positive cultures of respiratory specimens in ~30–70% of cases

childhood cases, systematically identifying features consistent with tuberculosis disease can enable its clinical diagnosis: the greater the number of features, the higher the probability that the child has tuberculosis. If the child has a positive therapeutic response to tuberculosis treatment, the likelihood is even higher. This systematic approach to the diagnosis of tuberculosis in children consists of four steps: (1) identifying clinical, radiographic, laboratory and/or endoscopic (when indicated) features suggestive of tuberculosis disease; (2) identifying findings supportive of tuberculosis as the etiology; (3) identifying risk factors for progression from tuberculosis infection to disease, and disease to death; and (4) carrying out follow-up evaluations to further support tuberculosis as the etiology (Table 9.2).

STEP 1: IDENTIFY FEATURES SUGGESTIVE OF TUBERCULOSIS DISEASE

Each intrathoracic clinical presentation of tuberculosis disease has its own constellation of clinical, radiological, laboratory, and endoscopic (if indicated) findings, although many may be shared by more than one clinical presentation. Furthermore, miliary lung disease may be accompanied by disease manifestations in potentially any organ system (Table 9.3).

Clinical Evaluation (History-taking and Physical Examination)

In young children, many of the clinical manifestations of intrathoracic tuberculosis result from a severe inflammatory reaction to a relatively low burden of organisms. There are no symptoms or signs that are pathognomonic for intrathoracic tuberculosis. The radiological abnormalities, especially the involvement of regional lymph nodes, are often more pronounced than the initial clinical findings, but there are combinations of historical features and physical findings that can be highly suggestive of intrathoracic tuberculosis and can help distinguish it from other causes with a similar presentation (Table 9.4).

LOCATIONS AND CHARACTERISTICS OF SYMPTOMS AND PHYSICAL SIGNS OF INTRATHORACIC TUBERCULOSIS

The localized symptoms and physical signs caused by intrathoracic tuberculosis depend on which

Table 9.2 Systematic Approach to the Diagnosis of Intrathoracic Tuberculosis in Children

Step 1: *Identify features suggestive of tuberculosis disease*

- Clinical evaluation: history and physical exam
- Imaging studies: chest radiography, CT, ultrasonography
- Laboratory studies: composite measures (cell count and chemistry) of body fluids (e.g., pleural fluid, pericardial fluid)
- Endoscopic studies: bronchoscopy

Step 2: *Identify findings supportive of tuberculosis as the etiology*

- Tuberculosis exposure history
- Immune-based tests: TST, IGRA
- Biochemical markers: ADA of body fluids (e.g., pleural fluid; pericardial fluid)
- Microbiological studies: NAAT, microscopy, mycobacterial culture
- Histopathological studies
- Ruling out alternative differential diagnoses

Step 3: *Screen for risk factors for progression from tuberculosis infection to disease, and disease to death*

- Immunocompromising conditions (e.g., immunological immaturity; HIV; malnutrition)
- Continued exposure to person(s) transmitting *M. tuberculosis*
- Drug-resistance

Step 4: *Carry out follow-up evaluations to further support tuberculosis as the etiology*

intrathoracic organs are involved: lung parenchyma, mediastinal lymph nodes, pleura, or pericardium. There are constitutional symptoms and physical signs that are frequently caused by all forms of intrathoracic tuberculosis. Well-defined symptoms and physical signs have higher specificity, but in children who are less than age 3 years, HIV-infected, or severely malnourished, these clinical findings have lower sensitivity and specificity.

Table 9.3 Organs That Can Be Affected by Tuberculosis

- **Respiratory system** (including chest): lungs, pleura, larynx, nasopharynx, sinuses.
- **Reticuloendothelial system**: lymph nodes, bone marrow, liver, spleen.
- **Cardiovascular system**: pericardium, myocardium.
- **Central nervous system** (including head, neck, ears, and eyes): meninges, brain, orbit, optic neuritis, retina, uvea, sclera, conjunctiva.
- **Musculoskeletal system**: bone, joint, bursa, muscle.
- **Urinary system**: kidneys, ureters, bladder.
- **Alimentary/digestive system** (including abdomen): oral cavity, esophagus, intestine, peritoneum, liver, gallbladder.
- **Endocrine system**: pancreatic, adrenal, thyroid, parathyroid, breast, pituitary, testicular, ovarian.
- **Reproductive/genital system**: uterine, oviduct, vulva, prostate, epididymis, penis.
- **Integumentary system**: skin.

Respiratory. Respiratory symptoms and signs depend on which anatomical part is involved, and on the degree of involvement (e.g., of airway obstruction). Cough is an important symptom, but there is a broad differential diagnosis for it (Table 9.5). The cough is nonspecific but is commonly persistent and unremitting (i.e., all day, every day, without improvement) for more than two weeks. It may be "dry" or "wet." When the airway is compressed by enlarged lymph nodes, there may be cough, wheezing, or stridor that may also be continuous and unrelenting, and do not respond to inhaled bronchodilators. Dyspnea and tachypnea are not common, and hemoptysis is extremely rare except in adolescents with adult-type disease.

Constitutional and Immunological. The systemic symptoms of tuberculosis appear early in the disease course and are related to pro-inflammatory cytokines (e.g., TNFα, IL-1, IL-6, IL-12, IFNγ) released by activated macrophages.[5] Fever is very common and is characteristically greater than 38.0°C, occurs daily, may be intermittent or persistent

throughout the day, and lasts more than one week[6,7]. Night sweats are uncommon and nonspecific, and significant only when so profuse that the child's clothes and/or bedsheets are drenched. Chills and rigors are rare except in miliary disease when there is hematogenous dissemination. Decreased appetite and associated wasting (cachexia) or failure to thrive are sensitive—albeit nonspecific—signs of more severe tuberculosis clinical presentation in young children.[8,9] Fatigue may be prominent, and subjective generalized weakness and malaise may manifest in young children as listlessness and in infants as apathy.

Lymphoid. Peripheral lymphadenopathy due to tuberculosis typically consists of a unilateral, enlarged, nonpainful, rubbery lymph node, sometimes with abscess formation, with or without a sinus tract. It is most often noted in the cervical or axillary regions and may be a component of a primary complex whose site of infection is in the lung (e.g., supraclavicular lymphadenopathy associated with a primary focus in the apex of the ipsilateral lung) or an intrathoracic lymph node.[10]

TEMPORAL PATTERN

Characterizing the temporal pattern, including the onset, progression, course, duration, timing, and chronology of symptoms can help the clinician recognize potential cases of pulmonary tuberculosis.

Subacute-to-Chronic. In most children whose tuberculosis infection progresses to intrathoracic disease, the symptoms have a gradual onset; a slow, insidious progression; and a persistent, unremitting course. A minimum duration of two to three weeks of the symptoms helps distinguish intrathoracic tuberculosis from most other causes, such as a viral respiratory infection or bacterial pneumonia.

Fulminant-to-Acute. However, in children who are more immunocompromised due to immune-immaturity or HIV-infection, the symptoms may have a more abrupt onset, rapid progression, and greater severity, as in the case of an acute tuberculous pneumonia and disseminated disease.[11]

Acute-on-Chronic. Another presentation is the child with undiagnosed pulmonary tuberculosis who has had several weeks or longer of cough and then has an acute exacerbation of respiratory symptoms due to a secondary bacterial pneumonia, often pneumococcal in origin. The secondary pneumonia will respond to appropriate antibiotics, but the underlying tuberculosis remains untreated unless the child is adequately followed and investigated.

Recurrent. There are also children who present with *recurrent* bacterial lower respiratory tract infections (pneumonia, bronchitis, or exacerbations of bronchiectasis) caused by infection distal to the bronchial obstruction created by enlarged or invasive tuberculous intrathoracic lymph nodes.

Imaging Studies (Reviewed in Detail in Chapter 8)

Chest imaging—including radiography, computed tomography (CT), and ultrasonography—is an essential diagnostic modality for detecting abnormalities consistent with intrathoracic tuberculosis. The spectrum of radiological abnormalities in intrathoracic tuberculosis in children is very broad, and none are specific enough to absolutely confirm the diagnosis. Nonetheless, certain radiological patterns or combinations of signs are highly suggestive of tuberculosis, especially when accompanied by clinical features consistent with tuberculosis disease and findings supportive of tuberculosis such as known recent exposure or a positive tuberculin skin test (TST) or interferon-gamma release assay (IGRA) test indicative of tuberculosis infection. Recognizing these radiological findings helps narrow the differential diagnosis (Figure 9.2 and Table 9.4).

Chest radiography, including both frontal (PA or AP in infants) and lateral views, is the first-line imaging modality when tuberculosis is suspected. The lateral view of the chest is very useful, as it can detect an additional 15–20% of abnormalities consistent with tuberculosis, especially intrathoracic lymphadenopathy in young children in whom the thymic silhouette may impede the ability to assess for adenopathy on the frontal view.[12,13]

Chest CT is not routinely indicated in the diagnostic evaluation of an asymptomatic child. However, it may provide helpful information for establishing, or suggesting, the correct diagnosis in a symptomatic child by demonstrating complicated intrathoracic lymph node or pleural disease, endobronchial lesions, bronchiectasis, or cavities that are not well revealed on plain radiographs.[14,15]

Chest ultrasonography is useful to evaluate mediastinal lymphadenopathy and pericardial effusions,

and is the preferred imaging modality for differentiating loculated from free-flowing pleural effusions.[16,17]

Laboratory Studies

Non-microbiological laboratory studies are not diagnostic of tuberculosis, but can be helpful when their results are consistent with tuberculosis disease.

CELL COUNT AND CHEMISTRY OF BODY FLUIDS

The cell count and chemistry of body fluids such as pleural or pericardial fluids can support the diagnosis of tuberculosis when the composite results are consistent with the disease. They do not confirm tuberculosis, because other diseases, including other mycobacterial and fungal infections, can be associated with similar results. Several features of pleural and pericardial fluid are consistent with tuberculosis: the cell count is usually predominantly lymphocytic at the time of diagnosis (but may be predominantly neutrophilic if detected within the first few days); the protein level is elevated (>3.0 g/dL; >0.5 of value in serum); the lactate dehydrogenase (LDH) level is elevated (>200 IU/L; >0.6 of value in serum); the glucose level is usually 60–100 mg/dL, higher than seen with effusions due to bacterial infection or rheumatoid arthritis; and lipid levels are normal unless the effusion is chylous.

HEMATOLOGICAL TESTS AND ACUTE PHASE REACTANTS

The complete blood count is of little value for diagnosing tuberculosis in children. The most common findings are anemia, neutrophilia, and monocytosis, but these abnormalities are found just as frequently in children with other respiratory infections.[18] Similarly, the erythrocyte sedimentation rate may be normal or elevated but is nonspecific, as are C-reactive protein and procalcitonin.

Endoscopic Studies

Although bronchoscopy is not routinely indicated in the diagnostic evaluation of intrathoracic tuberculosis in children, it may be useful in certain cases to better define the bronchial anatomy, such as with tracheobronchial disease.[19]

STEP 2: IDENTIFY FINDINGS SUPPORTIVE OF TUBERCULOSIS AS THE ETIOLOGY

The positive and negative predictive values of the tests discussed below depend on the prevalence of tuberculosis in the community, the child's specific clinical and radiographic findings, and, most importantly, whether the child has been exposed recently to a person with known or suspected contagious tuberculosis. The greater the likelihood that the child has been exposed recently, the higher the positive predictive value of these tests for helping diagnose tuberculosis disease.

Exposure History

Children are usually infected with *M. tuberculosis* by exposure to a person (the source case) with pulmonary tuberculosis whose sputum is positive for organisms by microscopy or culture, who is actively coughing, and with whom they share the same air space for a significant period of time. In children less than age 5 years with tuberculosis disease, the source case is most often from the same household, and the infection was usually acquired within the past year. As children and adolescents are exposed to the community outside the household, their risk of community-acquired infection increases. Inquiring about tuberculosis contacts, both confirmed cases and persons with chronic cough, is a critical part of the evaluation of a child for tuberculosis disease.[20] However, it is important to note that, because of the fairly short incubation period of tuberculosis in young children—the time between inhalation of organisms and the development of disease—the person from whom the child acquired the organism may not yet have been identified or diagnosed. If an ill contact of a child with suspected tuberculosis is discovered to have the disease, the likelihood that the child also has tuberculosis is raised significantly.

Immune-Based Tests

TUBERCULIN-SKIN TESTS (TST) AND INTERFERON-GAMMA RELEASE ASSAYS (IGRAS) (SEE ALSO CHAPTER 6)

These tests for tuberculosis infection, regardless of the degree of positivity of the result, cannot distinguish between tuberculosis infection and disease[21,22].

Also, they do not indicate immunity to *M. tuberculosis*, time of infection, or the extent of disease, and must be interpreted with caution in children with immunocompromising conditions in which the sensitivity is decreased. The TSTs and IGRAs are negative in up to 20% of children with culture-proven tuberculosis disease, and are more often negative with more severe forms of disease such as miliary and meningeal tuberculosis. They can be negative either because of immune compromise caused by tuberculosis or some other factor, or because the tuberculosis disease has developed faster than the time required for the tests to become positive. *A negative test result for tuberculosis infection NEVER rules out tuberculosis disease.* Repeating tests of infection after several weeks (4–8 weeks later) of treatment for tuberculosis often yields a positive result when the original result was negative.

SEROLOGICAL, ANTIBODY-BASED TESTS

At present, there are no accurate serological tests for the diagnosis of tuberculosis infection or disease, so they are *not* recommended by the World Health Organization.[23]

Biochemical Markers in Body Fluids

Depending on the cutoff levels used, biochemical markers can have a sensitivity and specificity sufficiently high to strongly support tuberculosis as the etiology of pleural or pericardial effusions. Most studies have been carried out in adults, but their results should be applicable to children.

ADENOSINE DEAMINASE (ADA)

In pleural tuberculosis, using 40 U/L as the cutoff, the sensitivity of ADA is approximately 90% and its specificity around 92%.[24,25] In pericardial tuberculosis, the sensitivity and specificity of ADA for values ≥40 U/L are approximately 88% and 83%, respectively.[26] The ADA is an underutilized test that can be very helpful in distinguishing tuberculosis from other causes of pleural effusion.

UNSTIMULATED INTERFERON-GAMMA (uIFNγ)

In the diagnosis of tuberculous pleuritis, using 44 pg/mL as the cutoff, uIFNγ has a sensitivity and specificity that tend to be slightly higher than that of

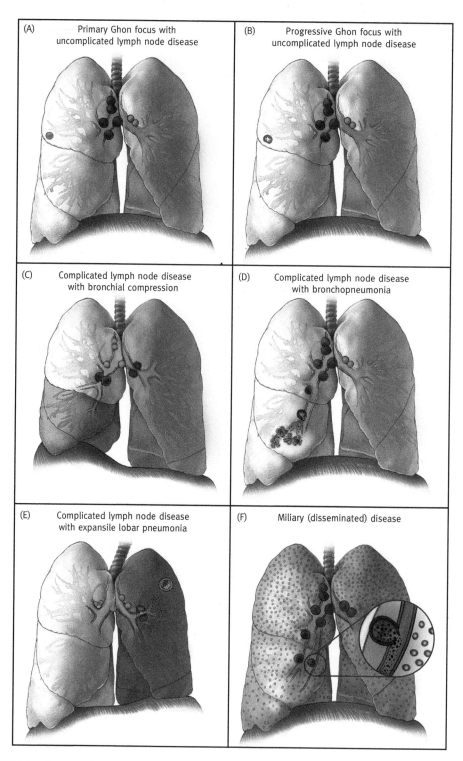

FIGURE 9.2   Continued

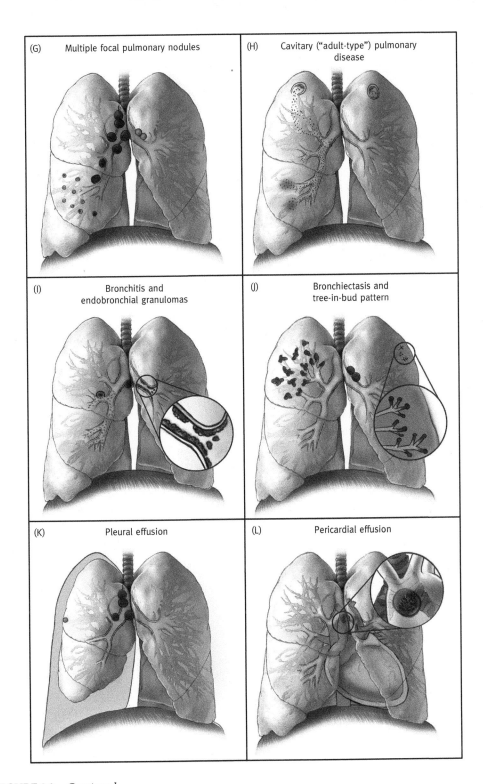

FIGURE 9.2   Continued

FIGURE 9.2   Illustrations of clinical-radiological syndromes caused by intrathoracic tuberculosis in children.

Panel A. *Primary Ghon focus with uncomplicated lymph node disease*

Shows hilar and mediastinal lymphadenopathy associated with an ipsilateral peripheral nodule, or "Ghon focus" (right lung); these nodules are often subpleural with an overlying pleural reaction.

Panel B. *Progressive Ghon focus with uncomplicated lymph node disease*

Shows a Ghon focus with cavitation (right lung), which is seen almost exclusively in infants and immunocompromised children; associated with hilar and mediastinal lymphadenopathy.

Panel C. *Complicated lymph node disease with bronchial compression*

Shows enlarged lymph nodes compressing the airway, causing either complete obstruction with lobar collapse (right middle and lower lobes), or partial obstruction with a ball-valve effect leading to hyperinflation (left upper and lower lobes).

Panel D. *Complicated lymph node disease with bronchopneumonia*

Shows necrotic lymph nodes erupting into bronchus intermedius, with endobronchial spread and patchy consolidation of the middle lobe (right lung).

Panel E. *Complicated lymph node disease with expansile lobar pneumonia*

Shows necrotic lymph nodes that compress and obstruct the left upper lobe bronchus and may infiltrate a phrenic nerve, causing hemidiaphragmatic palsy (left-sided); endobronchial spread causes dense consolidation of the entire lobe (left upper lobe), with displacement of the trachea and fissures and the formation of focal cavities.

Panel F. *Miliary (disseminated) disease*

Shows diffuse micronodules in both lungs, which may result from lymphohematogenous spread after recent primary infection, or from the infiltration of a necrotic lymph node or lung lesion into a blood vessel, leading to hematogenous spread.

Panel G. *Multiple focal pulmonary nodules*

Shows multiple focal pulmonary nodules involving the right middle lobe with enlargement of regional lymph nodes (right lung).

Panel H. *Cavitary ("adult-type") pulmonary disease*

Shows cavity formation in both upper lobes, with endobronchial spread to the right middle lobe. Nodules or cavities in apical lung segments are typical of adult-type disease.

Panel I. *Bronchitis and endobronchial granulomas*

Shows inflammation of the mucosa of mainstem bronchus with purulent secretions (left lung), and shows a necrotic lymph node that has eroded into the right middle lobe bronchus leading to endobronchial spread and subsequent development of endobronchial granulomas extending proximally to the bronchus intermedius and mainstem bronchus and distally to the lower lobe bronchus (right lung).

Panel J. *Bronchiectasis and tree-in-bud pattern*

Shows bronchiectasis that extensively involves the upper lobe (right lung), and shows tree-in-bud pattern observable on CT—reflecting dilated centrilobular bronchioles with mucoid impaction—involving the upper lobe (left lung).

Panel K. *Pleural effusion*

Shows a pleural effusion that is usually indicative of recent primary infection, with a hypersensitivity response to tuberculoprotein that leaked from a subpleural Ghon focus (often not visible) into the pleural cavity; in rare cases this effusion may also result from chylothorax.

Panel L. *Pericardial effusion*

Shows a pericardial effusion that occurs when tuberculoprotein leaks from a necrotic subcarinal lymph node (shown in "close-up" window) into the pericardial space; it may also occur after hematogenous spread.

Conceptualization and original sketches by Claudia L. Roya-Pabon, MD. Finished artwork by Mesa Schumacher, MA.

Table 9.4. Clinical-radiological presentations caused by intrathoracic tuberculosis, and their differential diagnosis

CLINICAL-RADIOLOGICAL PRESENTATION	DIFFERENTIAL DIAGNOSIS	
	INFECTIOUS	NON-INFECTIOUS
LYMPH NODE DISEASE		
Lymphadenopathies, Mediastinal/Hilar/ Paratracheal —Noncalcified —Calcified (Ranke)	*Mycobacteria*: NTM *Fungi: Histoplasma; Coccidioides* *Bacteria: B. pertussis, B. henselae* (cat scratch disease) *Viruses*: HIV; measles *Parasite: Toxoplasma*	*Tumors*: lymphoma (Hodgkin's & non-Hodgkin's); lymphangioma; lymphosarcoma; leukemia *Others*: sarcoidosis; hyperplastic thymus (or even normal thymus in infant); teratoma
PARENCHYMAL LUNG DISEASE		
Solitary pulmonary nodule —Noncalcified —Calcified	*Mycobacteria*: MAC *Fungi: Histoplasma; Aspergillus; Coccidioides*	*Malignant tumors*: sarcoma; lymphoma germ cell tumor *Others*: hamartoma; arteriovenous malformations
Multiple focal pulmonary nodules —Noncalcified —Calcified	*Mycobacteria*: MAC *Bacteria*: septic pulmonary emboli due to *S. aureus; Nocardia* *Atypical Bacteria: M. pneumoniae; Legionella; C. psittaci* *Fungi: Aspergillus; Cryptococcus; Histoplasma; Coccidioides; Candida* *Viruses*: CMV; VZV; HSV; HPV	*Malignant tumors*: sarcoma; lymphoma; Wilms' tumor *Autoimmune*: granulomatosis with polyangiitis (Wegener's) *Others*: hamartoma; recurrent pulmonary aspirations; hypersensitivity pneumonitis; pulmonary hemosiderosis
Diffuse pulmonary micronodules	*Bacteria*: streptococci & *Listeria* (esp. neonates) *Fungi: Aspergillus; Cryptococcus; Histoplasma; Coccidioides;* mucormycosis	*Malignant tumors*: sarcoma *Benign tumors*: inflammatory myofibroblastic tumor *Others*: toxic fume inhalation; alveolar hemorrhage syndrome
Acute lobar pneumonia	*Viruses*: RSV; influenza; parainfluenza; adenovirus; metapneumovirus *Bacteria: S. pneumoniae; S. aureus; S. pyogenes; H. influenzae; K. pneumoniae*	*Congenital malformations*: bronchopulmonary sequestration; bronchogenic cyst; tracheoesophageal fistula *Others*: pulmonary infarct
Subacute lobar pneumonia	*Atypical Bacteria: M. pneumoniae, C. pneumoniae* *Viruses*: adenovirus *Mycobacteria*: MAC; *M. abscessus*	*Aspiration syndromes*: aspiration pneumonia

(continued)

Table 9.4. Continued

CLINICAL-RADIOLOGICAL PRESENTATION	DIFFERENTIAL DIAGNOSIS	
	INFECTIOUS	NON-INFECTIOUS
Chronic lobar pneumonia	*Bacteria: Actinomyces; B. anthracis;* anaerobes *Atypical Bacteria: M. pneumoniae; C. pneumoniae; F. tularensis* *Mycobacteria:* MAC; *M. abscessus* *Fungi: Histoplasma; Coccidioides; Blastomyces; Cryptococcus* *Parasites: Paragonimus*	*Aspiration syndromes:* aspiration pneumonia; foreign body
Cavitary pulmonary disease —Solitary cavity —Multiple cavities	*Bacteria: S. aureus; K. pneumoniae; Actinomyces; Nocardia;* anaerobes *Fungi: Histoplasma; Coccidioides; Aspergillus; Pneumocystis* *Viruses:* HPV; influenza; measles *Parasites: Paragoniasis; E. histolytica; Ecchinococcus*	*Malignant tumors:* lymphoma *Benign tumors:* inflammatory pseudotumor *Autoimmune:* granulomatosis with polyangiitis (Wegener's) *Others:* cystic bronchiectasis; congenital; sarcoidosis; traumatic pneumatocele
AIRWAY DISEASE		
Subacute/Chronic bronchitis	*Virus:* post-viral reactive airways disease *Atypical Bacteria: M. pneumoniae; C. pneumoniae* *Bacteria:* protracted bacterial bronchitis (*H. influenzae; S. pneumoniae; M. catarrhalis*) *Fungi: Aspergillus* (e.g., ABPA)	*Obstructive airway diseases:* asthma; cystic fibrosis *Others:* bronchomalacia; gastroesophageal reflux; airway irritation by smoke or air pollution
Endobronchial granulomas	*Mycobacteria:* MAC *Viruses:* HPV	*Autoimmune:* eosinophilic granulomatosis with polyangiitis *Others:* sarcoidosis
Tree-in-bud pattern	*Mycobacteria:* MAC *Fungi: Aspergillus; Pneumocystis* *Viruses:* RSV; parainfluenza	*Mucociliary disorders:* cystic fibrosis; primary ciliary dyskinesia *Autoimmune:* rheumatoid arthritis
Bronchiectasis	Sequelae of chronic/severe airway infections due to the following: *Bacteria: S. aureus; K. pneumoniae; B. pertussis* *Mycobacteria:* MAC *Viruses:* influenza; RSV; adenovirus; measles *Fungi: Aspergillus*	*Mucociliary disorders:* cystic fibrosis; primary ciliary dyskinesia *Aspiration syndromes:* recurrent pulmonary aspiration; foreign body

(continued)

Table 9.4. Continued

CLINICAL-RADIOLOGICAL PRESENTATION	DIFFERENTIAL DIAGNOSIS	
	INFECTIOUS	NON-INFECTIOUS
PLEURAL DISEASE		
Pleural effusion	*Bacteria:* S. pneumoniae; S. aureus; H. influenzae; P. aeruginosa; Actinomyces *Atypical Bacteria:* M. pneumoniae *Virus:* adenovirus; influenza *Fungi:* Aspergillus; Histoplasma *Parasite:* Paragonimus	*Malignant tumors:* lymphoma *Autoimmune:* systemic lupus erythematosus *Vascular:* lymphatic disorders
Chylothorax	*Fungi:* Histoplasma (mediastinal lymph node disease)	*Malignant tumors:* lymphoma; teratoma; sarcoma; neuroblastoma *Others:* thoracic duct injury; congenital malformation; sarcoidosis
PERICARDIAL DISEASE		
Pericardial effusion	*Viruses:* enteroviruses; adenovirus; EBV; influenza, HIV *Bacteria:* S. aureus; S. pneumoniae; H. influenzae; Actinomyces; Nocardia *Atypical Bacteria:* C. psittaci; C. trachomatis; Legionella *Fungi:* Histoplasma; Aspergillus; Blastomyces; Coccidiodes	*Autoimmune:* rheumatic fever *Benign tumors:* teratoma; fibroma; leiomyoma *Malignant tumors:* Hodgkin's lymphoma; rhabdomyosarcoma *Metabolic:* hypothyroidism; uremia *Other:* trauma; drug-induced; radiation-induced

ADA.[27] In tuberculous pericarditis, the sensitivity is similar to that of ADA, but the specificity is superior (96%).[28] Unfortunately, this test is rarely available in the highest-burden settings.

Microbiological Studies (Considered in More Detail in Chapter 7)

In children with an intrathoracic clinical presentation consistent with tuberculosis, microbiological studies should always be pursued to the extent possible because they allow bacteriological confirmation of the diagnosis and antibiotic susceptibility and resistance testing; full advantage should be taken of the available resources for specimen collection and microbiological testing. However, attaining bacteriological confirmation may be challenging, for two main reasons.

First, currently available tests are not sensitive enough to detect the majority of cases of tuberculosis disease in children. In young children included in clinical research studies and having clinical *and* radiographic features consistent with tuberculosis disease associated with findings supportive of tuberculosis as the etiology, as many as 60–85% could not be confirmed bacteriologically by GeneXpert MTB/RIF and culture. Even in adults, 10–15% of cases of pulmonary tuberculosis are culture-negative.[29] Consequently, bacteriological confirmation cannot be a requirement for the diagnosis of intrathoracic tuberculosis, and treatment of children—especially those at risk for complications—should not be withheld when otherwise indicated just because the microbiological tests are negative. Second, as infants and young children tend to swallow their respiratory secretions, and older children often cannot effectively expectorate an adequate sample of spontaneous sputum, it is necessary to obtain alternative specimens, which require invasive procedures and some technical expertise to be carried out adequately. In children with pleural or pericardial effusion suspicious for tuberculosis, the histopathological and bacteriological yields from pleural and pericardial tissues are higher than from their respective serosal fluids, although their collection is very invasive.

SPECIMEN COLLECTION STRATEGIES

Bacteriological confirmation of pulmonary tuberculosis is dependent on the extent of disease, specimen collection strategy, and processing. *M. tuberculosis* can be detected from a variety of respiratory and alimentary tract specimens. Specimen collection should be carried out and submitted for microbiological studies *before* treatment is initiated in order for cultures to be optimally sensitive. The specimen collection strategy should take into account all of the factors that affect its yield, including the type of specimens collected; their quality, quantity, and number; and pooling of samples. Collecting more than one type of specimen, and more than one sample of each one, increases the overall bacteriological yield.

Respiratory Specimens. In children who can spontaneously expectorate sputum of adequate quality and volume after deep cough, sputum from the early morning is the specimen type of first choice. Some younger children are able to expectorate sputum of adequate quality and volume, but only with sputum induction techniques such as hypertonic saline nebulization (3–5%) and chest physiotherapy followed by coaching. In younger children unable to expectorate effectively, sputum induction techniques may allow for lower respiratory tract (LRT) secretions in the laryngopharynx to be suctioned. Alternatively, LRT secretions that have reached the nasopharynx can be suctioned (known as nasopharyngeal aspirate).

Young children tend to swallow their respiratory secretions. Swallowed respiratory secretions reaching the stomach traditionally have been collected by gastric aspiration or lavage. In addition, gastric contents can be captured in the esophagus using an intra-esophageal highly-absorbent nylon yarn (known as a "string test"), employing as a vehicle for its placement either a gelatin capsule

("entero-test") or a nasogastric tube ("combined nasogastric-tube-and-string-test" [CNGTST]). In cooperative children who can swallow a capsule (typically >4–6 y.o.), the conventional encapsulated string test is an alternative specimen collection method with minimal discomfort; in younger children who are unable to swallow a capsule, the CNGTST allows the collection of two specimens simultaneously, one gastric aspirate and one string test.

Bronchoalveolar lavage should be reserved for situations when the diagnosis is unclear and there is a need to explore the bronchial anatomy. It is not routinely recommended for the diagnosis of pulmonary tuberculosis in children because its bacteriological yield is lower than that from a series of gastric aspirates.[30,31]

Non-Respiratory Specimens. Stool may contain *M. tuberculosis* or some of its fragments derived from swallowed sputum. A NAAT applied to stool has been shown to detect only ~5% of clinically diagnosed cases of pulmonary tuberculosis. However, given that a stool NAAT can rapidly detect ~50% of those cases that later are confirmed by culture, and that its collection is not invasive, it may be worth including in a diagnostic evaluation.[32,33] In a child with suspected intrathoracic tuberculosis, an associated enlarged peripheral lymph node can undergo fine-needle aspiration or biopsy for cytopathological and histopathological studies, and microbiological testing, respectively.[34,35] Serosal fluids should be collected and submitted for biochemical markers, microbiological testing, and cytopathological studies. However, serosal tissue generally has a higher culture yield, and biopsy of the pleura or pericardium may be justified, especially when the diagnosis is in doubt or drug-resistant tuberculosis is suspected.

MICROBIOLOGICAL TESTS

Microbiological studies can be categorized into rapid tests (NAATs, microscopy, antigens) and cultures. Using respiratory specimens, the yield of cultures, NAATs, and microscopy correlates with the severity of parenchymal and airway disease noted on chest imaging, and is enhanced by the aforementioned specimen collection strategies, including an increased number of samples.[36,37] Currently available NAATs are less sensitive than liquid cultures, but more sensitive than microscopy.

Rapid Microbiological Tests: Microscopy, NAATs, and Antigen Detection

Microscopy. The yield of light and fluorescent microscopy of respiratory specimens from children with a clinical diagnosis of pulmonary tuberculosis is generally poor (3–6%), and false-positive results caused by environmental NTM may occur.[38–40] However, smear-microscopy positivity may be a useful indicator of transmission risk in older children who are coughing.[37]

NAATs. The overall yield of a commercial, fully automated, real-time polymerase chain reaction (RT-PCR) test such as GeneXpert MTB/RIF performed on respiratory specimens from children with a clinical diagnosis of pulmonary tuberculosis is poor (6–15%). The specificity is high (98–99%), and there is a high sensitivity (pooled estimate 95–96%) in microscopy-positive samples, with a moderate sensitivity (pooled estimate 55–62%) in microscopy-negative samples, both using culture as a reference standard.[41] For children, NAATs are approximately three to five times more sensitive than microscopy, and should be used as the initial rapid microbiological investigation.[17] Line probe assays such as GenoType MTBDR*plus* can detect *M. tuberculosis* in respiratory and nonrespiratory specimens of children suspected of having tuberculosis disease and are especially useful for simultaneously detecting isoniazid- and rifampin-resistance in microscopy-positive samples.[42–44] They also are useful in cases when rifampin-resistance has been detected by a NAAT and early determination of concomitant isoniazid resistance is critical in selecting an appropriate treatment regimen.[45]

Antigen Detection: Lipoarabinomannan (LAM). Urine tests for mycobacterial LAM are sensitive in adults and adolescents with advanced HIV disease having CD4+ T-cell counts lower than 100 cells/L.[46–48] However, in young children, the lateral flow LAM test has a low sensitivity (48%) and a poor specificity (61%) in both HIV-infected and HIV-uninfected children with culture-confirmed intrathoracic tuberculosis.[49]

Mycobacterial Culture. Mycobacterial cultures have the highest sensitivity and specificity for the bacteriological confirmation of intrathoracic tuberculosis in children. The levels of detection of liquid and solid media are 10–100 colony-forming units/mL and 50–150 CFU/mL, respectively (versus 100–200 CFU/mL for NAAT or 5000–10000 for microscopy).[50] In most prospective studies of children with a clinical diagnosis of pulmonary tuberculosis, cultures of respiratory specimens are positive in 10–30% of cases, but may be higher in infants with more severe disease. Studies reporting higher rates of culture confirmation tend to have been retrospective, to have included only quite ill children with extensive radiographic disease diagnosed through passive case-finding, and hospitalized children (probably due to greater severity of disease and better specimen-collection strategy).[36]

Histopathological Studies

Histopathological studies should be considered in clinical presentations compatible with tuberculosis disease but also with other causes, especially when bacteriological studies fail to confirm an etiology. Potentially useful tissues to biopsy in the setting of suspected intrathoracic tuberculosis are lymph nodes, pleura, pericardium, and lung. The classical findings include numerous granulomas in various stages of development, some with central caseous necrosis. However, granulomatous inflammation is not specific for the diagnosis of tuberculosis, especially in locales where environmental NTM or fungi are common. The differential diagnosis of granulomatous inflammation includes: bacterial infections (e.g., nontuberculous mycobacteria), fungal infections (e.g., histoplasmosis), helminthic infections (e.g., schistosomiasis), protozoal infections (e.g., toxoplasmosis), autoimmune diseases (e.g., Wegener's granulomatosis), idiopathic etiologies (e.g., sarcoidosis), and foreign bodies.

Ruling Out Alternative Differential Diagnoses

In infants and children, the clinical diagnosis of intrathoracic tuberculosis is not always clear, as other etiologies can present with similar clinical, radiological, and laboratory abnormalities or may present concomitantly (Table 9.4). Chronic cough, for example, has a broad differential diagnosis (Table 9.5). Failure to thrive and prolonged fever without localizing signs also have extensive differential diagnoses. Ruling out other causes can give weight to the *clinical* diagnosis of tuberculosis disease. It may be possible to rule out certain conditions using sensitive diagnostic tests. Also, a lack of response to a diagnostic-therapeutic trial may suggest an

Table 9.5. Differential diagnosis of chronic cough in children

CAUSE	NATURE OF COUGH	PRESENCE OF FEVER	NUTRITIONAL STATUS	OTHER ASSOCIATED FEATURES	RESPONSE TO THERAPY
INFECTIOUS DISEASES					
Pulmonary tuberculosis	Wet, persistent, & unremitting cough. Mucopurulent sputum; rarely bloody (with underlying bronchiectasis or cavitary disease).	Variable	Failure to thrive/malnutrition	Exposure to tuberculosis; fatigue or decreased activity/playfulness; mediastinal, hilar lymphadenopathies.	Significant improvement within weeks. Not resolved with an antibacterial trial.
Complicated lymph node tuberculosis (extrinsic compression of airway)	Dry, persistent, & unremitting cough.	Variable	Failure to thrive/malnutrition	Subacute onset; wheezing or stridor.	Responsive to corticosteroids plus appropriate antituberculosis drugs; no response to bronchodilators.
Recurrent viral respiratory tract infection	Acute-onset cough, initially dry, then wet	Recurrent	Normal	Especially infants; coryza, sore throat; improvement between episodes.	Delayed recovery, with back-to-back relapses; no response to antibacterials.
Bronchiolitis (e.g., respiratory syncytial virus)	Cough marked at onset, with steady improvement.	At onset, then resolves	Normal	Wheezing; infants.	Responsive to general supportive measures.
Pertussis-like syndrome (e.g., *Bordetella*; *Chlamydophila*; *Mycoplasma*; resp. viruses)	Intractable, loud, dry, paroxysmal cough; not always with inspiratory whoop. Small amounts of viscid, clear sputum.	At onset, then resolves	Normal	Not immunized; subconjunctival hemorrhages.	Resolves with appropriate antibiotics

Protracted bacterial bronchitis (e.g., *S. pneumoniae; H. influenzae; M. catarrhalis*)	Persistent wet-moist cough with delayed recovery. Mucopurulent sputum.	At onset, then resolves	Normal	Especially young children (<5 y.o.), who otherwise appear well.	Resolves with appropriate antibiotic.
Recurrent bacterial pneumonia	Acute-onset cough, then improvement, then relapse. Mucopurulent sputum.	Recurrent	Failure to thrive/malnutrition	Improvement between episodes; may be HIV-related.	Resolves with appropriate antibiotic.
Chronic bacterial rhinosinusitis	Persistent cough, worse when lying down.	At onset, then resolves	Normal	Postnasal drainage.	Resolves over 2–4 weeks with appropriate Tx (glucocorticoids & antibiotic & nasal washes)
ALLERGIC DISEASE					
Allergic chronic rhinosinusitis	Variable cough, worse when lying down.	Absent unless associated with secondary infection	Normal	Nasal congestion & postnasal drainage; frequent clearing of throat.	Can be controlled with ongoing combination of allergen avoidance, medications, immunotherapy.
Cough-dominant asthma	Recurrent episodes of cough, usually dry, worse at night. May be productive of thick/mucoid sputum.	Absent unless associated with secondary infection	Normal	May be accompanied by wheezing & dyspnea.	Responsive to bronchodilators & glucocorticoids
MUCOCILIARY DISORDERS					
Cystic fibrosis	Persistent wet cough. Copious, viscid, mucopurulent sputum.	Variable	Failure to thrive/malnutrition	Begins in early childhood; bronchiectasis; frequent wheezing; clubbing; generally Caucasian.	Acute exacerbations resolve with antibiotics; chronic cough ameliorated with daily pulmonary hygiene therapies.

(continued)

Table 9.5. Continued

CAUSE	NATURE OF COUGH	PRESENCE OF FEVER	NUTRITIONAL STATUS	OTHER ASSOCIATED FEATURES	RESPONSE TO THERAPY
Primary ciliary dyskinesia	Persistent moist cough. Mucoid or purulent sputum.	Absent (even sometimes during exacerbations).	Normal	Bronchiectasis; occasional wheezing; chronic rhinosinusitis, recurrent otitis media; may have situs inversus.	Acute exacerbations resolve with antibiotics; chronic cough ameliorated with daily pulmonary hygiene therapies.
ASPIRATION SYNDROMES					
Gastroesophageal reflux disease (GERD) with recurrent pulmonary aspiration	Dry cough with variable persistence, worse at night, sometimes associated with stridor and wheezing; hoarseness.	Absent unless associated with aspiration-related LRTI	Failure to thrive (especially in severe cases)	Children with neurological abnormalities are at greater risk for aspiration complications (pneumonitis/pneumonia).	Usually responsive to dietary and positioning and medical measures.
Oropharyngeal dysphagia with recurrent pulmonary aspiration	Cough or "wet breathing" during feeding (due to recurrent aspiration); recurrent wheezing, hoarseness.	Absent unless associated with aspiration-related LRTIs	Failure to thrive	Weak suck, gagging, choking, apnea, and cyanosis during feeding; recurrent pneumonias may cause bronchiectasis.	Responsive to swallow therapy; severe cases respond to gastrostomy.
Retained foreign body	Persistent cough.	Absent unless associated with secondary infection	Normal	Especially toddlers; choking episode at onset of aspiration.	Removal of aspirated foreign body by rigid bronchoscopy.

OTHERS

Lymphoid interstitial pneumonitis	Persistent cough.	Variable	Variable	HIV-infected; parotid enlargement; persistent generalized lymphadenopathy; clubbing.	Responsive to corticosteroids.
Tracheomalacia (TM)	Brassy cough, expiratory stridor, wheezing. Thin, clear, scarce sputum.	Absent unless associated with secondary infection	Normal	Laryngeal clefts, tracheoesophageal fistula, bronchomalacia.	Mild congenital TM improves as the infant grows. Severe TM requires surgical care.
Congestive heart failure	Persistent cough; worse at night. Thin, frothy sputum.	Absent unless associated with secondary infection	Failure to thrive/malnutrition	Pulmonary edema; exercise intolerance & easy fatigue; respiratory distress with tachypnea; hepatomegaly.	Depends on the underlying etiology.

alternative diagnosis such as tuberculosis. Examples include antibiotics for presumed bacterial lower respiratory tract infection, antimalarials for fever due to presumed malaria, and nutritional support for failure to thrive due to presumed undernutrition.

STEP 3: SCREEN FOR RISK FACTORS FOR PROGRESSION FROM TUBERCULOSIS INFECTION TO DISEASE, AND DISEASE TO DEATH

The presence of risk factors for progression from tuberculosis infection to disease are of some value in diagnosing intrathoracic tuberculosis and making the decision to begin treatment. They are important to take into account when assessing a child with suspected tuberculosis because they may: (a) compromise the immune response to the organism; (b) increase the "infecting dose" ("inoculum") of *M. tuberculosis*; and/or, (c) decrease the effectiveness of standard treatment (drug resistance risk factors). The identification of these risk factors is important for the following three reasons, because they should:

1. Increase the index of suspicion for the diagnosis of intrathoracic tuberculosis (both pulmonary and extrapulmonary);
2. Hasten the diagnostic evaluation; and,
3. Expedite the initiation of adequate tuberculosis treatment—immediately *after* collecting specimens for microbiological studies—if there are sufficient clinical and/or radiographic findings to even suspect the presence of intrathoracic tuberculosis.

Some of the typical features of intrathoracic tuberculosis in children are created by the child's immune response to the organism. Immunocompromising conditions can lead to acute presentations of intrathoracic tuberculosis that are atypical due to the absence of an adequate inflammatory response. Even in advanced disease states of tuberculosis, there may be few specific respiratory clinical manifestations, but prominent constitutional signs or symptoms. Radiological abnormalities may be atypical or even absent. Immune-based tests of infection may be negative. Immunocompromising risk factors include: immunological immaturity due to young age; HIV-infection; malnutrition; use of immunosuppressive medications; primary immunodeficiencies; diabetes mellitus; chronic kidney disease,

especially end-stage renal disease requiring hemodialysis; and recent measles or whooping cough.[51] HIV infection is such an important factor that it should be routinely tested for in every child suspected of having tuberculosis disease.[52]

Environmental risk factors (intensity, proximity, duration) for continued exposure to persons transmitting *M. tuberculosis*, especially having an adult in the household with smear-positive pulmonary tuberculosis who has not yet been effectively treated, also may increase the risk of progression from infection to disease.[53] Drug-resistance risk factors are important in assessing the potential response to standard tuberculosis-treatment regimens.

STEP 4: CARRY OUT FOLLOW-UP EVALUATIONS TO FURTHER SUPPORT TUBERCULOSIS AS THE ETIOLOGY

In very immunocompromised children, intrathoracic tuberculosis can present acutely; however, in otherwise immunocompetent children, it usually presents as a subacute or chronic illness. In the early stages of disease, there may not be sufficient findings to make a presumptive diagnosis, and, even if culture confirmation is achieved, it usually takes at least several weeks. In the typical case of childhood intrathoracic tuberculosis, all rapid microbiological tests are negative and the diagnosis is presumed or even in doubt. It is therefore critical to carry out follow-up evaluations to reassess the patient, whether or not treatment has been started, by continuing to reassess steps 1 and 2. On follow-up evaluations, failure to thrive may be more apparent, respiratory symptoms may become persistent or more apparent, chest radiography may reveal new abnormalities or evolution of previous findings, tests of infection may become positive, and microbiological studies may yield positive results.

Follow-up Evaluations of the Child Who *has not* Been Started on Tuberculosis Treatment

The vast majority (>90%) of children who go on to develop disease after infection do so within 3–12 months. It is therefore vital to reassess the child periodically during the first year after infection if treatment was not started because the index of suspicion for tuberculosis was low.

Follow-up Evaluations of the Child Who *has* Been Started on Tuberculosis Treatment

A good response to treatment retrospectively supports the diagnosis, but clinical improvement is usually slow, occurring over weeks to months. On the other hand, a poor response to seemingly adequate treatment does not rule out the diagnosis of tuberculosis. Unless tuberculosis was bacteriologically confirmed, the presence of drug-resistant tuberculosis and alternative diagnoses should be reconsidered, especially in immunocompromised children who may suffer from a variety of conditions and infections that can mimic tuberculosis. If tuberculosis has been confirmed or remains the most likely etiology for the child's clinical presentation, follow-up assessments are particularly important to follow clinical and radiographic improvement, be sure there are no significant adverse reactions to the medications, and to support good treatment adherence, especially as the child improves. If the child has reliable support, reassessments can take place two and four weeks after treatment initiation and then monthly thereafter.

STRUCTURED DIAGNOSTIC APPROACHES

Given the lack of a sensitive microbiological test for diagnosing intrathoracic tuberculosis in children, many structured clinical diagnostic approaches have been developed. Some are numerical scoring systems, some use hierarchical case definitions for classification, and others are binary (presence or absence of disease). Few have been validated against a gold standard.[54] Although some perform fairly well in advanced cases of tuberculosis, they perform less well in early or mild disease, in young children, and in individuals with immunocompromising conditions who are the ones most challenging to diagnose.[55,56] Commonly used approaches have poor agreement and result in widely disparate rates of reported disease, owing to differences such as: the purpose for which it was developed (screening versus diagnosis; patient care versus research versus epidemiological surveillance); healthcare setting (community versus hospital); disease severity (mild versus severe); and the prevalence of tuberculosis and/or HIV infection (low versus high).[7]

Clinical Case Definitions

Table 9.6 summarizes the clinical case definitions of tuberculosis exposure, infection, and possible, probable, and confirmed intrathoracic disease in children based on: clinical and radiographic features consistent with tuberculosis disease; additional findings supportive of tuberculosis as the etiology; and risk factors for progression from infection to disease.

CLINICAL SYNDROMES OF INTRATHORACIC TUBERCULOSIS

Intrathoracic Lymph Node Disease

Infection, inflammation, and enlargement of intrathoracic lymph nodes are the primal processes that determine most of the clinical and radiographic findings in intrathoracic tuberculosis in children. A hallmark of many presentations is the involvement of lymph nodes out of proportion to the lung parenchymal involvement. Because the radiographic density of lymph nodes is similar to that of the heart and lung consolidation, the exact extent of lymph node involvement may be difficult to discern from plain radiographs. Sometimes their presence is implied by their effects on the airways, such as narrowing or displacement. However, chest CT will clearly demonstrate the full extent of lymph node involvement if the anatomy is not clear from plain radiography.

ISOLATED INTRATHORACIC LYMPH NODE DISEASE

Tuberculosis may involve the hilar, mediastinal (frequently subcarinal), or paratracheal lymph nodes without radiological abnormalities in the pulmonary parenchyma to suggest a site of primary infection in the lung.

Features Suggestive of Tuberculosis Disease

Clinical Presentation. Children with isolated uncomplicated intrathoracic lymphadenopathy are usually asymptomatic. These children are discovered via active case-finding, such as during a contact investigation or the screening of high-risk children. This clinical-radiological presentation may be present in the early stages of progressive disease.

Table 9.6. Clinical case definitions of tuberculosis exposure, infection, and intrathoracic disease in children

TUBERCULOSIS DIAGNOSTIC CLASSIFICATION	DX STEP 1 FEATURES SUGGESTIVE OF TUBERCULOSIS DISEASE		DX STEPS 2 & 4 FINDINGS SUPPORTIVE OF TUBERCULOSIS AS THE ETIOLOGY				DX STEP 3 RISK FACTORS FOR PROGRESSION	MANAGEMENT
	CLINICAL MANIFESTATIONS[1] (SYMPTOMS & PHYSICAL SIGNS)	CHEST IMAGING ABNORMALITIES[2]	TUBERCULOSIS EXPOSURE	IMMUNE-BASED TESTING (TST/IGRA)	MICROBIOLOGICAL STUDIES (MICROSCOPY, NAAT, CULTURE)	CLINICAL RESPONSE TO TUBERCULOSIS TREATMENT	IMMUNO-COMPROMISING CONDITIONS	TREATMENT
Tuberculosis exposure *without* immune compromise	None	None	Yes	Negative	Negative	Not applicable	None	For children less than 5 years of age
Tuberculosis exposure *with* immune compromise	None	None	Yes	Negative	Negative	Not applicable	Yes	Treatment for tuberculosis infection
Tuberculosis infection	None	None, or *calcified lung nodules or lymph nodes*[3]	Yes	Positive	Negative	Not applicable	Yes or No	Treatment for tuberculosis infection
Possible intrathoracic tuberculosis disease	**Either** clinical findings[4] **or** chest imaging abnormalities		Yes	Positive (~90%), but may lag and initially be negative	Negative	Yes	Yes or No	Treatment for intrathoracic tuberculosis
Probable intrathoracic tuberculosis disease	**Both** clinical findings **and** chest imaging abnormalities		Yes	Positive (~90%), but may lag and initially be negative	Negative	Yes	Yes or No	Treatment for intrathoracic tuberculosis
Confirmed intrathoracic tuberculosis disease	Clinical findings **and/or** chest imaging abnormalities		Yes	Positive (~90%), but may lag and initially be negative	Positive	Yes	Yes or No	Treatment for intrathoracic tuberculosis

[1] Clinical manifestations compatible with intrathoracic tuberculosis:
—Respiratory: unremitting cough that persists more than 2 weeks; sputum production; wheezing unresponsive to bronchodilators.
—Constitutional/Immunological: unexplained fever (>38.0° C) that persists more than 1 week; failure to thrive; persistent unexplained fatigue.
—Lymphoid: peripheral lymphadenopathies greater than 1.5 cm diameter.

[2] Chest imaging abnormalities compatible with tuberculosis disease:
The following are consistent with active disease: enlarged lymph nodes (hilar/mediastinal/paratracheal); solitary pulmonary nodule; multiple focal pulmonary nodules; diffuse pulmonary micronodules; consolidation(s); solitary or multiple cavities; tree-in-bud pattern; bronchiectasis; endobronchial masses; pleural effusion; pericardial effusion.

[3] In the absence of clinical findings compatible with intrathoracic tuberculosis, calcified non-enlarged regional lymph nodes, dense nodules with calcifications, and/or pleural thickening (scarring) in an asymptomatic healthy child are generally considered to be due to previous tuberculosis disease that is now an inactive/latent infection.

[4] In active case finding, up to 50% of older children with pulmonary tuberculosis may have a normal physical exam.

Imaging Abnormalities. Chest radiography reveals one or more enlarged lymph nodes, most often in the right hilum. Subcarinal involvement leads to a splaying—increased angle—of the origin of two main bronchi. Chest CT is not recommended, but if done may reveal abnormalities in the lung parenchyma not detectable by plain chest radiography.

Findings Supportive of Tuberculosis as the Etiology. The TST or IGRA is usually positive. NAAT and culture of respiratory specimens are usually negative and often not performed.[57,58]

Airway (Tracheal or Bronchial) Compression: Atelectasis; Hyperinflation

Lymph node enlargement, occurring mostly in children less than 5 years of age, may lead to bronchial compression, which may be complete, leading to lung segment or lobar collapse, or may be partial with a ball-valve effect leading to air-trapping and hyperinflation. Enlarged paratracheal nodes cause partial obstruction and may lead to massive air-trapping or stridor.

Features Suggestive of Tuberculosis Disease
Clinical Presentation. Symptoms vary with the degree of bronchial or tracheal compression, from asymptomatic to: persistent cough; wheezing or stridor; or dyspnea and respiratory distress caused by extensive atelectasis or hyperinflation created by pressure from the node(s) on surrounding structures.
Imaging Abnormalities. Chest radiography, particularly a high kilo-voltage radiograph, or CT may reveal severe narrowing of a bronchus, leading to either collapse or hyperinflation, most commonly of the right upper lobe, the right middle lobe, and the left upper lobe.

Findings Supportive of Tuberculosis as the Etiology. If diseased tissue is limited to the lymph nodes and there is no associated parenchymal involvement, microbiological studies of respiratory specimens are likely to be negative, but nonetheless should be carried out.

Airway Disease

TRACHEOBRONCHIAL DISEASE

Endotracheal and endobronchial disease usually result from bronchogenic spread of tuberculosis after a diseased lymph node erodes into the airway, most commonly the left or right main bronchus, the bronchus intermedius, or the trachea, and can reach the small airways, leading to bronchiolar disease.[14,19] Disease may be diffuse (bronchitis) or localized (a mass), with the most common type of lesion being granulation tissue. The bronchial walls may be left with dilatations (i.e., bronchiectasis) after scarring or with bronchostenosis due to fibrosis and stricture.[51]

Features Suggestive of Tuberculosis Disease
Clinical Presentation. Tracheobronchial disease can have an acute, insidious, or delayed onset, with symptoms or signs of airway obstruction that depend on the location and severity of obstruction, including persistent cough, rhonchi, wheezing, stridor, and dyspnea.
Imaging Abnormalities. Chest radiography is not sensitive in detecting tracheobronchial disease unless it is marked or has an accompanying fibronodular appearance in the lung parenchyma. Bronchiolar disease is best seen on chest CT and may appear as a tree-in-bud pattern or as centrilobular nodules, consisting of dilated bronchioles that are thick-walled and filled with mucus. Bronchiectasis is also more easily seen on chest CT, which may reveal bronchial dilatation and wall-thickening as well as lack of tapering of bronchi.
Endoscopic Studies. Bronchoscopy may reveal findings consistent with tracheobronchial disease, ranging from nonspecific inflammation to highly suggestive findings, including: hyperemia, edema, ulcers, masses, fibrostenosis, granulation tissue, or caseous lesions.[59-61]

Findings Supportive of Tuberculosis as the Etiology. Then TST and IGRAs usually are positive. Endotracheal and endobronchial involvement is associated with higher rates of bacteriological confirmation, including acid-fast smear microscopy, NAAT, and culture of respiratory specimens.[51] Bronchoscopically collected specimens, including bronchoalveolar lavage, complement conventional specimens in the bacteriological confirmation.[61]

Parenchymal Lung Disease

NODULAR LUNG DISEASE: SOLITARY PULMONARY NODULE; FOCAL MULTIPLE PULMONARY NODULES

If inhaled *M. tuberculosis* bacilli are not immediately destroyed by the innate immune response, a small parenchymal focus of infection may develop and drain via local lymphatic vessels to regional lymph nodes. Most children with this form of disease have spontaneous resolution and are identified only by radiographic screening during contact investigations. Focal multiple pulmonary nodules may be seen on chest imaging in the early stages of a tuberculous bronchopneumonia.

Features Suggestive of Tuberculosis Disease

Clinical Presentation. A child with a solitary pulmonary nodule, with or without associated lymphadenopathy (primary complex), is usually asymptomatic.

Imaging Abnormalities. Chest radiography may reveal an isolated, non-cavitating, calcified parenchymal opacity that is round or oval, typically peripheral or surrounding the lobar fissures in either the lower part of an upper lobe or the upper part of a lower lobe or middle lobe. Ipsilateral thoracic lymph nodes may be slightly enlarged, and this combination of radiological signs is known as the primary/Ghon complex. When the associated lymphadenopathy is also calcified, it is known as a Ranke complex. Chest CT is more sensitive in the detection of small, ill-defined airspace nodules that tend to coalesce in some parts, but are different from the sharply defined micronodules that are separate from each other, as seen in miliary disease.

Findings Supportive of Tuberculosis as the Etiology. The TST and/or an IGRA usually are positive. Pulmonary tuberculosis presenting as small nodules is rarely bacteriologically confirmed.

PNEUMONIA: LOBAR PNEUMONIA, BRONCHOPNEUMONIA, AND EXPANSILE PNEUMONIA

When the primary infection is not well contained, mycobacteria replicate, and the initial lesion may enlarge. Hilar lymph nodes may also enlarge and sometimes compress or infiltrate contiguous bronchi, most commonly the right or left main bronchus, but also the bronchus intermedius.[14] Complications can occur when a necrotic hilar lymph node erupts into a bronchus and endobronchial spread leads to patchy or multifocal consolidation of the respective lobe, resulting in bronchopneumonia. When enlarged hilar lymph nodes also compress the bronchus, the endobronchial spread may cause distal expansion and dense consolidation of the entire lobe, resulting in an expansile pneumonia with

bowing of the lung fissure or displacement of the trachea and the formation of focal cavities.

Features Suggestive of Tuberculosis Disease

Clinical Presentation. Persistent cough, high fever, and significant weight loss are common. Rarely, this form of pulmonary tuberculosis can develop into an acute respiratory distress syndrome.

Imaging Abnormalities. The chest radiograph may reveal airspace consolidation and air bronchograms in any part of the lung parenchyma, more frequently on the right. Chest CT will demonstrate air-space disease, but also reveals the extrinsic bronchial compression that may lead to post-obstructive airspace disease with expansile pneumonia.

Findings Supportive of Tuberculosis as the Etiology. The TST or IGRA is positive in about 80% of cases. Bacteriological confirmation of tuberculous pneumonia from respiratory specimens, using culture and NAAT, depends on the extent of parenchymal involvement, but has been reported to be as high as 80%.[51]

CAVITARY PULMONARY DISEASE

Cavities are formed by several mechanisms. They can result from expulsion or drainage of the liquefaction of caseous lung parenchyma via the bronchial tree, with subsequent fibrosis. They also can occur as a result of aspiration from a caseous lymph node, which may be more common in children than cavitation caused by failure to contain the primary lung parenchymal focus. Cavitation is very uncommon in young children, occurring predominantly in infants with extensive lymph node involvement when the primary infection is not contained. Older children and adolescents may develop cavitation of lesions of their primary infection anywhere in the lung, or of lesions typically in the lung apices that resulted from the previous lymphohematogenous dissemination of bacteria known as "adult-type" or "reactivation" disease.

Features Suggestive of Tuberculosis Disease

Clinical Presentation. Young children with these forms of tuberculosis often present with chronic cough, fever, weight loss, fatigue, and may become very ill. Older children and adolescents with cavitary pulmonary disease typically have chronic cough, sputum production occasionally with hemoptysis, pleuritic chest pain, fever, night sweats, loss of appetite, weight loss, and fatigue.

Imaging Abnormalities. Chest radiography and CT in young children may reveal an oval-shaped lucency either isolated or within a consolidation or nodule, with walls that may be either thin or thick. In older children and adolescents, there may be multiple cavities, located typically in the apical segments of the upper lobes, often bilaterally, frequently in areas of consolidation or with surrounding infiltrates, and sometimes associated with pleural effusions.[3]

Findings Supportive of Tuberculosis as the Etiology. The TST and/or IGRAs are positive in the majority of cases. Given the high bacterial loads associated with cavities, cultures and NAATs usually allow bacteriological confirmation, and sputum or gastric aspirate microscopy is often positive as well.

MILIARY LUNG DISEASE

Miliary lung disease is the result of a tuberculous lesion infiltrating into a blood vessel, leading to hematogenous dissemination of millions of bacilli and seeding of the lungs and other organs, including the bone marrow, spleen, liver, central nervous system, and kidneys. This can occur within 2–6 months of the primary infection in immune-immature children—half of the cases occur in infants younger than 12 months of age—and in those with immunocompromising conditions, especially untreated HIV infection. Disseminated disease has the highest morbidity and mortality (10–15%).[56]

Features Suggestive of Tuberculosis Disease
Clinical Presentation. The temporal pattern of miliary disease is usually fulminant-to-acute, but it can also present with delayed onset. Although the word "miliary" refers to the common chest radiographic pattern, pulmonary involvement and respiratory symptoms often occur relatively late in the course. Given the multi-system involvement, presenting symptoms may include cough (72%), dyspnea, diarrhea and vomiting (33%), irritability, headache, convulsions, hepatomegaly (82%), splenomegaly (54%), lymphadenopathy (46%), subjective fever (61%), objective fever (39%), chills, loss of appetite and failure to thrive (40%), fatigue, generalized weakness, decreased activity, and malaise. Complications include acute respiratory distress syndrome, and the majority of untreated cases will terminate in meningitis.[56]

Imaging Abnormalities. Chest radiography may reveal innumerable rounded micronodules (≤3 mm in diameter) scattered diffusely throughout both lungs, but abnormalities are sometimes not apparent early on (9%).[51,56] Often these nodules are best seen on the lateral chest radiograph in the area behind the heart. Intrathoracic adenopathy is also a common finding and can help differentiate miliary tuberculosis from lymphoid interstitial hyperplasia in children with HIV infection.

Findings Supportive of Tuberculosis as the Etiology
Immune-Based and Laboratory Tests. As many as half of children with miliary tuberculosis have a negative TST or IGRA, and the likelihood of these tests being negative increases with progression of the disease. Bone marrow involvement may cause a normocytic anemia, thrombocytopenia, or a leukemoid reaction.
Microbiological Studies. Miliary/disseminated tuberculosis can be difficult to confirm microbiologically. Smear microscopy, NAAT, and culture of respiratory specimens are often negative. Other potential sources of positive culture or NAAT result include blood, urine, stool, and CSF. The organism occasionally can be isolated from the bone marrow or liver.

Pleural Disease

PLEURAL EFFUSION AND EMPYEMA

Pleural thickening is a common component of the primary infection but rarely results in a significant effusion. Overt pleural disease is uncommon in infants, is usually unilateral, and is seen more often in adolescents and older children. It typically occurs 3–6 months after the primary infection. Most tuberculous pleural effusions result from a delayed-type hypersensitivity reaction to *M. tuberculosis* antigens that leaked into the pleural space from a subpleural primary focus. These effusions rarely develop into an empyema.[62]

Features Suggestive of Tuberculosis Disease
Clinical Presentation. The child may present with pleuritic chest pain (58%), cough (80%), fever (67%), night sweats (7%), failure to thrive (29%), and fatigue, but is usually not severely ill and may even be asymptomatic (13%).[63] The presentation is

not significantly different from that caused by pleural effusions or even empyema caused by other bacteria such as the pneumococcus.

Imaging Abnormalities. Chest radiography demonstrates the homogeneously opacified fluid level of a nonloculated pleural effusion and, after drainage, often reveals lung parenchymal abnormalities and intrathoracic lymphadenopathy.[24] Reaccumulation of pleural fluid after initial drainage is common and not of prognostic significance. Chest ultrasonography is useful in determining the nature and quantity of the effusion and detecting early loculations and septations. Chest CT may be useful in cases of complicated pleural effusion, detecting associated parenchymal lesions and intrathoracic lymphadenopathy, and differentiating between pleural thickening and a chronic loculated effusion or empyema.

Laboratory Findings. Tuberculous pleural fluids are usually exudative with an elevated protein (>30 g/L) and LDH (>200 U/L), and have a predominantly lymphocytic pleocytosis. The pleural fluid may be grossly purulent, representing tuberculous empyema.[64] Because of the protein-rich nature of the fluid, one must be careful not to remove too much pleural fluid in a severely malnourished child, as this can acutely worsen the child's oncotic pressure.

Findings Supportive of Tuberculosis as the Etiology

Immune-based and Laboratory Tests. The TST or IGRA is positive in 80–90% of cases of pleural tuberculosis. Pleural fluid should be submitted for ADA (usually >35 U/L) or for uIFNγ (which has a sensitivity and specificity that is slightly higher than that of ADA), if available.[27] If the ADA is less than 40 U/L and pleocytosis is predominantly lymphocytic, bacterial empyema and rheumatoid pleuritis should be considered.[64]

Microbiological Studies. Pleural fluid is a suboptimal specimen for detecting *M. tuberculosis*, with culture yield less than 40%. NAAT is positive in less than 30% of cases, and microscopy is almost always negative. Pleural tissue has a much higher diagnostic yield than fluid; a pleural biopsy should be considered when there is moderate to high suspicion for pleural tuberculosis and results of testing pleural fluid and of respiratory specimens are not diagnostic, and/or there is an increased risk of a drug-resistant infection. Pleural tissue culture yields *M. tuberculosis* in up to 60% of cases.[65]

Histopathological Studies. Pleural tissue may demonstrate granulomatous inflammation, caseous necrosis, or positive microscopy in more than 50% of cases. When both microbiological and histopathological studies are done, the diagnostic yield increases to 60–95%.[65]

CHYLOTHORAX

Chylothorax is a type of pleural effusion caused by disruption or obstruction of the thoracic duct or its tributaries, resulting in leakage of lymphatic fluid (chyle) into the pleural space. It is a rare complication of pulmonary tuberculosis caused by the mediastinal lymphadenopathy externally compressing the thoracic duct or to diseased lymph nodes infiltrating into the thoracic duct.[66]

Features Suggestive of Tuberculosis Disease

Clinical Presentation. Children may present with a gradual onset of dyspnea on exertion and fatigue; however, fever and chest pain are rare. Depending on the size and location of the effusion, there may be decreased breath sounds and dullness to percussion.

Imaging Abnormalities. Chest radiography will reveal the pleural effusion, and a chest CT is helpful in looking for the site and cause of the chyle leakage.

Laboratory Findings. The pleural fluid typically has a milky white appearance, is predominantly lymphocytic (>80%), exudative, and has elevated levels of triglycerides.

Findings Supportive of Tuberculosis as the Etiology

Biochemical Markers. ADA of the chylous pleural fluid is elevated (>40 U/L).[67]

Microbiological Studies. NAAT and culture may detect *M. tuberculosis* from the chylous pleural fluid in a minority of cases.[67]

Pericardial Disease

PERICARDIAL EFFUSION

Tuberculosis is one of the most common causes of pericardial effusion in children in endemic countries, and approximately 1–4% of children with tuberculosis disease develop pericarditis.[68] It can arise from lymphohematogenous dissemination of mycobacteria but most often occurs as a result of an infected contiguous subcarinal lymph node infiltrating through the pericardium. There are three main presentations: (1) pericardial effusion (the most common); (2) constrictive pericarditis; and (3) a combination known as effusive-constrictive disease. HIV infection predisposes to disseminated disease and is associated with greater severity of pericardial tuberculosis.[69]

Features Suggestive of Tuberculosis Disease

Clinical Presentation. Children with tuberculous pericarditis may initially be asymptomatic, then develop symptoms and signs of heart failure, including persistent cough (70%), dyspnea (77%), chest pain (30%), hepatomegaly (77%), elevated jugular venous pressure (7%), soft heart sounds, and a pericardial friction rub (18%), in addition to subjective fever (63%), objective fever (52%), night sweats, failure to thrive (36%), fatigue, and malaise.[70]

Imaging Abnormalities. Chest radiography typically reveals cardiomegaly with a globular heart silhouette (91%), and often a concomitant pleural effusion (40%), pulmonary disease (40%), or mediastinal (especially subcarinal), lymphadenopathy (31%) consistent with pulmonary tuberculosis.[70] The electrocardiogram often shows diminished voltages or electrical alterans when the effusion is large or the constriction is great. Echocardiography is the most sensitive imaging study to confirm a pericardial effusion, and may reveal fibrinous strands suggestive of tuberculosis as the etiology. A chest CT may provide additional diagnostic information regarding associated mediastinal lymphadenopathy.

Laboratory Findings. Tuberculous pericardial fluids are typically exudative with an elevated protein level, and have a predominantly lymphocytic pleocytosis.

Findings Supportive of Tuberculosis as the Etiology

Immune-based Tests and Biochemical Markers. The TST or IGRA is positive in 60–80% of cases. Pericardial fluid should be submitted for ADA or preferably for uIFNγ, which has similar sensitivity and higher specificity.[28] The main differential diagnosis of elevated levels of ADA in pericardial fluid is bacterial pericarditis, which is distinguished by its predominantly neutrophilic effusion, positive Gram stain, and bacterial culture.

Microbiological Studies. In addition to culture, which has a sensitivity of about 40–50%, pericardial fluid should be submitted for NAAT such as GeneXpert MTB/RIF, which has been found to have a sensitivity of 64% in adults with pericardial tuberculosis.[28] Pericardial fluid microscopy has a very low sensitivity. NAAT and culture of respiratory specimens may confirm an underlying pulmonary tuberculosis that has disseminated.

Histopathological Studies. Biopsied samples of pericardial tissue do not always demonstrate granulomatous inflammation consistent with tuberculosis, even when the disease is bacteriologically confirmed from other specimens.

REFERENCES

1. Marais BJ, Graham SM. Childhood tuberculosis: a roadmap towards zero deaths. *J Paediatr Child Health*. 2014.
2. Marais B, Gie R, Schaaf H, Hesseling A, Enarson D, Beyers N. The spectrum of disease in children treated for tuberculosis in a highly endemic area [unresolved issues]. *Int J Tuberc Lung Dis*. 2006;10(7):732–738.
3. Marais BJ, Gie RP, Hesseling AH, Beyers N. Adult-type pulmonary tuberculosis in children 10–14 years of age. *Pediatr Infect Dis J*. 2005;24(8):743–744.
4. Wiseman CA, Gie RP, Starke JR, et al. A proposed comprehensive classification of tuberculosis disease severity in children. *Pediatr Infect Dis J*. 2012;31(4):347–352.
5. O'Garra A, Redford PS, McNab FW, Bloom CI, Wilkinson RJ, Berry MP. The immune response in tuberculosis. *Ann Rev Immunol*. 2013;31:475–527.
6. Achkar JM, Jenny-Avital ER. Incipient and subclinical tuberculosis: defining early disease states in the context of host immune response. *J Infect Dis*. 2011;204(Suppl 4):S1179–S1186.
7. Hatherill M, Hanslo M, Hawkridge T, et al. Structured approaches for the screening and diagnosis of childhood tuberculosis in a high prevalence region of South Africa. *Bull World Health Organ*. 2010;88(4):312–320.
8. Marais BJ, Gie RP, Hesseling AC, et al. A refined symptom-based approach to diagnose pulmonary tuberculosis in children. *Pediatrics*. 2006;118(5):e1350–e1359.
9. Boulware DR, Callens S, Pahwa S. Pediatric HIV immune reconstitution inflammatory syndrome. *Curr Opin HIV AIDS*. 2008;3(4):461–467.
10. Jawahar MS. Scrofula revisited: an update on the diagnosis and management of tuberculosis of superficial lymph nodes. *Indian J Pediatr*. 2000;67(2 Suppl):S28–S33.

11. Oliwa JN, Karumbi JM, Marais BJ, Madhi SA, Graham SM. Tuberculosis as a cause or comorbidity of childhood pneumonia in tuberculosis-endemic areas: a systematic review. *Lancet Respir Med.* 2015.

12. Smuts NA, Beyers N, Gie RP, et al. Value of the lateral chest radiograph in tuberculosis in children. *Pediatr Radiol.* 1994;24(7):478–480.

13. Andronikou S, Van der Merwe DJ, Goussard P, Gie RP, Tomazos N. Usefulness of lateral radiographs for detecting tuberculous lymphadenopathy in children—confirmation using sagittal CT reconstruction with multiplanar cross-referencing. *S African J Radiol.* 2012;16(3):87–90, 2.

14. Andronikou S, Joseph E, Lucas S, et al. CT scanning for the detection of tuberculous mediastinal and hilar lymphadenopathy in children. *Pediatr Radiol.* 2004;34(3):232–236.

15. Kim WS, Moon WK, Kim IO, et al. Pulmonary tuberculosis in children: evaluation with CT. *Am J Roentgenol.* 1997;168(4):1005–1009.

16. Daltro P, Nunez-Santos E, Laya BF. Pediatric tuberculosis. In: Garcia-Peña P, Guillerman RP, eds. *Pediatric Chest Imaging. Medical Radiology. Diagnostic Imaging.* 3rd ed. Berlin, Heidelberg: Springer-Verlag; 2014:285–304.

17. Graham S, Grzemska M, Hill S, Kedia T, Wong N. Guidance for national tuberculosis programmes on the management of tuberculosis in children. In: Programme GT, editor. 2 ed. Geneva: World Health Organization; 2014.

18. Wessels G, Schaaf HS, Beyers N, Gie RP, Nel E, Donald PR. Haematological abnormalities in children with tuberculosis. *J Trop Pediatr.* 1999;45(5):307–310.

19. Goussard P, Gie R. The role of bronchoscopy in the diagnosis and management of pediatric pulmonary tuberculosis. *Exp Rev Respir Med.* 2014;8(1):101–109.

20. Schaaf HS, Michaelis IA, Richardson M, et al. Adult-to-child transmission of tuberculosis: household or community contact? *Int J Tuberc Lung Dis.* 2003;7(5):426–431.

21. Starke JR, Committee on Infectious Diseases. Interferon-gamma release assays for diagnosis of tuberculosis infection and disease in children. *Pediatrics.* 2014;134(6):e1763–e1773.

22. Adetifa IM, Ota MO, Jeffries DJ, et al. Commercial interferon gamma release assays compared to the tuberculin skin test for diagnosis of latent *Mycobacterium tuberculosis* infection in childhood contacts in Gambia. *Pediatr Infect Dis J.* 2010;29(5):439–443.

23. Weyer K, Mirzayev F, van Gemert W, Gilpin C. *Commercial Serodiagnostic Tests for Diagnosis of Tuberculosis: Policy Statement.* Geneva: World Health Organization; 2011.

24. Merino JM, Carpintero I, Alvarez T, Rodrigo J, Sanchez J, Coello JM. Tuberculous pleural effusion in children. *Chest.* 1999;115(1):26–30.

25. Goto M, Noguchi Y, Koyama H, Hira K, Shimbo T, Fukui T. Diagnostic value of adenosine deaminase in tuberculous pleural effusion: a meta-analysis. *Ann Clin Biochem.* 2003;40(Pt 4):374–381.

26. Tuon FF, Litvoc MN, Lopes MI. Adenosine deaminase and tuberculous pericarditis—a systematic review with meta-analysis. *Acta Tropica.* 2006;99(1):67–74.

27. Greco S, Girardi E, Masciangelo R, Capoccetta GB, Saltini C. Adenosine deaminase and interferon gamma measurements for the diagnosis of tuberculous pleurisy: a meta-analysis. *Int J Tuberc Lung Dis.* 2003;7(8):777–786.

28. Pandie S, Peter JG, Kerbelker ZS, et al. Diagnostic accuracy of quantitative PCR (Xpert MTB/RIF) for tuberculous pericarditis compared to adenosine deaminase and unstimulated interferon-gamma in a high burden setting: a prospective study. *BMC Med.* 2014;12:101.

29. Kanagarajan K, Perumalsamy K, Alakhras M, Malli D, Gupta K, Krishnan P. Clinical characteristics and outcome of culture negative tuberculosis. *Chest.* 2003;124(4):108S.

30. Abadco DL, Steiner P. Gastric lavage is better than bronchoalveolar lavage for isolation of *Mycobacterium tuberculosis* in childhood pulmonary tuberculosis. *Pediatr Infect Dis J.* 1992;11(9):735–738.

31. Somu N, Swaminathan S, Paramasivan CN, et al. Value of bronchoalveolar lavage and gastric lavage in the diagnosis of pulmonary tuberculosis in children. *Tuberc Lung Dis.* 1995;76(4):295–299.

32. Walters E, Gie RP, Hesseling AC, Friedrich SO, Diacon AH, Gie RP. Rapid diagnosis of pediatric intrathoracic tuberculosis from stool samples using the Xpert MTB/RIF assay: a pilot study. *Pediatr Infect Dis J.* 2012;31(12):1316.

33. Nicol MP, Spiers K, Workman L, et al. Xpert MTB/RIF testing of stool samples for the diagnosis of pulmonary tuberculosis in children. *Clin Infect Dis.* 2013;57(3):e18–e21.

34. Wright CA, Warren RM, Marais BJ. Fine needle aspiration biopsy: an undervalued diagnostic modality in paediatric mycobacterial disease. *Int J Tuberc Lung Dis.* 2009;13(12):1467–1475.

35. Denkinger CM, Schumacher SG, Boehme CC, Dendukuri N, Pai M, Steingart KR. Xpert MTB/RIF assay for the diagnosis of extrapulmonary tuberculosis: a systematic review and meta-analysis. *Eur Respir J.* 2014;44(2):435–446.

36. Marais BJ, Hesseling AC, Gie RP, Schaaf HS, Enarson DA, Beyers N. The bacteriologic yield in children with intrathoracic tuberculosis. *Clin Infect Dis.* 2006;42(8):e69–e71.

37. Bolursaz MR, Mehrian P, Aghahosseini F, et al. Evaluation of the relationship between smear positivity and high-resolution CT findings in children with pulmonary tuberculosis. *Polish J Radiol.* 2014;79:120–125.

38. Gomez Pastrana Duran D, Torronteras Santiago R, Caro Mateo P, et al. [Effectiveness of smears and cultures in gastric aspirate samples in the diagnosis of tuberculosis]. *Anales Espanoles de Pediatria.* 2000;53(5):405–411.

39. Zar HJ, Hanslo D, Apolles P, Swingler G, Hussey G. Induced sputum versus gastric lavage for microbiological confirmation of pulmonary tuberculosis in infants and young children: a prospective study. *Lancet.* 2005;365(9454):130–134.

40. Laven GT. Diagnosis of tuberculosis in children using fluorescence microscopic examination of gastric washings. *Am Rev Respir Dis.* 1977;115(5):743–749.

41. World Health Organization. *Automated Real-Time Nucleic Acid Amplification Technology for Rapid and Simultaneous Detection of Tuberculosis and Rifampicin Resistance: Xpert MTB/RIF Assay for the Diagnosis of Pulmonary and Extrapulmonary TB in Adults and Children. Policy Update.* Geneva: World Health Organization, Programme GT; 2013. Contract No.: WHO/HTM/TB/2013.16.

42. World Health Organization. *Molecular Line Probe Assays for Rapid Screening of Patients at Risk of Multidrug-Resistant Tuberculosis (MDR-TB).* Geneva: 27 June 2008. Report No.

43. World Health Organization. *The Use of Molecular Line Probe Assay for the Detection of Resistance to Second-Line Anti-Tuberculosis Drugs: Expert Group Meeting Report.* Geneva: World Health Organization, February 2013. Report No.: WHO/HTM/TB/2013.01.

44. Sanchini A, Fiebig L, Drobniewski F, et al. Laboratory diagnosis of paediatric tuberculosis in the European Union/European Economic Area: analysis of routine laboratory data, 2007 to 2011. *Eur Commun Dis Bull.* 2014;19(11).

45. Barnard M, Gey van Pittius NC, van Helden PD, Bosman M, Coetzee G, Warren RM. The diagnostic performance of the GenoType MTBDR*plus* version 2 line probe assay is equivalent to that of the Xpert MTB/RIF assay. *J Clin Microbiol.* 2012;50(11):3712–3716.

46. Lawn SD, Kerkhoff AD, Vogt M, Wood R. High diagnostic yield of tuberculosis from screening urine samples from HIV-infected patients with advanced immunodeficiency using the Xpert MTB/RIF assay. *J Acq Immune Def Syn.* 2012;60(3):289–294.

47. Lawn SD, Dheda K, Kerkhoff AD, et al. Determine TB-LAM lateral flow urine antigen assay for HIV-associated tuberculosis: recommendations on the design and reporting of clinical studies. *BMC Infect Dis.* 2013;13:407.

48. Mutetwa R, Boehme C, Dimairo M, et al. Diagnostic accuracy of commercial urinary lipoarabinomannan detection in African tuberculosis suspects and patients. *Int J Tuberc Lung Dis.* 2009;13(10):1253–1259.

49. Nicol MP, Allen V, Workman L, et al. Urine lipoarabinomannan testing for diagnosis of pulmonary tuberculosis in children: a prospective study. *Lancet Global Health.* 2014;2(5):e278–e284.

50. Dunlap NE, Bass J, Fujimawara P, et al. Diagnostic standards and classification of tuberculosis in adults and children. *Am J Respir Clin Care Med.* 2000;161(4 Pt 1):1376–1395.

51. Marais BJ, Gie RP, Schaaf HS, et al. The natural history of childhood intra-thoracic tuberculosis: a critical review of literature from the pre-chemotherapy era. *Int J Tuberc Lung Dis.* 2004;8(4):392–402.

52. Sculier D, Getahun HG. *WHO Policy on Collaborative TB/HIV Activities: Guidelines for National Programmes and Other Stakeholders.* Geneva: Department ST; 2012. Contract No.: WHO/HTM/TB/2012.1. WHO/HIV/2012.1.

53. Grzybowski S, Barnett GD, Styblo K. Contacts of cases of active pulmonary tuberculosis. *Bull Int Union Against Tuberc.* 1975;50(1):90–106.

54. Hesseling AC, Schaaf HS, Gie RP, Starke JR, Beyers N. A critical review of diagnostic approaches used in the diagnosis of childhood tuberculosis. *Int J Tuberc Lung Dis.* 2002;6(12):1038–1045.

55. Graham SM. The use of diagnostic systems for tuberculosis in children. *Indian J Pediatr.* 2011;78(3):334–339.

56. Hussey G, Chisholm T, Kibel M. Miliary tuberculosis in children: a review of 94 cases. *Pediatr Infect Dis J.* 1991;10(11):832–836.

57. Gwee A, Pantazidou A, Ritz N, et al. To X-ray or not to X-ray? Screening asymptomatic children for pulmonary TB: a retrospective audit. *Arch Dis Child.* 2013;98(6):401–404.

58. Lapphra K, Sutthipong C, Foongladda S, et al. Drug-resistant tuberculosis in children in Thailand. *Int J Tuberc Lung Dis.* 2013;17(10):1279–1284.

59. de Blic J, Azevedo I, Burren CP, Le Bourgeois M, Lallemand D, Scheinmann P. The value of flexible bronchoscopy in childhood pulmonary tuberculosis. *Chest.* 1991;100(3):688–692.

60. Chung HS, Lee JH. Bronchoscopic assessment of the evolution of endobronchial tuberculosis. *Chest.* 2000;117(2):385–392.

61. Cakir E, Uyan ZS, Oktem S, et al. Flexible bronchoscopy for diagnosis and follow up of childhood endobronchial tuberculosis. *Pediatr Infect Dis J.* 2008;27(9):783–787.

62. Fischer GB, Andrade CF, Lima JB. Pleural tuberculosis in children. *Paediatric Respir Rev.* 2011;12(1):27–30.

63. Cruz AT, Ong LT, Starke JR. Childhood pleural tuberculosis: a review of 45 cases. *Pediatr Infect Dis J.* 2009;28(11):981–984.

64. Light RW. *Pleural Diseases.* 6th ed. Philadelphia: Wolters Kluwer Health; 2013.

65. Gopi A, Madhavan SM, Sharma SK, Sahn SA. Diagnosis and treatment of tuberculous pleural effusion in 2006. *Chest.* 2007;131(3):880–889.

66. Grobbelaar M, Andronikou S, Goussard P, Theron S, Mapukata A, George R. Chylothorax as a complication of pulmonary tuberculosis in children. *Pediatr Radiol.* 2008;38(2):224–226.

67. Karapolat S, Sanli A, Onen A. Chylothorax due to tuberculosis lymphadenopathy: report of a case. *Surg Today.* 2008;38(10):938–941.

68. Weber S. Tuberculosis and pericarditis in children. *Trop Doctor.* 1999;29(3):135–138.

69. Mayosi BM, Wiysonge CS, Ntsekhe M, et al. Clinical characteristics and initial management of patients with tuberculous pericarditis in the HIV era: the Investigation of the Management of Pericarditis in Africa (IMPI Africa) registry. *BMC Infect Dis.* 2006;6:2.

70. Hugo-Hamman CT, Scher H, De Moor MM. Tuberculous pericarditis in children: a review of 44 cases. *Pediatr Infect Dis J.* 1994;13(1):13–18.

10

DIAGNOSIS OF THE MOST COMMON FORMS OF EXTRATHORACIC TUBERCULOSIS IN CHILDREN

H. Simon Schaaf and Anthony J. Garcia-Prats

HIGHLIGHTS OF THIS CHAPTER

- Extrathoracic tuberculosis occurs, with or without intrathoracic manifestation, in 30–60% of children with tuberculosis disease.
- It is more common in children with immune compromise, including children with poorly controlled HIV infection.
- Peripheral lymph node tuberculosis is the most common form of extrathoracic tuberculosis in children and adolescents and is most often found in the anterior cervical region.
- Some forms of extrathoracic tuberculosis, such as renal disease, are more common in older children and adolescents.
- Culture confirmation of most forms of extrathoracic tuberculosis is difficult as they are paucibacillary forms of disease.
- The diagnosis of extrathoracic tuberculosis is often suggested by a consistent history and physical examination, recent contact with a contagious tuberculosis case, a positive test of tuberculosis infection (TST or IGRA), lack of response to treatment for other possible etiologies, and, when available, histopathology demonstrating granulomas and/or bacteriological confirmation.

TUBERCULOSIS is primarily considered a pulmonary (lung) disease, but hematogenous dissemination of *Mycobacterium tuberculosis* occurs early after infection, and organisms can seed and affect any part of the body. Tuberculosis outside of the lungs is commonly referred to as extrapulmonary tuberculosis; however, in children it is often called extrathoracic tuberculosis, which is disease outside of the chest cavity, to exclude miliary tuberculosis (in the lungs), pleural effusion, and mediastinal lymphadenopathy.

Extrapulmonary tuberculosis (including all forms of tuberculosis except lung and mediastinal lymph node disease), with or without pulmonary tuberculosis, occurs in 30–60% of tuberculosis cases in children.[1,2] Many childhood tuberculosis cases will have features of both extrapulmonary and pulmonary tuberculosis. The World Health Organization (WHO) reports all pulmonary cases that also have extrapulmonary manifestations as pulmonary tuberculosis; therefore, the true prevalence of extrapulmonary tuberculosis is not reflected in WHO reports. Table 10.1 displays a general overview of the types of extrathoracic tuberculosis. Given how common extrathoracic tuberculosis is, clinicians caring for children must be aware of the possible clinical presentations and best diagnostic approaches for most of these forms.

This chapter will concentrate on the diagnosis of extrathoracic tuberculosis in children, excluding tuberculous meningitis, which will be covered in Chapter 11.

PERIPHERAL LYMPHADENITIS

Overview

Peripheral lymphadenitis is the most common form of extrathoracic tuberculosis. In tuberculosis high-burden regions, 8–10% of cases in children present with peripheral lymphadenitis caused by *M. tuberculosis*. In our experience, 8% of culture-confirmed tuberculosis cases have only peripheral lymphadenopathy without pulmonary changes on chest radiograph, while 22% of all culture-confirmed tuberculosis cases have peripheral lymphadenopathy (60% are therefore associated with pulmonary disease). Of these, 90–95% are in the cervical region (cervical, submandibular, pre- and post-auricular, and supraclavicular), approximately 1–2% are inguinal, 2% axillary (excluding *M. bovis* BCG complications), and 1% of cases have generalized lymphadenopathy (unpublished data, HS Schaaf).

Table 10.1. Types of extrathoracic tuberculosis in children

TYPE OF EXTRATHORACIC TUBERCULOSIS	COMMENT
Peripheral lymphadenopathy	Mainly (95%) in cervical area; most common form of extrathoracic tuberculosis
Osteoarticular	50% of osteoarticular tuberculosis is in the spine; tuberculous arthritis, mainly in large, weight-bearing joints, is the second most common presentation
Abdominal	Different forms of abdominal tuberculosis occur. Abdominal lymphadenopathy and peritoneal involvement are the commonest in children, but intestinal tuberculosis and solid viscera tuberculosis do occur
Cutaneous	Many different clinical forms, mainly based on the route of infection, the host's prior contact with *M. tuberculosis*, and the host's immune status
Urogenital	Rare in children, as it represents reactivation of a focus in the kidney(s) >5–8 years after primary infection. Urine culture positive for *M. tuberculosis* in young children usually indicates a bacteremic phase of primary tuberculosis rather than urogenital disease
Ear, nose, and throat	Mastoiditis, chronic middle ear infection, and tonsillar tuberculosis are the most common forms in children
Eye involvement	Hypersensitivity reaction (phlyctenular conjunctivitis) and true tuberculosis of the eye

Tuberculous lymphadenitis usually develops within several weeks to 6–12 months of primary infection with *M. tuberculosis*. Lymphadenitis mainly follows lymphatic spread from a primary focus in the lung, tonsils, oropharynx, or from a site of distal skin implantation of the organism (as with *M. bovis* BCG).[3] Often the primary focus has resolved by the time lymphadenopathy presents. Hematogenous spread may lead to rare cases of generalized lymphadenitis. Inguinal lymphadenopathy may be associated with a psoas abscess and spinal tuberculosis.

In tuberculosis low-burden countries, nontuberculous mycobacteria (NTM)—mainly *M. avium* complex (MAC) in up to 80% of cases, but also *M. scrofulaceum* (United States and Australia) and *M. malmoense* and *M. haemophilum* in the United Kingdom, Scandinavia, and Northern Europe—are the most common mycobacteria causing peripheral lymphadenitis.[4–6] The increase in NTM-associated lymphadenitis in developed countries where BCG vaccination was discontinued suggests that BCG may have a protective effect in development of NTM-related lymphadenitis.[7,8] Where *M. bovis* (bovine TB) is not well controlled, *M. bovis* may cause substantial lymphadenitis in children. *M. bovis* BCG lymphadenitis as an adverse effect of BCG presenting mainly in the ipsilateral axillary area of where the BCG was administered, is common in infants and children less than 2 years of age in South Africa, especially in HIV-infected children.[9]

A differential diagnosis for peripheral lymphadenitis is summarized in Table 10.2.

Pathogenesis

Tuberculous lymphadenitis starts with granuloma formation and lymphoid hyperplasia, which may progress to caseation and necrosis. Usually more than one lymph node is involved, although one node may be more prominent. Nodes become matted due to periadenitis. If left untreated, nodes will undergo liquefaction, leading to one or more cold abscesses. These are fluctuant nodes, often with violaceous discoloration of the overlying skin. Spontaneous drainage with sinus formation may follow (scrofuloderma). If still not treated, nodes may come and go, with fluctuation, drainage, and scarring occurring over a long period of even years before final (scarred) healing or calcification occurs.

Table 10.2. Differential diagnosis for peripheral lymphadenitis

Infective causes

Acute suppurative: Pyogenic bacteria (usually painful, warm, and red)

Chronic granulomatous:

Mycobacteria: *M. tuberculosis, M. bovis, M. bovis* BCG, nontuberculous mycobacteria (NTM)

Fungi: Histoplasmosis, coccidioidomycosis, actinomycosis

Other infective causes: Toxoplasmosis, brucellosis, cat scratch disease (*Bartonella* species), sarcoidosis (rare)

Reactive hyperplasia: Viral—Infectious mononucleosis (Epstein Barr virus), HIV, cytomegalovirus

Idiopathic (undetermined cause)

Malignancy
Lymphoma, Kaposi's sarcoma, Hodgkin's disease, neuroblastoma, rhabdomyosarcoma, histiocytosis X

Congenital malformations
Branchial, thyroglossal, and/or dermoid cysts

Deep cavernous hemangioma

Diagnosis

CLINICAL PRESENTATION

Painless and non-tender swelling of peripheral nodes in the neck area, not responding to antibiotic therapy and with no other local cause for lymphadenopathy, usually more than 2x2 cm in diameter and often matted, are the clues to suspect mycobacterial infection. The lymph nodes are initially firm to hard, but may become fluctuant (cold abscess) and eventually present with sinus formation and draining pus.[3]

This can occur in any age group. A history of close contact with an infectious source case is found in only 50% of cases. The setting is important (*M. tuberculosis* vs. NTM), and age of the child and location of the lymphadenitis may also suggest the cause, as in *M. bovis* BCG adverse reaction. Constitutional symptoms are present in only 50–60% of cases. A positive tuberculin skin test (TST) is common and suggestive chest radiograph changes are seen—the latter, which are present in less than 50% of cases, may suggest *M. tuberculosis* as the cause, but in a non-endemic setting with no BCG received, a TST reaction less than 10 mm of induration could suggest NTM lymphadenitis. With NTM lymphadenitis, the same neck nodes are affected, are usually unilateral, with slow onset and rarely with any systemic symptoms or other organ involvement.

In a tuberculosis high-burden setting, a clinical algorithm in which children had persistent (>4 weeks) cervical adenopathy greater than 2x2 cm in size without a visible cause or response to antibiotic treatment was highly sensitive and specific for tuberculosis.[10]

IMAGING

Chest radiography should be done to show signs of pulmonary tuberculosis; however, absence of pulmonary findings does not rule out a diagnosis of peripheral tuberculous lymphadenitis. Ultrasound imaging of lymphadenitis will rarely add substantially to a clinical and bacteriological diagnosis. Computed tomography (CT) to determine the extent of disease may be indicated in deep-seated cervicofacial lymphadenitis.

BACTERIOLOGY AND HISTOLOGY

Confirmation of the diagnosis is by bacteriology and/or histology/cytology. Pus can be sent for culture of mycobacteria if there is a draining sinus. Fine-needle aspiration (FNA) is the method of choice for obtaining specimens for culture and histology/cytology.[9] FNA is a safe and well-tolerated procedure, which can be implemented in most settings, and the specimens can aid in making a definitive diagnosis of tuberculosis when submitted for culture or molecular tests.[11,12] This may be particularly important in low-burden settings where other diagnoses may predominate, and in settings where there is a high prevalence of drug-resistant tuberculosis. Molecular-based methods, which identify mycobacterial DNA, are increasingly utilized for the diagnosis of extrathoracic tuberculosis. Examples, such as GeneXpert MTB/RIF (GeneXpert; Cepheid, Sunnyvale, California) and line-probe assays, such as Genotype MTBDR*plus* (Hain Lifescience, Nehren, Germany), identify *M. tuberculosis* complex, which includes several species, including *M. bovis* and *M. bovis* BCG. If a BCG adverse effect is clinically suspected, further differentiation of species is indicated, which can be done by requesting a polymerase chain reaction (PCR) assay identifying the absence of the Region of Difference 1 (RD1), which is absent in all *M. bovis* BCG strains and present in *M. tuberculosis*.[13] We have used the rapid MPT64 commercial test kit to differentiate between *M. bovis* BCG and *M. tuberculosis* in the Copenhagen (Danish) BCG strain, as MBP64 (similar to MPT64 in *M. tuberculosis hominis*) is absent in some *M. bovis* BCG strains.[14] If cytology or staining of specimens show acid-fast bacilli (AFB) and an GeneXpert MTB/RIF or line-probe assay is negative, NTM is the likely cause, as both tests are highly sensitive for *M. tuberculosis* complex in AFB-positive specimens.

Complications

Peripheral lymphadenitis may develop draining abscesses and scarring. Lesions can infiltrate bone and nerves and cause compression of upper airways. In some patients, a paradoxical reaction may occur, with lymph nodes increasing in size or new lymph nodes appearing during and even after completion of treatment. This can be part of an immune reconstitution syndrome, but poor adherence to therapy, drug resistance, or incorrect diagnosis also should be considered in these cases.

OSTEOARTICULAR TUBERCULOSIS

Osteoarticular tuberculosis (OA-TB) is uncommon, occurring in only 1–4% of all tuberculosis cases and 10–20% of all extrapulmonary tuberculosis cases.[15–17] In endemic areas, children are more likely than adults to be affected. Fifty percent of all OA-TB is spinal tuberculosis, also known as tuberculous spondylitis or Pott's disease. The thoracic spine and lumbosacral spine are equally affected, while the cervical spine is affected the least.[18] The next commonly affected by OA-TB are the weight-bearing joints, usually single joints, such as the hips (50%), knees (20%), and ankle/foot (10%).[15] Elbow and shoulder joints are affected in 10–15% of cases. Any bone or joint can be affected; in 5–10% of cases, other bones, such as the skull, ribs, fingers, and toes, and sometimes multiple sites are affected. Multiple site involvement is almost exclusively found in young infants. The sites of OA-TB in children are summarized in Table 10.3.

Table 10.3. Sites of osteoarticular tuberculosis involvement in children

Spinal tuberculosis (50%)

Extra-spinal tuberculosis (40%):

—arthritis (synovial disease)

—osteomyelitis

—bursitis / tendon sheath (rare)

Uncommon forms (10%):

—Multiple cystic tuberculosis

—Disseminated skeletal tuberculosis

—Multiple diaphysitis

—Tuberculous dactylitis

PATHOGENESIS OF OA-TB

M. tuberculosis is the most common mycobacterium causing OA-TB, although *M. bovis* BCG, *M bovis, M. africanum,* and some NTM can also cause osteitis and/or arthritis.[15] The main route of osteoarticular infection is through hematogenous spread from a primary infection in the lungs, tonsils, or alimentary track. Chest radiographic changes are, however, only seen in approximately 50% of cases. Lymphatic spread, directly from the pleura into bone or direct infection through the skin, is rare but possible. A history of previous injury to the affected joint or soft tissue is often obtained.[15,17] Spread of the mycobacterial infection can be primarily to the metaphyses or to the synovium.

Spinal Tuberculosis

In spinal tuberculosis, mycobacteria are deposited via the end arterioles in the vertebral body adjacent to the anterior aspect of the vertebral end plate, therefore, the anterior inferior half of the vertebral body is most commonly involved.[16,17] Collapse of one or more anterior vertebral bodies results in gibbus deformity of the spine. Intervertebral disc spaces are usually affected late; the preservation of the intervertebral disc spaces is an important diagnostic feature of spinal tuberculosis. Subligamentous spread of infection may lead to multiple contiguous or skip vertebral body lesions. Extension of infection into adjacent soft tissue to form paravertebral or epidural abscesses is common. Epidural abscesses may cause neurological complications, such as cord compression.[16]

DIAGNOSIS OF SPINAL TUBERCULOSIS

Spinal tuberculosis usually has an insidious onset with slow progression, with back pain being the most common complaint. Young children may not be able to complain, but they often stop walking because of back pain or weakness. Hip pain with flexure contracture may indicate the development of a psoas abscess. Constitutional symptoms, such as fever, fatigue, weight loss, and night sweats may be present, but their absence does not rule out the diagnosis. A stiff or rigid spine due to muscle spasm is common. Acute onset of kyphosis with visible gibbus formation is common in children and can become very severe if not managed urgently. Neurological signs of weakness and/or paralysis may occur early. Complete paraplegia usually occurs late, due to missed diagnosis. Cold abscesses and sinus formation may occur in distant locations because pus can dissect along tissue planes. Cervical spine tuberculosis may present with torticollis, retropharyngeal abscess, cervical lymphadenopathy, and hoarseness.[15–17]

SPECIAL INVESTIGATIONS

Plain radiography of the whole spine (anteroposterior and lateral) remains the first special investigation in spinal tuberculosis.[17] The classical picture is destruction of two, usually adjacent, vertebral bodies with sparing of the disc space, with gibbus formation with or without a paravertebral abscess. In tuberculosis low-prevalence areas, it may be difficult to distinguish tuberculosis from other causes such as pyogenic and other infections and malignancies. Typical features of tuberculosis on radiography, if present, are involvement of the posterior elements of vertebra, calcification, and late preservation of the adjacent intervertebral disc(s). On chest radiography, features of pulmonary tuberculosis are present in approximately 50% of cases, and paraspinal abscesses may be seen in thoracic spine disease as a fusiform opacification adjacent to the spine (Figure 10.1) and in cervical spine tuberculosis as a nest-shaped opacification.

CT scans show bone destruction earlier than magnetic resonance imaging visualizing the disco-vertebral lesions and paravertebral abscesses. Smaller lesions than can be seen on plain radiography can be identified on CT, but soft-tissue spread such as epidural extension of the disease is not defined as well as with MRI.[19]

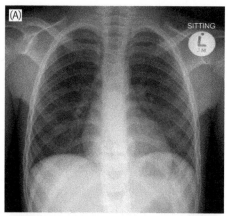

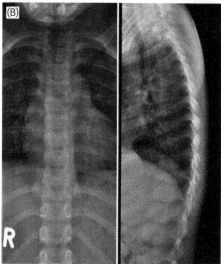

FIGURE 10.1 An 8-year-old girl. Mother has pulmonary tuberculosis. Child complained of hip pain, but hip radiograph was normal. Child lost weight, and did not want to walk or play. She had a rigid back on examination. *A.* Chest radiograph (antero-posterior) did not show any lung pathology, but fusiform opacification can be seen behind the heart shadow, indicating a paraspinal abscess. *B & C.* Fusiform opacification *(B)* and collapse of 10th thoracic vertebra can be seen *(B & C).*

MRI of the whole spine remains the investigation of choice. This is best done with gadolinium-diethylenetriamine pentaacetic acid (Gd-DTPA) enhancement.[20] This yields information on the condition of the spinal cord, spread of the disease to the soft tissues, and the extent of spinal cord involvement.[18] Pathology is visible on MRI before plain radiographs; for example, intravertebral abscess

formation can be seen before vertebral collapse occurs, and noncontiguous (skip) lesions are identified much more commonly with MRI (in 16–70% of spinal tuberculosis cases) than on plain spinal radiography.[19,21]

Bacteriological (by culture and/or molecular methods) and histological confirmation should be aimed for, both to confirm the diagnosis and for drug susceptibility testing (DST). Biopsies or FNA can be technically difficult and require the assistance of experienced surgeons. Radiological assistance, as with CT or fluoroscopic-guided FNA, may limit the need for open biopsies in some cases.[19,22] History of the source case DST is important, and the child should be treated according to the DST of the known source case's *M. tuberculosis* isolate. Drug-resistant tuberculosis of the spine may be associated with delayed diagnosis, advanced disease, and frequent complications,[23] so efforts to make a bacteriological diagnosis are especially important where the prevalence of drug-resistant tuberculosis is high or when drug-resistant disease is suspected.

COMPLICATIONS OF SPINAL TUBERCULOSIS

The most important complication, which should be prevented if at all possible, is paraplegia due to a thoracic or lower spinal lesion, or quadriplegia due to cervical spine tuberculosis. Early-onset paraplegia may be caused by mechanical pressure on the spinal cord by an abscess, tubercular debris, and caseous tissue, or by mechanical instability caused by subluxation or dislocation. Tuberculomas, tuberculous myelitis, tuberculous arachnoiditis, or infective spinal artery thrombosis may also lead to paraplegia.[17,18] Late-onset paraplegia (even many years after treatment completion) may be caused by transection of the spinal cord by a bony bridge or severe kyphotic deformity, or by fibrosis of the dura.[17,18] Immune reconstitution syndrome associated with onset of antiretroviral therapy may also cause acute paraplegia due to new or worsening pathology, in our experience. Table 10.4 lists indications for surgery in spinal tuberculosis.

In addition to the physical deformity caused by severe kyphosis, severe thoracic spine kyphosis may also impair lung function. Extension of infection along the ilio-psoas muscle may result in psoas abscesses and discharging sinuses in unusual

Table 10.4. Indications for surgery in the management of spinal tuberculosis

Absolute indications:

- Marked neurological deficit (due to surgically correctable causes)
- Large abscess causing respiratory distress
- Neurological deficit worsening despite adequate tuberculosis treatment
- Progression of kyphosis or spinal instability, despite adequate tuberculosis treatment

Relative indications:

- To obtain adequate material for culture and drug susceptibility testing for diagnosis
- Persistence of pain or spasticity due to demonstrable mechanical block
- Pain related to spinal instability
- To drain paraspinal or psoas abscesses if not responding to adequate tuberculosis treatment

General indications from the literature:

- Uncertain diagnosis (etiology)
- Draining of large abscesses
- Failure of conservative treatment (antituberculosis therapy)
- Progression of neurological deficit
- Impeding or progressive kyphosis

Adapted from Storm M, Vlok GJ. Musculoskeletal and spinal tuberculosis in adults and children. In: *Tuberculosis: A Comprehensive Clinical Reference.* Schaaf HS and Zumla AI, eds. London: Saunders, Elsevier Publishers; 2009:494–503.

locations, such as the buttocks, groin, or chest. In cervical spine tuberculosis, paravertebral abscesses may occur in retropharyngeal locations and may cause upper airway obstruction.

Tuberculous Arthritis

Tuberculosis involving the synovial joints is the second most common form of OA-TB after spinal disease.[15,16] More than 90% of tuberculous arthritis is monoarthritis, with the hip or knee affected in the majority of cases, although any joint may be involved.

PATHOGENESIS

The bacilli are almost always spread by hematogenous route from a primary focus to the bone or joint. Joints become involved either by transphyseal spread from a primary/reactivated metaphyseal osteomyelitis (granulomas) crossing the epiphyseal plate into the joint space, or by seeding of the synovium directly via the bloodstream causing tuberculous synovitis, which may then spread transphyseally to the metaphysis.[15,16]

DIAGNOSIS OF TUBERCULOUS ARTHRITIS

A high index of suspicion is needed to make the diagnosis. Chest radiography may be suggestive of tuberculosis in up to 50% of cases, and can assist in the diagnosis. Imaging of affected joints may strengthen the suspicion and is helpful, but the final diagnosis is by positive bacteriology.

Tuberculosis usually causes a monoarthritis in large, weight-bearing joints but occasionally may involve other joints or multiple joints. The clinical symptoms and signs usually have an insidious course. There frequently is a history of previous trauma, and in such cases, symptoms may develop more rapidly. Pain (80%), loss of function (80%), swelling (30%), sinus tract formation (20%), and (cold) abscess formation (20%) are all relatively common findings but develop over time. Tuli describes the natural history of tuberculous arthritis as progressing through five stages (Table 10.5).[24]

Plain radiography is usually done first. Radiographic findings vary with the site and age of the lesion, and may be difficult to distinguish from other infectious and inflammatory causes of arthritis.[25] Initial radiographic imaging may be normal, but the imaging findings are progressive in nature, usually starting off with periarticular soft-tissue swelling, joint effusion (initial widening of joint space), osteopenia, subchondral cystic erosion (lytic lesions), and eventually progressing to joint-space narrowing, collapse, and sclerosis with deformity and, finally, ankyloses (Figure 10.2). The Phemister's triad is described as characteristic of tuberculous arthritis: (1) juxtarticular osteopenia, (2) peripheral osseous erosions, and (3) gradual narrowing of joint space.

Other helpful diagnostic imaging methods in tuberculous arthritis are:

—Ultrasound: may demonstrate joint effusions, synovitis (thickened synovium), associated

Table 10.5. Tuli's classification of the natural history of tuberculous arthritis progressing through 5 stages

STAGE OF TUBERCULOUS ARTHRITIS	CLINICAL FINDINGS	RADIOGRAPHIC FINDINGS	EXPECTED OUTCOME
Stage I Sinovitis	Soft-tissue swelling with 75% motion preserved	Soft-tissue swelling and osteopenia	Normal or minimal residual joint problem
Stage II Early arthritis	Soft-tissue swelling with 25–50% loss of motion	Soft-tissue swelling, marginal joint erosions, and diminution in joint space	50–70% joint mobility
Stage III Advanced arthritis	75% loss of motion	Marginal erosions, cysts, and significant loss of joint space	Stable, painless joint after salvage, with or without motion
Stage IV Advanced arthritis	75% loss of motion plus subluxation or dislocation	Joint destruction	Stable, painless joint after salvage
Stage V Ankylosis	Ankylosis (fixed joint)	Ankylosis	Stable, painless joint

Adapted from Tuli SM. General principles of osteoarticular tuberculosis. *Clin Orthop Relat Res.* 2002;(398):11–19.

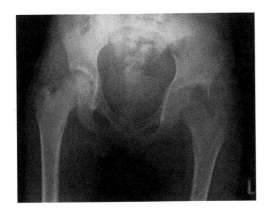

FIGURE 10.2 A 10-yr-old girl with a history of injury of left hip and thigh, but pain not improving. On plain radiography, lytic lesions are seen in the left acetabulum as well as osteopenia and a narrowed joint space.

soft-tissue masses and tendon sheath involvement, but is unlikely to distinguish from other causes of arthritides.[26] It also aids the aspiration of these effusions for mycobacterial culture and DST.[16]

—CT: may demonstrate the extent of bone destruction and extension into the surrounding tissue and may differentiate between tuberculous arthritis and neoplasm.

—MRI: where available, MRI is the imaging modality of choice. It demonstrates bone marrow changes, joint effusion, synovitis, pannus and erosions of cartilage and bone, but these findings are still nonspecific.[16,25]

The microbiological diagnosis of tuberculous arthritis is achieved by joint aspiration or synovial biopsy. Specimens (synovial tissue and synovial fluid) should be sent for cytology/histology and bacteriological confirmation of mycobacterial infection, as well as for DST. GeneXpert MTB/RIF or other molecular tests may be very helpful in confirming the diagnosis early on synovial fluid, as culture of synovial fluid gives positive mycobacterial yield in up to 80%, while smear-microscopy for AFB has a yield of only 20–40%.[15,27] The gold standard remains mycobacterial culture of tissue and/or fluid, preferably on liquid media by automated method, which is more rapid than the solid media methods.

Chronic Tuberculous Rheumatism (Poncet's Disease)

Poncet's disease is a rare condition that presents as a polyarthritis associated with tuberculosis elsewhere in the body, usually extrapulmonary (including mediastinal lymph nodes and pleural effusion). There is no evidence of bacteriological involvement of the joints, so it is considered a reactive arthritis. Once the diagnosis has been made, treating the tuberculosis disease usually rapidly resolves the arthritis.[15]

Tuberculous Osteomyelitis

PATHOGENESIS

Tuberculous osteomyelitis occurs in only 3–11% of OA-TB cases in children.[15,16] It is most commonly found in bones of the extremities, especially tubular and flat bones such as the small bones of the hands and feet, and the skull, but it can affect any bone. The mycobacteria usually implant in the medulla of the metaphysis or, less often, in the diaphysis. A granulomatous lesion is formed and enlarges, with eventual caseation and liquefactive necrosis.[26] Transphyseal spread to the joint or erosion through the cortex with formation of a paraosseous mass may occur. Single lesions are the majority, but multifocal lesions may occur, especially in young children.

DIAGNOSIS OF TUBERCULOUS OSTEOMYELITIS

Clinical presentation: Symptoms and signs most commonly associated with tuberculous osteomyelitis are pain, swelling, erythema (redness), and refusal to bear weight. Associated pulmonary disease is found in less than 50% of cases.

Plain radiographs show mainly soft-tissue swelling, some periosteal reaction (which can be extensive in infants with multiple bone lesions or dactylitis), osteolysis with minimal reactive change, periarticular osteopenia, and erosions. Some unusual forms of osteomyelitis are: closed cystic tuberculosis, which presents as well-defined cystic lesions in bone; multiple (cystic) bone lesions or disseminated bone tuberculosis (mainly infants); tuberculous dactylitis; and closed multiple diaphysitis. Dactylitis can present as spina ventosa, which is a spindle-shaped expansion with multiple layers of subperiosteal new bone and occurs in the short tubular bones of the hands and feet. MRI may demonstrate intraosseous lesions earlier than with other imaging modalities, but cannot generally distinguish tuberculosis from other causes.[26]

Given the nonspecific clinical and imaging findings, obtaining a sample for histology and microbiology is critical to making a diagnosis of tuberculous osteomyelitis.[16] Microbiological diagnosis may require sampling of other sites such as the lungs, if affected. Though data are limited, newer molecular techniques may be important contributors to the diagnosis and are an option where available.[27,28]

ABDOMINAL TUBERCULOSIS

Abdominal tuberculosis is relatively unusual in children, although underestimation is likely, as abdominal ultrasound is not routinely done in children with tuberculosis in high-burden settings. In one study, 11 out of 47 (23%) children with confirmed pulmonary tuberculosis either had abdominal lymphadenopathy or other lesions of abdominal tuberculosis found on ultrasound.[29] The majority of abdominal tuberculosis occurs in adults, with only 10–20% occurring in children. Abdominal tuberculosis may occur as early as the first weeks of life, due to congenital spread of *M. tuberculosis*, which may present as a primary focus (granuloma) in the liver, intra-abdominal lymphadenopathy, and peritoneal spread with ascites.[30] Although abdominal tuberculosis can present at any age in children, it is expected that the majority of cases will present in those younger than 5 years of age because this is the peak age of childhood disease. However, many reports claim the majority of children to be older, which is most likely because of missed diagnosis in younger children. Because of its nonspecific presentation, diagnosis is often delayed, leading to increased morbidity and mortality.

Epidemiology, Pathogenesis, and Etiology

The classification of abdominal tuberculosis is not consistent in the literature; therefore, the reported prevalence varies from <1% to approximately 10% of childhood tuberculosis cases.[31] Some authors define abdominal tuberculosis as only intestinal or peritoneal disease with associated lymphadenitis, while others include peritonitis, intestinal disease, abdominal lymphadenopathy, and tuberculosis of solid viscera (mainly liver and spleen). These sites can be involved independently or in combination. Taking all of these sites together, abdominal tuberculosis constitutes approximately 12% of extrapulmonary disease and 1–3% of all tuberculosis in children.[32,33]

Abdominal tuberculosis is caused mainly by *M. tuberculosis*. In children, the majority of cases follow hematogenous and/or lymphatic spread from a primary focus elsewhere, mainly pulmonary. Retrograde lymphatic spread from intrathoracic disease to abdominal lymph nodes may occur. A rare form in children is primary intestinal infection caused by swallowing of infected sputum, which is more likely in older children with cavitary pulmonary disease. *M. bovis* will also cause primary intestinal and mesenteric lymph node disease in children in regions where *M. bovis* infection is present and infected milk is not pasteurized.[34] NTM, especially *M. avium intracellulare*, is a rare cause of intra-abdominal lymphadenitis occurring in severely immunocompromised children and should be considered especially in HIV-infected children with CD4 T-cell counts <50/μL.

Peritonitis and Lymph Node Tuberculosis

Peritoneal and nodal disease are more common in children than intestinal tuberculosis. Tuberculous peritonitis results from lymphohematogenous spread (recent, or reactivation of old focus), or contiguous spread from a mesenteric lymph node or an intestinal focus.[35–37] Peritoneal tuberculosis occurs in three types: (1) wet type with ascites—the most common form; (2) encysted or loculated type with localized abdominal swelling; and (3) a fibrotic type with abdominal masses composed of matted and thickened mesenterium, omentum, and intestinal loops felt as lump(s) in the abdomen.[35,39] Both visceral and parietal peritoneal layers are affected with the formation of multiple tuberculous nodules and ascites, often associated with intra-abdominal lymphadenopathy.[36,39]

Intestinal Tuberculosis

Ingestion of mycobacteria (infected sputum, unpasteurized milk products) is the most common route of infection. The distal ileum and cecum are most often affected, but any part of the intestine can be involved, with the proximal small bowel the least affected. Mucosal thickening (hypertrophic form), mucosal ulceration (ulcerative form), or a combination (ulcerohypertrophic form) may occur, and lesions may be circumferential.

Visceral Tuberculosis

Although any solid viscera in the abdomen can be affected, the liver and spleen are most commonly involved. Tuberculosis in these viscera can occur as miliary lesions, nodular lesions (granuloma), or solitary abscess forms. Except for miliary spread to these viscera in young children, the other types are extremely rare. Splenic microabscesses seen on ultrasonography, mainly in immunocompromised children, may be due to tuberculosis.

Diagnosis of Abdominal Tuberculosis

CLINICAL PRESENTATION

The clinical features of abdominal tuberculosis are varied and nonspecific. A high index of suspicion should be maintained in children with unexplained abdominal disease or fever of unknown origin. In high-burden areas, abdominal tuberculosis should be considered in any child presenting with nonspecific constitutional symptoms and long-standing abdominal complaints, which may be present from weeks to months (before and after presentation to health care facilities). Although the majority of these children will present with chronic or acute on chronic onset of symptoms, a few children present with an apparent acute abdomen, often mimicking an acute appendicitis or intestinal obstruction.

Commonly presenting symptoms and signs vary widely between studies. In eight studies with a total of 467 children with abdominal tuberculosis, the following were the most common symptoms and signs:[31,33,39–44] abdominal pain 44–100%, abdominal distension 35–92%, fever (often low grade) 34–90%, failure to thrive or loss of weight 30–78%, malnutrition 28–90%, abdominal mass 12–56%, ascites 7–44%, diarrhea or constipation (almost equal) 15–30%, and peripheral lymphadenopathy 8–49%. Less frequent symptoms are vomiting, gastrointestinal hemorrhage, and hematochezia. Although a "doughy" abdomen on palpation is a well-known clinical sign, it is not common: present in only 4–28% of these cases.

Evidence of close contact with a tuberculosis source case was reported in only 31–65% of cases. TST was positive in only 33–68% of children in four studies.[31,33,41,42] The TST may be negative because of severe illness or malnutrition and does not exclude the disease.

IMAGING STUDIES

Evidence of pulmonary tuberculosis on chest radiography, current or past, is found in 20–60% of children with abdominal tuberculosis and may alert the clinician to the correct diagnosis. However, children may present without specific respiratory complaints, and therefore chest radiography is often not requested.

Abdominal radiography is of little value, but it may show intestinal obstruction, suggest ascites, and in rare cases show evidence of intestinal perforation or calcification of lymph nodes or granulomas in solid viscera.[38] Bowel contrast studies are not usually performed in children.[45]

Abdominal ultrasound is often the initial investigation of choice and widely available. It may demonstrate enlarged para-aortic, porta hepatis, and mesenteric lymph nodes. Ultrasound is better than CT for detecting ascites, and may demonstrate fibrin strands, loculations, and debris, which if present are more indicative of tuberculosis. Other possible findings on ultrasound are bowel wall thickening (often obscured by bowel gas), omental mass, focal lesions (single or multiple nodular abscess) in the liver and spleen, and psoas abscess (retroperitoneal).[46]

Abdominal CT scan (and MRI) perform better than ultrasound in identifying intra-abdominal lymphadenopathy and may show the characteristic appearance of tuberculous lymph nodes with ring-enhancement and low-density centers.[45] Inflammatory masses composed of bowel loops, adherent omentum, and lymphadenopathy are demonstrated as omental cakes immediately deep to the abdominal wall. Solid visceral lesions appear as low-density single or multifocal areas in the liver or spleen, and rarely in the pancreas; these lesions may calcify over time. A combination of the above CT features, especially when lymphadenopathy is rim-enhancing or calcified, is highly suggestive of abdominal tuberculosis.[45]

LABORATORY INVESTIGATIONS

Few laboratory investigations other than mycobacterial confirmation add to the diagnosis of abdominal tuberculosis. TST or IGRAs may confirm tuberculosis infection, but do not confirm abdominal tuberculosis disease.

Ascitic fluid should be obtained if present. Chemistry usually shows an exudate (and rarely chyle) with a high albumin (>25 g/L) and a low serum-ascites albumin gradient of less than 11 g/L. Lymphocytes usually predominate (>70%) and in combination with a high adenosine deaminase (ADA) level of >35 U/L are highly suggestive of tuberculosis. However, normal or low ADA levels may occur with low-protein ascites and with HIV infection; therefore a low ADA does not exclude tuberculosis.[35,38]

Bacteriological confirmation of mycobacterial disease should be attempted. Culture and/or molecular-based (polymerase chain reaction [PCR]) bacteriology of extra-abdominal specimens such as sputum, gastric aspirates, and peripheral lymph node FNA are helpful if positive for *M. tuberculosis*, but do not confirm abdominal tuberculosis. Smear microscopy for AFB has an extremely low yield of <5% on ascitic fluid, and culture is positive in <20% of cases. GeneXpert MTB/RIF, although less sensitive than culture, gives an immediate result and may detect some cases in which culture is negative, and should therefore be performed when available.[28] Stool specimens for GeneXpert MTB/RIF could possibly also be used for intestinal tuberculosis.[47,48]

Laparoscopy has confirmed value in the diagnosis of abdominal tuberculosis. Visualization of the peritoneal space with ascites, fibrous bands, and adhesions of the peritoneum and omentum; yellow-white nodules on peritoneal surfaces; enlarged lymph nodes; edematous and distended bowel loops allows a presumptive diagnosis of abdominal tuberculosis. Histology and bacteriology of biopsied material (peritoneal, lymph node, omental) often provide confirmation of the diagnosis and exclude other pathology.[38] Ultrasound or CT-guided percutaneous biopsies of peritoneal, omental, or solid viscera lesions for both histology and bacteriological confirmation are possible, but rarely done in children.[49]

If intestinal tuberculosis is suspected, colonoscopy may be a valuable investigation, even in children. Ulcers are the most common finding; these are typically transverse and superficial with irregular edges and mainly situated in the ileocecal region. Biopsies for histology and bacteriology should be obtained to confirm the diagnosis.[38]

The diagnosis is often confirmed when a laparotomy is done for complications such as intestinal obstruction, perforation, or possible appendicitis. Biopsies can be done, and consistent features, as with laparoscopy, can be observed. In some cases, laparotomy needs to be done to confirm the diagnosis if all other methods of confirmation have failed.[38]

In the absence of sophisticated investigations or ability to confirm the diagnosis, a trial of therapy remains an option, but such management should be closely monitored, as lymphoma is one of the most important differential diagnoses.[38,39]

Complications

Intestinal complications such as bowel obstruction due to inflammatory process, strictures, or adhesions may occur. Ulcerations and bowel perforation may occur. Fistulas may form to the skin or other bowel segments. Malabsorption with resultant malnutrition is common with long-standing intestinal tuberculosis. Intestinal lymphangiectasis may develop, as well as chyloperitoneum. Rare vascular complications include portal vein thrombosis and mesenteric artery aneurysms.[50,51]

CUTANEOUS TUBERCULOSIS

Cutaneous tuberculosis, which includes a diverse spectrum of dermatological manifestations involving the skin, occurs in <1% of all tuberculosis cases and in 1–4% of all extrathoracic tuberculosis in children.[52–54] Cutaneous tuberculosis is mainly caused by *M. tuberculosis*, but can also be caused by *M. bovis* and *M. bovis* BCG. In some regions, NTM may cause cutaneous lesions more often than *M. tuberculosis* complex. The clinical picture of cutaneous tuberculosis is similar in adults and in children. In our experience, scrofuloderma is the most common form, although it is usually reported according to the underlying lesion of either lymph node or bone tuberculosis, rather than as cutaneous disease.

Pathogenesis

Cutaneous tuberculosis presents in different clinical and pathological forms, although there may be substantial overlap.[55] The form of cutaneous disease that develops is dictated by the route of infection (exogenous or endogenous), the patient's prior contact (infection) with *M. tuberculosis* complex, the effectiveness of the patient's immune system, as well as the number and virulence of the infecting organisms.[55,56] Different classifications of cutaneous tuberculosis have been proposed, but current classifications are based on the route of infection and the number of organisms in the lesions. Table 10.6 summarizes the classification, basic pathology, clinical features, and usual outcome of TST, and bacteriological test results of cutaneous tuberculosis.

The histological hallmark of cutaneous tuberculosis is granulomatous inflammation, which may vary from sarcoidal or tuberculoid to necrotizing, suppurative, or palisading granulomas. Necrotizing vasculitis may be present in some forms such as the tuberculids. The epidermis may be atrophic, hyperplastic, or ulcerated, and scarring may vary from mild to severe. Histopathological findings may indicate the diagnosis, but they should be supported by the clinical picture and identification of *M. tuberculosis* organisms in skin lesions or other organs. The identification of *M. tuberculosis* in the lesion depends on the form of cutaneous disease, the adequacy of the tissue sample obtained, and the methods of identification (microscopy/culture/PCR) available.

Clinical Presentation

The classification of clinical forms of cutaneous tuberculosis is summarized in Table 10.6. The more common forms seen in children are presented below.[52,55,56]

Scrofuloderma (Figure 10.3) is the most common form of cutaneous tuberculosis in children. It develops from contiguous spread of peripheral lymph node disease at any site, mostly in the cervicofacial region, but also from a tuberculous focus in the bones, joints, testes, breasts, lacrimal glands, and, rarely, abdomen. It starts as a painless subcutaneous swelling, which over time becomes fluctuant with violaceous discoloration of overlying skin, and eventually forms an ulcer or draining sinus. Lesions can be multiple and widespread. It may heal spontaneously over months to years, leaving scars. Pulmonary or other systemic tuberculous involvement is found in approximately 50% of cases. Diagnosis is by FNA of the lesion before ulceration occurs or by skin biopsy from the edge of the sinus for histology/cytology and bacteriological confirmation. A pus swab from the lesion often yields a positive smear for AFB and/or positive culture for *M. tuberculosis*.

Lupus vulgaris (Figures 10.4 and 10.5) mainly follows hematogenous or lymphatic spread but can also be caused by contiguous spread or exogenous inoculation in patients previously infected with *M. tuberculosis*. The main sites of these lesions are the head and neck, but in some countries, the lower extremities and gluteal area are more often affected in children due to inoculation tuberculosis.[52] It

is a slowly progressive form of cutaneous disease starting as asymptomatic papules and plaques. The plaques form as a result of coalescing granulomatous papules that have been described as resembling apple-jelly nodules on applying pressure with a glass slide (diascopy).[52,55] Enlarging plaques show active peripheral margins with redness and infiltration, and central atrophy and scarring. If it is allowed to progress, severe fibrosis, joint contractures, and mutilation may follow in some children. Constitutional symptoms are usually absent, but underlying tuberculosis may be present in lymph nodes or lungs. Biopsy from the active margin shows tuberculoid granulomas and epidermal hyperplasia with no necrosis. Ziehl-Neelsen stains are mostly negative, but culture of biopsied material may be positive for *M. tuberculosis*.

Tuberculous verrucosa cutis (Figure 10.6) follows exogenous inoculation of *M. tuberculosis* into the skin of mainly the hands and feet in patients previously infected with *M. tuberculosis*. It is relatively common in children with lesions more often in the lower limbs. It starts as a warty, indurated nodule or papule, which extends to a verrucous (warty) plaque. Constitutional symptoms are absent, but lymph nodes may be enlarged. Skin biopsy should be taken from the least keratotic area and be deep enough to include the underlying indurated lesion.[52] Pathological findings include caseating granulomas in the dermis, but Ziehl-Neelsen staining of tissue usually reveals only sparse bacilli.[55]

Tuberculous gumma (metastatic tuberculous abscess) follows hematogenous dissemination from a primary focus in children with lowered immunity. One or several subcutaneous nodules form, which become fluctuant due to necrosis and may eventually ulcerate or form sinus tracts. Biopsies show granulomatous inflammation with caseous necrosis mainly in the subcutaneous tissue, which extends to the dermis. Ziehl-Neelsen stains of pus swab or biopsy specimens show bacilli.

Tuberculous chancre (Figure 10.7) is rare in children. It occurs after penetrating skin trauma, such as ear piercing, ritual scarring, or tattooing, and can be an adverse effect after BCG vaccination. The lesion develops at the site of inoculation in a naïve host. An indurated papulonodular lesion forms at the site of trauma within weeks, which subsequently ulcerates, with or without regional lymphadenitis. Bacilli are easily demonstrated in pus or biopsy by Ziehl-Neelsen stain or mycobacterial culture.

Table 10.6. Classification of cutaneous tuberculosis and associated findings

ROUTE OF INFECTION	DISEASE FORM	HOST IMMUNITY AND BACILLARY LOAD	CLINICAL APPEARANCE	TST RESULT	IDENTIFICATION OF M. TUBERCULOSIS COMPLEX	PATHOLOGY AND SITES OF LESIONS
EXOGENOUS						
Direct inoculation	Tuberculous chancre	Naïve host, primary infection. Also after BCG vaccination. Multibacillary	Painless papulonodule, ulcerates +/– lymphadenopathy.	±	ZN+/Culture +	Papulonodular lesion, forms ulcer. Primary granulomatous focus/ complex, ++ bacilli. Face or limbs (e.g., skin or ear piercing).
Direct inoculation	Tuberculosis verrucosa cutis (warty tuberculosis)	High immunity Previous infection. Paucibacillary	Initial warty nodule, expands to verrucous plaque with caseating center.	+	ZN ±, culture ±	Epidermal hyperkeratosis & papillomatosis. Dermal tuberculoid granuloma +/– bacilli. Typically hands or feet.
Direct inoculation	Lupus vulgaris (some cases)	Moderate immunity. Previous/current tuberculosis. BCG vaccination. Paucibacillary	Plaque type: gelatinous (apple-jelly nodule); hypertrophic type: soft nodule; ulcerative type: necrosis; vegetative type: papule with ulceration/ necrosis.	+	Culture ±	Intradermal tuberculoid granuloma with little/ no necrosis +/– bacilli. Head & neck (esp. nose), less commonly limbs, feet, gluteal area and trunk.
ENDOGENOUS						
Hematogenous, lymphatic, contiguous	Lupus vulgaris	Moderate–high immunity. Paucibacillary	See Lupus vulgaris above.	+	Culture ±	See Lupus vulgaris above.
Contiguous	Scrofuloderma	High immunity. Multibacillary.	Painless, reddish purple nodule over tuberculous lymph node or bone/joint tuberculosis, suppurate, ulcerates ± sinus tract.	+	ZN+, culture+	Necrosis, abscess, scarring, +bacilli. Neck and submandibular, but any site overlying TB lesion.

Route	Type	Immunity	Clinical features	TST	ZN/Culture	Histology
Hematogenous	Miliary tuberculosis	Low immunity. Multibacillary.	Profuse discrete pinpoint papules, pustules.	±, but often –	ZN±, culture+	Microabscesses and necrosis, bacilli ++.
Hematogenous	Tuberculous gumma/metastatic abscess	Low immunity. Multibacillary.	Subcutaneous nodules, necrosis, and ulcerate. Simulate scrofuloderma.	±	ZN+, culture+	Necrosis, abscess, ulcerate, bacilli++.
Autoinoculation	Orificial tuberculosis	Very low immunity. Multibacillary.	Red-yellow nodules break down, painful punched-out ulcers.	Often –	ZN+, culture+	Tuberculoid granuloma, bacilli++. Mucosa/skin around orifices.
			TUBERCULIDS			
Hematogenous	Lichen scrofulosorum	High immunity.	Numerous tiny perifollicular lichenoid papules.	+	Culture–	Granulomatous perifolliculitis, no bacilli Trunk, mainly children.
Hematogenous	Papulonecrotic tuberculid	High immunity.	Recurring crops skin-colored/red papules with central necrosis, ulceration, crusts, and pustules.	+	Culture–, PCR±	Wedge-shaped necrosis upper dermis. Ears, extensor surfaces limbs, buttocks.
Hematogenous	Erythema induratum of Bazin (EIB)	High immunity.	Red violaceous nodules on the calves, often painful, may ulcerate and heal with scarring.	±	Culture–	Granuloma, necrosis, panniculitis, vasculitis. Posterior calves.
Hematogenous	Nodular/phlebitis tuberculid	High immunity.	Few/many dull red or bluish-red non-tender nodules 1 cm —non-ulcerating.	+	Culture–, PCR±	Granulomas, necrosis, some vasculitis in superficial dermis. Anteromedial aspects legs of children.

PCR = polymerase chain reaction; TST = tuberculin skin test; ZN = Ziehl-Neelsen stain for acid-fast bacilli; + = positive; − = negative; ± = positive or negative.

Adapted from Barbagallo J, Tager P, Ingleton R, Hirsch RJ, Weinberg JM. Cutaneous tuberculosis: diagnosis and treatment. *Am J Clin Dermatol.* 2002;3:319–328. With added information from: Sethuraman G, Ramesh V. Cutaneous tuberculosis in children. *Pediatr Dermatol.* 2013;30:7–16; Jordaan HF, Scneider JW. Dermatological manifestations of tuberculosis in adults and children. In: *Tuberculosis: A Comprehensive Clinical Reference.* Schaaf HS and Zumla AI, eds. London: Saunders, Elsevier Publishers; 2009:484–493.

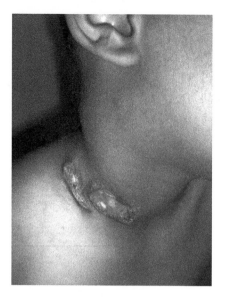

FIGURE 10.3   Scrofuloderma in cervical region from contiguous spread from underlying tuberculous lymph nodes.

Courtesy of Dr. W. I. Visser, Division of Dermatology, Stellenbosch University

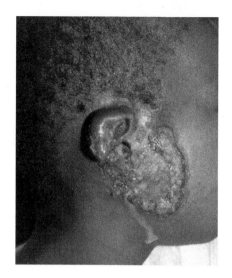

FIGURE 10.5   Lupus vulgaris of the ear and right cheek.

Courtesy of Dr. W. I. Visser, Division of Dermatology, Stellenbosch University

Miliary cutaneous TB may rarely accompany underlying miliary disease as a result of hematogenous spread. It presents as widespread small erythematous papules, pustules, or vesicles. Skin biopsy shows numerous micro-abscesses, and Ziehl-Neelsen stain and culture demonstrate mycobacteria.

Tuberculids are mostly referred to as delayed-type hypersensitivity reactions to *M. tuberculosis* in patients with good immunity and underlying and often subclinical tuberculosis elsewhere in the body. Although Ziehl-Neelsen stain for bacilli and culture for *M. tuberculosis* are always negative, *M. tuberculosis* DNA can be shown by PCR in a quarter to half of the patients.[55] Tuberculids are divided into different groups, but classifications often do not fully agree, demonstrating that it is most likely a spectrum of clinico-pathological manifestations of cutaneous tuberculosis. *Lichen scrofulosorum* (Figure 10.8) is

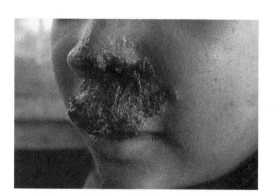

FIGURE 10.4   Lupus vulgaris of the nose and upper lip.

Courtesy of Dr. W. I. Visser, Division of Dermatology, Stellenbosch University

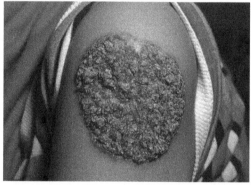

FIGURE 10.6   Tuberculosis verrucosa cutis of the shoulder.

Courtesy of Dr. W. I. Visser, Division of Dermatology, Stellenbosch University

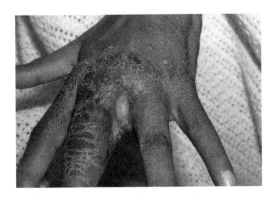

FIGURE 10.7 Primary tuberculous chancre of the hand.

Courtesy of Dr. W. I. Visser, Division of Dermatology, Stellenbosch University

the most superficial of these lesions and most commonly reported tuberculid in children. The lesions consist of asymptomatic, tiny yellow to red follicular and parafollicular papules on the trunk that usually heal without scarring. *Papulonecrotic tuberculids* (Figures 10.9 and 10.10) are situated in the upper dermis and epidermis and present as recurring crops of skin-colored to red papules that often show central necrosis, ulceration, crusts, and pustules that heal in time with small, depressed scars. The lesions may be symmetrical and widespread or localized, and typically involve the ears and extensor surfaces of the limbs, but also occur on the face or buttocks.

Phlyctenular conjunctivitis has been associated with papulonecrotic tuberculids in one series.[57] *Nodular tuberculids* (Figure 10.11) are lesions situated in the superficial dermis and show features of both papulonecrotic tuberculids and erythema induratum of Bazin. The lesions present as red to bluish-red non-tender nodules approximately 1 cm in diameter on the legs of children. *Erythema induratum of Bazin* (Figure 10.12) is a panniculitis that presents as red violaceous nodules that classically occur on the calves/lower legs, mainly in female patients. The nodules may be painful and undergo ulceration, with prolonged healing and scarring.

Diagnosis

As with other forms of tuberculosis, a high index of suspicion in cutaneous TB is necessary, and considering tuberculosis in the differential diagnosis of cutaneous lesions remains important; if this is followed, a clinical diagnosis of cutaneous tuberculosis can be made with reasonable confidence in most cases.[55] The diagnosis should be confirmed whenever possible by histology/cytology and by mycobacterial culture or PCR-based techniques. PCR-based techniques are increasingly being used to confirm a diagnosis and appear to have good sensitivity and specificity for many forms of cutaneous tuberculosis, with the added advantage of a more rapid result.[58,59] DST should also be done

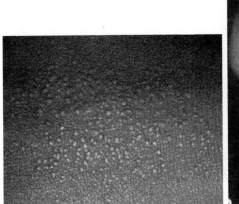
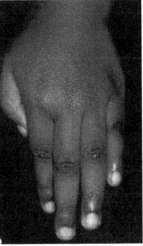

FIGURE 10.8 Lichen scrofulosorum on the trunk and hand of two different patients.

Courtesy of Dr. W. I. Visser, Division of Dermatology, Stellenbosch University

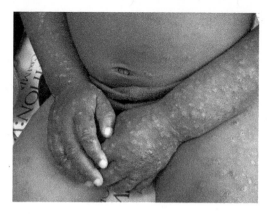

FIGURE 10.9   Papulonecrotic tuberculids on the extensor surfaces of the hands and legs of a child.

Courtesy of Dr. W. I. Visser, Division of Dermatology, Stellenbosch University

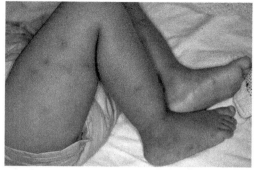

FIGURE 10.11   Nodular tuberculids on the legs of a young child.

Courtesy of Dr. W. I. Visser, Division of Dermatology, Stellenbosch University

when possible, particularly in settings with a high burden of drug resistance, as multidrug-resistant cutaneous tuberculosis is possible and may influence the response to treatment.[60,61] Specimens for identification of *M. tuberculosis* can be obtained by skin biopsy and/or FNA of associated lymphadenopathy. In cases of open ulcers or draining sinuses, Ziehl-Neelsen staining of smears from pus swabs may identify acid-fast bacilli, and mycobacterial cultures can be performed.

Cutaneous tuberculosis may be the first clinical manifestation of underlying systemic disease, so it is essential that a full clinical evaluation be performed, including a history of onset of both systemic and cutaneous lesions, contact with a tuberculosis case, a full clinical examination, and special investigations such as a TST, chest radiograph, and possibly other imaging, and bacteriological confirmation from other sites of infection such as the lungs and bones.

TUBERCULOSIS OF THE KIDNEY AND URINARY TRACT

Renal tuberculosis in children is very rare, as it usually does not develop before five or more years after primary infection in immune-competent children;

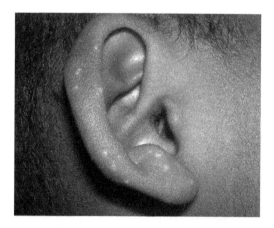

FIGURE 10.10   Papulonecrotic tuberculids on the pinna of the ear.

Courtesy of Dr. W. I. Visser, Division of Dermatology, Stellenbosch University

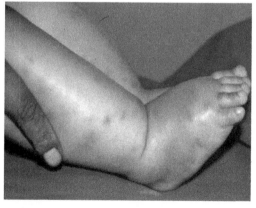

FIGURE 10.12   Erythema induratum of Bazin on lower legs and feet of an infant.

Courtesy of Dr. W. I. Visser, Division of Dermatology, Stellenbosch University

however, it has been described to occur in young children in the context of HIV infection.[62–65]

Pathogenesis

Renal tuberculosis is a late complication rarely seen in childhood, despite the fact that tubercle bacilli can often be recovered from the urine of children with recent primary infection following hematogenous spread. Granulomas develop in the glomeruli of the renal cortex, which for unknown reasons become manifest only years later.[64] Further progression to caseation and breaching of the collecting parenchyma leads to dissemination of the bacilli throughout the urinary tract.[66] Whereas renal tuberculosis develops from reactivation of a focus from hematogenous spread to the kidney, tuberculosis of the urinary tract, bladder, and genital tract almost always follows contiguous spread from the kidney. The disease breaks through to the rest of the kidney and eventually to the ureters from the cortical granulomas, which may be unilateral or bilateral. In rare cases, the kidneys are relatively unaffected, with spread mainly to the urogenital tract. Hematogenous spread to the epididymis and prostate may also occur in boys.[62]

Diagnosis

Dysuria, hematuria, and sterile pyuria are the most common presenting features of urogenital tuberculosis. Constitutionally associated with tuberculosis, recurrent urinary tract infection (with often no organism identified) and scrotal mass may be seen in children.[66] In HIV-infected children, severe proteinuria in the nephrotic range with low serum albumin has been observed.[65] Renal tuberculosis often presents at an advanced stage, as it has an insidious, relatively symptom-free nature, and only becomes known as a result of lumbar pain and symptoms of spread to the bladder. As such, tuberculosis can be a cause of end-stage renal failure, especially in adults.[62] History or evidence of previous or current tuberculosis is rarely found, because of the long interval between the primary infection and reactivation of renal disease. Tuberculosis of the epididymis presents as a scrotal swelling, and caseation necrosis may lead to the development of sinuses. [66]

Imaging is useful in demonstrating renal, urethral, and bladder involvement. Plain radiography may show calcifications, especially in the renal parenchyma. Ultrasound is most often used as the primary screening method for possible renal and urinary tract abnormalities. It may show hydronephrosis as well as features of advanced disease, such as pelvicalyceal dilatation, perinephric abscesses, and extensive calcifications, but it is less sensitive than intravenous urography (IVU). IVU, whose use has diminished lately, still remains the best modality to diagnose calyceal irregularity of early tuberculosis.[67] IVU identifies the earliest finding in tuberculosis, which is caliectasis with a feathery contour, later appearing as a phantom calyx or a cavity communicating with a deformed calyx. These findings can also be seen on CT. With progression of renal disease, granulomas coalesce, forming mass-like lesions (tuberculoma), which may rupture into the pelvi-calyceal system.[67] Fibrosis follows, leading to infundibular stenosis. Ureteric involvement may manifest as hydronephrosis, urethral strictures and obstructions, and fibrosis of the bladder (small capacity), all of which can be seen on imaging. CT scan demonstrates similar pathology to ultrasound and IVU and is most likely the current imaging method of choice.[64,67]

Cystoscopy provides the opportunity to do biopsies for histology and culture, visualization of the ureteric orifice, configuration of bladder capacity, and determination of the affected renal unit if purulent efflux is seen.[66]

Diagnosis is confirmed by culture, mainly from urine, but culture yield is moderate to poor.[66] GeneXpert MTB/RIF or other PCR methods may assist in earlier confirmation.[68] It should be remembered that early in primary tuberculosis in children, a positive urine culture for *M. tuberculosis* most likely reflects hematogenous dissemination and not urogenital or renal disease.

EAR, NOSE, AND THROAT TUBERCULOSIS

Tuberculosis of the head and neck area, excluding tuberculous meningitis, often presents as ear, nose, and throat (ENT) disease. True ear, mastoid, nose, oropharynx, and laryngeal involvement by tuberculosis is very rare, representing <1% of all cases.[69] Ear and mastoid tuberculosis are the most common of these infections in children, although mostly only case reports are available.

Over a 10-year period (March 2003–Feb 2013), we documented 33 (2.1%) cases of culture-confirmed ear/mastoid tuberculosis among 1,581 confirmed tuberculosis cases in children less than 13 years of age. Of these, 11 had mastoiditis with or without chronic otorrhea, 21 had chronic otorrhea, and one had acute otorrhea associated with miliary disease. Cervicofacial lymphadenitis was present in 11 (33%), tuberculous meningitis in 6 (18%), facial palsy in 2 (6%), and parotid node tuberculosis in 1 (3%) child (unpublished data, HS Schaaf).

In adults, laryngeal tuberculosis is the second most common form after ear/mastoid tuberculosis, but it is exceedingly rare in children. Tonsilar and oropharyngeal tuberculosis is rarely seen, although it may present as cervico-facial lymphadenitis without the primary lesion's ever being diagnosed, as the primary focus is usually painless and therefore not noticed. Because other sites of ENT tuberculosis are very rare in children, only tuberculosis of the ear and mastoids is discussed here.

Tuberculosis of the Ear and Mastoids

PATHOGENESIS

M. tuberculosis can enter the middle ear through three different routes: spread through the Eustachian tube, hematogenous spread from another focus, or direct implantation through the tympanic membrane.[70] Tuberculous mastoiditis is usually a complication of unrecognized and untreated tuberculosis of the middle ear.[71]

DIAGNOSIS

The classical picture of multiple perforations of the tympanic membrane and pale granulation tissue in the middle ear is less commonly seen now, most likely due to the frequent use of ear drops containing antibiotics such as aminoglycosides and fluoroquinolones that have activity against *M. tuberculosis*.[70] The most common current presentation of tuberculosis of the ear is the same as chronic otitis media, with chronic tympanic membrane perforation, refractory otorrhea, and hearing loss.[71] Acute otitis media with otorrhea also has been described.[72] Tuberculous mastoiditis can present with pain, with or without postauricular swelling. Clinical features that should raise the suspicion of tuberculous ear or mastoid disease are: a chronically discharging ear with no response to antibiotic treatment, especially in an HIV-infected child or with tuberculosis affecting another site;[73] pale granulation tissue in the middle ear or in a mastoid cavity; a postauricular

abscess; or a facial paralysis associated with chronic otitis media.[70,71]

Imaging is mainly by CT scan, which shows mastoiditis with or without temporal bone destruction.

Mycobacteria in the ear are usually sparse. Ear swabs of a purulent discharge are in some cases positive for *M. tuberculosis* and therefore should be done, but a negative culture does not exclude tuberculosis of the ear.[73] If surgery is performed, tissue and pus should be sent for histology (granulomas) and culture and/or PCR molecular tests for the identification of mycobacteria. DST should be done where possible; 7 of 33 (21%) of our cases described above had drug-resistant tuberculosis.

COMPLICATIONS

Hearing loss is common. Facial nerve palsy is often seen in children but can be reversible. The most serious complication is tuberculous meningitis or tuberculomas. Post-aural fistula, involvement of the temporo-mandibular joint, and lateral (sigmoid) sinus thrombosis are rare complications.[74]

CONCLUSION

Extrathoracic forms of tuberculosis as a group are common in children, although some forms, such as peripheral lymphadenitis and tuberculous meningitis, dominate, while other forms, such as abdominal tuberculosis and OA-TB, are less common; all other forms are rare. We have not discussed tuberculosis of the eye or the endocrine system other than mentioning some entities in passing; for example, phlyctenular conjunctivitis and tuberculous pancreatic cyst. However, it should be remembered that *M. tuberculosis*, through either lympho-hematogenous spread, contiguous spread, or by direct inoculation from outside, can affect literally any organ in the body.

REFERENCES

1. Schaaf HS, Marais BJ, Whitelaw A, et al. Culture-confirmed childhood tuberculosis in Cape Town, South Africa: a review of 596 cases. *BMC Infectious Diseases.* 2007;7:140.
2. Jain SK, Ordonez A, Kinikar A, et al. Pediatric tuberculosis in young children in India: a prospective study. *Biomed Res Int.*

2013;2013:783698. doi: 10.1155/2013/783698. Epub 2013 Dec 10.

3. Marais BJ, Graham SM. Tuberculosis lymphadenitis and involvement of the reticuloendothelial system in children. In: *Tuberculosis: A Comprehensive Clinical Reference*. Schaaf HS and Zumla AI, eds. London: Saunders, Elsevier Publishers; 2009:391–396.

4. Amir J. Non-tuberculous mycobacterial lymphadenitis in children: diagnosis and management. *Isr Med Assoc J*. 2010;12:49–52.

5. Piersimoni C, Scarparo C. Extrapulmonary infections associated with nontuberculous mycobacteria in immunocompetent persons. *Emerg Infect Dis*. 2009;15:1351–1358.

6. Tortoli E. Clinical manifestations of nontuberculous mycobacteria infections. *Clin Microbiol Infect*. 2009;15:906–910.

7. Katila ML, Brander E, Backman A. Neonatal BCG vaccination and mycobacterial cervical adenitis in childhood. *Tubercle*. 1987;68:291–296.

8. Marras TK, Daley CL. Epidemiology of human pulmonary infection with nontuberculous mycobacteria. *Clin Chest Med*. 2002;23:553–567.

9. Wright CA, Warren RM, Marais BJ. Fine needle aspiration biopsy: an undervalued diagnostic modality in paediatric mycobacterial disease. *Int J Tuberc Lung Dis*. 2009;13:1467–1475.

10. Marais BJ, Wright CA, Schaaf HS, et al. Tuberculous lymphadenitis as a cause of persistent cervical lymphadenopathy in children from a tuberculosis-endemic area. *Pediatr Infect Dis J*. 2006;25:142–146.

11. Ligthelm LJ, Nicol MP, Hoek KG, et al. Xpert MTB/RIF for rapid diagnosis of tuberculous lymphadenitis from fine-needle-aspiration biopsy specimens. *J Clin Microbiol*. 2011;49:3967–3970.

12. Coetzee L, Nicol MP, Jacobson R, et al. Rapid diagnosis of pediatric mycobacterial lymphadenitis using fine needle aspiration biopsy. *Pediatr Infect Dis J*. 2014;33:893–896.

13. Reddington K, O'Grady J, Dorai-Raj S, Niemann S, van Soolingen D, Barry T. A novel multiplex real-time PCR for the identification of mycobacteria associated with zoonotic tuberculosis. *PLoS ONE*. 2011;6(8):e23481. doi: 10.1371/journal.pone.0023481

14. Li H, Ulstrup JC, Jonassen TO, Melby K, Nagai S, Harboe M. Evidence for absence of the MPB64 gene in some substrains of *Mycobacterium bovis* BCG. *Infect Immun*. 1993;61:1730–1734.

15. Malaviya AN, Kotwal PP. Arthritis associated with tuberculosis. *Best Pract Res Clin Rheumatol*. 2003;17:319–343.

16. Teo HE, Peh WC. Skeletal tuberculosis in children. *Pediatr Radiol*. 2004;34:853–860.

17. Storm M, Vlok GJ. Musculoskeletal and spinal tuberculosis in adults and children. In: *Tuberculosis: A Comprehensive Clinical Reference*. Schaaf HS and Zumla AI, eds. London: Saunders, Elsevier Publishers; 2009:494–503.

18. Garg RK, Somvanshi DS. Spinal tuberculosis: a review. *J Spinal Cord Med*. 2011;34:440–454.

19. Jain AK. Tuberculosis of the spine: a fresh look at an old disease. *J Bone Joint Surg Br*. 2010;92:905–913.

20. Andronikou S, Jadwat S, Douis H. Patterns of disease on MRI in 53 children with tuberculous spondylitis and the role of gadolinium. *Pediatr Radiol*. 2002;32:798–805.

21. Kaila R, Malhi AM, Mahmood B, Saifuddin A. The incidence of multiple level noncontiguous vertebral tuberculosis detected using whole spine MRI. *J Spinal Disord Tech*. 2007;20:78–81.

22. Francis IM, Das DK, Luthra UK, et al. Value of radiologically guided fine needle aspiration cytology (FNAC) in the diagnosis of spinal tuberculosis: a study of 29 cases. *Cytopathology*. 1999;10:390–401.

23. Seddon JA, Donald PR, Vlok GJ, Schaaf HS. Multidrug-resistant tuberculosis of the spine in children—characteristics from a high burden setting. *J Trop Pediatr*. 2012;58:341–347.

24. Tuli SM. General principles of osteoarticular tuberculosis. *Clin Orthop Relat Res*. 2002;(398):11–19.

25. Andronikou S, Bindapersad M, Govender N, et al. Musculoskeletal tuberculosis—imaging using low-end and advanced modalities for developing and developed countries. *Acta Radiol*. 2011;52:430–441.

26. De Backer AI, Mortelé KJ, Vanhoenacker FM, Parizel PM. Imaging of extraspinal musculoskeletal tuberculosis. *Eur J Radiol*. 2006;57:119–130.

27. Agashe V, Shenai S, Mohrir G, et al. Osteoarticular tuberculosis—diagnostic solutions in a disease endemic region. *J Infect Dev Ctries*. 2009;3:511–516.

28. Scott LE, Beylis N, Nicol M, et al. Diagnostic accuracy of Xpert MTB/RIF for extrapulmonary tuberculosis specimens: establishing a laboratory testing algorithm for South Africa. *J Clin Microbiol*. 2014;52:1818–1823.

29. Scheepers S, Andronikou S, Mapukata A, Donald P. Abdominal lymphadenopathy in children with tuberculosis presenting with respiratory symptoms. *Ultrasound*. 2011;19:134–139.

30. Schaaf HS, Collins A, Bekker A, Davies PDO. Tuberculosis at extremes of age. *Respirology*. 2010;15:747–763.

31. Shah I, Uppuluri R. Clinical profile of abdominal tuberculosis in children. *Indian J Med Sci*. 2010;64:204–209.

32. Sheer TA, Coyle WJ. Gastrointestinal tuberculosis. *Curr Gastroenterol Rep*. 2003;5:273–278.

33. Basu S, Ganguly S, Chandra PK, Basu S. Clinical profile and outcome of abdominal tuberculosis in Indian children. *Singapore Med J*. 2007;48:900–905.

34. Ridaura-Sanz C, López-Corella E, Lopez-Ridaura R. Intestinal/peritoneal tuberculosis in children: an analysis of autopsy cases. *Tuberc Res Treat*. 2012;2012:230814. doi: 10.1155/2012/230814. Epub 2012 Dec 19.

35. Sharma MP, Ahuja V. Abdominal (gastrointestinal tract) tuberculosis in adults. In: *Tuberculosis: A Comprehensive Clinical Reference*. Schaaf HS and Zumla AI, eds. London: Saunders, Elsevier Publishers; 2009:425–431.

36. Dinler G, Sensoy G, Helek D, Kalayci AG. Tuberculous peritonitis in children: report of nine patients and review of the literature. *World J Gastroenterol*. 2008;14:7235–7239.

37. Cruz AT, Starke JR. Clinical manifestations of tuberculosis in children. *Paediatr Respir Rev*. 2007;8:107–117.

38. de la Rey Nel E. Abdominal tuberculosis in children. In: *Tuberculosis: A Comprehensive Clinical Reference*. Schaaf HS and Zumla AI, eds. London: Saunders, Elsevier Publishers; 2009:432–437.

39. Talwar BS, Talwar R, Chowdhary B, Prasad P. Abdominal tuberculosis in children: an Indian experience. *J Trop Pediatr*. 2000;46:368–370.

40. Johnson CA, Hill ID, Bowie MD. Abdominal tuberculosis in children. A survey of cases at the Red Cross War Memorial Children's Hospital, 1976–1985. *S Afr Med J*. 1987;72:20–22.

41. Davies MR. Abdominal tuberculosis in children. *S Afr J Surg*. 1982;20:7–19.

42. Saczek KB, Schaaf HS, Voss M, Cotton MF, Moore SW. Diagnostic dilemmas in abdominal tuberculosis in children. *Pediatr Surg Int*. 2001;17:111–115.

43. Veeragandham RS, Lynch FP, Canty TG, Collins DL, Danker WM. Abdominal tuberculosis in children: review of 26 cases. *J Pediatr Surg*. 1996;31:170–175; discussion, 175–176.

44. Lin YS, Huang YC, Lin TY. Abdominal tuberculosis in children: a diagnostic challenge. *J Microbiol Immunol Infect*. 2010;43:188–193.

45. Andronikou S, Wieselthaler N. Modern imaging of tuberculosis in children: thoracic, central nervous system and abdominal tuberculosis. *Pediatr Radiol*. 2004;34:861–875.

46. Sheikh M, Moosa I, Hussein FMY, Qurttom MAF, Behbehani AI. Ultrasonographic diagnosis in abdominal tuberculosis. *Australas Radiol*. 1999;43:175–179.

47. Walters E, Hesseling AC, Friedrich SO, Diacon AH, Gie RP. Rapid diagnosis of pediatric intrathoracic tuberculosis from stool samples using the Xpert MTB/RIF assay: a pilot study. *Pediatr Infect Dis J*. 2012;31:1316.

48. Nicol MP, Spiers K, Workman L, et al. Xpert MTB/RIF testing of stool samples for the diagnosis of pulmonary tuberculosis in children. *Clin Infect Dis*. 2013;57:e18–e21.

49. Wang J, Gao L, Tang S, et al. A retrospective analysis on the diagnostic value of ultrasound-guided percutaneous biopsy for peritoneal lesions. *World J Surg Oncology*. 2013;11:251.

50. Bhalla AS, Hari S, Chandrashekhara SH, Sinha A, Makharia G, Gupta R. Abdominal lymphatic tuberculosis and portal hypertension. *Gastroenterol Clin Biol*. 2010;34:696–701.

51. Kahn SA, Kirschner BS. Massive intestinal bleeding in a child with superior mesenteric artery aneurysm and gastrointestinal tuberculosis. *J Pediatr Gastroenterol Nutr*. 2006;43:256–259.

52. Sethuraman G, Ramesh V. Cutaneous tuberculosis in children. *Pediatr Dermatol*. 2013;30:7–16.

53. Lai-Cheong JE, Perez A, Tang V, Martinez A, Hill V, Menagé HduP. Cutaneous manifestations of tuberculosis. *Clin Exp Dermatol*. 2007;32:461–466.

54. Frankel A, Penrose C, Emer J. Cutaneous tuberculosis. A practical case report and review for the dermatologist. *J Clin Aesthet Dermatol*. 2009;2:19–27.

55. Jordaan HF, Schneider JW. Dermatological manifestations of tuberculosis in adults and children. In: *Tuberculosis: A Comprehensive Clinical Reference*. Schaaf HS and Zumla AI, eds. London: Saunders, Elsevier Publishers; 2009:484–493.

56. Barbagallo J, Tager P, Ingleton R, Hirsch RJ, Weinberg JM. Cutaneous tuberculosis: diagnosis and treatment. *Am J Clin Dermatol*. 2002;3:319–328.

57. Jordaan HF, Schneider JW, Schaaf HS, et al. Papulonecrotic tuberculid in children: a report of eight patients. *Pediatr Dermatopathol*. 1996;18:172–185.

58. Abdalla CM, de Oliveira ZN, Sotto MN, Leite KR, Canavez FC, de Carvalho CM. Polymerase chain reaction compared to other laboratory findings and to clinical evaluation in the diagnosis of cutaneous tuberculosis and atypical mycobacteria skin infection. *Int J Dermatol*. 2009;48:27–35.

59. Negi SS, Basir SF, Gupta S, Pasha ST, Khare S, Lal S. Comparative study of PCR, smear examination and culture for diagnosis of cutaneous tuberculosis. *J Commun Dis*. 2005;37:83–92.

60. Ramesh V, Sen MK, Nair D, Singla R, Sengupta A. Cutaneous tuberculosis caused by multidrug-resistant tubercle bacilli: report of three cases. *Int J Dermatol*. 2011;50:300–303.

61. Nanda S, Rajpal M, Reddy BS. Multidrug-resistant cutaneous tuberculosis: response to therapy. *Pediatr Dermatol*. 2003;20:545–547.

62. Figueiredo AA, Lucon AM, Junior RF, Srougi M. Epidemiology of urogenital tuberculosis worldwide. *Int J Urol*. 2008;15:827–832.

63. Carrol ED, Clark JE, Cant AJ. Non-pulmonary tuberculosis. *Paediatr Respir Rev*. 2001;2:113–119.

64. Eastwood JB, Corbishley CM. Tuberculosis of the kidney and urinary tract. In: *Tuberculosis: A Comprehensive Clinical Reference*. Schaaf HS and Zumla AI, eds. London: Saunders, Elsevier Publishers; 2009:438–449.

65. Nourse PJ, Cotton MF, Bates WD. Renal manifestations in children co-infected with HIV and disseminated tuberculosis. *Pediatr Nephrol*. 2010;25:1759–1763.

66. Nerli RB, Kamat GV, Alur SB, Koura A, Vikram P, Amarkhed SS. Genitourinary tuberculosis in pediatric urological practice. *J Pediatr Urol*. 2008;4:299–303.

67. Das CJ, Ahmad Z, Sharma S, Gupta AK. Multimodality imaging of renal inflammatory lesions. *World J Radiol*. 2014;6:865–873.

68. Hemal AK, Gupta NP, Rajeev TP, Kumar R, Dar L, Seth P. Polymerase chain reaction in clinically suspected genitourinary tuberculosis: comparison with intravenous urography, bladder biopsy, and urine acid fast bacilli culture. *Urology*. 2000;56:570–574.

69. Vaamonde P, Castro C, García-Soto N, Labella T, Lozano A. Tuberculous otitis media: a significant diagnostic challenge. *Otolaryngol Head Neck Surg*. 2004;130:759–766.

70. Cho YS, Lee HS, Kim SW, et al. Tuberculous otitis media: a clinical and radiologic analysis of 52 patients. *Laryngoscope*. 2006;116:921–927.

71. Jonas NE, Prescott CAJ. Ear, nose, and throat tuberculosis in adults and children. In: *Tuberculosis: A Comprehensive Clinical Reference*. Schaaf HS and Zumla AI, eds. London: Saunders, Elsevier Publishers; 2009:463–468.

72. Mustafa A, Debry C, Wiorowski M, Martin E, Gentine A. Treatment of acute mastoiditis: report of 31 cases over a ten year period. *Rev Laryngol Otol Rhinol (Bord)*. 2004;125:165–169.

73. Schaaf HS, Geldenhuys A, Gie RP, Cotton MF. Culture-positive tuberculosis in human immunodeficiency virus type 1-infected children. *Pediatr Infect Dis J*. 1998;17:599–604.

74. Saunders NC, Albert DM. Tuberculous mastoiditis: when is surgery indicated? *Int J Pediatr Otorhinolaryngol*. 2002;65:59–63.

11

CENTRAL NERVOUS SYSTEM TUBERCULOSIS IN CHILDREN

Ronald van Toorn

HIGHLIGHTS OF THIS CHAPTER

- Tuberculosis meningitis (TBM) is the most common cause of death and morbidity as a result of tuberculosis in children.
- Negative cultures or tests for tuberculosis infection *never* rule out TBM.
- Delayed diagnosis and institution of appropriate treatment is the main cause of clinical deterioration and death as a result of TBM in children.
- Because the incubation period of TBM can be very long, the person from whom the child acquired *M. tuberculosis* may not yet be identified.
- Tuberculous meningitis should be suspected and empirical therapy for it started for any child with meningitis and no apparent etiology (negative Gram stain and/or bacterial culture of cerebrospinal fluid) who also has any of the following: cranial nerve involvement, basilar inflammation shown by imaging, hydrocephalus, or evidence of ischemia or a stroke.
- When TBM is suspected, all appropriate attempts should be made to isolate the organism to confirm the diagnosis and determine the drug susceptibility pattern.
- TBM can be prevented by the timely institution of treatment for young children in contact with contagious tuberculosis cases.

TUBERCULOUS MENINGITIS (TBM) continues to be an important cause of neurological disability, especially in resource-poor countries. It accounts for only approximately 1% of all disease caused by *Mycobacterium tuberculosis* but kills or disables more children than any other form of tuberculosis.

According to World Health Organization (WHO) estimates, there were 550,000 TB cases in children in 2013 and 80,000 deaths among children who were HIV-uninfected [WHO 2014]. The true worldwide burden of childhood TBM remains unknown. Epidemiological studies report a good correlation between the incidence of TBM in children 0–4 years of age per 100,000 population and the annual rate of tuberculosis infection (ARTI) multiplied by 5 [Shimao T 1983] [Styblo K 1982]. The ARTI in Southern African townships has been reported to be as high as 4% per year [Wood R 2010]. This implies an annual childhood TBM incidence in these townships of 20 per 100,000 children. A study in the Western Cape of South Africa highlighted the importance of TBM by finding it to be the commonest type of pediatric bacterial meningitis [Wolzak NK 2012].

PATHOGENESIS

A century and a quarter after the discovery of *M. tuberculosis*, the exact pathogenesis of TBM is still not fully understood. Much of the current understanding is based on the work by Arnold Rich and Howard McCordock, who demonstrated upon autopsy that the majority of TBM patients displayed a small granuloma in the brain parenchyma or the meninges [Rich and McCordock 1933]. They postulated that meningitis occurred once bacteria contained within these granulomas (Rich foci) were released into the subarachnoid space, months or years after the initial bacteremia. Rich and McCordock dissociated miliary tuberculosis from a role in the pathogenesis of TBM, a concept that has been challenged by epidemiological studies and more recently by an MRI study demonstrating meningo-cerebral granulomata in 88% of childhood TBM cases [Janse van Rensburg P 2008]. It is thus likely that miliary tuberculosis, especially in young children, plays an integral part in the pathogenesis of TBM, by establishing the cortical and meningeal foci that lead to TBM [Donald P 2005]. Experimental animal studies do not incorporate the long time interval required for tuberculous meningeal granulomas to form and caseate, and thus represent artificial models of TBM infection.

The mechanism(s) by which the bacilli initially invade the blood–brain barrier (BBB) are still to be elucidated. No TBM animal study has yet achieved an immediate breach of the BBB from experimental systemic infection, as is the case in natural human infection. In contrast to other bacteria, tubercle bacilli do not enter the cerebrospinal fluid (CSF) via the choroid plexus, and TBM most often only develops three to six months after the primary infection has occurred [Wallgren A 1934].

The release of *M. tuberculosis* into the subarachnoid space following rupture of a Rich focus triggers a robust inflammatory T-cell response. The importance of T cells to the protective immune response against tuberculosis is highlighted by their contribution to the generation of granulomas in which aggregated macrophages that have engulfed *M. tuberculosis* are surrounded by a cuff of lymphocytes, including the CD4+ and CD8+ T cells. Immunity to mycobacterial infections is associated with Th1 cell activity; in particular production of tumor necrosis factor alpha (TNF-α), interferon-γ, and interleukin (IL)-12 [Tobin DM 2012]. TNF-α is required for control of bacillary growth and the protective granulomatous response but may cause immunopathology. More studies are required to improve our understanding of the role of cytokines in TBM and their relationship with clinical outcome. A better understanding of how *M. tuberculosis* invades the central nervous system (CNS) and how it manages to survive initially will be essential to developing better preventative and treatment strategies.

CLINICAL COURSE

TBM may present at any age but is less common at the extremes of life. The age of peak incidence in children is from two to four years [van Well GT 2009]. Early clinical diagnosis is notoriously difficult and often delayed, with disastrous consequences. Very young infants and children living in non-tuberculosis endemic regions are at the highest risk for delayed diagnosis.

TBM usually manifests as a subacute meningitic illness and seems in some cases to be precipitated by a viral infection, a fall, or a blow to the head. Rarely, the onset is abrupt and marked by convulsions or rapid progression of neurological deficits. The onset is mostly insidious (days to weeks), and the early symptoms such as cough, low-grade fever, vomiting, anorexia, irritability, and general listlessness are nonspecific. Young children in the early stages often miss or lose developmental milestones. These nonspecific signs and symptoms can usually be recognized as due to tuberculous meningitis only in retrospect. Neck stiffness is often absent during early disease in children. Vomiting without preceding nausea should alert physicians to the possibility of raised intracranial pressure (ICP). An important factor that differentiates the symptoms of TBM from common illnesses such as influenza is their persistence, although this feature is often missed if a patient does not see the same health professional consistently [Smith HV 1964]. Over days to weeks, the full-blown clinical picture of meningitis develops, and the neurological picture can be ascribed to the combined effects of meningeal irritation, raised ICP, and infarction. Loss of consciousness, stiff neck, raised intracranial pressure (ICP), papillary abnormalities, convulsions, and motor and cranial nerve palsies (especially of cranial nerves III, VI, and VII) occur commonly. In older patients, headache, personality changes, and vomiting are often the major complaints, until a devastating neurological event occurs. Hemiplegia may occur at the onset of disease or at a later stage but usually correlates with ischemic infarction in the territory of the middle cerebral artery. Quadriplegia occurs only in advanced cases after bilateral infarctions or severe generalized edema have occurred. Monoplegia is uncommon and is caused by a small vascular lesion that occurs at an early stage of disease. Rare cases of tuberculous meningitis are dominated early by abnormal movements such as choreiform or hemi-ballistic movements, athetosis, tremors, myoclonic jerks, or ataxia.

Some of the specific aspects of the correlation between the pathophysiology and clinical presentation are discussed below. In summary, *tuberculous meningitis should be suspected and empirical therapy for it started for any child with meningitis and no apparent etiology (negative Gram stain and/or bacterial culture of CSF) who also has any of the following: cranial nerve involvement, basilar inflammation shown by imaging, hydrocephalus, or evidence of ischemia or a stroke.*

COMPLICATIONS OF TUBERCULOSIS MENINGITIS

Tuberculous Hydrocephalus and Raised Intracranial Pressure

Central to the pathology of TBM is the florid, basal meningeal exudate that obliterates the basal cisterns and encases the brainstem, cerebral arteries, cranial nerves, and spinal roots. Hydrocephalus results whenever the basal exudate blocks the flow of CSF. In about 70% of cases, CSF can exit the fourth ventricle but is prevented from moving past the tentorium by the exudate blocking the basal cisterns (communicating hydrocephalus) [van Well G 2009]. In the remainder, obstruction of the outlet foramina of the fourth ventricle results in non-communicating hydrocephalus. Occasionally, hydrocephalus results from obstruction of the foramen of Munro or the aqueduct of Sylvius.

Tuberculous hydrocephalus is often complicated by raised ICP, which may be life-threatening. Diagnosing raised ICP in children with TBM can be challenging, as tuberculous infection itself can mimic many of the signs of raised ICP, including depressed level of consciousness, cranial nerve palsies, absent brainstem responses, and decerebration. The clinical signs of raised ICP are often unreliable, especially in children with closed anterior fontanels, and the value of computed tomography (CT) is limited by the poor correlation that exists between the degree of hydrocephalus (ventricular size) and the severity of ICP [Schoeman JF 1997]. Lumbar CSF pressure measurement in TBM accurately reflects intracranial pressure in children with communicating tuberculous hydrocephalus [van Toorn R 2013]. Many noninvasive techniques of measuring ICP (including transcranial Doppler imaging) in children with TBM have been evaluated; none have been found reliable enough to replace invasive procedures [van Toorn R 2013].

Tuberculous Cerebrovascular Disease

The poor outcome from TBM is mainly a manifestation of the extent of the ischemic brain injury. Vessel pathology appears to be a consequence of its immersion in the basal cisternal meningeal reaction [Lammie GA 2009]. Infiltrative, proliferative and necrotizing vessel pathology has been described, but the relative contributions of each and of luminal thrombosis to brain damage remains unclear [Lammie GA 2009].

About a third of all children with advanced TBM will develop stroke [van Well G 2009]. Most of these strokes are due to infarcts located in the middle cerebral artery (MCA) territories, particularly in the so-called "TB zone" of the medial lenticulostriate and thalamo-perforating vessels [Misran UK 2011]. Bilateral symmetrical basal ganglia infarcts are particularly characteristic of TBM. There is some evidence that vasospasm may mediate strokes early in the course of the disease, and proliferative intimal disease causes later strokes [Lammie GA 2009]. Recently, a transcranial Doppler imaging (TCDI) study on children with TBM reported abnormally high blood-flow velocities in all the basal cerebral arteries in the majority (70%) of the children [van Toorn R 2014]. The high blood-flow velocities persisted for longer than seven days, suggesting the presence of stenosis due to vasculitis, rather than functional vasospasm.

Antituberculosis treatment appears to be relatively ineffective in preventing vascular complications, suggesting an underlying immune mechanism. Corticosteroids do not affect the incidence of basal ganglia infarcts, or the extent of residual hemiplegia in children [Schoeman JF 1997].

TBM Immune Reconstitution Syndrome (IRIS)

Clinical and neuroradiological deterioration may occur in children with TBM despite adequate treatment. This phenomenon, the result of IRIS, is often more severe in the setting of HIV co-infection and may be life-threatening. In resource-limited settings, the diagnosis of TBM-IRIS is based on clinical and radiological signs and its temporal relationship to the initiation of antiretroviral therapy (ART); no specific predictive or diagnostic test exists for this condition [Meintjies G 2008].

The prevalence and mortality of TBM IRIS in children is unknown; adult studies report a prevalence of 12% and mortality of 13–75% [Marais S 2013]. In most cases, TBM-IRIS in HIV-infected children occurs within the first three months after ART initiation, and neurological signs and symptoms include headache, seizures, meningeal irritation, ataxia, and focal neurological deficit [van Toorn R 2012]. Manifestations of TB-IRIS at other organ sites, especially the lungs (new pulmonary infiltrates, mediastinal lymph node enlargement), are also supportive of a diagnosis of TBM-IRIS.

The immune pathogenesis of TBM-IRIS remains poorly understood. It is thought that hypercytokinemia contributes to the pathology of TBM-IRIS [Tadokera R 2011]. Recently, a combination of high CSF TNF-α and low interferon (IFN)-γ concentrations was found to be predictive of TBM-IRIS [Marais S 2013]. Other risk factors for subsequent TBM-IRIS in patients with TBM include severe CD4 T-cell lymphopenia prior to ART initiation, high baseline CSF mycobacterial load (reflected by *M. tuberculosis* culture positivity), high CSF neutrophil counts, and shorter interval from initiation of tuberculosis treatment to ART initiation

[Marais 2013]. Larger prospective studies are needed to elucidate the predictive and diagnostic value of IRIS biomarkers in children with TBM and advance them to clinical practice.

The optimal time to initiate ART in children with HIV-associated TBM is unknown. A randomized double-blind placebo-controlled trial of immediate versus deferred ART in adult Vietnamese patients showed that HIV-associated TBM was associated with a poor prognosis regardless of the timing of ART [Lawn SD 2011]. In this study, early initiation of ART was not associated with an increased risk of TBM-IRIS [Torok ME 2011]. However, there were significantly more grade 4 adverse events in the immediate ART arm, providing some support for delaying the initiation of ART in HIV-associated TBM by four to six weeks [Torok ME 2011].

Adjunctive corticosteroid treatment is associated with symptomatic improvement in non-TBM-related IRIS [Meintjies G 2010]. Corticosteroid therapy has little effect on CSF cytokine concentrations in patients with TBM and TBM-IRIS [Marais S 2013]. These findings suggest a possible role for the use of more potent and specific immune-modulatory agents. Other immune-modulatory agents that have been used to treat TBM-IRIS in a limited number of children include thalidomide, chloroquine, mycophenolatemofetil, and cyclosporine [van Toorn R 2012]. Interruption of ART should be reserved for children who develop life-threatening complications.

TUBERCULOUS MASS LESIONS (TUBERCULOMAS AND TUBERCULOUS PSEUDO-ABSCESSES)

Tuberculomas of the central nervous system may occur in isolation or in association with TBM. The clinical presentation of a tuberculoma depends on the location and size of the lesion. Intracranial tuberculomas are often silent and unsuspected; a focal seizure in an otherwise normal child is the most common mode of presentation in tuberculosis-endemic populations. Tuberculomas may also manifest with focal neurological signs or raised intracranial pressure due to obstruction of CSF pathways. Headache, seizures, paralysis, personality changes, and other focal neurological problems occur frequently. Children are more prone to developing infratentorial lesions, so ataxia and sudden onset of

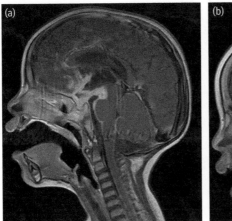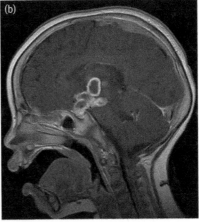

FIGURE 11.1   MRI sagittal T1-weighted post-gadolinium on admission in a 4-year-old HIV-uninfected male infant with tuberculous meningitis (TBM). *A*: Shows severe extensive inflammatory exudates covering the brainstem and suprasellar cistern. *B*: Shows the appearance of multiple ring-enhancing tuberculous granulomas following two months of antituberculosis treatment. This represents paradoxical TB-IRIS.

severe neurological dysfunction are more common in children than adults. Clinical diagnosis is made on the basis of neuroimaging, as the CSF findings and culture are usually negative. Most tuberculomas will resolve on antituberculosis treatment and corticosteroids; paradoxically, enlarging tuberculomas (secondary to IRIS) may require longer treatment (Figure 11.1) [Afghani B 1994]. Duration of therapy is guided by radiological response; the degree of contrast enhancement on follow-up CT or MRI reflects the activity of a tuberculoma. Late radiological changes include calcification and atrophy of surrounding brain parenchyma.

In contrast, tuberculous pseudo-abscesses tend to have a more accelerated clinical course and are unresponsive to standard chemotherapy. Drainage and excision may offer the only chance of cure, but lesion location within the basal cisterns and inadequate neurosurgical facilities usually combine to preclude surgical management [Schoeman JF 2006]. Tuberculous pseudo-abscesses have been shown to be responsive to adjunctive thalidomide, a potent TNF-α inhibitor [Schoeman JF 2006, van Toorn R 2015].

THE INFLUENCE OF HIV INFECTION

The clinical, laboratory and radiological features of TBM are similar in HIV-infected and HIV-uninfected children. Tuberculomas may be more common in HIV-infected children and can occur as a manifestation of IRIS even in children without previous evidence of CNS tuberculosis [van der Weert 2006]. The diagnostic work-up for TBM and tuberculoma should therefore always include an HIV test.

DIAGNOSIS OF TUBERCULOSIS MENINGITIS

Early diagnosis of TBM is notoriously difficult due to its inconsistent clinical presentation and lack of a rapid, sensitive, and specific test. Once a diagnosis of TBM is considered, the following features are supportive of the diagnosis: weight faltering, documented as crossing of weight percentiles (90%); household contact with a person who has tuberculosis (53%); positive tuberculin skin test or interferon-γ release assay (60%); chest radiography suggestive of pulmonary tuberculosis (44%); and positive culture from sputum or gastric lavage (18%) [van Well GTJ 2009].

The CSF in TBM is usually macroscopically clear due to the relatively low cell count. In cases with very high protein count (e.g., spinal block), the appearance becomes xanthochromatic. CSF analysis characteristically shows a predominance of lymphocytes, decreased CSF glucose (CSF: plasma ratio <0.5 or absolute CSF glucose <2.2 mmol/L) and increased CSF protein (0.5–5.0 g/L) [Donald PR 1991]. It should be noted that, misleadingly, in a minority of cases, a predominance of polymorpho-nuclear leucocytes may be found in the CSF if an unusually large amount of tuberculoprotein is discharged into the CSF [Patel VB 2008].

As the CSF in both TBM and aseptic (usually viral) meningitis is clear and lymphocyte-predominant, distinguishing between the two at times can be difficult. Failure of the CSF to improve/normalize within a week of starting appropriate chemotherapy suggests that the diagnosis of TBM is correct. Collecting adequate CSF volumes (at least 6 ml) for culture and microscopy has been shown to improve diagnostic yield [Thwaites G 2004]. Ziehl-Neelsen (ZN) or auramine O microscopy staining of the CSF is the most widely applied rapid diagnostic technique; however, its sensitivity for TBM rarely exceeds 20%. The clinical value of mycobacterial cultures is limited by the one to four weeks it takes to yield a positive result, and negative results cannot exclude a TBM diagnosis. Studies to identify useful biomarkers for TBM in CSF, blood, and urine are ongoing. A 2010 meta-analysis on the diagnostic value of adenosine deaminase (ADA) in the CSF of TBM patients reported a sensitivity of 79% and specificity of 91% [Xu HB 2010]. Raised CSF ADA activity also occurs in a number of other CNS infections, and thus is not recommended as a routine diagnostic test for TBM. Detection of urinary *M. tuberculosis* antigens such as lipoarabinomannan (LAM) is of little value in children with TBM [Blok N 2014].

Few studies have examined the diagnostic value of interferon-γ release assays (IGRA) on the CSF for the diagnosis of TBM; low sensitivities (50–70%) have been reported, and the results may depend on the CSF volume tested [Kim SH 2010, Vidhate MR 2011]. The smaller CSF volumes obtained in children with TBM therefore limit the use of IGRAs.

A 2003 systematic review and meta-analysis concluded that first-generation commercial nucleic acid amplification tests (NAATs) can confirm TBM (98% specificity) but cannot rule it out (56% sensitivity) [Pai 2003]. A 2013 meta-analysis on the diagnostic accuracy of the newer commercial NAATs similarly concluded high specificity (98%) with suboptimal sensitivity (64%) [Solomons RS 2014].

In 2010, the WHO endorsed the GeneXpert MTB/RIF test for the diagnosis of pulmonary tuberculosis [WHO 2011]. The GeneXpert MTB/RIF is a closed-cartridge-based real-time polymerase chain reaction (PCR) test that is cheap ($10), easy to operate by minimally trained staff, and gives a result in approximately two hours. Another advantage is that it simultaneously determines susceptibility to rifampicin, which can be used as a surrogate marker for multidrug resistance (MDR). The diagnostic accuracy of CSF GeneXpert MTB/RIF has been evaluated in three TBM studies; sensitivities of 67–85% and specificities of 99% were obtained [Tortoli 2012, Patel 2013, Nhu NT 2014]. As the Xpert test system depends on the capture and lysis of whole bacilli, adequate volumes of CSF are crucial to achieving high sensitivities.

Neuroimaging plays an important role in the rapid and early diagnosis of TBM, as well as for detection of complications and monitoring of disease progression (see Chapter 8 for more detail). Computed tomography (CT) is more readily available in resource-poor countries than MRI, and a combination of pre-contrast hyperintense exudates, basal meningeal enhancement, basal ganglia infarctions, and hydrocephalus is highly suggestive [Andronikou S 2004]. A normal CT scan, as encountered in one-third of early stage I TBM cases, does not exclude TBM [van Toorn R 2013].

Gadolinium-enhanced magnetic resonance imaging (MRI) is diagnostically superior to CT in identifying basal meningeal enhancement and miliary leptomeningeal nodules, which have been reported to be present in 88% of children with TBM [Pienaar M 2009; Janse van Rensburg P 2008]. Prognostically, diffusion-weighted MRI is useful at detecting early, subtle infarcts, especially in the brainstem [Pienaar M 2009]. Therapeutically, MRI assists with identification of tuberculous optochiasmic arachnoiditis, which requires urgent immune-modulation to reduce the risk of blindness [Schoeman JF 2010] (Figure 11.2, *A* and *B*). In children compromised by tuberculous pseudo-abscesses, serial T2-weighted MRI plays a critical role in identifying the nature of the necrotizing process, and evaluating treatment response and duration of thalidomide therapy [van Toorn R 2015](Figure 11.3, *A–F*). Magnetic resonance spectroscopy (MRS) is helpful at differentiating tubercular from pyogenic abscesses by demonstration of a lipid peak [Luthra G 2007]. Magnetic resonance imaging (MRA) allows identification of tuberculous vasculitis, which most commonly involves the terminal portions of the internal carotid arteries and the proximal parts of the middle and anterior cerebral arteries.

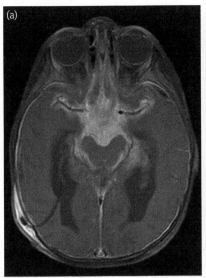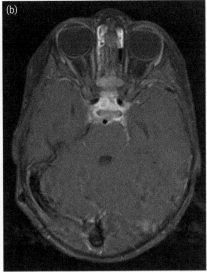

FIGURE 11.2   MRI axial T1WI post-gadolinium images of a 2-year-old boy with visual impairment secondary to tuberculous optochiasmic arachnoiditis. *A*: The extensive suprasellar enhancing exudates involving the optic chiasm and proximal optic nerves. *B*: Repeat MRI after three months of thalidomide shows marked interval improvement, with reduction in the extent of the exudates.

TREATMENT OF TUBERCULOSIS MENINGITIS

Fluid Management

Hyponatremia occurs in up to 85% of children with TBM and is independently associated with a poorer outcome [van Well GT 2009]. It occurs secondary to either the syndrome of inappropriate antidiuretic hormone (SIADH) or cerebral salt wasting (CSW). Distinction between the two conditions is very difficult and not of clinical relevance, as treatment for severe hyponatremia associated with intracranial disease should be hypertonic saline in all cases [Figaji A 2010]. Maintenance of adequate cerebral perfusion pressure is of critical importance in children with TBM, to reduce the risk of cerebral ischemia and cerebral venous thrombosis; systemic hypotension needs to be addressed immediately. Fluid restriction is potentially harmful as it may precipitate hypovolemia, which adversely affects cerebral perfusion pressure with an increased the risk of cerebral ischemia.

Antimicrobial Therapy

Childhood TBM treatment duration and regimens are based on expert opinion rather than randomized controlled trials [Woodfield J 2008]. Current WHO guidelines advocate treatment with RHZE (comprising rifampicin [R], isoniazid [H], pyrazinamide [Z] and ethambutol [E] for two months, followed by two-drug therapy [HR] for 10 months [WHO 2010] (Table 11.1) Some experts substitute ethionamide for ethambutol because of its better penetration into the CSF.

Studies evaluating length of childhood TBM therapy report similar relapse rates when comparing 6-months treatment with 12-months treatment [Woodfield 2008, Donald 1998]. Recently, short intensified treatment (6 months RHZE for HIV-uninfected and 9 months RHZE for HIV-infected children) was found to be safe and effective in a large study of children with drug-susceptible TBM (van Toorn R 2015). In this study, the mortality at completion of therapy was 3.8%, and 80% of children had a good outcome [van Toorn R 2015]. This compares favorably with the 19.3% risk of death and 53.9% risk of neurological sequelae recently reported in a systematic review and meta-analysis of childhood TBM treatment outcomes [Chiang SS 2014]. Table 11.1 shows the WHO and Tygerberg Children's Hospital first-line treatment regimens for TBM in children [WHO 2010; van Toorn R 2014.

Table 11.2 shows the pharmacokinetic activity, suggested daily dosages, and CSF penetration of

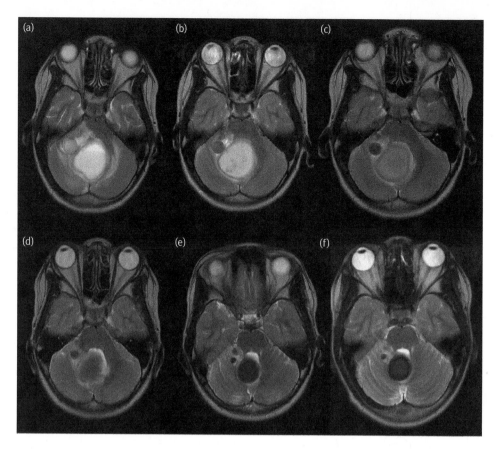

FIGURE 11.3 *A*: MRI axial T2-weighted imaging on admission (pretreatment) in a 9-year-old ataxic female with a large cerebellar tuberculous abscess surrounded by smaller abscesses. *B*: Reduction in perilesional edema after three months of thalidomide. *A–F*: Demonstrate gradual loss of T2 signal and reduction in lesion size after 6, 10, 31, and 41 months. The patient was asymptomatic within three months, and thalidomide and antituberculosis drugs were stopped after six months. *A–F*: Demonstrate the gradual evolution, on sequential studies, of all these abscesses to homogenous hypointense lesions with reduction in size and perilesional edema.

first-line and second-line anti-TBM drugs [Donald PR 2010]. Increasing the dose of rifampicin, a key drug with poor CSF penetration, may result in higher mycobacteriocidal activity in the brain and possibly greater survival. The potential benefit of intensified anti-TBM treatment was recently explored in two adult, randomized, controlled trials. In an open-label, phase II trial with a factorial design, patients with TBM were randomly assigned to receive, according to a computer-generated schedule, rifampicin standard dose (450 mg, about 10 mg/kg) orally, or high dose (600 mg, about 13 mg/kg) intravenously, and oral moxifloxacin 400 mg, moxifloxacin 800 mg, or ethambutol 750 mg once daily [Ruslami R 2013]. All patients were given standard-dose isoniazid, pyrazinamide, and adjunctive corticosteroids. After 14 days of treatment, all patients continued with standard treatment for tuberculosis. Intensified treatment was associated with lower 6-month mortality (35 versus 65%) without increased toxicity, which could not be explained by HIV status or severity of disease at the time of presentation. Unfortunately, no comparable trials have been reported for children with TBM.

Fluoroquinolones possibly offer an alternative option to ethionamide, as they demonstrate *in vitro* activity, tolerability, good bioavailability, relatively good CSF penetration, and ease of administration [Thwaites GE 2011]. The preliminary findings from adult TBM studies highlight the need for childhood randomized controlled trials, evaluating alternative, more palatable antituberculosis drugs with fewer adverse effects but with at least similar efficacy to the regimen the WHO currently advocates.

Table 11.1. WHO and Tygerberg Children's Hospital first-line treatment regimens for TBM in children

ANTITUBERCULOSIS AGENT	WHO REGIMEN			TYGERBERG CHILDREN'S HOSPITAL REGIMEN		
	RECOMMENDED DOSE (MG/KG/DAY)	MAXIMUM DOSE (MG/DAY)	DURATION	RECOMMENDED DOSE (MG/KG/DAY)	MAXIMUM DOSE (MG/DAY)	DURATION
Isoniazid	10–20	500	12 months	20	400	6 months
Rifampicin	10–20	600	12 months	20	600	6 months
Pyrazinamide	15–30	2000	2 months	40	2000	6 months
Ethambutol	15–20	1000	2 months	not recommended		
Ethionamide	not recommended			20	750	6 months

Table 11.2. Pharmacokinetic activity, suggested daily dose, and CSF penetration of first-line and second-line antituberculosis drugs

ANTITUBERCULOSIS 1ST-LINE AGENTS	ACTIVITY	SUGGESTED DAILY DOSE FOR CHILDREN	ESTIMATED RATIO OF CSF TO PLASMA CONCENTRATION
Isoniazid	bactericidal	15 mg/kg	90–95%
Rifampicin	bactericidal	20 mg/kg	5–25%
Pyrazinamide	bactericidal	40 mg/kg	90–100%
Ethambutol	bacteriostatic	25 mg/kg	20–30%
Streptomycin	bacteriostatic	Not recommended	10–20%
Levofloxacin	bactericidal	20 mg/kg	70–80%
Moxifloxacin	bactericidal	10–15 mg/kg	50–60%
ANTITUBERCULOSIS 2ND-LINE AGENTS			
Ethionamide	bactericidal	20 mg/kg	80–90%
Terizidone	bactericidal	15–20 mg/kg	50–60%
Linezolid	bactericidal	20 mg/kg	40–70%
p-Aminosalicyclic acid	bacteriostatic	200 mg/kg	20%
Clofazimine	bactericidal	3–5 mg/kg	20%
Amikacin	bactericidal	15 mg/kg IV	10–25%

Multidrug-resistant (MDR) TBM in children has a poor clinical outcome and is associated with death [Seddon J 2012]. Diagnosis of drug resistance depends on the recognition of risk factors (e.g., multidrug-resistant contact) and, when available, the results of susceptibility testing (molecular or conventional methods) on the organism isolated from the child or the likely source case. Treatment regimens are determined by drug susceptibility results and include the addition of second-line antituberculosis agents. However the additional use of second-line agents should not be delayed in the event of reasonable suspicion of MDR or XDR tuberculosis (see Table 11.1). The spread of MDR and extensively drug-resistant (XDR) tuberculosis necessitates the use of every possible avenue to obtain a culture of *M. tuberculosis* from the child for susceptibility determination and to detection of the source case for the child's infection.

Long-term in-hospital TBM treatment is seldom feasible in resource-poor countries, due to bed shortages and budget constraints. Home-based anti-TBM treatment, after initial in-hospital stabilization, is a viable option, provided that patients are carefully selected and meticulously followed up by a dedicated health team [Schoeman J 2009].

Treatment of Tuberculous Hydrocephalus

Treatment of tuberculous hydrocephalus depends on the level of CSF obstruction, which determines the type of hydrocephalus. In both communicating and non-communicating hydrocephalus, pan-ventricular dilatation is observed on neuroimaging, and differentiation between the two types is not possible. In the absence of MRI with CSF flow cytometry, air-encephalography is the only reliable way of determining the level of CSF obstruction [Bruwer E 2004] (Figure 11.4).

Medical therapy consisting of acetazolamide (50 mg/kg/day) and furosemide (1 mg/kg/day)

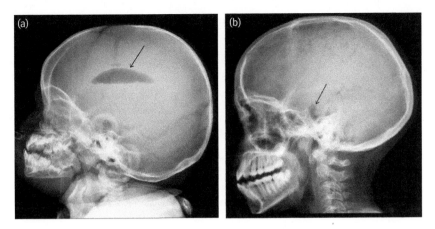

FIGURE 11.4   A: The lateral skull X-ray shows air in the basal cistern and lateral ventricles. This indicates communicating hydrocephalus (arrow) due to basal cistern obstruction to the flow of cerebrospinal fluid. B: The lateral skull X-ray shows only air at the level of the basal cistern (arrow). This indicates non-communicating hydrocephalus due to obstruction of the 4th ventricle outlet foramen.

has been shown to normalize raised ICP within seven days in children with communicating hydrocephalus [van Toorn 2014](Figure 11.5). Carbonic anhydrase inhibitors (acetozolamide) and loop diuretics (furosemide) exert their effect on ICP by reducing CSF production at the choroid plexus. Inhibition of CSF flow occurs once 99.5% of choroid plexus carbonic anhydrase is inhibited [McCarthy KD 1974].

Children with non-communicating hydrocephalus are preferably treated surgically because of the risk of cerebral herniation. Endoscopic third ventriculostomy (ETV) offers the benefits of CSF diversion without the risk of shunt complications. However, careful patient selection is important, as thick, tuberculous basal exudates may obscure important anatomical landmarks (vertebrobasilar artery) beneath the floor of the third ventricle.

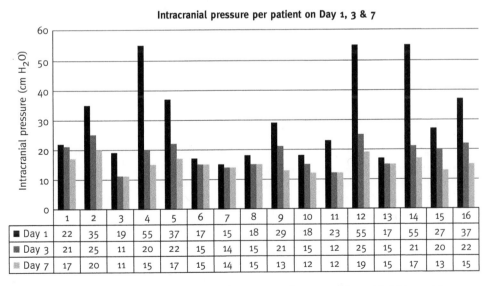

Intracranial pressure per patient on Day 1, 3 & 7

	1	2	3	4	5	6	7	8	9	10	11	12	13	14	15	16
■ Day 1	22	35	19	55	37	17	15	18	29	18	23	55	17	55	27	37
■ Day 3	21	25	11	20	22	15	14	15	21	15	12	25	15	21	20	22
■ Day 7	17	20	11	15	17	15	14	15	13	12	12	19	15	17	13	15

FIGURE 11.5   Illustrates the change in intracranial pressure on days 1, 3, and 7 in 16 children with tuberculous meningitis and communicating hydrocephalus following medical therapy consisting of acetazolamide and furosemide.

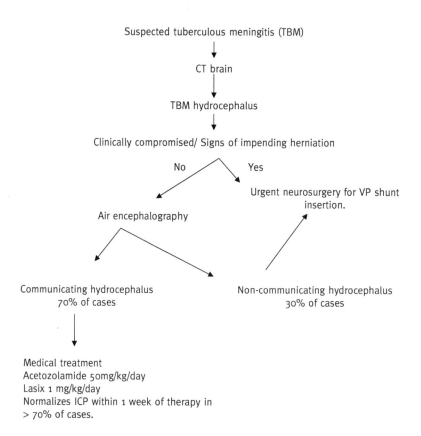

Suspected tuberculous meningitis (TBM)

↓

CT brain

↓

TBM hydrocephalus

↓

Clinically compromised/ Signs of impending herniation

No ╱ ╲ Yes

Urgent neurosurgery for VP shunt insertion.

Air encephalography

Communicating hydrocephalus
70% of cases

Non-communicating hydrocephalus
30% of cases

↓

Medical treatment
Acetozolamide 50mg/kg/day
Lasix 1 mg/kg/day
Normalizes ICP within 1 week of therapy in
> 70% of cases.

FIGURE 11.6   Tygerberg Children's Hospital management algorithm for tuberculous hydrocephalus.

Abbreviations: ICP = intracranial pressure; VPS = ventriculoperitoneal shunt.

Figure 11.6 illustrates the Tygerberg Children's Hospital (TCH) treatment algorithm for children with tuberculous hydrocephalus.

Adjuvant Anti-inflammatory Therapy

Many of the sequelae of TBM can be attributed to the severity of the intracranial inflammatory immune response. Studies have shown that the host immune system is a critical factor for both the containment and the cure of M. tuberculosis infection. Augmentation or dampening of pro-inflammatory responses may thus be of value in the treatment of children who experience inflammation-induced complications.

CORTICOSTEROIDS

A Cochrane systematic review of seven clinical trials found that corticosteroids reduce the risk of death (relative risk 0.78, 95% CI: 0.67–0.91) or disabling neurological deficit (relative risk 0.82, 95% CI: 0.70–0.97) in HIV-uninfected patients with TBM [Prasad K 2008]. There is currently insufficient evidence to either support or refute treating HIV-infected TBM patients with corticosteroids [Prasad K 2008]. The exact mechanism of action of corticosteroids in TBM remains unclear. Recently, a functional single-nucleotide polymorphism (SNP) was identified in a gene (LTA4H locus) which controls the balance of pro- and anti-inflammatory eicosanoids [Tobin DM 2012]. In TBM patients, the SNP (LTA4H-high genotype) was associated with inflammatory cell recruitment, increased TNF-α production, and patient survival [Tobin DM 2012]. In this study, only those patients with the LTA4H-high genotype benefited from adjunctive corticosteroids. The impact of LTA4H genotype on corticosteroid effect requires further exploration. If validated, it opens up the exciting prospect of genotype-directed adjunctive therapy.

Table 11.3. The refined MRC score stages, mean development quotient (DQ), and percentage of children with TBM in each stage developing a spastic quadriplegia

REFINED MRC SCALE		MEAN DQ	% WITH QUADRIPARESIS
Stage 1	GCS score of 15 with no focal neurological deficits	78.6	0%
Stage 2a	GCS score of 15 with neurological deficit, or a GCS of 13–14 with or without neurological deficit	68.3	3.3%
Stage 2b	GCS score of 10–12 with or without neurological deficit	58.3	23.3%
Stage 3	GCS score <10	44.3	73.3%

ASPIRIN

Two studies explored the value of aspirin's anti-thrombotic, anti-ischemic, and anti-inflammatory properties in TBM. Misra et al. reported a significant reduction in mortality after three months in adult TBM patients [Misra UK 2010]. In contrast, a randomized controlled trial in children reported no significant benefit in morbidity or mortality at six months [Schoeman JF 2011]. Further studies are needed before aspirin can be advocated as routine therapy.

THALIDOMIDE

TNF-α is an important cytokine involved in the protective cell-mediated immune response to mycobacteria. The immunopathological effects are dose-dependent [Bekker LG 2000]. Insufficient TNF-α production delays granuloma formation, which is essential for control of bacillary growth; while excessive production leads to tissue necrosis and cachexia [Tsenova L 1999]. In adult TBM studies, elevated CSF levels of TNF-α were associated with persistence of CNS inflammation and higher risk of developing TBM-IRIS [Marais S 2013].

Adjuvant thalidomide (3–5 mg/kg/day), a potent TNF-α inhibitor, has been shown to be effective in uncontrolled studies in children with visual compromise due to tuberculous opto-chiasmic arachnoiditis and large, tuberculous pseudo-abscesses in the brain and spinal cord [Schoeman JF 2010; van Toorn R 2015] (Figures 11.2, 11.3). Duration of therapy is guided by serial MRI, and clinical improvement often precedes regression in lesion size. Loss of MRI T2-weighted hyperintensity on serial MRI is a marker of cure (Figure 11.3, A–F).

Thalidomide can be used safely in HIV-infected children with TBM as it has been shown to enhance HIV-specific CD8 T-cell function without affecting the viral load [Reves-Teran G 1996]. An additional benefit is reduction of HIV-associated wasting [Kaplan G 2000]. Prolonged thalidomide therapy can cause sensory axonal neuropathy, which may be exacerbated by the combined use of antituberculosis drugs and ART [Zara G 2008].

OUTCOME IN CHILDHOOD TUBERCULOSIS MENINGITIS

Accurate prediction of outcome in childhood TBM is difficult, due to the protracted course of the disease, diversity of underlying pathological mechanisms, unpredictability of injury-induced cerebral plasticity, and variation in host immunity. Prognosis is related directly to the clinical stage of disease. Other factors associated with a poor outcome include MDR tuberculosis and HIV co-infection. Table 11.3 illustrates the "refined Medical Research Council (MRC) scale after 1 week," which has been shown to have the highest predictive value of all TBM-staging systems [van Toorn R 2012]. The importance of early diagnosis in TBM is emphasized by the 10-point reduction in developmental quotient associated with every change to lower stage and the 73% risk of quadriplegia in children who progress to stage III [van Toorn R 2012].

REFERENCES

Afghani B, Lieberman JM. Paradoxical enlargement or development of intracranial tuberculomas during therapy: case report and review. *Clin Infect Dis.* 1994;19:1092–1099.

Andronikou S, Smith B, Hatherhill M, et al. Definitive neuroradiological features of tuberculous meningitis in children. *Pediatr Radiol.* 2004;34:876–885.

Bekker LG, Moreira AL, Bergtold A, et al. Immunopathologic effects of tumour necrosis factor alpha in murine mycobacterial infection are dose dependent. *Infect Immun.* 2000;68:6954–6961.

Blok N, Visser DH, Solomons R, et al. Lipoarabinomannan enzyme-linked immunosorbent assay for early diagnosis of childhood tuberculous meningitis. *Int J Tuberc Lung Dis.* 2014;18:205–210.

Bruwer GE, van der Westhuizen S, Lombard CJ, Schoeman JF. Can CT predict the level of CSF block in tuberculous hydrocephalus? *Childs Nerv Syst.* 2004;20:183–187.

Chiang SS, Khan FA, Milstein BM, et al. Treatment outcomes of childhood tuberculous meningitis; a systematic review and meta-analysis. *Lancet Infect Dis.* 2014;10:947–957.

Donald PR, Schoeman JF, Coton M, van Zyl LE. Cerebrospinal fluid investigations in tuberculous meningitis. *Ann Trop Paediatr.* 1991;11:241–246.

Donald PR, Schaaf HS, Schoeman JF. Tuberculous meningitis and miliary tuberculosis: the Rich focus revisited. *J Infect.* 2005;50:193–195.

Figaji AA, Fieggen AG. The neurosurgical and acute management of tuberculous meningitis: evidence and current practise. *Tuberculosis.* 2010;90:393–400.

Janse van Rensburg P, Andronikou S, van Toorn R, Pienaar M. Magnetic resonance imaging of the central nervous system in children with tuberculous meningitis. *Pediatr Radiol.* 2008;38:1306–1313.

Kaplan G, Thomas S, Fierer DS, et al. Thalidomide for the treatment of AIDS-associated wasting. *AIDS Res Hum Retroviruses.* 2000;16:1345–1355.

Kim SH, Cho OH, Park SJ. Rapid diagnosis of tuberculous meningitis by T-cell-based assays on peripheral blood and cerebrospinal fluid mononuclear cells. *Clin Infect Dis.* 2010;50:1349–1358.

Lammie GA, Hewlett RH, Schoeman JF, Donald PR. Tuberculous cerebrovascular disease: a review. *J Infect.* 2009;59:156–166.

Lawn SD, Wood R. Poor prognosis of HIV-associated tuberculous meningitis regardless of timing of antiretroviral therapy. *Clin Infect Dis.* 2011;52:1384–1387.

Luthra G, Parihar A, Nath K, et al. Comparative evaluation of fungal, tubercular, and pyogenic brain abscesses with conventional and diffusion MR imaging and proton MR spectroscopy. *AJNR Am J Neuroradiol.* 2007;28:1332–1338.

Marais S, Meintjies G, Pepper DJ, et al. Frequency, severity, and prediction of tuberculous meningitis immune reconstitution inflammatory syndrome. *Clin Infect Dis.* 2013;56:450–460.

McCarthy KD, Reed DJ. The effect of acetazolamide and furosemide on CSF production and carbonic anhydrase activity. *J Pharmacol Exp Ther.* 1974;189:194–201.

Meintjies G, Lawn SD, Scano F, et al. Tuberculosis-associated immune reconstitution inflammatory syndrome: case definitions for use in resource-limited settings. *Lancet Infect Dis.* 2008;8:516–523.

Meintjies G, Wilkinson RJ, Morroni C, et al. Randomized placebo-controlled trail of prednisone for paradoxical tuberculosis-associated immune reconstitution inflammatory syndrome. *AIDS.* 2010;24:2381–2390.

Misra UK, Kalita J, Nair PP. Role of aspirin in tuberculous meningitis: a randomized open label placebo controlled trial. *J Neurol Sci.* 2010 15;293:12–17.

Nhu NT, Heemskerk D, Thu do DA, et al. Evaluation of GeneXpert MTB/RIF for diagnosis of tuberculous meningitis. *J Clin Microbiol.* 2014;52:226–233.

Pai M, Flores LL, Pai N, et al. Diagnostic accuracy of nucleic acid amplification tests for tuberculous meningitis: a systematic review and meta-analysis. *Lancet Infect Dis.* 2003;3:633–643.

Patel VB, Burger I, Connolly C. Temporal evolution of cerebrospinal fluid following initiation of treatment for tuberculous meningitis. *S Afr Med J.* 2008;98:610–613.

Pienaar M, Andronikou S, van Toorn R. MRI to demonstrate features and complications of TBM not seen with CT. *Childs Nerv Syst.* 2009;25:941–947.

Prasad K, Singh MB. Corticosteroids for managing tuberculous meningitis. *Cochrane Database Syst Rev.* 2008;1:CD002244.

Reyes-Teran G, Sierra-Madero JG, Martinez del Cerro V, et al. Effects of thalidomide on HIV-associated wasting syndrome: a randomized, double-blind, placebo controlled clinical trial. *AIDS*. 1996;10:1501–1507.

Rich AR, McCordock HA. The pathogenesis of tuberculous meningitis. *Bull Johns Hopkins Hosp*. 1933;52:5–38.

Ruslami R, Ganiem AR, Dian S. Intensified regimen containing rifampicin and moxifloxacin for tuberculous meningitis: an open-label randomised controlled phase 2 trial. *Lancet Infect Dis*. 2013;13:27–35.

Schoeman JF, Janse van Rensburg A, Laubsher JA, Springer P. The role of aspirin in childhood tuberculous meningitis. *J Child Neurol*. 2011;26:956–962.

Schoeman JF, Van Zyl LE, Laubscher JA, Donald PR. Effect of corticosteroids on intracranial pressure, computed tomographic findings, and clinical outcome in young children with tuberculous meningitis. *Pediatrics*. 1997;99:226–231.

Schoeman JF, Fieggen G, Seller N, et al. Intractable intracranial tuberculous infection responsive to thalidomide: report of four cases. *J Child Neurol*. 2006;21:301–308.

Schoeman J, Malan G, van Toorn R, et al. Home-based treatment of childhood neurotuberculosis. *J Trop Pediatr*. 2009;55:149–154.

Schoeman JF, Andronikou S, Stefan DC, et al. Tuberculous meningitis-related optic neuritis: recovery of vision with thalidomide in 4 consecutive cases. *J Child Neurol*. 2010;25:822–828.

Seddon JA, Visser DH, et al. Impact of drug resistance on clinical outcome in children with tuberculous meningitis. *Pediatr Infect Dis J*. 2012;31:711–716.

Shimao T. Surveillance of tuberculosis. *Bull Int Union Tuberc*. 1983;58:48–52.

Smith HV. Tuberculous meningitis. *Int J Neurol*. 1964;4:134–157.

Solomons RS, van Elsland SL, Visser DH, et al. Commercial nucleic amplification tests in tuberculous meningitis: a meta-analysis. *Diagn Microbiol Infect Dis*. 2014;78:398–403.

Styblo K, Sutherland I. The epidemiology of tuberculosis in children. *Bull Int Union*. 1982;57:133–139.

Tadokera R, Meintjies G, Skolimowska KH, et al. Hypercytokinaemia accompanies HIV-tuberculosis immune reconstitution inflammatory syndrome. *Eur Respir J*. 2011;37:1248–1259.

Tsenova L, Bergtold A, Freedman VH, et al. Tumor necrosis factor alpha is a determinant of pathogenesis and disease progression in mycobacterial infection in the central nervous system. *Proc Natl Acad Sci USA*. 1999;96:5657–5662.

Thwaites GE, Bhavnani SM, Chau TT, et al. Randomized pharmacokinetic and pharmacodynamic comparison of fluoroquinolones for tuberculous meningitis. *Antimicrob Agents Chemother*. 2011;55:3244–3253.

Tobin DM, Roca FJ, Oh SF, et al. Host genotype-specific therapies can optimize the inflammatory response to mycobacterial infections. *Cell*. 2012;148:434–446.

Torok ME, Yen NT, Chau TT, et al. Timing of initiation of antiretroviral therapy in human immunodeficiency virus (HIV)-associated tuberculous meningitis. *Clin Infect Dis*. 2011;52:1374–1383.

van der Weert EM, Hartgers NM, Schaaf HS, et al. Comparison of diagnostic criteria of tuberculous meningitis in human immunodeficiency virus-infected and uninfected children. *Pediatr Infect Dis J*. 2006, 25:65–69.

van Toorn R, Springer P, Laubscher JA, et al. Value of different staging systems for predicting neurological outcome in childhood tuberculous meningitis. *Int J Tuberc Lung Dis*. 2012;16:628–632.

van Toorn R, Rabie H, Dramowski A, et al. Neurological manifestations of TB-IRIS: a report of 4 children. *Eur J Paediatr Neurol*. 2012;16:676–682.

van Toorn R, Schaaf HS, Laubscher JA, et al. Short intensified treatment in children with drug-susceptible tuberculous meningitis. *Pediatr Infect Dis J*. 2014;33:248–252.

van Toorn R, Schaaf HS, Solomons R, et al. The value of transcranial Doppler imaging in children with tuberculous meningitis. *Childs Nerv Syst*. 2014;30:1711–1716.

Vidhate MR, Singh MK, Garg RK, et al. Diagnostic and prognostic value of Mycobacterium tuberculosis complex specific interferon gamma release assay in patients with tuberculous meningitis. *J Infect*. 2011;62:400–403.

Wallgren A. Some aspects of tuberculous meningitis and the possibility of prevention. *J Pediatr*. 1934;5:291–298.

Wait JW, Schoeman JF. Behavioural profiles after tuberculous meningitis. *J Trop Pediatr*. 2010;56:166–171.

Wood R, Johnson-Robertson S, Uys P. Tuberculosis transmission in young children in a South African community: modeling household and community infection risks. *Clin Infect Dis*. 2010;51:401–408.

Woodfield J, Argent A. Evidence behind the WHO guidelines: Hospital care for children: what is the most appropriate treatment for tuberculous meningitis? *J Trop Pediatr.* 2008;54(4):220–224.

World Health Organization. Automated Real Time Nucleic Acid Amplification Technology for Rapid and Simultaneous Detection of Tuberculosis and Rifampicin Resistance: Xpert MTB/RIF System. Policy Statement. WHO/HTM/TB/2011.4. Geneva: World Health Organization; 2011.

Wolzak NK, Cooke ML, Orth H, et al. The changing profile of pediatric meningitis at a referral centre in Cape Town, South Africa. *J Trop Pediatr.* 2012;58:491–495.

Xu HB, Jiang RH, Li L, et al. Diagnostic value of adenosine deaminase in cerebrospinal fluid for tuberculous meningitis: a meta-analysis. *Int J Tuberc Lung Dis.* 2010;14:1382–1387.

Zara G, Ermani M, Rondinone R, et al. Thalidomide and sensory neurotoxicity: a neurophysiological study. *J Neurol Neurosurg Psychiatry.* 2008;79:1258–1261.

12

TUBERCULOSIS IN ADOLESCENTS

Andrea T. Cruz

HIGHLIGHTS OF THIS CHAPTER

- Determining the true burden of tuberculosis disease in adolescents is challenging because of varying age definitions and patterns of care in different countries.
- Certain forms of tuberculosis, such as pleural, renal, and ocular disease, are more common in adolescents than younger children.
- While the treatment regimens used for tuberculosis in adolescents are the same as for younger children, adolescents often develop more adverse effects and have more interruptions in treatment.
- Infection control considerations are important for adolescents with tuberculosis as they can develop adult-type disease with positive acid-fast sputum smears, and can infect many others in schools and social circles.

"ADOLESCENCE" IS from the Latin *adolescere*, "to grow up." The transitory nature of adolescence makes this period hard to define uniformly across cultures and time, and there is no one widely accepted age range for adolescence. The World Health Organization (WHO) defines adolescents as persons between 10 and 19 years of age, but states that adolescence is better defined by acquisition of developmental experiences than by chronological age. From the standpoint of tuberculosis, adolescence is a time when patients have started to transition from childhood forms of tuberculosis, most of

which are not contagious, to adult-type tuberculosis, which has more infection-control ramifications for their contacts and healthcare workers.

Unfortunately, the immunological maturity associated with findings more characteristic of adult-type tuberculosis may not be mirrored by psychosocial maturity. Pediatricians may feel less comfortable broaching subjects such as sexual activity and substance use/abuse with patients for whom they have been caring for years. Adult providers, on the other hand, may have no qualms about discussing these subjects, but may be frustrated by the chasm between knowledge and behavior that can characterize adolescence. It is this mixture of findings of both younger children and adults that can be vexing to the providers caring for adolescents, and makes this population worthy of special consideration.

EPIDEMIOLOGY

Determining the burden of tuberculosis disease in adolescents is challenging. For many years, all pediatric cases (<15 years old) were reported together by the WHO. Beginning in 2006, pediatric data were disaggregated into cases under 5 years old and cases 5–14 years old.[1] While this was hugely beneficial to evaluating the specific impact of TB mortality in the under-5 population, this modification does not alter the ability to describe the burden of adolescent tuberculosis. Currently, adolescents can be included either with the school-aged children or with adults. As a consequence, most data specific to adolescents stem from single-center or national studies. For example, in the United States, where children (<18 years of age) compose 5–6% of all tuberculosis cases, adolescents 13–17 years of age accounted for between 19% (in US-born children) and 52% (in foreign-born children) of all pediatric cases.[2] In one large series from an urban Brazilian city, 37% of pediatric cases occurred in children 11–15 years of age.[3] For reasons that are unclear, the risk of progression from infection to disease is higher in adolescents (10–20%) than in primary school–aged children, and this risk is 2–6 times higher in adolescent girls than in adolescent boys. In both genders, the highest risk occurs during the peak of the adolescent growth spurt.

The prevalence of tuberculosis infection in adolescents is unclear, as in many high-burden communities, identification of infection has not been prioritized. One study in a region with high prevalence of both tuberculosis and human immunodeficiency virus (HIV) found that tuberculosis infection prevalence was 45% in secondary school students and was more common in older students and in boys.[4] These associations were thought to be due to increased contact with tuberculosis cases outside of the home. The social networks of adolescents more closely resemble those of adults. A social mixing study in adolescents living in a South African township found that 80% of their time was spent indoors, where tuberculosis can be most readily transmitted.

The median number of daily contacts peaked at 40 contacts in late adolescence (15–19 years old), with most of these contacts outside the home, including contact while riding public transportation.[5] This has significant implications for contact investigations based on an index case identifying their contacts. Consequently, adolescents are more likely to be discovered while already symptomatic, as opposed to being identified via active surveillance.[6] It is important to ask adolescents with tuberculosis, "Where do you go?" in addition to, "Who have you been with?" With broader social networks, unconventional public health measures may be needed. One example is using social media sites to find cases with mutual friends.[7] Even in some high-burden countries, a significant proportion of adolescents have access to cell phones and computers.

Another aspect of tuberculosis epidemiology unique to adolescents is the increasing prevalence of chronic conditions or adult-type diseases in childhood. Globally, the incidence of non-insulin-dependent diabetes mellitus is increasing in late childhood and adolescence, and diabetes is one of the most common risk factors for tuberculosis in adults in many nations. In addition, as adolescents take responsibility for insulin administration for juvenile-onset diabetes, adherence may wane, with resultant loss of glycemic control and an increased risk of progression to disease proportional to increases in glycosylated hemoglobin (Hgb A1c) levels.[8] Also, horizontal acquisition of HIV infection may first be noted in the adolescent who is dually infected with HIV and tuberculosis.

CLINICAL MANIFESTATIONS

The most frequent forms of tuberculosis disease are intrathoracic tuberculosis and peripheral lymphadenitis, similar to that seen in younger children (Table 12.1).[9,10] "Intrathoracic" tuberculosis refers to pulmonary parenchymal findings, pleural disease, and intrathoracic adenopathy. Extrathoracic disease accounts for 20–30% of all adolescent tuberculosis cases, with both intra- and extrathoracic tuberculosis seen in up to 20% of cases.[3,9,10]

The most common symptoms of pulmonary parenchymal and pleural disease in adolescents are described in Table 12.2. Classic symptoms seen in adults, such as night sweats and hemoptysis, are found less commonly in adolescents, even in those with cavitary disease. While many of the symptoms

Table 12.1. Most common sites of tuberculosis in adolescents*

SITE	DE PONTUAL ET AL. (2006; N = 52) FRANCE[9] %	CRUZ ET AL. (2013, N = 145) UNITED STATES[6] %
Intrathoracic	52	78
Pulmonary parenchymal	44	56
Intrathoracic adenopathy	58	22
Pleural	21	15
Extrathoracic	17	19
Peripheral lymphadenitis	8	7
Abdominal	10	1
Skeletal	6	2
Meningitis	8	4
Genitourinary	2	0
Ocular	0	2
Pericardial	0	0.6
Laryngeal	0	0.6
Intrathoracic and extrathoracic disease	31	3

*May not sum to 100% due to rounding and because some children had >1 manifestation.

will be the same in younger children and adolescents, the latter can better describe their symptoms. In low-incidence nations with active surveillance for tuberculosis, a sizeable percentage of adolescents with early tuberculosis disease may be asymptomatic or minimally symptomatic at time of diagnosis.

Peripheral lymphadenitis is seen most commonly in cervical nodes (in up to 75% of adolescents), followed by axillary and inguinal lymphadenitis. Relatively painless nodes, often lacking overlying skin discoloration, are noted. Most patients have constitutional or pulmonary findings; in one large series of patients of all ages, only 4% had isolated lymphadenitis. Weight loss, night sweats, and fever were seen in over 80%, and cough was reported in almost one-third of patients.[10]

In addition to intrathoracic disease and peripheral tuberculous lymphadenitis, providers caring for adolescents need to be cognizant of the manifestations of extrathoracic tuberculosis (see Chapter 10) with long incubation periods, which more commonly present during adulthood. These include genitourinary and ocular disease. Genitourinary tuberculosis accounts for over one-quarter of extrathoracic tuberculosis cases in adults, and is the second most common site of extrathoracic disease after peripheral lymphadenitis. Symptoms include dysuria, urgency, and frequency; some patients note hematuria.[11] Bilateral renal disease is seen in a minority. It is thought that genitourinary tuberculosis begins in the kidneys and spreads distally. Involvement of the uterus and Fallopian tubes may also be seen, resulting in infertility, unusual patterns of uterine bleeding, or recurrent miscarriages. Although it is unlikely that adolescents will seek evaluation for infertility, their disease may start during this time; tuberculosis has been found in up to 6% of women evaluated for infertility and is one of the more common causes of infertility in developing nations.[12]

Ocular tuberculosis occurs in adolescents and can be either a manifestation of miliary or

Table 12.2. Most common symptoms in adolescents with intrathoracic tuberculosis*

SYMPTOM	FREQUENCY (%)
CONSTITUTIONAL	
Fever	63–77
Malaise	26–71
Weight loss	30–73
PULMONARY	
Cough	54–88
Hemoptysis	8–24
Dyspnea	25–28
Asymptomatic	20**

*Data from.[6,9,14,15]

**From industrialized nation with active tuberculosis surveillance and targeted testing for latent tuberculosis infection.[6]

meningeal disease or an isolated finding. Posterior or pan-uveitis are the most common sites of disease, with manifestations including floaters and loss of visual acuity. Ophthalmological examination can demonstrate vasculitis, uveitis, "snowball" lesions in the vitreous, iridocyclitis, or retinal detachment. Loss of the red reflex (leukocoria) can be seen and confused with retinoblastoma.[13] While tuberculous meningitis peaks in children in the first few years of life, meningitis is seen in between 4% and 8% of adolescents with tuberculosis.[9,10] The clinical manifestations are similar to those of the younger child (see Chapter 11), but unusual neurological and psychiatric manifestations are more common. Diagnosis may be delayed if clinicians fail to consider the diagnosis in the older child or adolescent with unusual behavior, signs of increased intracranial pressure, or meningitis with cranial nerve involvement or signs of a stroke.

DIAGNOSIS

Intrathoracic Tuberculosis

Intrathoracic disease is the most common site of tuberculosis among adolescents. The incidence of cavitary disease increases with patient age, and cavities are seen in up to one-third of older adolescents.[14] The most common radiographic findings in adolescents with intrathoracic tuberculosis are described in Table 12.3, based on four series where adolescent data were disaggregated from data in younger children.[9,10,14,15] In contrast to the findings in younger children, intrathoracic adenopathy is somewhat less common among adolescents, but more likely if they have been infected recently. Radiographic findings, such as collapse-consolidation patterns, and symptoms (e.g., fixed wheezing unresponsive to beta agonists) seen commonly in younger children will be less common in adolescents given their larger airway diameters. Predominance of apical disease, as is seen in adult reactivation tuberculosis, has been reported variably in adolescents. While some series have shown that almost 60% of adolescents have apical lesions, up to one-third have had multilobar involvement.[16]

Given the nonspecific radiographic findings of non-cavitary intrathoracic tuberculosis, several scoring systems have been derived to differentiate tuberculosis from other etiologies in children and adults. One symptom-based approach from South Africa found that in children younger than 13 years of age, presence of a non-remitting cough of at least two weeks' duration, documented failure to thrive in the preceding three months, and fatigue had a sensitivity and specificity of 63% and 90%, respectively, for tuberculosis disease in HIV-uninfected children older than two years of age. However, this scoring system was insensitive in younger children and HIV-infected children of any age, and was not evaluated fully in adolescents.[17] The Brazilian National Ministry of Health scoring system for pediatric and adolescent tuberculosis uses a combination of clinical manifestations (fever, cough, malaise, expectoration, weight loss, diaphoresis), radiographic findings, and risk factors (tuberculosis contact, tuberculin skin test [TST] results, malnutrition) to stratify patients into three groups: highly likely, possible, and unlikely to be tuberculosis disease. This scoring system seemed to correlate well in both HIV-infected and HIV-uninfected children and adolescents who had positive cultures or a response to tuberculosis treatment.[18] A recent systematic review detailed the findings in adults of 13 scoring systems (9 derived in low-incidence nations) utilizing radiographic components in adults and found that cavitary lesions and apical involvement were significantly associated with intrathoracic

Table 12.3. Common radiographic findings for adolescents with intrathoracic tuberculosis*

FINDING	DE PONTUAL ET AL. (2006; N = 43) FRANCE[9] %	WONG ET AL. (2010; N = 78) TAIWAN[16] %	SANT'ANNA ET AL. (2011; N = 850) BRAZIL[14] %	CRUZ ET AL. (2013, N = 118) UNITED STATES[6] %
Consolidation	54	78	53	34
Cavity	33	58	32	26
Intrathoracic adenopathy	70	22	2	27
Pleural effusion	26	18	9	19
Miliary disease	14	N/A	1	8
Bilateral lesions	N/A	78	29	27

*Some studies[9,10] included adolescent with intra- and extrathoracic disease; the data reported here are only for those patients with thoracic involvement. Percentages may not sum to 100% due to rounding and because some children had >1 manifestation.

N/A: not available.

tuberculosis. While sensitivities of the scoring systems were high (>90%), specificities were poor.[19] It has been difficult to generalize results across settings due to differences in HIV prevalence and in tuberculosis incidence, which affect the pre-test probability of disease. None of these studies adequately evaluated the scoring systems in adolescent patients.

The diagnostic yield of microbiological, molecular, and immunological tests for tuberculosis in adolescents, where available, is compared to existing data for children and adults in Table 12.4. This was done in part because, for many diagnostic assays, it is not possible to differentiate data for adolescents alone. Unlike younger children, many adolescents with intrathoracic tuberculosis can expectorate sputum. Expectoration should occur in an outdoor setting or in a negative-pressure room to avoid transmission to health care personnel or other patients. One study in Ugandan adolescents found that adding an early-morning sputum specimen to specimens obtained at other times of the day resulted in a 10% and 43% increased culture yield for Lowenstein-Jensen and mycobacterium growth indicator tube (MGIT) methods, respectively.[20] Sputum induction—using heated saline to cause the younger adolescent patient to cough more vigorously and deeply—increases culture yield compared with passively collected sputum. Another study noted that, after controlling for age, induced sputum specimens in children less than 15 years old were more than four times more likely to be GeneXpert MTB/RIF–positive than non-induced sputum specimens,[21] potentially indicating the suboptimal nature of passively obtained sputum specimens even in older patients who can expectorate. Other studies have noted that obtaining multiple specimens per day was equivalent in diagnostic yield to obtaining specimens over several days,[22] which would make specimen collection easier. In contrast to infants and young children, in whom gastric aspirates often are culture-positive with miliary disease, adolescents with miliary tuberculosis often have negative sputum smears and cultures. As with adults, broncho-alveolar lavage or lung biopsy may be required to obtain microbiological confirmation of the disease.

Pleural effusions are common in adolescents, either in isolation or with concomitant parenchymal lung disease; the latter occurs in 20–40% of cases. Effusions usually are free-flowing and will layer out on decubitus radiographs. Bedside ultrasonography will not demonstrate the septations or debris that would be seen in pyogenic empyemas. Pleural fluid is exudative with elevated protein (>30 g/dL) and has an initial neutrophilic response, with lymphocytic predominance occurring later. An adenosine

Table 12.4. Sensitivity of tests in adolescents* treated for intrathoracic tuberculosis or tuberculosis lymphadenitis, as compared to younger children and to adults

TEST	CHILDREN (%)	ADOLESCENTS (%)[‡]	ADULTS (%)
IMMUNOCOMPETENT			
TST	70–90	83–89	31–84
IGRA	75–92	N/A	32–100
Smear microscopy: respiratory	27–38	25–38	45–82
Smear microscopy: lymph node	20–43	38	25–40
AFB culture: respiratory	8–30	17–54	57–72
AFB culture: lymph node	40–75	0–45	60–90
Xpert MTB/RIF: respiratory, smear-positive specimens	22–100	N/A	74–100
Xpert MTB/RIF: respiratory, smear-negative specimens	49–70	N/A	47–100
Xpert MTB/RIF: lymph node	80–84	N/A	78–99
IMMUNOCOMPROMISED			
TST	11–46	39	25–85
IGRA	12–55	11–47	64–91
Smear microscopy: respiratory	16–20	N/A	36–64
Smear microscopy: lymph node	35–53	N/A	10–24
AFB culture: respiratory	27–50	N/A	37–72
AFB culture: lymph node	73–88	N/A	42–92
Xpert MTB/RIF: respiratory, smear-positive specimens	36–84	N/A	67–100
Xpert MTB/RIF: respiratory, smear-negative specimens	67–100[†]	N/A	43–67
Xpert MTB/RIF: lymph node	N/A	N/A	75–100

Abbreviations: AFB = acid-fast bacilli; IGRA = interferon-gamma release assay; MTB = *Mycobacterium tuberculosis*; N/A = data not available (because either not published or not disaggregated from data from other age groups); RIF = rifampicin; TST = tuberculin skin test.

*Studies in which adolescent-specific data could not be disaggregated from pediatric or adult data were not included. Similarly, studies in which immunocompromised and immunocompetent children's data could not be disaggregated also were excluded. This resulted in a bias toward including studies in immunocompetent children from industrialized nations where the incidence of human immunodeficiency virus (HIV) is lower.

[‡]From references.[6,9,14,15,31,32]

[†]Small case series.

deaminase (ADA) level in pleural fluid greater than 40 IU/L has a sensitivity approaching 90%; the sensitivity of this test makes it highly desirable. Pleural punch biopsy has a higher yield for acid-fast stain and culture than pleural fluid alone, and histopathology performed on the biopsy specimen has a sensitivity of approximately 80%. The sensitivity of PCR for *M. tuberculosis* performed on pleural fluid in adolescents has varied widely (from 20–80%).[23] In one series of pleural tuberculosis, gastric aspirates or sputum culture were acid-fast smear or culture positive in one-third of adolescents and children with pleural effusions who had no apparent parenchymal lung lesions on chest radiography;[24] thus, upper respiratory cultures should be attempted in children with suspected pleural tuberculosis even if no lung parenchymal lesions are noted.

Extrathoracic Tuberculosis

For clinicians in low-incidence nations, differentiating tuberculosis and nontuberculous mycobacterial (NTM) lymphadenitis can be challenging. Studies have indicated that NTM adenitis is more common in preschool-aged children, children with normal chest radiographs, and children from low tuberculosis incidence areas who lack epidemiological risk factors for tuberculosis. In contrast, *M. tuberculosis* adenitis is more common in the school-aged child or adolescent, in those with abnormal chest radiographs, and in those with tuberculosis risk factors.[25] In one study performed in a region of South Africa with a very high tuberculosis incidence, Marais and colleagues found that tuberculous lymphadenitis could be diagnosed by fine-needle aspirate with acid-fast stain and mycobacterial culture in 94% of children with persistent (>4 weeks) cervical lymphadenopathy unresponsive to routine antibiotics, lymph node size ≥ 2 × 2 cm, and no visible skin lesion in a region drained by that node. Sensitivity of FNA was 89%, specificity was 98%, and positive predictive value was 93%.[26] FNA may be more feasible in the adolescent, who may not require sedation for the procedure. In one study of children and adolescents, FNA culture and GeneXpert MTB/RIF results had sensitivities of 63% and 80%, respectively.[27] The yield of smear microscopy can be enhanced by centrifugation of lymph node aspirates, with one study showing an increase in smear positivity from 34% to 66%.[28]

The diagnosis of other forms of extrathoracic tuberculosis that are more common in adolescents than younger children remains challenging. The hallmark finding of renal tuberculosis on urinalysis is sterile pyuria, but proteinuria and microscopic hematuria can also be seen. Renal biopsy may show caseating granulomas, papillary necrosis, and fibrosis. Distal spread can result in ureteral stenosis, hydroureter, and urinary reflux or obstruction. Imaging may show hydronephrosis, ureters with both dilated and stenotic regions, and renal atrophy (the latter occurring in late disease). Culture of urine is frequently positive but often requires a large volume to increase sensitivity. Tuberculosis in the female genital tract can result in a beaded or cobblestoned appearance to the Fallopian tubes on imaging due to strictures; calcified adnexal nodes; or endometrial adhesions.[29] Culture yield is low, even with laparoscopy (approximately 30%), and few specimens are AFB smear-positive. PCR for *M. tuberculosis* performed on biopsied tissue is 85–95% sensitive in uterine tuberculosis.[30] TB should be considered for any adolescent with uveitis. Diagnosis rarely is microbiologically confirmed, but instead is based upon a positive test for tuberculosis infection (TST or IGRA), exclusion of other conditions, and clinical response to antituberculosis therapy.

Immunological Tests

Performance characteristics of TSTs and IGRAs for adolescents are summarized in Table 12.4.[6,9,14,15,31,32] The predictive value of a positive TST or IGRA for the development of tuberculosis disease during adolescence is unclear, especially for patients in whom infection occurred years before. In contrast, recent conversion from a negative to positive result of IGRAs in adolescents is associated with an eightfold higher risk of progression to disease within two years when compared to IGRA nonconverters.[31] Compared with adults, the predictive value of IGRAs appears to be higher for adolescents, in whom the pooled positive predictive values of IGRAs are 1.8-fold higher than for TSTs.[33] Thus, IGRAs, more so than the TST, may allow for risk-stratification of adolescents who would most benefit from treatment of tuberculosis infection. There are few data on sensitivity and specificity of IGRAs in adolescents with suspected tuberculosis disease. The WHO does not recommend using IGRAs in low- and middle-income nations due to cost, uncertain advantages, and the need for laboratory infrastructure.

TREATMENT

The treatment regimens are no different for adolescents than for younger children or adults. For pediatricians accustomed to writing medications in milligrams per kilogram, it is important that the doses prescribed do not exceed the maximum doses used for adults (see Chapter 15). Few data exist on optimal dosing of tuberculosis medications in obese adolescents; some experts recommend dosing based on ideal body weight as opposed to total body weight.[34] The care of the patient dually infected with HIV and tuberculosis is discussed in Chapter 14.

The rate of adverse events in adolescents is difficult to discern, as data in studies and organization reports often are not disaggregated from those of younger children or adults. Using cohorts of young adults as proxies, one large study of goldminers found rates of hepatotoxicity of 0.07%, hypersensitivity reactions (0.25%), and peripheral neuropathy (0.21%) with isoniazid treatment of tuberculosis infection.[35] Smaller single-center studies in adolescents receiving multidrug therapy for tuberculosis disease found that 4% of patients complained of abdominal pain, but this was rarely associated with elevated liver transaminases or with synthetic hepatic dysfunction.[6] Asymptomatic elevation in transaminases may be seen in up to 15% of adolescents receiving treatment for disease, but these often return to normal levels during continued treatment.[9] The decision on whether to obtain baseline transaminases before starting adolescents on antituberculosis medication(s) should be informed by any medical comorbidities (particularly liver abnormalities), concomitant medication usage, substance use (see below), and rates of viral hepatitis in the community.

Adherence to treatment for adolescents has been best studied longitudinally in patients with chronic diseases, such as diabetes, cystic fibrosis, and HIV infection. For many of these conditions, adherence wanes in adolescence as the patients begin taking more control over their disease management. While adherence is less of a concern for patients with tuberculosis disease who are receiving directly observed therapy (DOT), it is a significant consideration for patients with tuberculosis infection or disease taking medications that are administered by the patient or family. Educational interventions have been useful in increasing completion of therapy for tuberculosis infection.[36] Other strategies to increase adherence include having families remind the patient to take medications, setting cellular phone alarms or making calendar reminders to prompt medication administration, and linking medication administration to something else the patient does daily. For many adolescents, taking medication in the morning may be easier than afternoon administration, as the morning schedule when the adolescent is in school is usually more consistent. Providers need to be cognizant that only 50% of children and adolescents with tuberculosis infection whose families administer the medication for regimens lasting six months or longer will actually complete therapy. Therefore, if an adolescent is at high risk for progression to disease, providers should consider determining if tuberculosis infection therapy can be administered under DOT. This has been shown in one low-incidence setting to result in completion rates of over 95%.[37]

Immune reconstitution inflammatory syndrome (IRIS) is signaled either by new symptoms or by worsening of existing TB symptoms after the patient started antituberculosis medications. While it has been best described in HIV-infected patients, where IRIS occurs in up to 20% of children and adolescents with tuberculosis disease after starting antiretroviral therapy,[38] IRIS has also been seen in HIV-uninfected adolescents. In these patients, the most common presentation is an increase in respiratory symptoms and worsening of existing intrathoracic lymphadenopathy or lung parenchymal disease. IRIS is often more common in adolescents than younger children, males, patients with multifocal disease, and patients with low body weight,[39] but these associations have not been seen uniformly.[40]

End-of-therapy chest radiographs may be abnormal in 50–60% of adolescents with intrathoracic involvement. Findings may include scarring, residual hilar or mediastinal lymphadenopathy, calcifications, bronchiectasis, or small residual pleural effusions. Adolescents who have cavitary disease and who continue to have positive acid-fast sputum smears after three months of treatment or whose six-month chest radiograph continues to demonstrate cavitary lesions should have therapy extended to nine months (for drug-susceptible isolates) to decrease the risk of relapse, similar to what is done for adult patients.

CONCOMITANT SUBSTANCE AND MEDICATION USE

Abuse of commercially available substances, illicit drugs, and prescription medications often begins in late childhood or early adolescence. For example, over 10% of smokers begin smoking before 10 years of age;[41] consequently, providers caring for adolescents with tuberculosis need to obtain a tobacco history for the child as well as the family. Smoking can impact transmission within the home and patient outcomes. One study found that smoking by the index case was associated with a 1.5-fold increase of tuberculosis infection among household contacts.[42] In addition, exposure to secondary smoke in household contacts resulted in an almost threefold increased risk of development of childhood tuberculosis disease.[43] Smokers are more likely to have delayed sputum-culture conversion[44] and higher rates of adverse events, relapse, and mortality.[45]

Alcohol is one of the most common substances used and abused by adolescents, with an estimated prevalence of up to 50% in some cultures, and binge drinking is common in adolescents. As an example, the age at first consumption of alcohol averages 12–13 years in Brazil.[46] Providers should consider obtaining baseline hepatic transaminases before starting antituberculosis therapy in adolescents admitting to substance use. Because of possible adverse effects on the liver, heavy substance use/abuse may change the risk/benefit ratio for the treatment of tuberculosis infection, making treatment less safe. When counseling adolescents with substance abuse who are about to start taking antituberculosis medications, it is unreasonable for providers to think that the patient will suddenly stop taking all the substances. While not condoning their substance use, it is important for providers to have a frank discussion with the adolescent about which substances would be relatively more and less harmful to them while they are taking TB medications.

It is also important to ask the adolescent about their use of drugs, including marijuana, which the adolescent may not consider when asked about "smoking," when the family/caregiver is not in the room. Certain behaviors associated with marijuana use may make M. tuberculosis transmission easier. These include "hotboxing," when marijuana is smoked inside of a closed car with multiple people repetitively inhaling exhaled smoke,[47] and the use of water pipes (bongs).[48] In one study, sharing bongs with an index case with cavitary disease was associated with a sixfold increased risk of transmission of M. tuberculosis.[49] "Shotgunning" is the practice of inhaling smoke and exhaling it into the mouths of others; this has been described with

smoking marijuana, heroin, and crack cocaine,[50] and is another possible route of tuberculosis transmission.

One cross-sectional study of South African tuberculosis patients (older adolescents and young adults) found that anxiety and depression were seen in up to 80% at diagnosis or while on treatment.[51] As many depressed patients may self-medicate with alcohol or other substances, and concomitant substance use may increase their risk of hepatotoxicity, adolescents with tuberculosis disease should be screened for depression. Providers should also be cognizant of the risk of intentional overdoses, particularly with isoniazid, which can cause benzodiazepine-refractory seizures which can only be stopped with administration of intravenous pyridoxine. For any adolescent who presents with new-onset unexplained refractory seizures, obtaining the history that someone in the house is taking isoniazid may be the clue to finding the cause.

In comparison with younger children, adolescent patients may be more likely to be receiving medications for chronic health conditions. Health care personnel need to be sure that there are no drug interactions if adolescents receiving antituberculosis medications are to be started on psychotropic or other agents. While selective serotonin reuptake inhibitors (SSRIs) do not interact with rifampicin, lamotrigine (used for bipolar disorder) and some atypical antipsychotic drugs may require dosage adjustments when rifamycins are also taken. Finally, providers need to discuss alternative contraceptive options (e.g., barrier protection, intrauterine devices) with post-menarchal females who are sexually active and receiving estrogen- or progesterone-based contraceptives if they are to be starting rifampicin-based regimens.

INFECTION CONTROL

While most young children with intrathoracic tuberculosis are not infectious, this is not the case for adolescents. The higher rates of cavitary disease and a more robust tussive force in adolescents make tuberculosis transmission easier. Risk factors for AFB sputum-smear positivity in adolescents, the best predictor of infectiousness, include presence of cavitary lesions, cough of greater than four weeks' duration, and lower lobe involvement.[16] If possible, adolescents with suspected pulmonary tuberculosis undergoing medical evaluation should be placed in a negative-pressure room in a high-resource setting or a highly ventilated room with open windows in a lower resource setting until the results of chest radiographs and sputum smears are available. If this is not feasible, patients should wear simple surgical facemasks, as this has been shown to reduce transmission over the short term.[52] At most children's hospitals in low tuberculosis-burden settings, transmission of M. tuberculosis is uncommon even for adolescents. In one case series, only 12% of children and adolescents had radiographic findings consistent with contagious tuberculosis (miliary disease, cavities, or extensive apical disease), and these patients accounted for all of the positive AFB sputum smears in the series. In the same series, chest radiographs performed during the child's hospitalization revealed that 17% of the family caregivers for these patients had previously undiagnosed pulmonary tuberculosis and were the likely source for the child's disease and a potential risk for other patients and hospital staff.[53]

OTHER CONSIDERATIONS

In addition to the medical challenges of treating adolescents with tuberculosis, providers must also be aware of social challenges that these patients often face. Adolescents may need to be isolated at home after the initiation of treatment until they are rendered noninfectious by chemotherapy. While it is a necessary public health measure in some instances, isolation has substantial ramifications for the adolescent. Some adolescents work at a job, and the loss of income to the family while the child is isolated can have significant consequences. Being held out of school can have academic implications for students, and providers should work with families to see that, when possible, schools send home work for the student to decrease the academic impact of school absenteeism. Isolation from peers is difficult for most adolescents. While social media sites can alleviate some of this isolation and enable continued contact with peers, adolescents should be cautioned about what information to share on social media so as to not make the social stigma that sometimes accompanies tuberculosis more widespread. Certain infection-control measures within the home are considered more palatable than others. In one study of adult TB patients in a rural region of South Africa, while almost 90% of patients accepted wearing face masks in health care facilities, only 66% accepted wearing face masks in their home.[54]

Recognition of poor adherence with this recommendation should affect the decision on when to screen household contacts. Frequently obtaining sputum specimens for smear microscopy can allow an adolescent to safely return to activities in an efficient time frame.

Another social consideration is the impact of school-based contact investigations. While unnecessary for most young children, these investigations may be necessary for adolescent patients with infectious intrathoracic tuberculosis. Given the percentage of waking hours that most children spend in schools, substantial transmission has been reported in schools when the index case was a secondary school student.[55] School-based contact investigations should strive to maintain patient confidentiality and be minimally disruptive of educational endeavors. Early communication with school stakeholders (school administration, teachers, and organizers of parental organizations), educational sessions at the school for students and their families, and clear explanation of necessary public health steps may alleviate concerns and increase participation in investigations.

PREVENTION

Treatment of tuberculosis infection is described in Chapter 16. One treatment regimen that has been more thoroughly studied in adolescents than in younger children is isoniazid/rifapentine given weekly for three months (3HP). This regimen has the advantage of a shortened duration, and the rates of completion were much higher for this regimen than for nine months of isoniazid (9H); adverse event rates were comparable to those with 9H.[56] One barrier to more widespread use is that 3HP is currently given only by directly observed therapy, which may limit use in certain regions. However, prior studies have indicated that older adolescents receiving six to nine months of self-administered isoniazid were significantly less likely to complete therapy than younger children were.[57] Failure to complete therapy was associated with development of hepatitis or symptoms of adverse events. Another option for treatment of tuberculosis infection is four months of rifampicin. When administered to one cohort of adolescents, 88% completed therapy, and only 5% experienced any symptoms; none developed hepatitis.[58] Given the historically higher rates of progression from infection to disease in adolescents compared with school-aged children, and that an adolescent with intrathoracic tuberculosis is more likely to be contagious than a younger child, optimizing adherence for the treatment of tuberculosis infection in this population is critical.

REFERENCES

1. World Health Organization. *Global Tuberculosis Report 2014*. Geneva: World Health Organization; 2014.

2. Winston CA, Menzies HJ. Pediatric and adolescent tuberculosis in the United States, 2008–2010. *Pediatrics*. 2012 Dec;130(6):e1425–e1432.

3. Franco R, Santana MA, Matos E, Sousa V, Lemos AC. Clinical and radiological analysis of children and adolescents with tuberculosis in Bahia, Brazil. *Braz J Infect Dis*. 2003 Feb;7(1):73–81.

4. Middelkoop K, Bekker LG, Liang H, et al. Force of tuberculosis infection among adolescents in a high HIV and TB prevalence community: a cross-sectional observational study. *BMC Infect Dis*. 2011 Jun;11:156. doi:10.1186/1471-2334-11-156

5. Wood R, Racow K, Bekker LG, et al. Indoor social networks in a South African township: potential contribution of location to tuberculosis transmission. *PLoS One*. 2012 Jun;7(6):e39246. doi:10.1371/journal.pone.0039246

6. Cruz AT, Hwang KM, Birnbaum GD, Starke JR. Adolescents with tuberculosis: a review of 145 cases. *Pediatr Infect Dis J*. 2013 Sep;32(9):937–941.

7. Thomas TA, Heysell SA, Houpt ER, Moore JL, Keller SJ. Outbreak of pyrazinamide-monoresistant tuberculosis identified using genotype cluster and social media analysis. *Int J Tuberc Lung Dis*. 2014 May;18(5):552–558.

8. Webb EA, Hesseling AC, Schaaf HS, et al. High prevalence of *Mycobacterium tuberculosis* infection and disease in children and adolescents with type 1 diabetes mellitus. *Int J Tuberc Lung Dis*. 2009 Jul;13(7):868–874.

9. De Pontual L, Balu L, Ovetchkine P, et al. Tuberculosis in adolescents: a French retrospective study of 52 cases. *Pediatr Infect Dis J*. 2006 Oct;25(10):930–932.

10. Biadglegne F, Tesfaye W, Sack U, Rodloff AC. Tuberculous lymphadenitis in northern Ethiopia: in a public health and microbiological perspective. *PLoS One*. 2013 Dec;8(12):e81918. doi:10.1371/journal.pone.0081918.

11. Daher Ede F, da Silva GB Jr, Barros EJ. Renal tuberculosis in the modern era. *Am J Trop Med Hyg*. 2013 Jan;88(1):54–64.

12. Chavhan GB, Hira P, Rathod K, et al. Female genital tuberculosis: hysterosalpingographic appearance. *Br J Radiol*. 2004 Feb;77(914):164–169.

13. Wroblewski KJ, Hidayat AA, Neafie RC, Rao NA, Zapor M. Ocular tuberculosis: a clinicopathologic and molecular study. *Ophthalmology*. 2011 Apr;118(4):772–777.

14. Sant'Anna CC, Schmidt CM, March Mde F, Pereira SM, Barreto ML. Radiologic findings of pulmonary tuberculosis in adolescents. *Braz J Infect Dis*. 2011 Jan–Feb;15(1):40–44.

15. Sant'Anna C, March MF, Barreto M, Pereira S, Schmidt C. Pulmonary tuberculosis in adolescents: radiographic features. *Int J Tuberc Lung Dis*. 2009 Dec;13(12):1566–1568.

16. Wong KS, Huang YC, Lai SH, Chiu CY, Huang YH, Lin TY. Validity of symptoms and radiographic features in predicting positive acid-fast bacilli smears in adolescents with tuberculosis. *Int J Tuberc Lung Dis*. 2010 Feb;14(2):155–159.

17. Marais BJ, Gie RP, Hesseling AC, et al. A refined symptom-based approach to diagnose pulmonary tuberculosis in children. *Pediatrics*. 2006 Nov;118(5):e1350–e1359.

18. Pedrozo C, Sant'Anna CC, March Mde F, Lucena SC. Efficacy of the scoring system, recommended by the Brazilian National Ministry of Health, for the diagnosis of pulmonary tuberculosis in children and adolescents, regardless of their HIV status. *J Bras Pneumol*. 2010 Jan-Feb;36(1):92–98.

19. Pinto LM, Pai M, Dheda K, Schwartzman K, Menzies D, Steingart KR. Scoring systems using chest radiographic features for the diagnosis of pulmonary tuberculosis in adults: a systematic review. *Eur Respir J*. 2013 Aug;42(2):480–494.

20. Ssengooba W, Kateete DP, Wajja A, et al. An early morning sputum sample is necessary for the diagnosis of pulmonary tuberculosis, even with more sensitive techniques: a prospective cohort study among adolescent TB suspects in Uganda. *Tuberc Res Treat*. 2012 Dec;2012:970203. doi:10.1155/2012/970203

21. Rachow A, Clowes P, Saathoff E, et al. Increased and expedited case detection by Xpert MTB/RIF assay in childhood tuberculosis: a prospective cohort study. *Clin Infect Dis*. 2012 May;54(10):1388–1396.

22. Al-Aghbari N, Al-Sonboli N, Yassin MA, et al. Multiple sampling in one day to optimize

smear microscopy in children with tuberculosis in Yemen. *PLoS One.* 2009 Apr;4(4):e5140. doi:10.1371/journal.pone.005140

23. Fischer GB, Andrade CF, Lima JB. Pleural tuberculosis in children. *Paediatr Respir Rev.* 2011 Mar;12(1):27–30.

24. Cruz AT, Ong LT, Starke JR. Childhood pleural tuberculosis: a review of 45 cases. *Pediatr Infect Dis J.* 2009 Nov;28(11):981–984.

25. Carvalho AC, Codecasa L, Pinsi G, et al. Differential diagnosis of cervical mycobacterial adenitis in children. *Pediatr Infect Dis J.* 2010 Jul;29(7):629–633.

26. Marais BJ, Wright CA, Schaaf HS, et al. Tuberculous lymphadenitis as a cause of persistent cervical lymphadenitis in children from a tuberculosis-endemic area. *Pediatr Infect Dis J.* 2006 Feb;25(2):142–146.

27. Coetzee L, Nicol MP, Jacobson R, et al. Rapid diagnosis of pediatric mycobacterial lymphadenitis using fine needle aspiration biopsy. *Pediatr Infect Dis J.* 2014 Sep;33(9):893–896.

28. Tadesse M, Abebe G, Abdissa K, et al. Concentration of lymph node aspirate improves the sensitivity of acid-fast smear microscopy for the diagnosis of tuberculous lymphadenitis in Jimma, southwest Ethiopia. *PLoS One.* 2014 Sep;9(9):e106726. doi:10.1371/journal.pone.0106726

29. Ahmadi F, Zafarani F, Shahrzad G. Hysterosalpingographic appearances of female genital tract tuberculosis: Part II: Uterus. *Int J Fertil Steril.* 2014 Apr;8(1):13–20.

30. Sankar MM, Kumar P, Munawwar A, et al. Usefulness of multiplex PCR in the diagnosis of genital tuberculosis in females with infertility. *Eur J Clin Microbiol Infect Dis.* 2013 Mar;32(3):399–405.

31. Machingaidze S, Verver S, Mulenga H, et al. Predictive value of recent QuantiFERON conversion for tuberculosis disease in adolescents. *Am J Respir Crit Care Med.* 2012 Nov;186(10):1051–1056.

32. Stavri H, Ene L, Popa GL, et al. Comparison of tuberculin skin test with a whole-blood interferon gamma release assay and ELISA, in HIV positive children and adolescent with TB. *Roum Arch Microbiol Immunol.* 2009 Jan–Mar;68(1):14–19.

33. Diel R, Loddenkemper R, Nienhaus A. Predictive value of interferon-gamma release assays and tuberculin skin testing for progression from latent TB infection to disease state: a meta-analysis. *Chest.* 2012 Jul;142(1):63–75.

34. Geiseler PJ, Manis RD Jr, Maddux MS. Dosage of antituberculosis drugs in obese patients. *Am Rev Respir Dis.* 1985 Jun;131(6):944–946.

35. Grant AD, Mngadi KT, van Halsema CL, Luttig MM, Fielding KL, Churchyard GJ. Adverse events with isoniazid preventive therapy: experience from a large trial. *AIDS.* 2010 Nov;24(Suppl 5):S29–S36.

36. M'imunya JM, Kredo T, Volmink J. Patient education and counselling for promoting adherence to treatment for tuberculosis. *Cochrane Database Syst Rev.* 2012 May;16:5:CD006591. doi:10.1002/14651858.CD006591.pub2

37. Cruz AT, Starke JR. Increasing adherence for latent tuberculosis infection therapy with health department-administered therapy. *Pediatr Infect Dis J.* 2012 Feb;31(2):193–195.

38. Wang ME, Castillo ME, Montano SM, Zunt JR. Immune reconstitution inflammatory syndrome in human immunodeficiency virus-infected children in Peru. *Pediatr Infect Dis J.* 2009 Oct;28(10):900–903.

39. Thampi N, Stephens D, Rea E, Kitai I. Unexplained deterioration during antituberculous therapy in children and adolescents: clinical presentation and risk factors. *Pediatr Infect Dis J.* 2012 Feb;31(2):129–133.

40. Olive C, Mouchet F, Toppet V, Haelterman E, Levy J. Paradoxical reaction during tuberculosis treatment in immunocompetent children: clinical spectrum and risk factors. *Pediatr Infect Dis J.* 2013 May;32(5):446–449.

41. Everett SA, Warren CW, Sharp D, Kann L, Husten CG, Crossett LS. Initiation of cigarette smoking and subsequent smoking behavior among U.S. high school students. *Prev Med.* 1999 Nov;29(5):327–333.

42. Godoy P, Cayla JA, Carmona G, et al., & Grupo de Trabajo de Estudios de Contactos de Tuberculosis de Cataluña. Smoking in tuberculosis patients increases the risk of infection in their contacts. *Int J Tuberc Lung Dis.* 2013 Jun;17(6):771–776.

43. Patra S, Sharma S, Behera D. Passive smoking, indoor air pollution, and childhood tuberculosis: a case control study. *Indian J Tuberc.* 2012 Jul;59(3):151–155.

44. Nijenbandring de Boer R, Oliveira e Souza Filho JB, Cobelens F, et al. Delayed culture conversion due to cigarette smoking in active pulmonary tuberculosis patients. *Tuberculosis (Edinb).* 2014 Jan;94(1):87–91.

45. Bonacci RA, Cruz-Hervert LP, Garcia-Garcia L, et al. Impact of cigarette smoking on rates and clinical prognosis of pulmonary tuberculosis in Southern Mexico. *J Infect.* 2013 Apr;66(4):303–312.

46. Malta DC, Machado IE, Porto DL, et al. Alcohol consumption among Brazilian adolescents

according to the National Adolescent School-based Health Survey (PeNSE 2012). *Rev Bras Epidemiol*. 2014;17(Suppl 1):203–214.

47. Oeltmann JE, Oren E, Haddad MB, et al. Tuberculosis outbreak in marijuana users, Seattle, Washington, 2004. *Emerg Infect Dis*. 2006 Jul;12(7):1156–1159.

48. Munckhof WJ, Konstantinos A, Wamsley M, Mortlock M, Gilpin C. A cluster of tuberculosis associated with use of a marijuana water pipe. *Int J Tuberc Lung Dis*. 2003 Sep;7(9):860–865.

49. Thu K, Hayes M, Miles S, Tierney L, Foy A. Marijuana "bong" smoking and tuberculosis. *Intern Med J*. 2013 Apr;43(4):456–458.

50. Perlman DC, Perkins MP, Paone D, et al. "Shotgunning" as an illicit drug smoking practice. *J Subst Abuse Treat*. 1997 Jan–Feb;14(1):3–9.

51. Peltzer K, Naidoo P, Matseke G, Louw J, Mchunu G, Tutshana B. Prevalence of psychological distress and associated factors in tuberculosis patients in public primary care clinics in South Africa. *BMC Psychiatry*. 2012 Jul;12:89. doi:10.1186/1471-244X-12-89

52. Dharmadhikari AS, Mphahlele M, Stoltz A, et al. Surgical facemasks worn by patients with multidrug-resistant tuberculosis: impact on infectivity of air on a hospital ward. *Am J Respir Crit Care Med*. 2012 May;185(10):1104–1109.

53. Cruz AT, Medina D, Whaley EM, Ware KM, Koy TH, Starke JR. Tuberculosis among families of children with suspected tuberculosis and employees at a children's hospital. *Infect Control Hosp Epidemiol*. 2011 Feb;32(2):188–190.

54. Gonzalez-Angulo Y, Geldenhuys H, Van As D, et al. Knowledge and acceptability of patient-specific infection control measures for pulmonary tuberculosis. *Am J Infect Control*. 2013 Aug;41(8):717–722.

55. Trollfors B, Stangebye-Nielsen R, Karlsson E, Jonsson B, Dotevall L. Spread of tuberculosis in a high school. *Acta Paediatr*. 2013 Mar;102(3):e140–e141.

56. Sterling TR, Villarino ME, Borisov AS, et al., & TB Trials Consortium PREVENT TB Study Team. *N Engl J Med*. 2011 Dec 8;365(23):2155–2166.

57. Chang SH, Eitzman SR, Nahid P, Finelli ML. Factors associated with failure to complete isoniazid therapy for latent tuberculosis infection in children and adolescents. *J Infect Public Health*. 2014 Mar–Apr;7(2):145–152.

58. Daskalaki I, Byun J, Dogbey MC, Tolbert-Warren C, Watson BM. Tolerability of rifampin monotherapy for latent tuberculosis infection in children. *Pediatr Infect Dis J*. 2011 Nov;30(11):1014–1015.

13

TUBERCULOSIS IN NEONATES AND INFANTS

Adrie Bekker

HIGHLIGHTS OF THIS CHAPTER

- Any unwell tuberculosis-exposed infant, regardless of the mother's infectious status, needs urgent evaluation for tuberculosis disease.
- Treatment initiation is urgent in any infant with tuberculosis. If an infant is symptomatic, start treatment as soon as appropriate specimens have been obtained for culture and determination of drug-susceptibility.
- If at all possible, an infant with tuberculosis should remain in close contact with the mother and every effort made to enable her to continue breastfeeding.
- Remain vigilant for drug toxicity in the very young infant where enzyme immaturity and varying body constitution may affect antituberculosis and antiretroviral drug exposure and toxicity.
- Undiagnosed infectious tuberculosis may occur in any health facility, but it is particularly dangerous in congregate neonatal settings such as "kangaroo" care units; continual vigilance for symptoms and signs of tuberculosis in patients and staff is essential.

TUBERCULOSIS IS a global health problem and adversely affects both pregnant women and their offspring. In 2013, the World Health Organization (WHO) estimated there were 3.3 million new cases of tuberculosis in women, resulting in 510,000 deaths, of which 180,000 (35%) were in HIV-infected women.[1] Non-obstetric infection-related deaths, including tuberculosis, now account for 28% of maternal deaths worldwide.[2]

Tuberculosis in pregnancy is associated with unfavorable perinatal and infant outcomes. Increases in pre-eclampsia and vaginal bleeding have been observed, as well as a twofold risk of delivering premature and low birthweight infants, and a sixfold increase in perinatal infant deaths.[3,4] Table 13.1 refers to definitions for maternal-infant tuberculosis used in this chapter. Tuberculosis in pregnant and post-partum women, especially if untreated, can

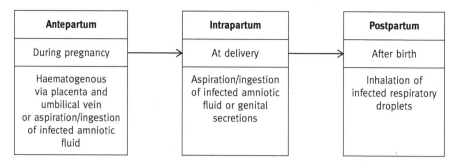

FIGURE 13.1   Transmission modes for perinatal tuberculosis.

result in transmission of *Mycobacterium tuberculosis* to the fetus and newborn (Figure 13.1). *In utero* transmission, hematogenously via the placenta or aspiration, or ingestion of infected amniotic fluid before or during birth, results in *congenital* tuberculosis; respiratory droplet spread from an infectious source case, usually the mother, after birth results in *postnatal* tuberculosis. *Perinatal tuberculosis* is the preferred term, combining the entities of congenital (ante- and intra-partum transmission) and postnatal (post-partum transmission) tuberculosis.

Tuberculosis disease progression is highest in the first year following infection, affecting particularly the very young, when immune immaturity is present. Without appropriate treatment, up to 50% of infected infants will develop tuberculosis disease, 30% of whom will have progressive pulmonary or disseminated disease.[5] In Pune, India, a fourfold increase in mortality was reported among infants with maternal HIV-associated tuberculosis,[6] while among South African infants, a 24% mortality was observed in those aged less than three months with culture-confirmed tuberculosis.[7] The outcome of isolated pulmonary tuberculosis can be good in the young, however, if treatment is initiated early.[8] Increased awareness and early diagnosis and treatment are vital to improve outcomes of tuberculosis in infants.

A high index of suspicion by health care providers for tuberculosis in pregnancy and post-partum is imperative in order to identify and treat the disease early. Appropriate assessment of the tuberculosis-exposed newborn is essential, considering the high risk of progression to disease following infection. Signs and symptoms of tuberculosis in the newborn and infant must be recognized early and acted upon rapidly. In infants, the time elapsing between infection and disease can be of shorter duration and disease presentation more acute than in older children. Optimal treatment in newborns

and infants is essential for improved outcomes. In high-burden tuberculosis/HIV settings, HIV testing should be offered to all persons with suspected tuberculosis, including mothers and infants, and combination antiretroviral therapy (ART) initiated if indicated. Integrated maternal and infant tuberculosis care strategies are key to control this disease and improve overall outcomes in these vulnerable populations.

TUBERCULOSIS IN PREGNANCY

The global burden of tuberculosis disease among pregnant women remains undefined, but 216,500 cases of tuberculosis were estimated worldwide in 2011.[9] Although relatively rare, a resurgence of tuberculosis in pregnancy has occurred as a result of the start of the HIV epidemic, the increase in drug-resistant tuberculosis, changes in socio-economic conditions, and increased migration. Data from selected populations show a prevalence of tuberculosis in pregnant women ranging from 0.06–0.53% in HIV-uninfected women to 1–11% in HIV-infected women.[10]

Potential risk factors for developing tuberculosis in pregnancy include HIV infection, prior close contact with a case of contagious tuberculosis, and a past history of tuberculosis. A high index of suspicion for tuberculosis in pregnancy is also needed for individuals emigrating from endemic regions to the developed world. Current WHO guidelines for tuberculosis infection-screening differ between tuberculosis low- and high-burden countries. In areas of low prevalence, screening, which includes a tuberculin skin test (TST) or interferon-gamma-release assay (IGRA), is recommended for high-risk individuals only, followed by treatment of infected individuals after tuberculosis disease has been excluded.[11] In high-burden settings, routine screening is not

Table 13.1. Definitions for maternal-infant tuberculosis used in this chapter

Neonate or newborn	First 28 days of life
Prematurity	Born at less than 37 weeks' gestational age
Low birth weight	Birth weight of less than 2500 grams
Infant	Less than 12 months
Congenital tuberculosis	Newborn presenting with tuberculosis disease at birth or shortly thereafter. Tuberculosis infection took place *in utero* or during birth
Postnatal tuberculosis	Infection occurs post-partum and disease presents shortly after birth
Perinatal tuberculosis	Combined congenital and postnatal tuberculosis
Perinatal period	Period around birth (5 months before and 1 month after)
Close contact	Someone sharing an enclosed space with the index case for extended daily periods*
Tuberculosis-exposed newborn	A newborn in close contact with someone with infectious tuberculosis, normally the mother or another caregiver
Tuberculosis screening	A systematic process to establish the diagnosis or its exclusion in someone with clinical signs and symptoms suggestive of tuberculosis disease
Tuberculosis infection	No symptoms or signs of tuberculosis, but the person is infected with tubercle bacilli, following exposure
Tuberculosis disease	Illness that occurs in someone infected with *M. tuberculosis*, characterized by clinical symptoms and signs, with or without laboratory or radiological evidence*
Treatment for tuberculosis infection	Treatment offered to contacts who are at risk of developing tuberculosis disease, following exposure to an infectious person, in order to reduce that risk*
Tuberculosis treatment	A 2-month intensive phase with 3 or 4 antituberculosis drugs, followed by a 4-month continuation phase with 2 drugs

*Adapted from the WHO's *Guidance for National Tuberculosis Programmes on the Management of Tuberculosis in Children.* 2nd ed. Geneva: WHO; 2014.

recommended, with the exception of HIV-infected individuals and children below 5 years of age with a known contact.[11] Divergent results have been reported for the TST, with earlier studies suggesting diminished tuberculin sensitivity in pregnancy,[12] while more recent studies showed no difference.[13,14] In an Indian study performed in pregnant women, an IGRA resulted in more positive results than the TST; of the 401 women included, 150 (37%) had a positive IGRA, compared to 59 (14%) positive TST results ($p < 0.005$) among a background prevalence of tuberculosis infection of 35–40% in the population.[15] A potential decrease in the sensitivity of both TST and the IGRAs during pregnancy is postulated

to be caused by increasing levels of progesterone, favoring a Th2-type immune response, and suppressing the cell-mediated Th1 immune response, which must be intact for both the TST and the IGRA assays to function properly.[16]

Increased awareness for diagnosing tuberculosis in pregnancy is required during the ante-, intra-, and post-partum period, as symptoms are often vague and nonspecific. The recommended tuberculosis symptom-screening tool (cough, fever, night sweats, and weight loss) does not perform well in pregnancy as poor weight gain is an unreliable predictor for the disease in pregnant women. Confounding matters further is the fact that additional symptoms of tuberculosis, like tiredness and fatigue, frequently occur with pregnancy, potentially leading to delayed diagnosis. The tuberculosis symptom-screening tool has high specificity of between 84–90.9%, but its sensitivity is very poor, ranging from 28–54.5%, as shown by two recent studies reporting on tuberculosis screening in HIV-infected pregnant women.[17,18] Despite this low reported sensitivity, the tuberculosis symptom-screening tool is currently the best one available when deciding upon further evaluation for tuberculosis in a pregnant woman. Noteworthy is the finding from a recent large United Kingdom cohort that women in the early post-partum period are twice as likely to develop tuberculosis as non-pregnant women.[19] Health care providers caring for mothers need to have a high index of suspicion for tuberculosis in the puerperal period, a period of extremely high risk for transmission of *M. tuberculosis* to the newborn. If any tuberculosis-related symptoms are present in a pregnant or post-partum woman, a thorough history, a clinical examination, with or without shielded chest radiology, and other special investigations to exclude tuberculosis disease should be conducted.

The clinical presentation of tuberculosis in pregnancy varies widely. Women can be asymptomatic, or develop typical pulmonary tuberculosis (PTB), but they may also present with more severe forms of tuberculosis, including disseminated disease. PTB is the most common form of disease, but extrapulmonary tuberculosis (EPTB) occurs in 5–10% of pregnant women with tuberculosis.[20] However, EPTB has become more frequent since the start the HIV epidemic, presenting more commonly in immune-compromised individuals. The type of perinatal tuberculosis in the fetus or newborn—congenital or postnatal—depends mainly on the type of tuberculosis in the mother (Figure 13.2). *In utero* and at-birth transmission (congenital) are more likely in pregnant

women with primary tuberculosis, presenting with pleural effusion, disseminated disease (miliary tuberculosis or meningitis), or other EPTB that has a bacillemic phase; postnatal transmission is more likely in post-partum women with typical cavitating PTB.[21,22] Regardless of the mode or time of transmission, the approach to a tuberculosis-exposed newborn is the same.

Tuberculosis-Exposed Newborn

A tuberculosis-exposed newborn is a neonate who has been in direct contact with a tuberculosis source case, most often the mother, who may pose an infectious risk irrespective of the type of tuberculosis or sputum acid-fast smear or mycobacterial culture results. Previous studies have shown a 60–80% risk of transmission to infants from a close acid-fast sputum smear-positive contact, and 30–40% from an acid-fast sputum smear-negative contact.[23] More pronounced adverse perinatal outcomes have been reported when the mother has advanced pulmonary lesions and when tuberculosis is either treated late in pregnancy or incompletely treated.[24] In South Africa, a high-burden setting, the Southern African Society for Paediatric Infectious Diseases (SASPID) defined a potentially infectious mother as someone who has received less than two months of effective treatment for tuberculosis disease at the time of delivery, or whose sputum smear has not yet become negative or is unknown at the time of birth.[25]

Guidelines regarding the management of the tuberculosis-exposed newborn vary widely across different countries, with little evidence to support current practices.[26] The approach to a tuberculosis-exposed newborn depends largely on clinical circumstances and available resources. We therefore propose a strategy used within a tuberculosis high-burden setting, based on clinical experience

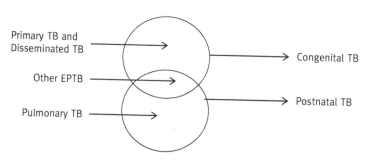

Primary TB and Disseminated TB → Congenital TB

Other EPTB →

Pulmonary TB → Postnatal TB

FIGURE 13.2   Types of maternal tuberculosis associated with perinatal tuberculosis.

and expert opinion, realizing that this may not suit all settings, and cases may need to be individualized. In this strategy, two issues are key to ensuring appropriate management: (1) Establish whether the newborn is well or unwell; (2) determine whether the possible source case is infectious. The risk for disease progression in a newborn may vary following infection with *M. tuberculosis* (see Figure 13.3).

An unwell newborn is defined as a tuberculosis-exposed newborn with symptoms and signs suggestive of tuberculosis disease, which may include respiratory distress, hepatosplenomegaly, or fever. Any unwell tuberculosis-exposed newborn, regardless of the mother's infectious status, needs urgent newborn care, as well as evaluation for tuberculosis disease. After stabilization of the newborn, testing should be conducted in the maternal-infant pair, including a tuberculosis symptom-screening tool given to the mother, chest radiography for the mother, and a clinical examination and tuberculosis-directed special investigations for the newborn. *If tuberculosis in the newborn is suspected or present, appropriate treatment should be initiated immediately*, as delay in treatment will worsen prognosis. Once tuberculosis has been excluded in the newborn and mother, and the underlying condition treated in the newborn, regular follow-up visits should ensue to monitor the well-being of the infant.

In the case of a well tuberculosis-exposed newborn whose mother does not have infectious tuberculosis disease or who has received more than two months of appropriate tuberculosis treatment and is responding well, a more conservative approach may be advised. In this scenario, no treatment is indicated for the infant while the child remains asymptomatic, but a BCG vaccine should be given where this is standard practice. Routine management and regular follow-up of the newborn is paramount in this setting. The infant should be evaluated for symptoms and signs of tuberculosis at each well-child visit, and promptly investigated for tuberculosis if indicated.

In the case of a mother with potentially contagious tuberculosis, the approach to a tuberculosis-exposed newborn at risk for *M. tuberculosis* infection and disease progression becomes more challenging, and the strategy in Figure 13.4 is proposed.

"Unwell" (symptoms and signs suggestive of tuberculosis) and "well and high-risk" tuberculosis-exposed newborns who are diagnosed with confirmed or probable tuberculosis disease should receive at least six months of treatment with three or four antituberculosis drugs in the intensive phase, and two drugs during the continuation phase. Other facets of care are important, including regular follow-up, weight checks, and drug-dose adjustments according to weight gain. A "well and high-risk" tuberculosis-exposed newborn who has had tuberculosis excluded, and a "well and low-risk" exposed newborn should receive six to nine months of isoniazid for possible tuberculosis infection. Monthly follow-up visits should be conducted for the duration of treatment, and isoniazid dosage adjusted according to weight gain. At each visit, screening for symptoms and signs suggestive of tuberculosis should be performed, and an infant who develops these should be evaluated for tuberculosis disease. Some guidelines recommend performing a TST toward the end of treatment—if the result is negative, a single dose of a BCG vaccine is given when it is standard practice, or where the risk of exposure to additional cases of tuberculosis is high.[27] BCG vaccine protects against the more severe types of disseminated tuberculosis, miliary and meningitis disease, but is contraindicated in HIV-infected newborns. Careful follow-up of the tuberculosis-exposed newborn should continue for a period of at least two years.

Where the health system makes use of "Road to Health" cards, it is essential that the diagnosis and steps taken for treatment and management be briefly noted.

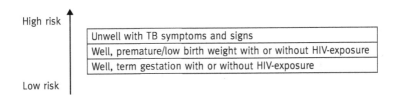

FIGURE 13.3   Risk for a tuberculosis-exposed newborn to develop tuberculosis disease.

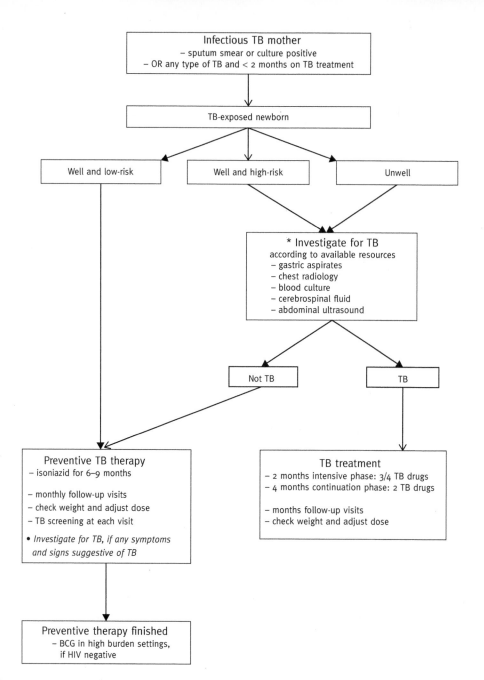

FIGURE 13.4   Approach to a tuberculosis-exposed newborn from a potentially infectious mother.

PERINATAL AND INFANT TUBERCULOSIS

Tuberculosis disease in the young is not a single entity; it represents a continuum of disease, with many overlapping symptoms and signs. The term "perinatal tuberculosis" encompasses both congenital and postnatal disease (Figure 13.5), where the exact time point and mode of infection with *M. tuberculosis* is difficult to determine, and the clinical and radiological presentations overlap. Newborns can also be infected with *M. tuberculosis* later in infancy, via droplet spread from an infectious contact. "Infant tuberculosis" refers to children diagnosed in the first year of life. Early diagnosis of tuberculosis may be difficult, with neonates and infants

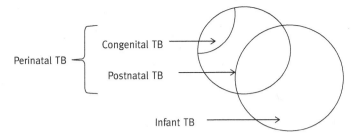

FIGURE 13.5   Tuberculosis disease terminology in neonates and infants.

often being asymptomatic, and symptoms and signs only becoming apparent in the late neonatal period and early infancy. TST and IGRA are insensitive for neonates and infants and are more often negative in these children than in older children with tuberculosis infection or disease.[28] In the following section, important differences between the earlier (mainly congenital) and later (mainly postnatal and infant) presentations of tuberculosis are highlighted.

Early Presentation of Tuberculosis in Infancy

True congenital tuberculosis is rare, with fewer than 300 cases reported in the literature prior to 1994.[22] Since the recognition of HIV infection, and with more women of childbearing age developing tuberculosis, an increase in vertical transmission of *M. tuberculosis* has been observed. In Durban, South Africa, prior to the routine use of ART in HIV-pregnant women, a 16% vertical transmission rate of *M. tuberculosis* was documented in tuberculosis-exposed newborns, from both HIV-infected and HIV-uninfected pregnant women.[29] Maternal tuberculosis in HIV-infected women is also a risk factor for increased vertical HIV transmission.[30] The revised Cantwell's criteria from 1994 define true congenital tuberculosis as disease diagnosed in any infant with a tuberculous lesion *and* one or more of the following: (i) the lesion being present in the first week of life; (ii) a primary hepatic complex or caseating hepatic granuloma; (iii) infection of the placenta or endometrial tuberculosis in the mother; or (iv) exclusion of the possibility of postnatal transmission by excluding tuberculosis in other contacts.[22]

Symptoms and signs of congenital tuberculosis may be present at birth, but they often occur in the first weeks of life, and mainly involve the lung and liver. Combined data from 75 individual congenital tuberculosis cases demonstrated a median age of presentation at 2–3 weeks and reported the following symptoms and signs: respiratory distress (including tachypnea), hepatomegaly, splenomegaly, fever (low-grade), prematurity, and low birthweight occurred in more than 40% of cases; cough (acute or chronic), poor feeding, failure to thrive, abdominal distention (including ascites) in 25–40% cases; and irritability, peripheral lymphadenopathy, and sepsis syndrome in 10–25% of cases. Less than 10% of these cases presented with tuberculous meningitis, obstructive jaundice, skin lesions, otorrhea or mastoiditis, wheeze or stridor, apnea or cyanosis attacks, facial nerve palsy, or shock.[21] Chest radiography was available for 53 of the 75 infants, with miliary disease (30%), bronchopneumonia (32%), and lobar opacification (34%) being the most common radiological presentations.

A mycobacterial blood culture should be performed in suspected disseminated tuberculosis cases. Placental histology and culture and post-partum endometrial biopsy may be of value in confirming tuberculosis in the mother and congenital infection of the neonate. However, finding evidence of *M. tuberculosis* in the placenta does not confirm congenital infection, nor does its absence rule out infection of the neonate. Abdominal ultrasound should be performed in all suspected cases of congenital tuberculosis, as hypodense lesions may be observed in both the liver and spleen of the infant. In a review of 170 congenital tuberculosis cases from the literature, caseating hepatic granulomas were found in 15 infants subjected to liver biopsy, and a primary hepatic complex was found in two infants, probably pathognomic of congenital infection.[31]

Late Presentation of Tuberculosis in Infancy

PTB, also referred to as "intrathoracic tuberculosis" that includes hilar and mediastinal lymphadenopathy, is present in up to 90% of infants with tuberculosis: EPTB occurs in 15–30% of cases.[8,21] In a case series of 47 infants, the most common symptoms and signs for infant tuberculosis included cough (79%), fever (64%), poor feeding (43%), localized rales or wheezing (38%), and decreased breath sounds.[8] These clinical features relate to the pathophysiology of PTB disease in the infant, which involves marked hilar and mediastinal lymphadenopathy. Enlarged glands can easily compress the airways of infants, which are of small caliber. Partial compression of the large airways may present with stridor, whereas compression of the smaller airways leads to signs of air trapping, including wheezing and focal decreased breath sounds. Progressive obstruction may cause a "ball-valve" effect, which can lead to hyperinflation of parts of the lungs or even an entire lung. Complete obstruction can result in collapse of certain sections of the lung. Enlarged lymph nodes are also known to erode into the bronchus, spreading caseous material to the lungs, which in turn may create segmental parenchymal lesions. A parenchymal lesion in the lung can also enlarge and cause widespread opacification in a segment or lobe of the lung, presenting with symptoms and signs similar to pneumonia. In the case series of 47 infants, 44 had parenchymal disease, and one infant had hilar adenopathy only. The majority of infants (86%) had radiologically confirmed segmental lesions associated with hilar adenopathy.[8] A similar report showed radiological evidence of air-trapping (56%), lobar or segmental opacification (52%), lymphadenopathy (52%), and large airway compression (48%) in 27 younger infants with PTB.[32] Pleural effusions do not occur commonly in infants,[21] although slight thickening of the pleura near a primary focus is not uncommon.

Gastric aspirates for acid-fast smear, GeneXpert MTB/RIF, and culture are routinely recommended when investigating young infants for tuberculosis disease. Sputum induction may also be successfully conducted in older infants. Although tuberculosis disease in children is paucibacillary in nature, studies have reported that more than 70% of clinically suspected cases in infants can be confirmed by culture.[8,21,33] This higher microbiological yield may be partially explained by the often-late diagnosis in the young, as well as the infants' immature immune system, which allow for uncontrolled multiplication of the tubercle bacilli.[21] In a study performed in a tuberculosis-endemic region, peripheral lymphadenopathy, mainly cervical, occurred less frequently

in infants than older children.[34] Prior to the universal use of ART in HIV-infected infants, axillary lymphadenopathy was a frequent adverse event in HIV-infected infants receiving BCG vaccination at birth. Tuberculous meningitis is unusual in infants less than three months of age, probably because of the time needed (several weeks or months) for the spread of *M. tuberculosis* infection from the primary focus to the brain and the establishment of a "Rich focus" close to the meninges.[35]

ANTITUBERCULOSIS DRUGS IN PREGNANCY AND INFANTS

This section highlights specific drug issues and matters related to pregnancy, neonates, and infants. The focus is on first-line drugs, as limited data are available for second-line drugs within these vulnerable populations.

First-line Antituberculosis Drugs in Pregnancy

First-line antituberculosis drugs—isoniazid (INH), rifampicin (RMP), ethambutol (EMB), and pyrazinamide (PZA)—are used in the treatment of drug-susceptible tuberculosis. They are safe and widely used in pregnancy, with no evidence associating them with increased human fetal malformations.[36] Streptomycin and other injectable drugs, however, are contraindicated in pregnancy because of the potential risk for fetal ototoxicity.[37]

INH as a single drug is recommended for the treatment of tuberculosis infection, both in low-burden settings and for HIV-infected individuals in high-burden settings. Due to the potential risk of INH hepatotoxicity, health care workers are hesitant to administer this drug in pregnancy or the immediate post-partum period, and many defer treatment until after delivery of the baby. Preexisting liver disease and the use of other hepatotoxic drugs may predispose to liver injury in pregnant women; therefore, baseline transaminases should be performed prior to starting treatment with INH. Regular monitoring of transaminases should be conducted in pregnant women taking INH, and the development of symptoms that may be referrable to the liver or an increase of serum transaminases of 3–5 times more than the upper limit of normal in an asymptomatic pregnant woman should prompt immediate cessation of any potentially hepatotoxic drug, including

INH.[38,39] A large randomized international trial is underway with the aim of establishing the safety of antepartum-initiated INH versus deferred or post-partum initiated INH among HIV-infected women in tuberculosis high-burden settings. Results from this study will guide future use of INH during pregnancy and the post-partum period. Pyridoxine supplementation is indicated in most patients taking INH, including pregnant women, to prevent the development of peripheral neuropathy.

Recommended first-line tuberculosis treatment regimens for pregnant women differ between countries, with many recommending the standard adult regimen (two-month intensive phase of INH, RMP, EMB, and PZA, followed by four months of INH and RMP).[40] In the United States, PZA is currently not recommended for use in pregnancy because of lack of specific teratogenicity studies in animals, and an alternative regimen of INH, RMP, and EMB for two months, followed by seven months of INH and RMP, is recommended. RMP induces the cytochrome P450 microsomal hepatic enzymes, which play an important role in the metabolism of several drugs, and can lead to lower drug-exposures of certain concomitant drugs. Because bleeding tendencies have been observed with RMP, giving prophylactic vitamin K to the newborn of a mother being treated for tuberculosis is of paramount importance to prevent hemorrhagic disease of the newborn. All of the first-line drugs cross the placenta, and minimal amounts are excreted into breast milk. Breastfeeding is recommended and should be encouraged for mothers being treated for tuberculosis who are no longer infectious.[40]

Second-line Antituberculosis Drugs in Pregnancy

Globally, the proportion of new cases with multidrug-resistant tuberculosis (MDR-TB), resistant to INH and RMP, was 3.5% in 2013.[1] Limited data are available for the use of second-line antituberculosis drugs in pregnancy, and it is largely unknown to what extent they cross the placenta or are excreted in the breast milk. Most second-line drugs have a greater incidence of adverse effects in the mother and/or an increased risk to the fetus in pregnancy.[36] Injectable drugs can cause neurosensory hearing loss in the fetus. The safety of the fluoroquinolones in pregnancy has not been established, and there are no data in this regard for newer drugs such as linezolid. However, untreated or poorly treated tuberculosis in the pregnant woman is associated with many poor fetal outcomes, including prematurity and stillbirth. The benefits of treating tuberculosis disease in pregnancy usually outweigh the risks of the specific drugs for the fetus, but the advice of a specialist in tuberculosis should be obtained when managing drug-resistant tuberculosis in pregnant women.

Antituberculosis Drugs in Infants with Tuberculosis Disease

INH, RMP, and PZA, with or without EMB, remain the cornerstones of first-line tuberculosis drug regimens in children of all ages (Table 13.2). The recommended standard regimen for PTB and peripheral lymphadenitis in the young consists of six months of treatment; three or four drugs (INH, RMP, PZA, and EMB) for two months (intensive phase), followed by two drugs (INH and RMP) for the following four months.[27] Ethionamide (ETH), a second-line drug, is sometimes preferred to EMB in the very young because of good CNS penetration in tuberculous meningitis, and due to the difficulty in monitoring for ocular toxicity that is caused rarely by EMB in this age group. However, in a literature review of EMB in children, the drug was stopped due to fears about possible ocular toxicity in only two of 3,811 patients.[41,42] A dose of 15–20 mg/kg/day is recommended for ETH use.[43]

In 2009, the WHO recommended higher doses of all first-line drugs for children than previously

Table 13.2. Revised WHO-recommended tuberculosis drug-dosing guidelines for children[27]

FIRST-LINE ANTITUBERCULOSIS DRUGS	DAILY DOSE
INH	10 mg/kg (range 7–15 mg/kg)
RMP	15 mg/kg (range 10–20 mg/kg)
PZA	35 mg/kg (range 30–40 mg/kg)
EMB	20 mg/kg (range 15–25 mg/kg)

recommended: INH 10 mg versus 5 mg/kg/day, RMP 15 mg versus 10 mg/kg/day, PZA 35 mg versus 25 mg/kg/day, and EMB 20 mg versus 15 mg/kg/day.[44] These recommendations were based on evidence from pharmacokinetic (PK) studies involving mainly older children, which showed that higher milligram-per-kilogram dosing is necessary to achieve target drug concentrations that correlate with efficacy in adults. The effect of these higher doses on young infants, with immature organ systems and who are more prone to drug injury, remains largely unknown. Limited PK and safety data are available for neonates and infants for first-line drugs, with none available for long-term use of second-line drugs. Fortunately, adverse reactions to first-line drugs are seen less frequently in infants and children than in adults.[45] A transient increase in transaminases may occur with the hepatotoxic drugs, but clinically significant hepatitis is rare and documented in only 0.1% of children.[46] As older children generally tolerate first-line drugs well, routine laboratory monitoring of safety data is not standard of care in the otherwise healthy older child receiving first-line drugs.

However, caution about hepatotoxicity may be advised in neonates and infants with immature organ systems, and many experts recommend biochemical monitoring in this age group. Young infants have unique developmental and physiological changes that may influence the absorption, metabolism, and excretion of specific drugs. For INH, both *N-acetyltransferase 2* (*NAT2*) genotyping and enzyme maturation determine INH serum concentration. The rate of INH elimination shows genetic polymorphism, with individuals classified as homozygous fast (FF), heterozygous fast (FS), or homozygous slow (SS) acetylators, depending on their ability to eliminate this drug. Despite genetic differences influencing the rate of elimination of INH, evidence suggests that *NAT2* expression phenotypically matures with age as enzyme maturation develops, with faster acetylators metabolizing INH more rapidly with increasing age. The exact time of enzyme maturation remains unclear, with full maturity of the enzymatic pathways responsible for INH metabolism only reached at an estimated 2–4 years of age.[47] Genetically determined fast acetylators may therefore behave like slow acetylators in the very young with reduced clearance and relatively higher serum concentrations of INH. In a study conducted in 20 low-birthweight infants receiving 10 mg/kg/day of INH (dosed at the lower end of the WHO-recommended dosing guideline), all 20 LBW infants achieved at least adult INH target values, and some were much higher, cautioning against the use of high-dose INH in the neonate or infant.[48] Some of the infants were monitored with periodic measurement of alanine transaminases (ALT); most results were normal, but one asymptomatic infant had a three times elevated value of ALT, which normalized at six months of age with continued treatment. The high serum concentrations of INH achieved in this group require further investigation, and careful safety monitoring is imperative in the very young.

Rifampicin is a strong inducer of cytochrome CYP3A4, and since large numbers of medications are CYP3A4 substrates, RMP use leads to reduced concentrations and, in some cases, reduced effectiveness of other drugs. In HIV high-prevalence settings, potential interactions may occur with specific ART drugs, leading to decreased serum levels of these drugs in neonates and infants. The protease inhibitor lopinavir/ritonavir (LPV/r) and the non-nucleoside reverse transcriptase inhibitor nevirapine (NVP), used in prevention of mother to child transmission, have been documented to have lower serum concentrations in the presence of RMP co-administration.[49] Overlapping toxicity of antituberculosis drugs and other concomitant drugs may increase the risk of adverse events. RMP is also known for its large inter-individual variation in serum concentrations, with some evidence suggesting lower RMP exposures in the young.[50] Whether higher doses of RMP should be considered when treating disseminated tuberculosis disease (high bacillary load), HIV co-infection (drug–drug interactions), and also within a background of rising INH resistance, remains uncertain. Genotyping may influence RMP exposures, with recent data indicating that a single-nucleotide polymorphism (SNP) in *SLCO1B1* is associated with rifampicin plasma concentrations.

The treatment of neonatal and infant tuberculosis remains a challenge due to the paucity of PK and safety data on the use of antituberculosis drugs in this age group. Ongoing PK studies will inform future guidelines for the optimal dosing of first- and second-line drugs in the young.

INFECTION CONTROL

General Principles for Maternal-Infant Pairs

Mothers with tuberculosis disease and their newborns should preferably *not* be separated from each other. The mother with undiagnosed PTB or recently started PTB treatment poses the highest infectious risk to other people, including her own baby. Transmission of M. tuberculosis depends the degree and duration of exposure to the infectious individual. Patients with acid-fast sputum smear-positive PTB are more likely to transmit the organism than sputum smear-negative, culture-positive patients, although both carry an infectious risk. Breastfeeding should be encouraged, especially within resource-constrained settings, where it may be essential for infant survival. The recent WHO guidelines recommend breastfeeding, irrespective of the tuberculosis status of the mother,[27] while the American Academy of Pediatrics recommends that women with tuberculosis who have been treated appropriately for two weeks or more and who are not contagious may breastfeed.[51] It is evident that the mother should start appropriate treatment as soon as the diagnosis of tuberculosis disease is made, which will decrease her infectious risk. The mother should wear a protective mask during breastfeeding, and treatment for the newborn considered, depending on the likely contagiousness of the mother. The risk of transmission through breast milk is negligible, and only small amounts of antituberculosis drugs are excreted in breast milk. Management of drug-resistant tuberculosis cases should be discussed with a specialist familiar with treating these cases.

Isolation of potentially infectious tuberculosis cases should be facilitated within a health care facility, for both mother and newborn, to offer protection to fellow patients and other health care providers. Good ventilation strategies within the isolation facility will reduce transmission risk, with negative-pressure ventilation the preferred option. PTB patients initiated on treatment can safely leave isolation once the following criteria are met: at least two consecutive sputum acid-fast smear microscopy samples negative for mycobacteria; evidence of clinical improvement; and adherence to an adequate treatment regimen for two weeks or more.[52]

Undiagnosed PTB may potentially occur in any patient or health care provider, and caution is advised, especially in resource-constrained congregate settings where mothers share facilities; for example, during "kangaroo mother care" practices (skin–skin contact and nursing of premature babies). Heyns et al.[53] reported four infants that were infected and developed tuberculosis disease following exposure to a different mother with undiagnosed tuberculosis, illustrating that nosocomial transmission of M. tuberculosis may occur within a kangaroo mother care unit. In tuberculosis high-burden settings, symptom screening is advised for all rooming-in mothers, and a high index of suspicion for tuberculosis is essential, including for health care providers.

In the unfortunate event of a new drug-susceptible PTB diagnosis within a neonatal care setting, immediate steps should to be taken to assist the index case and protect all exposed individuals. If babies are exposed to tuberculosis in the neonatal care setting, appropriate testing and treatment should always be carried out. The index case should be started on appropriate treatment as soon as possible, and remain home until noninfectious. Health care providers are known to be at higher risk for tuberculosis disease in high-burden settings. In a recent study from South Africa, 133 primary health care facilities were reviewed, showing an incidence ratio of acid-fast smear-positive tuberculosis in primary health care workers of more than double that of the general population.[54] In low-burden settings, asymptomatic exposed individuals may be offered TST or IGRA assays, and if results are positive and conversion happened recently, treatment of tuberculosis infection is recommended. In high-burden settings, adults exposed to the index case usually will be followed without treatment. After a detailed history and clinical examination, regular follow-up should be conducted to identify suggestive symptoms and signs for tuberculosis disease. However, it could be argued that health care providers who care for neonates and infants and have been infected recently with M. tuberculosis should always be offered treatment to ensure that transmission to the young patients does not occur. Treatment of tuberculosis infection is recommended for HIV-infected individuals in all settings.

Optimal management of tuberculosis-exposed maternal-infant pairs requires integration of maternal and infant health services, which relies on good communication between those caring for the pregnant mother and those responsible for the newborn.

REFERENCES

1. World Health Organization. *Global Tuberculosis Report, 2014*. Geneva: WHO; 2014.
2. Say L, Chou D, Gemmill A, et al. Global causes of maternal death: a WHO systematic analysis. *Lancet Global Health*. 2014;2(6):e323–e333.

3. Bjerkedal T, Bahna SL, Lehmann EH. Course and outcome of pregnancy in women with pulmonary tuberculosis. *Scand J Respir Dis.* 1975;56(5):245–250.

4. Jana N, Vasishta K, Jindal SK, Khunnu B, Ghosh K. Perinatal outcome in pregnancies complicated by pulmonary tuberculosis. *Int J Gynaecol Obstet.* 1994;44(2):119–124.

5. Marais BJ, Gie RP, Schaaf HS, et al. The natural history of childhood intra-thoracic tuberculosis: a critical review of literature from the pre-chemotherapy era. *Int J Tuberc Lung Dis.* 2004;8(4):392–402.

6. Gupta A, Nayak U, Ram M, et al. Postpartum tuberculosis incidence and mortality among HIV-infected women and their infants in Pune, India, 2002–2005. *Clin Infect Dis.* 2007;45(2):241–249.

7. Schaaf HS, Marais BJ, Whitelaw A, et al. Culture-confirmed childhood tuberculosis in Cape Town, South Africa: a review of 596 cases. *BMC Infect Dis.* 2007;7:140.

8. Vallejo JG, Ong LT, Starke JR. Clinical features, diagnosis, and treatment of tuberculosis in infants. *Pediatrics.* 1994;94(1):1–7.

9. Sugarman J, Colvin C, Moran AC, Oxlade O. Tuberculosis in pregnancy: an estimate of the global burden of disease. *Lancet Global Health.* 2014;2(12):e710–e716.

10. Mathad JS, Gupta A. Tuberculosis in pregnant and postpartum women: epidemiology, management, and research gaps. *Clin Infect Dis.* 2012;55(11):1532–1549.

11. World Health Organization. *Guidelines on the Management of Latent Tuberculosis Infection, 2015.* Geneva: WHO; 2015.

12. Finn R, Ward DW, Mattison ML. Immune suppression, gliomas, and tuberculosis. *Br Med J.* 1972;1(5792):111.

13. Nolan TE, Espinosa TL, Pastorek JG 2nd. Tuberculosis skin testing in pregnancy: trends in a population. *J Perinatol.* 1997;17(3):199–201.

14. Mofenson LM, Rodriguez EM, Hershow R, et al. Mycobacterium tuberculosis infection in pregnant and nonpregnant women infected with HIV in the Women and Infants Transmission Study. *Arch Intern Med.* 1995;155(10):1066–1072.

15. Mathad JS, Bhosale R, Sangar V, et al. Pregnancy differentially impacts performance of latent tuberculosis diagnostics in a high-burden setting. *PLoS One.* 2014;9(3):e92308.

16. Munoz-Suano A, Hamilton AB, Betz AG. Gimme shelter: the immune system during pregnancy. *Immunol Rev.* 2011;241(1):20–38.

17. Hoffmann CJ, Variava E, Rakgokong M, et al. High prevalence of pulmonary tuberculosis but low sensitivity of symptom screening among HIV-infected pregnant women in South Africa. *PLoS One.* 2013;8(4):e62211.

18. Gupta A, Chandrasekhar A, Gupte N, et al. Symptom screening among HIV-infected pregnant women is acceptable and has high negative predictive value for active tuberculosis. *Clin Infect Dis.* 2011;53(10):1015–1018.

19. Zenner D, Kruijshaar ME, Andrews N, Abubakar I. Risk of tuberculosis in pregnancy: a national, primary care-based cohort and self-controlled case series study. *Am J Respir Crit Care Med.* 2012;185(7):779–784.

20. Wilson EA, Thelin TJ, Dilts PV, Jr. Tuberculosis complicated by pregnancy. *Am J Obstet Gynecol.* 1973;115(4):526–529.

21. Schaaf HS, Collins A, Bekker A, Davies PD. Tuberculosis at extremes of age. *Respirology.* 2010;15(5):747–763.

22. Cantwell MF, Shehab ZM, Costello AM, et al. Brief report: congenital tuberculosis. *N Engl J Med.* 1994;330(15):1051–1054.

23. Marais BJ, Gie RP, Schaaf HS, et al. The clinical epidemiology of childhood pulmonary tuberculosis: a critical review of literature from the pre-chemotherapy era. *Int J Tuberc Lung Dis.* 2004;8(3):278–285.

24. Figueroa-Damian R, Arredondo-Garcia JL. Pregnancy and tuberculosis: influence of treatment on perinatal outcome. *Am J of Perinatol.* 1998;15(5):303–306.

25. Moore DP, Schaaf HS, Nuttall J, Marais BJ. Childhood tuberculosis guidelines of the Southern African Society for Paediatric Infectious Diseases. *South Afr J Epidemiol Infect.* 2009;24:57–68.

26. Mittal H, Das S, Faridi MM. Management of newborn infant born to mother suffering from tuberculosis: current recommendations and gaps in knowledge. *Indian J Med Res.* 2014;140(1):32–39.

27. World Health Organization. *Guidance for National Tuberculosis Programmes on the Management of Tuberculosis in Children.* 2nd ed, 2014. Geneva: WHO; 2014.

28. Nicol MP, Davies MA, Wood K, et al. Comparison of T-SPOT. TB assay and tuberculin skin test for the evaluation of young children at high risk for tuberculosis in a community setting. *Pediatrics.* 2009;123(1):38–43.

29. Pillay T, Sturm AW, Khan M, et al. Vertical transmission of *Mycobacterium tuberculosis* in

KwaZulu-Natal: impact of HIV-1 co-infection. *Int J Tuberc Lung Dis.* 2004;8(1):59–69.

30. Gupta A, Bhosale R, Kinikar A, et al. Maternal tuberculosis: a risk factor for mother-to-child transmission of human immunodeficiency virus. *J Infect Dis.* 2011;203(3):358–363.

31. Peng W, Yang J, Liu E. Analysis of 170 cases of congenital TB reported in the literature between 1946 and 2009. *Pediatr Pulmonol.* 2011;46(12):1215–1224.

32. Schaaf HS, Gie RP, Beyers N, Smuts N, Donald PR. Tuberculosis in infants less than 3 months of age. *Arch Dis Child.* 1993;69(3):371–374.

33. Starke JR, Taylor-Watts KT. Tuberculosis in the pediatric population of Houston, Texas. *Pediatrics.* 1989;84(1):28–35.

34. Marais BJ, Wright CA, Schaaf HS, et al. Tuberculous lymphadenitis as a cause of persistent cervical lymphadenopathy in children from a tuberculosis-endemic area. *Pediatr Infect Dis J.* 2006;25(2):142–146.

35. Donald PR, Schaaf HS, Schoeman JF. Tuberculous meningitis and miliary tuberculosis: the Rich focus revisited. *J Infect.* 2005;50(3):193–195.

36. Bothamley G. Drug treatment for tuberculosis during pregnancy: safety considerations. *Drug Safety.* 2001;24(7):553–565.

37. Varpela E, Hietalahti J, Aro MJ. Streptomycin and dihydrostreptomycin medication during pregnancy and their effect on the child's inner ear. *Scand J Respir Dis.* 1969;50(2):101–109.

38. Joint Tuberculosis Committee of the British Thoracic Society. Chemotherapy and management of tuberculosis in the United Kingdom: recommendations, 1998. *Thorax.* 1998;53(7):536–548.

39. Bass JB Jr., Farer LS, Hopewell PC, et al. Treatment of tuberculosis and tuberculosis infection in adults and children. American Thoracic Society and the Centers for Disease Control and Prevention. *Am J Respir Crit Care Med.* 1994;149(5):1359–1374.

40. World Health Organization. *Treatment of Tuberculosis Guidelines.* 4th ed, 2009. Geneva: 2009.

41. Trebucq A. Should ethambutol be recommended for routine treatment of tuberculosis in children? A review of the literature. *Int J Tuberc Lung Dis.* 1997;1(1):12–15.

42. Graham SM, Daley HM, Banerjee A, Salaniponi FM, Harries AD. Ethambutol in tuberculosis: time to reconsider? *Arch Dis Child.* 1998;79(3):274–278.

43. World Health Organization. *Guidelines for the Programmatic Management of Drug-Resistant Tuberculosis: Emergency Update, 2008.* Geneva: WHO; 2008.

44. World Health Organization. *Dosing Instructions for the Use of Currently Available Fixed-Dose Combination TB Medicines for Children, 2009.* Geneva: WHO, 2009. Available at http://www.who.int/tb/challenges/interim_paediatric_fdc_dosing_instructions_sept09.pdf. Accessed January 2015.

45. Frydenberg AR, Graham SM. Toxicity of first-line drugs for treatment of tuberculosis in children: review. *Trop Med Int Health.* 2009;14(11):1329–1337.

46. Kopanoff DE, Snider DE Jr., Caras GJ. Isoniazid-related hepatitis: a U.S. Public Health Service cooperative surveillance study. *Am Rev Respir Dis.* 1978;117(6):991–1001.

47. Pariente-Khayat A, Rey E, Gendrel D, et al. Isoniazid acetylation metabolic ratio during maturation in children. *Clin Pharm Ther.* 1997;62(4):377–383.

48. Bekker A, Schaaf HS, Seifart HI, et al. Pharmacokinetics of isoniazid in low-birth-weight and premature infants. *Antimicrob Agents Chemother.* 2014;58(4):2229–2234.

49. McIlleron H, Meintjes G, Burman WJ, Maartens G. Complications of antiretroviral therapy in patients with tuberculosis: drug interactions, toxicity, and immune reconstitution inflammatory syndrome. *J Infect Dis.* 2007;196(Suppl 1):S63–S75.

50. Donald PR, Maritz JS, Diacon AH. The pharmacokinetics and pharmacodynamics of rifampicin in adults and children in relation to the dosage recommended for children. *Tuberculosis.* 2011;91(3):196–207.

51. American Academy of Pediatrics. Tuberculosis. In: Pickering LK, ed. *Red Book: Report of the Committee on Infectious Diseases.* 29th ed. Elk Grove Village, IL: American Academy of Pediatrics; 2012:736–756.

52. Dramowski A. Tuberculosis. In: *Infection Prevention and Control: A Guide for Healthcare Workers in Low-Resource Settings.* Cape Town, South Africa: Bettercare, 2014:141.

53. Heyns L, Gie RP, Goussard P, Beyers N, Warren RM, Marais BJ. Nosocomial transmission of *Mycobacterium tuberculosis* in kangaroo mother care units: a risk in tuberculosis-endemic areas. *Acta Paediatr.* 2006;95(5):535–539.

54. Claassens MM, van Schalkwyk C, du Toit E, et al. Tuberculosis in healthcare workers and infection control measures at primary healthcare facilities in South Africa. *PLoS One.* 2013;8(10):e76272.

14

TUBERCULOSIS IN HIV-INFECTED AND EXPOSED INFANTS, CHILDREN, AND ADOLESCENTS

Helena Rabie and Mark F. Cotton

HIGHLIGHTS OF THIS CHAPTER

- Tuberculosis is a very important opportunistic infection in HIV-infected infants, children, and adolescents and can be the presenting complaint. All children with tuberculosis should have an age-appropriate HIV test.
- In high-burden settings, HIV-infected children are frequently exposed to tuberculosis.
- Timely access to combination antiretroviral therapy (cART) for HIV-infected children and adults is the most important strategy to prevent tuberculosis.
- There are conflicting data about giving universal isoniazid preventive therapy (IPT) to all children with HIV infection living in a high tuberculosis-burden setting, but preventing tuberculosis through IPT in children with known exposure is very important.
- Diagnosis is made more difficult by overlapping symptoms and signs of other HIV-related conditions, and conducting a careful history and assessment remain important.
- The use of the tuberculin skin test, laboratory and imaging tools are the same as for HIV-uninfected children, but interpretation of findings should consider HIV-related organ damage and other opportunistic infections.
- Intra- and extra-thoracic tuberculosis may occur simultaneously in HIV co-infected children.
- Rifampicin is the most commonly used rifamycin in co-infected children, despite drug–drug interactions. Checking that the child is on the appropriate cART regimen is extremely important.
- Early initiation of cART in co-infected children not yet on cART is appropriate except in meningitis where delaying initiation for four weeks to avoid paradoxical IRIS is appropriate.
- In children developing incident tuberculosis on cART, viral and immunological response to cART must be ensured during and after co-treatment.
- Tuberculosis treatment outcomes have improved with access to cART, but early morbidity and mortality are still reported. This may not be related only to tuberculosis.

EPIDEMIOLOGY OF TUBERCULOSIS AND RISK FACTORS FOR INFECTION AND DISEASE IN HIV-INFECTED INFANTS, CHILDREN, AND ADOLESCENTS

In 2011, an estimated 34 million people were HIV-infected worldwide, with 3.4 million younger than age 15 years, while an additional 330,000 children acquired HIV infection. Female adolescents and young adults carry a disproportionate burden of HIV. Scaling up prevention of mother-to-child transmission (PMTCT) programs resulted in a 40% reduction in perinatal transmission compared to 2009.[1] Breastfeeding has become safer through continuing combination antiretroviral therapy (cART) in the mother and providing nevirapine to infants for at least the first six weeks of life.[2] However, there is still incomplete access to cART for many woman, especially in sub-Saharan Africa and India. Perinatally infected infants and children have high morbidity and mortality in the absence of cART, with 50% dying by the age of two years in low-resource settings.[3] Increasing numbers of perinatally infected children are diagnosed for the first time in adolescence, and slow-progressing infection may allow survival for many years without treatment.[4]

In high-resource settings, perinatal transmission has been almost completely prevented, with rates of less than 5 per 1,000 cases recently reported from the United Kingdom.[5] However, adolescents and youth in high-risk categories still can acquire HIV through sexual and shared-needle routes.

Tuberculosis is an important opportunistic infection in children living with HIV. High rates of tuberculosis disease were reported in the pre-cART era. One early study from 2000 found that 47% of children diagnosed with tuberculosis at a large hospital in Soweto in South Africa were also HIV-infected.[6] Despite subsequent improvements in care and programs, tuberculosis remains an important cause of hospitalization and mortality in HIV-infected children and adolescents.[7,8] There is a wide range of incidence of tuberculosis in African studies of HIV infection in children, reflecting either true differences or regionally varying ability to diagnose tuberculosis and access

cART.[9] Also, many studies from low-resource settings poorly represent very young infants who are at particularly high risk of tuberculosis disease with increased severity due to their young age. Reports focusing on infants with HIV infection report high rates of all forms of tuberculosis.[10] Among HIV-infected infants in South Africa, up to 1,595 cases of tuberculosis per 100,000 population are reported annually, more than 24 times the rate reported at the same time for HIV-unexposed infants.[10] Among HIV-infected infants with access to cART in South Africa, the tuberculosis incidence is 121 per 1,000 child-years. In the same setting, a high tuberculosis burden was also identified among HIV-exposed-uninfected children (41 cases per 1,000 child-years), indicating a high rate of tuberculosis in their close contacts.[11] High tuberculosis rates are also reported in older HIV-infected children from the same high-burden setting: 53 cases per 100 patient years in the absence of cART, but declining to 6.4 per 100 patient years after initiating cART in patients in the same cohort.[12]

In low-burden tuberculosis settings, although the overall risk is much lower, tuberculosis still occurs. For example, 3–5.5% of children attending HIV services in the United Kingdom between 1991 and 2006 and in New York City between 1989 and 1995 had tuberculosis disease.[13,14] Reinfection and recurrence of tuberculosis in HIV-infected children is well documented in the pre- and post-cART eras.[15]

WHY ARE HIV-INFECTED INFANTS, CHILDREN, AND ADOLESCENTS AT SUCH HIGH RISK FOR TUBERCULOSIS INFECTION AND DISEASE?

BCG Vaccination

Although Bacille Calmette Guérin (BCG) vaccines do not prevent many cases of pulmonary tuberculosis, meta-analysis shows their efficacy in preventing disseminated disease and meningitis.[16] HIV-infected infants have far higher rates of all forms of tuberculosis, including disseminated tuberculosis.[10] However, the role of BCG vaccines in preventing tuberculosis in HIV-infected infants remains unclear.

There are concerns regarding severe adverse effects of BCG in HIV-infected infants. Retrospective studies from low-resource settings and a prospective South African study indicate a high risk of disseminated BCG disease in HIV-infected infants vaccinated at birth.[17,18] Poor access to early cART was almost certainly contributory to the results of these older studies. Although the World Health Organization (WHO) now recommends that BCG vaccine not be administered to infants with confirmed HIV infection, this advice is difficult to implement, as BCG vaccine is usually given at birth when the HIV status of the infant is still unknown. Therefore, in high-prevalence settings, all HIV-exposed infants still receive BCG vaccine.[19] With early infant diagnosis of HIV infection and early administration of cART, the risk of adverse events caused by BCG vaccines is significantly reduced. For example, in a prospective study of 451 HIV-infected infants receiving early cART and BCG vaccine, none developed disseminated BCG disease.[20] Immune reconstitution inflammatory syndrome (IRIS) associated with BCG causing local or regional disease remains a problem in HIV-infected infants, but the incidence is reduced substantially by early administration of cART.[20,21]

High Risk of Exposure to Tuberculosis Source Cases That Are HIV-Infected

Many HIV-infected children live in communities with high rates of tuberculosis and in households with many potential source cases. HIV-infected adults not taking cART are 21–34 times more likely to develop tuberculosis than HIV-uninfected adults in the same setting, accounting for 25% of all HIV-related mortality.[22] In some settings, the annual case-notification rate for tuberculosis now exceeds 1,400 per 100,000.[23] These adults are also at risk of developing recurrent disease, especially if not taking effective cART.

Woman of childbearing age bear the brunt of both tuberculosis and HIV.[23] Infants are therefore at high risk of exposure to both pathogens. Where adult diagnosis relies on acid-fast smear-positive sputum microscopy, tuberculosis diagnosis in HIV-infected adults is often delayed.[24] In low-burden settings, acid-fast smear-negative tuberculosis accounts for 10–20% of transmission at a community level.[25] In high-burden settings, a large number of patients with HIV infection

and tuberculosis disease have a negative acid-fast smear of sputum, and the resulting diagnostic delay is likely to contribute significantly to transmission. In a study from Cape Town, where more than 25% of severely immunocompromised HIV-infected adults presenting for care also had disease caused by *M. tuberculosis*, 80% of these patients were acid-fast sputum smear-negative. In the absence of rapid molecular diagnostics, the time to their tuberculosis diagnosis exceeded three weeks.[26]

This high tuberculosis disease burden in dually infected adults leads to high rates of *M. tuberculosis* exposure in both HIV-exposed and HIV-unexposed infants and young children. If tuberculosis in an HIV-infected pregnant women is missed, the infant is not only at risk for tuberculosis but has a threefold higher HIV acquisition rate.[27] The impact of transmission of *M. tuberculosis* from adults among young children who are not living in the same household should not be underestimated.[28,29] In a study of isoniazid preventative therapy (IPT) in high tuberculosis-burden settings, 10% of HIV-exposed infants had contact with potential tuberculosis source cases by the age of 14 weeks, some of whom did not live with the child.[8] Infection can also occur among adolescents outside the home in social and school settings.

Poor penetration of cART programs contributes to the community tuberculosis risk. When cART is delayed in adults until the CD4 count is below 200 cells per mm^3, the lifetime risk of tuberculosis remains increased, as tuberculosis is often one of the earliest manifestations of HIV infection. With good access to cART in adults, the risk of pulmonary tuberculosis declines for both HIV-infected and -uninfected children. For example, in Johannesburg, South Africa, cART access in adults increased from 21.5% in 2005 to 68.2% in 2009. During the same period, the annual rate of tuberculosis in HIV-uninfected children declined from 18.7 to 11.0 per 100,000.[30]

Immunosuppression, Clinical Disease, and Access to Antiretroviral Therapy in Children

In children with HIV infection and poor nutritional status (stunting, wasting, and reduced mid-upper arm circumference), advanced immune suppression, anemia, and delayed access to cART, the risk for developing tuberculosis increases. School attendance or prior hospitalization are also associated with transmission of *M. tuberculosis* and subsequent development of disease, reflecting poor ventilation in schools in low-resource settings.[31]

Young age is poorly studied as an independent risk factor for tuberculosis in HIV-infected children in resource-limited settings, but as many as 33% of infants starting cART at a median age of eight months are already on tuberculosis therapy.[32] Early administration of cART in young infants effectively decreases tuberculosis rates. In the Children with HIV Early Antiretroviral (CHER) trial, tuberculosis disease occurred in the first year of life in 8.3 % of children receiving early cART but in 20% in whom cART administration was delayed. In older children initiating cART, the decline of both microbiologically confirmed and clinically diagnosed cases of tuberculosis is well documented; this decline in case detection relates to the duration on cART therapy,[33] and reductions in tuberculosis case rates of between 32% and 70% can be achieved by cART. Nevertheless, in high-burden settings, HIV-infected children continue to have more tuberculosis than their uninfected peers.

Despite a better understanding of the need for early treatment of HIV infection and improved access to drugs, many children in high tuberculosis-burden settings still start cART only after becoming severely immunocompromised. Data from Asia, Africa, and North and South America in 2010 document this delayed start of cART in 77% of HIV-infected children in low-income countries, 66% in low-middle income countries, and 58% in upper-middle income countries.[34] Data from low-resource settings show an increase in tuberculosis diagnosis in the first three months of cART.[7,35] This is a particularly challenging time for these children, with high rates of death and hospitalization often caused by respiratory infections.[36,37] This increase in tuberculosis diagnosis early in cART may represent previously missed cases, exposure to tuberculosis just before initiation of cART, or, if the clinical features are unusual or severe, unmasking IRIS.[38] The lack of effective rapid screening and diagnostic protocols for tuberculosis in children presents a specific challenge to preventing this phenomenon.

Isoniazid Preventive Therapy

Recent *M. tuberculosis* infection is a risk factor for rapid progression to disease; therefore, isoniazid preventive therapy (IPT) is an integral component of tuberculosis prevention in HIV-infected children. Giving post-exposure treatment with isoniazid (INH) for six months to HIV-infected children regardless of age, although not fully studied, has been effective in young children.[11,32] In a retrospective cohort of 494 children in Cape Town initiating cART prior to two years of age, 127 courses of post-exposure IPT were provided, with only two children developing confirmed drug-susceptible tuberculosis.[32]

Studies of routine longer-term preventive therapy without specific exposure—also called pre-exposure preventive therapy—have produced conflicting results. In one multicenter study, pre-exposure prevention had no effect on tuberculosis incidence in either HIV-exposed-uninfected or -infected infants.[11] However, a prospective clinical study that enrolled mostly older infants and young children found significant reductions both in all-cause mortality (16% in the placebo arm vs. 8% in the IPT arm) and incident tuberculosis (9.9% with placebo vs. 3.8% with IPT).[39] Subsequent analysis of this cohort illustrated that combining IPT with cART was more effective than either strategy alone to prevent tuberculosis.[40]

The 2014 WHO Guidelines recommend giving IPT for 6 months to all HIV-infected children older than 12 months unless they have tuberculosis disease, suggestive symptoms (poor weight gain, fever, and cough), or a tuberculosis contact history that requires adequate investigation before starting IPT. However, "adequate investigation" is not further defined, as access to diagnostic tests varies.[41] The yield for further investigation of children who have only a single symptom of tuberculosis also has not been evaluated. The WHO Guidelines also recommend that HIV-infected children treated for tuberculosis disease with a good response should receive an additional six months of INH at the end of their of antituberculosis therapy,[41] but this also has not been studied in children. Unlike for adults, there are no data from children on the utility of tuberculosis skin testing prior to administering IPT.

No studies of IPT have been conducted in adolescents as a target population. In the HIV-uninfected population the risk of tuberculosis increases sharply during adolescence, and HIV-infected adolescents with confirmed *M. tuberculosis* infection and no disease should receive treatment with at least six months of isoniazid.

Having a contact with drug-resistant tuberculosis may be a major factor in patients' failing INH treatment. In the only pre-exposure prevention study published thus far, all HIV-infected children developing culture-confirmed tuberculosis while taking INH had multidrug-resistant disease. It could not be determined if giving INH contributed to the resistance profile, but none of the HIV-infected children developed INH mono-resistance.[42]

When a child develops tuberculosis disease while on or after taking IPT, a careful review of the contacts' therapeutic history and drug-resistance profile should be done. When possible, respiratory and other specimens should be taken from the child for culture and drug-susceptibility testing prior to beginning tuberculosis therapy. Also, the child's clinical response to the selected tuberculosis treatment regimen must be monitored carefully.

CLINICAL PRESENTATION, DIAGNOSIS, AND DIFFERENTIAL DIAGNOSIS

Because tuberculosis is common in HIV-infected children, health care workers must maintain a high index of suspicion for its diagnosis. A careful history and clinical assessment for tuberculosis should be done at each visit. The general approach to the diagnosis of tuberculosis for children is similar in the HIV-infected and -uninfected child: asking about a history of contact and suggestive symptoms, seeking proof of infection and evidence of disease, and attempting to isolate the organism when appropriate (Figure 14.1).

However, when HIV-infected children first come to attention for possible tuberculosis, especially if they are not on cART, the symptoms and signs may be difficult to interpret because poor weight gain, fever, cough, hepatosplenomegaly, and adenopathy are common in children with inadequately treated HIV infection. Also, when children are significantly immunosuppressed and have concomitant pulmonary disease, a vast array of opportunistic and common childhood infections and HIV-associated conditions require consideration. For example, children with lymphoid interstitial pneumonitis and/or bronchiectasis often have a chronic cough and are susceptible to developing both tuberculosis and other pulmonary infections.

It is also important to remember that HIV-infected children may present to the health service with tuberculosis but without a prior diagnosis of HIV infection. *All children suspected of having tuberculosis disease require HIV testing, regardless of setting.* In studies performed in the United Kingdom and the United States of HIV-infected children co-infected with *M. tuberculosis*, the HIV diagnosis occurred after tuberculosis was diagnosed in 30% and 44% of children, respectively.[13,14] According to the pediatric WHO clinical staging system, tuberculosis is an AIDS-defining illness: stage 3 for pulmonary tuberculosis or stage 4 for extrapulmonary and disseminated tuberculosis.[43]

Important Clinical Issues

A history of tuberculosis contact: This remains one of the most important diagnostic tools for clinicians. Obviously, all children with tuberculosis infection or disease must have had a contact at some time, whether or not the specific contact can be determined. In studies of microbiologically confirmed tuberculosis disease, up to 40% of HIV-infected and -uninfected children had a known contact.[12,44] It is valuable to interview the child's caretaker carefully to elicit this history. In addition, a history of symptoms in the mother or another adult in the home and an assessment for tuberculosis in adults close to the child is often of great clinical value; tuberculosis disease can develop rapidly in a child, and the adult contact is often identified only after the child is evaluated for tuberculosis because of suggestive symptoms or signs.[45] Close-contact HIV-infected adults not on cART with symptoms suggestive of tuberculosis but a negative acid-fast sputum-smear should undergo further evaluation, including at least two GeneXpert MTB/RIF tests. If unavailable, a chest radiograph should be done and the local algorithm for the evaluation of acid-fast smear-negative adult tuberculosis followed. There are two additional important points: first, the clinicians and the caretaker may not have the same definition of a "household." Often many families live on the same plot of land, sometimes renting a room in the house or in the yard. Families may share cooking or ablution facilities.[28,46] Second, although this situation is not common, the tuberculosis contact may have occurred many months or occasionally years before the child's presentation. Therefore, it is prudent to also ask about household contacts at least 12 months prior to the current presentation. Adult contacts of hospitalized children potentially pose an infection risk to staff and other patients; infection prevention and control measures should be implemented.

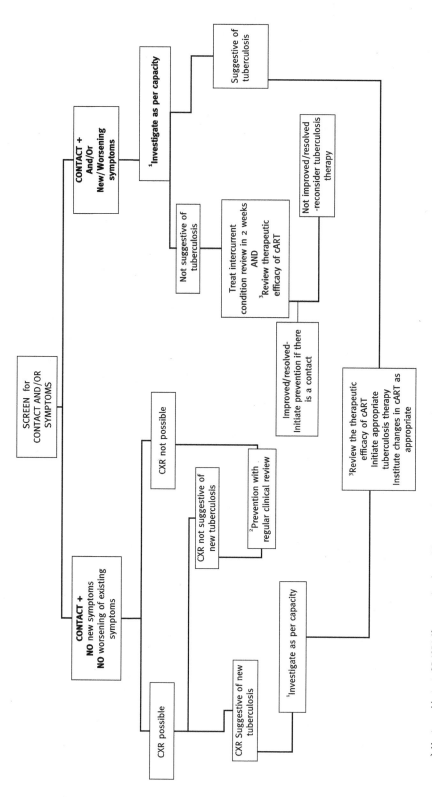

SCREEN for CONTACT AND/OR SYMPTOMS

**CONTACT +
NO new symptoms
NO worsening of existing symptoms**

**CONTACT +
And/Or
New/Worsening symptoms**

CXR possible

CXR not possible

CXR Suggestive of new tuberculosis

CXR not suggestive of new tuberculosis

¹Investigate as per capacity

²Prevention with regular clinical review

³Review the therapeutic efficacy of cART
Initiate appropriate tuberculosis therapy
Institute changes in cART as appropriate

¹Investigate as per capacity

Not suggestive of tuberculosis

Suggestive of tuberculosis

Treat intercurrent condition review in 2 weeks AND
³Review therapeutic efficacy of cART

Improved/resolved-
Initiate prevention if there is a contact

Not improved/resolved
-reconsider tuberculosis therapy

1) Mantoux skin test OR IGRA if not previously positive or confirmed tuberculosis; CXR and Other appropriate imaging as per site suspected; specimens for rapid diagnosis, culture and histology

2) Can do IGRA or mantouxto confirm infection but must still provide preventative therapy

3) Clinical review with CD4 and viral load where possible

FIGURE 14.1   Approach to tuberculosis screening for patients attending antiretroviral therapy clinics and on antiretroviral therapy.

Pulmonary tuberculosis in children can present with acute pneumonia: This scenario is well-documented in prospective cohort studies of acute respiratory infection and necropsy studies of children dying from acute respiratory infection in Africa, where up to 43% of children with tuberculosis had an acute respiratory tract infection.[47] In a necropsy study from Zambia, tuberculosis was documented in 18% of HIV-infected children.[48] These data suggest that tuberculosis must be considered as the cause of acute pneumonia in HIV-infected children presenting to hospitals and clinics, especially if they are not on cART. In addition, acute bacterial or viral pneumonia can present at the same time as tuberculosis, making the clinical picture more confusing and difficult.

Risk factors for tuberculosis disease in HIV-infected children are the absence of cART, low CD4 + T-cell count, and malnutrition: Unlike in HIV-uninfected children in high-burden settings, using symptoms to diagnose tuberculosis in HIV-infected children has a poor predictive value.[49,50] However, the most common symptoms in HIV-infected children treated for tuberculosis are weight loss or failure to thrive (61.2–65.7%), cough >2–4 weeks (36.5–52.2%), and intermittent fever >1 week (31.4–73.1%).[6,12] This constellation of symptoms should prompt an assessment for tuberculosis regardless of contact history. In addition, any child with a respiratory infection not responding adequately to antibiotics requires further investigation.

Pulmonary tuberculosis remains the most common form of tuberculosis in HIV-infected children: Regardless of cART status, pulmonary tuberculosis is the most common form of presentation, occurring in up to 78% of cases. There are conflicting data on the risk for extrapulmonary tuberculosis in HIV-infected children. In some HIV cohorts, few cases of extrapulmonary tuberculosis are reported; while others from both high and low tuberculosis-burden settings have high rates—up to 42%—of extrapulmonary disease. However, the reports from high-burden settings suggest that in 22% of children, *intra- and extrathoracic disease occur simultaneously*.[6,12,44,51] In infants and children with poor or delayed access to cART, disseminated disease accounts for 11–16% of cases and meningitis for 9–14%.[10,12,32,44,51,52] Therefore, when tuberculosis is suspected, one should consider that the disease may be present in more than one organ system. For instance, one should always obtain a chest radiograph for children with suspected tuberculous meningitis or abdominal tuberculosis. With

tuberculous meningitis, HIV-infected children are more likely to have features of tuberculosis on chest radiography than are HIV-uninfected children.[53] Similarly, doing fine-needle aspiration of accessible pathological lymph nodes in HIV-infected children may assist in confirming the diagnosis of tuberculosis, establishing the drug susceptibility profile, and excluding other conditions such as lymphoma. Tuberculosis should always be considered in HIV-infected children despite unusual presentations. For example, tuberculosis presenting as a psoas abscess, chronic otorrhea, renal disease, or with parotid gland involvement have all been documented in HIV-infected children.[54]

Serial clinical assessment and physical examination, with careful documentation of findings, are very important and may suggest a diagnosis other than tuberculosis. Careful documentation of the child's nutritional status at baseline and during follow-up evaluations is absolutely essential. Digital clubbing and parotid enlargement suggest lymphoid interstitial pneumonia or bronchiectasis, while clubbing without parotid enlargement suggests bronchiectasis. Although hepatomegaly and splenomegaly are features of HIV infection, having them as a new finding may indicate tuberculosis. Enlarged lymph nodes, similarly, are often present in HIV-infected children and are usually symmetrically distributed and do not rapidly enlarge. Occasionally, large masses are present on abdominal palpation and are always abnormal, the most common considerations being tuberculosis and lymphoma. Similarly, cardiac, neurodevelopmental, and neurological dysfunction may complicate pulmonary illness and require ongoing assessment. Measuring and plotting the head circumference may allow for the differentiation between encephalopathy and meningitis. HIV encephalopathy can also present with focal neurological signs and seizures. Chronicity is an important clue and these children usually have normal levels of consciousness. In contrast, children with tuberculous meningitis usually have a depressed level of consciousness with focal neurological signs. *Cryptococcus neofomans* infection of the brain, lungs, and even skin can also be confused with tuberculosis but can usually be diagnosed rapidly with an appropriate antigen test, histological examination, or culture. Tuberculosis can occur at the same time as other opportunistic pathogens and HIV-associated illnesses, so lack of complete response to treatment for one infection or condition should lead to evaluation for others. The approach to the child who is

Table 14.1. Approach to the child with a poor clinical response to, or deterioration while on, tuberculosis therapy

ACTION	
Reconsider the diagnosis	Consider the differential diagnosis, especially in children where tuberculosis was not confirmed by culture.
	When acid-fast smear was positive but no culture or molecular diagnosis was available, consider non-tuberculous mycobacteria and other acid-fast-positive organisms.
	Positive acid-fast smear with negative molecular testing would support the diagnosis of nontuberculous mycobacteria.
Consider drug resistance	Review the drug resistance profile of the child's organism and/or that from known contacts if no testing available for the child.
	Review the clinical progress of the possible contact(s). In adults, drug resistance is commonly associated with clinical deterioration and the IRIS phenomena in those with HIV co-infection
	Always re-culture patients; include fine-needle aspirates of nodes and all other possible sites.
Review dosing and drugs	Ensure that the correct dosing is used for the type of tuberculosis disease noted in the child.
Adherence	Review adherence. In older children and adolescents, ensure that they are actually swallowing the tablets.
Review cART	Ensure that the child has initiated cART and, for children on cART, ensure that the dosing is correct and the child is adherent to therapy.
	For children on cART for more than 6 months, ensure that there is an appropriate response.
Absorption and drug interactions and metabolism	Consider malabsorption, especially for abdominal tuberculosis or when there is chronic diarrhea.
	Consider determining drug levels if possible; if not possible, ensure optimized doses.
Consider IRIS	If features are suggestive, consider IRIS and decide if corticosteroids are needed. Even if IRIS is considered, always culture at appropriate sites and investigate and manage other possible suspected diagnoses

not responding or deteriorating while on treatment is outlined in Table 14.1.

THE ROLE OF CONFIRMING INFECTION WITH SKIN TESTING AND INTERFERON GAMMA RELEASE ASSAYS

Positive and negative tuberculin skin test (TST) results have the same implications regardless of HIV status. However, the TST is considered positive at ≥5 mm in children with HIV infection. Positive TST results are noted in up to 60% of HIV-infected children with microbiologically confirmed tuberculosis.[44] Unfortunately, children with untreated HIV infection are more likely to have a negative TST than are HIV-uninfected children.[6]

Interferon gamma release assays (IGRAs) provide results that are similar to the TST's, and it is unclear if these tests offer any advantage in high-burden settings. Many studies have found that the rates of indeterminate/invalid results from IGRAs are higher in HIV-infected children.

IMAGING

The chest radiograph remains one of the most important diagnostic tools for intrathoracic tuberculosis in HIV-infected children, despite the known caveats of interpretation and inter-observer variability. In HIV-infected children, the chest radiographic appearance of tuberculosis is generally the same as in the HIV-uninfected child. However, alveolar opacification and cavitary disease are more common.[6,44] An additional difficulty with interpretation is that other opportunistic infections must be considered, as many HIV-infected children have significant underlying lung disease. Lymphoid interstitial pneumonitis can look exactly like miliary disease, except that enlarged perihilar lymph nodes rarely cause bronchial compression in lymphoid interstitial pneumonitis. For paratracheal adenopathy without hilar adenopathy, malignancy should be excluded with care. When possible, all available radiographs should be reviewed, as the change in appearance over time and correlating it with symptoms can aid making the correct diagnosis.

Ultrasound is an effective method to detect abdominal, pleural, and pericardial tuberculosis in HIV-infected children. To expedite care and overcome the lack of access to specialized imaging centers, the Focused Assessment with Sonography for HIV/TB (FASH) has been developed. In adults it is increasingly seen as an important adjunct to strengthen the diagnosis of extrapulmonary tuberculosis in high-burden settings. Front-line clinicians are taught to use the ultrasound probe in six positions. The basic assessment identifies pathological effusions in body cavities. In the FASH Plus assessment, enlarged lymph nodes and micro-abscesses of the liver and spleen are identified and suggest hematogenous spread.[55] Visualizing multiple enlarged abdominal lymph nodes is 97% (CI, 94–99%) specific for tuberculosis with a positive likelihood ratio of 11 (CI, 4–30). Pathology identified with ultrasound must be interpreted contextually. Prospective studies using FASH in children are not yet published, but it is clear that, where available, ultrasound is an important tool. Pediatric studies suggest that ultrasound can effectively detect mediastinal nodes and may detect nodes in children not seen on chest radiography.[56]

The modalities of CT and MRI are reserved in low-resource settings for central nervous system tuberculosis, although they can be useful in all types of tuberculosis. However, the CT features of meningitis such as obstructive hydrocephalus and basal enhancement are significantly less prominent in HIV-infected children.[53]

MICROBIOLOGICAL DIAGNOSIS

Children with HIV infection face the same issues as HIV-uninfected children regarding microbiological confirmation of tuberculosis:

1. Difficulty in collecting respiratory specimens in young children
2. Paucibacillary disease
   • Decreased yield in smear positivity
   • Decreased in yield in molecular diagnostic tests
   • Decreased culture positivity

In addition, a number of opportunistic infections may complicate the diagnosis. For example, nontuberculous mycobacteria, BCG, and *Nocardia* are acid-fast and can cause positive sputum smears. Distinction can only be made through culture or molecular techniques. Understanding the contexts in which these occur and the differences in their diagnosis and management is absolutely essential. An example is disseminated nontuberculous mycobacterial disease that usually will not occur unless the child is severely immune-compromised, reflected by a CD4+ T-cell count below 100.

MANAGING TUBERCULOSIS IN INFANTS, CHILDREN AND ADOLESCENTS WITH HIV INFECTION

When co-treating tuberculosis and HIV infection the following should be considered:

Treating the tuberculosis: In low-resource settings, changing the cART regimen as a consequence of commencing tuberculosis treatment occurs as commonly as changing for adverse effects[57] due to the drug interactions between antituberculosis drugs, especially rifampicin (RMP) and cART. RMP is a strong inducer of the cytochrome (CYP) p450 system, thus increasing metabolism for cART components. RMP also increases expression of transporter proteins like p-glycoprotein (limiting oral bioavailability and increasing elimination), multiple drug-resistance protein 2, and organic-anion transporting polypeptide. Furthermore, RMP induces phase II metabolism by inducing UDP-glucouronyltransferase and sulphotransferase.[58] CYPp450 is fully induced by one week and only returns to baseline around two weeks after stopping RMP.[58] Although INH inhibits some components of the CYPp450 system, all inhibitory effects are overcome by RMP's strong induction affecting metabolism of all classes, but especially nevirapine, a non-nucleoside reverse transcriptase inhibitor (NNRTI), and key protease inhibitors (PI) such as lopinavir, darunavir, and atazanavir.

Replacing RMP with rifabutin (RIF, a less potent CYPp450 inducer) does not eradicate this problem. RIF is metabolized by CYP3A4, and dose adjustments are needed if co-treating with PIs. Combining RIF with lopinavir-ritonavir (LPV/r) has led to severe RIF-induced neutropenia in children and insufficient exposure when given at 5 mg/kg three times per week.[59] Two-way interactions are complex to manage, and RIF is very costly with no fixed dose combinations available. In low-resource settings where a public health approach is needed, RIF is not presently a feasible intervention. Rifapentine, a long-acting rifamycin, has been associated with the development of RMP mono-resistant tuberculosis in adults and is not recommended.[60]

Replacing rifamycins with other antituberculosis drugs such as fluoroquinolones can be considered in selected cases where drug interactions are complex; however, there are no prospective cohort data for their routine use in children. Regimens that make this substitution probably require a longer treatment period than when including rifamycins.

The standard additional drugs for treating tuberculosis disease are the same as for uninfected children: INH and pyrazinamide (PZA). Most guidance recommends adding a fourth drug, usually ethambutol (EMB), for all forms of pulmonary tuberculosis in HIV-infected children regardless of disease severity.[41]

Data from HIV-infected adults suggest that malabsorption of antituberculosis drugs occurs in some individuals.[61] Data for HIV-infected children are scarce but suggest that adequate serum levels of antituberculosis drugs are achieved with the doses recommended in current WHO guidelines. However, malabsorption should be considered if there is a poor clinical response to what should be adequate therapy. Children with HIV infection may have malabsorption without overt symptoms, especially when concomitant abdominal tuberculosis is present.

The duration of tuberculosis therapy for HIV-infected children is generally the same as for HIV-uninfected children, but with a strong emphasis on confirming clinical improvement with the possibility of extending the continuation phase, if needed. Severely immunocompromised children may require a longer period of treatment. Tuberculous meningitis is an exception, with the intensive phase extended to a minimum of nine months in HIV-infected children. Some centers replace EMB as the fourth drug with ethionamide (ETH), which has better CSF penetration and may also be of value in the presence of INH-resistance due to *katG* mutations that give rise to high-level INH resistance. HIV-infected children should not be treated with intermittent regimens but should receive daily therapy for the entire course.

Initiation of cART: The timing of cART initiation in children not yet on therapy has never been studied prospectively in children with tuberculosis. Adult data strongly support initiating cART within the first eight weeks of tuberculosis treatment.[62] In observational pediatric cohorts, delaying therapy for more than two months was associated with an increased risk of virological failure and mortality.[63] The presence of tuberculous meningitis is a notable exception where clinical deterioration due to paradoxical IRIS caused by reconstitution of the immune system can be devastating. In the adult literature, IRIS is associated more disseminated forms of the disease and positive culture for *M. tuberculosis* in the CSF. This form of IRIS has high morbidity and up to 30% mortality in children and adults.[32,64-66] The adult data for tuberculous meningitis suggest that the outcomes are determined by severity of the meningitis rather than timing of cART.[66] However, for children, the usual recommendation for tuberculous meningitis is to give at least four weeks of effective tuberculosis therapy prior to beginning cART to avoid IRIS.[64] The role of corticosteroids in preventing and treating IRIS has not been assessed, but it is common practice to initiate cART while these children are still on corticosteroids used for treating the tuberculous meningitis.

Paradoxical deterioration: There is very little published data on paradoxical IRIS, but children at highest risk are those with severe immunosuppression

Table 14.2. Features suggestive of paradoxical IRIS

Abdominal tuberculosis	Enlarging nodes
	New or worsening ascites including chylous ascites
	Malabsorption and diarrhea
Chest	New or increasing alveolar opacification
	New cavitation
	New pleural or pericardial effusion
	New or worsening nodal obstruction
Brain	New or enlarging granuloma (tuberculoma) or tuberculous abscess
	New worsening hydrocephalus
	New neuritis or vasculitis
Peripheral adenopathy	Enlarging nodes often filled with pus that may rupture spontaneously

and disseminated tuberculosis[67] (Table 14.2). In general, IRIS is much less common in high-resource settings due to a lower burden of opportunistic infections and earlier initiation of cART. Tuberculosis is the most common cause of paradoxical deterioration in older children in high-burden settings, occurring in up to 7% of children following treatment initiation.[7,68] Prior to diagnosing paradoxical IRIS, other causes of deterioration such as drug resistance, non-adherence, drug side effects, and other infections or cancers must be considered. In high-resource settings, confirming a reduction in viral load and an increase in CD4+ T-cell count is also part of the diagnosis.[69] In low-resource settings this may not be possible, but a careful review of adherence and cART dosing must be performed.[70]

Developing tuberculosis while on cART: Children initiating cART remain at high risk for tuberculosis, especially in the initial period of cART, with a gradual drop in the risk thereafter.[71] If tuberculosis develops in the initial three months of cART, unmasking IRIS should be considered, especially with severe or unusual presentations.[72] These children can present with very severe tuberculosis manifestations and are at high risk of death, with a mortality rate of 10.8 deaths

per 100 person-years.[7,12,21,32,73] The risk for tuberculosis declines as the duration on cART increases.[71] When children develop tuberculosis after the first six months on cART, checking treatment adherence and excluding virological failure are crucial aspects of assessment. Failing children with severe immunosuppression may require a change in cART regimen.

Deciding on the appropriate antiretroviral regimen: Planning the cART regimen can be challenging. Drug interactions between nucleoside reverse transcriptase inhibitors (NRTI) and RMP are not considered clinically significant. The difficulty is to manage the NNRTI or PI components of cART. Not all therapy requires dose adjustment or drug switching. When managing these children, clinicians must consider the age and weight of the child, availability of antiretroviral drugs, possible resistance due to PMTCT, and other prior drug exposure. In young children LPV/r has emerged as the better third drug in children, regardless of previous nevirapine (NVP) or efavirenz (EFV) exposure through PMTCT.[74,75] As LPV/r levels are also significantly affected by RMP, adding ritonavir (RTV) to alter the ratio from a 1:4 to 1:1 (so called "super boosting") overcame this RMP effect in a small study of 15 children.[76] In adults, double dosing LPV/r also works, but this strategy does not overcome the RMP effect in children.[77] Explanations include characteristics of the formulation as well as the metabolism of the drug. Based on the currently available information, super boosting is the preferred strategy. The additional ritonavir should be given for two weeks after stopping RMP. It is not clear at which age double dosing with solid LPV/r formulations can be adopted.

Boosted atazanavir and darunavir cannot be used with RMP due to a lack of information regarding the management of the possible drug interactions.

EFV is the preferred NNRTI. EFV dosing was not available in children younger than three years until recently. When mothers received NVP- or EFV-containing cART during pregnancy and, or if, infants received NVP postnatally, NNRTI resistance was likely. Initial data showed low EFV exposure in children regardless of RMP co-treatment, leading to increasing EFV dosage.[78] Recent data suggest that no further adjustment of EFV dose is required when RMP is used. This may be due to INH blocking accessory metabolic pathways for EFV, especially in slow-metabolizing phenotypes, thus counteracting RMP effects.[79]

NVP is a commonly used NNRTI in low-resource settings where it is incorporated in fixed-dose tablets. However, with RMP co-treatment, there is a very significant risk of under-dosing even if giving NVP at more than 260 mg/m² per day.[80] The period of initiating NVP-containing cART using daily NVP for 14 days may be particularly risky in children also on RMP for tuberculosis therapy. Avoiding the induction dosing in all children younger than two years when only fixed-dose combinations are available has been suggested.[81] Also, when NVP use cannot be avoided, a dose of 200 mg/m²/dose twice daily should be used.[41] There are no published data on virological outcomes in these situations. When possible, children should be switched from NVP to EFV if requiring RMP. Also when they are above three years of age and already suppressed on LPV/r, a switch to EFV can be considered for children developing incident tuberculosis. In this scenario, the viral load should be determined within 8–12 weeks to ensure that virological suppression is maintained.

The WHO recommends three NRTIs as a preferred strategy in HIV-infected children age over three years needing RMP co-treatment based on data from the Antiretroviral Research for Watoto (ARROW) study.[57] In this study, three NRTIs were used as an intensive induction and a maintenance strategy when combined with NNRTIs. Children were placed on a three-drug NRTI maintenance regimen at 48 weeks after initial therapy included an NNRTI; this was compared with a control cohort. Fifty-nine of the 1,143 children required a drug alteration for tuberculosis, which included stopping or replacing NVP. Triple NRTI was effective at 36 weeks but not at 144 weeks.[57] More data are needed to support this strategy.

There are currently no data available for co-treatment with integrase inhibitors, but in adults, raltegravir requires double dosing when an RMP-based tuberculosis regimen is being used.[82]

When should corticosteroids be considered? The indications for corticosteroids are the same as for HIV-uninfected children. An unexpected finding from a study in South African adults evaluating corticosteroids for pericardial tuberculosis was an association with malignancy when compared to placebo, but this needs further exploration.[83] Prospective data for corticosteroid use in IRIS are not available for children, but short courses of systemic corticosteroids are often used to manage moderate to severe IRIS symptoms.

Supportive care should include adequate nutritional support, and although there is little evidence for them, vitamin supplements including pyridoxine are usually given. Micronutrient deficiency is common in HIV-infected children with or without tuberculosis and is not corrected with antituberculosis therapy only.[84] Co-trimoxazole preventative therapy should be given to all children regardless of CD4+ T-cell count. Adult data from the pre-cART era show clearly that patients receiving co-trimoxazole have better outcomes and possibly an associated reduction in the risk of incident tuberculosis.

Drug-related adverse events could complicate therapy: Antituberculosis and antiretroviral therapy have overlapping adverse effects. Clinical monitoring is essential and includes review for rash, jaundice, and other signs and symptoms of hepatitis, bone marrow suppression, and peripheral neuropathy. Laboratory monitoring includes liver function evaluation for hepatitis and possibly full blood count and renal function tests. Adverse events occur in approximately 9% of co-treated children in routine care, with drug-induced liver injury (DILI) being the most common.[12] It should be noted that a transient, mild, asymptomatic transaminitis is not uncommon and does not require drug interruption. When events require stopping therapy for moderate to severe DILI, all drugs must be interrupted, and unlike with antituberculosis drugs, **antiretrovirals must never be introduced at a reduced dose or in a staged fashion or drug resistance may be induced.** Tuberculosis of the liver, and opportunistic and other infections such as hepatitis A must be considered when hepatotoxicity occurs. When the cause of transaminitis is not DILI, interruption or modification of therapy may still be required to avoid exacerbating the hepatitis.

Children with HIV infection may be at an increased risk of toxicity to second-line antituberculosis drugs, although published data are limited.[85,86]

What are the clinical outcomes for children with tuberculosis and HIV? In the pre-cART era, mortality of more than 50% during antituberculosis therapy was reported from high-burden settings.[6,47,51] Fortunately, cART has changed these outcomes. In the majority of children treated for tuberculosis based on a clinical diagnosis, cure cannot always be documented. However, in general, children have favorable outcomes if cART is started. Better outcomes are reported for children who develop tuberculosis once on cART for more than six months.[7,12,32] Mortality does occur, particularly in children diagnosed with tuberculosis prior to cART initiation, with most deaths occurring within first two months of cART. These deaths are not necessarily related to tuberculosis, but may be due to other complications of HIV and immune suppression or IRIS.

Does rifampicin co-treatment alter the viral load outcomes? In a number of cohorts, particularly from South Africa where LPV/r is the preferred initial therapy in children under three years and where viral load monitoring is available, high degrees of viral suppression are achieved in children receiving LPV/r 1:1. However, concurrent tuberculosis therapy may be a risk factor for failure but not LPV resistance.[87–90] A likely explanation is the robust resistance profile of the LPV, but great care should be taken to ensure dosing accuracy and appropriate addition of ritonavir. Ritonavir at full dose should not be used as mono-PI therapy as it is associated with the highest risk of failure and development of PI resistance.[91,92] No difference in suppression is seen with EFV-based therapies.

CONCLUSION

Despite the increase in knowledge about the epidemiology of tuberculosis in HIV-infected children, it remains the most important opportunistic infection in high-burden settings. A multipronged approach including cART access and IPT will reduce the epidemic. Although there are significant diagnostic challenges, history and clinical assessment with a chest radiograph can contribute significantly to suggesting the diagnosis of tuberculosis in HIV-infected children. Whenever possible, microbiological testing should be performed. Attending to drug interaction between RMP and cART is essential to the management of co-treated children. With access to cART, there is a reduction in the mortality and morbidity of HIV-infected children with tuberculosis.

REFERENCES

1. World Health Organization. *Global Update on the Health Sector Response to HIV, 2014.* Geneva: World Health Organization; 2014.
2. World Health Organization. *Consolidated Guidelines on the Use of Antiretroviral Drugs for Treating and Preventing HIV Infection: Recommendations for a Public Health Approach.* Geneva: World Health Organization; 2013 June.
3. Newell ML, Coovadia H, Cortina-Borja M, Rollins N, Gaillard P, Dabis F. Mortality of infected and uninfected infants born to HIV-infected mothers in Africa: a pooled analysis. *Lancet.* 2004;364:1236–1243.
4. Ferrand RA, Corbett EL, Wood R, et al. AIDS among older children and adolescents in Southern Africa: projecting the time course and magnitude of the epidemic. *AIDS.* 2009;23:2039–2046.
5. Townsend CL, Byrne L, Cortina-Borja M, et al. Earlier initiation of ART and further decline in mother-to-child HIV transmission rates, 2000–2011. *AIDS.* 2014;28:1049–1057.
6. Madhi SA, Huebner RE, Doedens L, Aduc T, Wesley D, Cooper PA. HIV-1 co-infection in children hospitalised with tuberculosis in South Africa. *Int J Tuberc Lung Dis.* 2000;4:448–454.
7. Orikiiriza J, Bakeera-Kitaka S, Musiime V, Mworozi EA, Mugyenyi P, Boulware DR. The clinical pattern, prevalence, and factors associated with immune reconstitution inflammatory syndrome in Ugandan children. *AIDS.* 2010;24:2009–2017.
8. Lowenthal ED, Bakeera-Kitaka S, Marukutira T, Chapman J, Goldrath K, Ferrand RA. Perinatally acquired HIV infection in adolescents from sub-Saharan Africa: a review of emerging challenges. *Lancet Infect Dis.* 2014;14:627–639.
9. Venturini E, Turkova A, Chiappini E, Galli L, de Martino M, Thorne C. Tuberculosis and HIV co-infection in children. *BMC Infect Dis.* 2014;14(Suppl 1):S5. doi:10.1186/1471-2334-14-S1-S5
10. Hesseling AC, Cotton MF, Jennings T, et al. High incidence of tuberculosis among HIV-infected infants: evidence from a South African population-based study highlights the need for improved tuberculosis control strategies. *Clin Infect Dis.* 2009;48:108–114.
11. Madhi SA, Nachman S, Violari A, et al. Effect of primary isoniazid prophylaxis against tuberculosis in HIV-exposed children. *N Engl J Med.* 2011;365:21–31.
12. Walters E, Cotton MF, Rabie H, Schaaf HS, Walters LO, Marais BJ. Clinical presentation and outcome of tuberculosis in human immunodeficiency virus infected children on antiretroviral therapy. *BMC Pediatr.* 2008;8:1. doi:10.1186/1471-2431-8-1
13. Thomas P, Bornschlegel K, Singh TP, et al. Tuberculosis in human immunodeficiency virus-infected and human immunodeficiency virus-exposed children in New York City. The New York City Pediatric Spectrum of HIV Disease Consortium. *Pediatr Infect Dis J.* 2000;19:700–706.

14. Cohen JM, Whittaker E, Walters S, Lyall H, Tudor-Williams G, Kampmann B. Presentation, diagnosis and management of tuberculosis in HIV-infected children in the UK. *HIV Med.* 2008;9:277–284.

15. Schaaf HS, Krook S, Hollemans DW, Warren RM, Donald PR, Hesseling AC. Recurrent culture-confirmed tuberculosis in human immunodeficiency virus-infected children. *Pediatr Infect Dis J.* 2005;24:685–691.

16. Colditz GA, Brewer TF, Berkey CS, et al. Efficacy of BCG vaccine in the prevention of tuberculosis. Meta-analysis of the published literature. *JAMA.* 1994;271:698–702.

17. Hesseling AC, Marais BJ, Gie RP, et al. The risk of disseminated Bacille Calmette-Guerin (BCG) disease in HIV-infected children. *Vaccine.* 2007;25:14–18.

18. Hesseling AC, Rabie H, Marais BJ, et al. Bacille Calmette-Guerin vaccine-induced disease in HIV-infected and HIV-uninfected children. *Clin Infect Dis.* 2006;42:548–558.

19. Hesseling AC, Cotton MF, Fordham van Reyn C, Graham SM, Gie RP, Hussey GD. Consensus statement on the revised World Health Organization recommendations for BCG vaccination in HIV-infected infants. *Int J Tuberc Lung Dis.* 2008;12:1376–1379.

20. Rabie H, Violari A, Duong T, et al. Early antiretroviral treatment reduces risk of bacille Calmette-Guérin immune reconstitution adenitis. *Int J Tuberc Lung Dis.* 2011;15:1194–1200.

21. Smith K, Kuhn L, Coovadia A, et al. Immune reconstitution inflammatory syndrome among HIV-infected South African infants initiating antiretroviral therapy. *AIDS.* 2009;23:1097–1107.

22. Lawn SD, Churchyard G. Epidemiology of HIV-associated tuberculosis. *Curr Opin HIV AIDS.* 2009;4:325–333.

23. Lawn SD, Bekker LG, Middelkoop K, Myer L, Wood R. Impact of HIV infection on the epidemiology of tuberculosis in a peri-urban community in South Africa: the need for age-specific interventions. *Clin Infect Dis.* 2006;42:1040–1047.

24. Dimairo M, MacPherson P, Bandason T, et al. The risk and timing of tuberculosis diagnosed in smear-negative TB suspects: a 12 month cohort study in Harare, Zimbabwe. *PloS One.* 2010;5:e11849. doi:10.1371/journal.pone.0011849.

25. Tostmann A, Kik SV, Kalisvaart NA, et al. Tuberculosis transmission by patients with smear-negative pulmonary tuberculosis in a large cohort in the Netherlands. *Clin Infect Dis.* 2008;47:1135–1142.

26. Lawn SD, Edwards D, Wood R. Tuberculosis transmission from patients with smear-negative pulmonary tuberculosis in sub-Saharan Africa. *Clin Infect Dis.* 2009;48:496–497.

27. Gupta A, Bhosale R, Kinikar A, et al. Maternal tuberculosis: a risk factor for mother-to-child transmission of human immunodeficiency virus. *J Infect Dis.* 2011;203:358–363.

28. Cotton MF, Schaaf HS, Lottering G, Weber HL, Coetzee J, Nachman S. Tuberculosis exposure in HIV-exposed infants in a high-prevalence setting. *Int J Tuberc Lung Dis.* 2008;12:225–227.

29. Wood R, Johnstone-Robertson S, Uys P, et al. Tuberculosis transmission to young children in a South African community: modeling household and community infection risks. *Clin Infect Dis.* 2010;51:401–408.

30. Dangor Z, Izu A, Hillier K, et al. Impact of the antiretroviral treatment program on the burden of hospitalization for culture-confirmed tuberculosis in South African children: a time-series analysis. *Pediatr Infect Dis J.* 2013;32:972–977

31. Wood R, Morrow C, Ginsberg S, et al. Quantification of shared air: a social and environmental determinant of airborne disease transmission. *PloS One.* 2014;9(9):e106622. doi: 10.1371/journal.pone.0106622

32. Walters E, Duvenhage J, Draper HR, et al. Severe manifestations of extrapulmonary tuberculosis in HIV-infected children initiating antiretroviral therapy before 2 years of age. *Arch Dis Child.* 2014;99(11):998–1003.

33. Violari A, Cotton MF, Gibb DM, et al. Early antiretroviral therapy and mortality among HIV-infected infants. *N Engl J Med.* 2008;359:2233–2244.

34. Koller M, Patel K, Chi BH, et al. Immunodeficiency in children starting antiretroviral therapy in low-, middle-, and high-income countries. *J Acquir Immune Defic Syndr.* 2015 Jan 1;68:62–72.

35. Bakeera-Kitaka S, Conesa-Botella A, Dhabangi A, et al. Tuberculosis in human immunodeficiency virus infected Ugandan children starting on antiretroviral therapy. *Int J Tuberc Lung Dis.* 2011;15:1082–1086.

36. Bolton-Moore C, Mubiana-Mbewe M, Cantrell RA, et al. Clinical outcomes and CD4 cell response in children receiving antiretroviral therapy at primary health care facilities in Zambia. *JAMA.* 2007;298:1888–1899.

37. Puthanakit T, Aurpibul L, Oberdorfer P, et al. Hospitalization and mortality among

HIV-infected children after receiving highly active antiretroviral therapy. *Clin Infect Dis.* 2007;44:599–604.

38. Meintjes G, Lawn SD, Scano F, et al. Tuberculosis-associated immune reconstitution inflammatory syndrome: case definitions for use in resource-limited settings. *Lancet Infect Dis.* 2008;8:516–523.

39. Zar HJ, Cotton MF, Strauss S, et al. Effect of isoniazid prophylaxis on mortality and incidence of tuberculosis in children with HIV: randomised controlled trial. *BMJ.* 2007;334:136.

40. Frigati LJ, Kranzer K, Cotton MF, Schaaf HS, Lombard CJ, Zar HJ. The impact of isoniazid preventive therapy and antiretroviral therapy on tuberculosis in children infected with HIV in a high tuberculosis incidence setting. *Thorax.* 2011;66:496–501.

41. WHO. *Guidance for National Tuberculosis Programmes on the Management of Tuberculosis in Children.* 2nd ed. Geneva: World Health Organization; 2014.

42. Hesseling AC, Kim S, Madhi S, et al. High prevalence of drug resistance amongst HIV-exposed and -infected children in a tuberculosis prevention trial. *Int J Tuberc Lung Dis.* 2012;16:192–195.

43. World Health Organization. *WHO Case Definitions of HIV for Surveillance and Revised Clinical Staging and Immunological Classification for HIV-Related Disease in Adults and Children.* Geneva: World Health Organization; 2006.

44. Schaaf HS, Marais BJ, Whitelaw A, et al. Culture-confirmed childhood tuberculosis in Cape Town, South Africa: a review of 596 cases. *BMC Infect Dis.* 2007;7:140. doi:10.1186/1471-2334-7-140

45. Maritz E, Liu L, Montepierda G, Mitchelle C, Madhi S, Bobat R, Hesseling AC, Cotton MF. Timing of tuberculosis source case contact information and tuberculosis in HIV-infected and HIV-exposed non-infected children from southern Africa: IMPAACT 1041. 43rd Union World Conference on Lung Health 2012 Nov 13–17; Kuala Lumpur, Malaysia. Abstract PC 640 17.

46. Van Wyk SS, Mandalakas AM, Enarson DA, Gie RP, Beyers N, Hesseling AC. Tuberculosis contact investigation in a high-burden setting: house or household? *Int J Tuberc Lung Dis.* 2012;16:157–162.

47. Jeena PM, Pillay P, Pillay T, Coovadia HM. Impact of HIV-1 co-infection on presentation and hospital-related mortality in children with culture proven pulmonary tuberculosis in Durban, South Africa. *Int J Tuberc Lung Dis.* 2002;6:672–678.

48. Chintu C, Mudenda V, Lucas S, et al. Lung diseases at necropsy in African children dying from respiratory illnesses: a descriptive necropsy study. *Lancet.* 2002;360:985.

49. Marais BJ, Gie RP, Hesseling AC, et al. A refined symptom-based approach to diagnose pulmonary tuberculosis in children. *Pediatrics.* 2006;118:e1350–e1359.

50. Marais BJ, Gie RP, Obihara CC, Hesseling AC, Schaaf HS, Beyers N. Well defined symptoms are of value in the diagnosis of childhood pulmonary tuberculosis. *Arch Dis Child.* 2005;90:1162–1165.

51. Hesseling AC, Schaaf SH, Westra AE, et al. Outcome of HIV-infected children with culture-confirmed tuberculosis. *Arch Dis Child.* 2005;90:1171–1174.

52. Schaaf HS, Geldenduys A, Gie RP, Cotton MF. Culture-positive tuberculosis in human immunodeficiency virus type 1-infected children. *Pediatr Infect Dis J.* 1998;17:599–604.

53. van der Weert EM, Hartgers NM, Schaaf HS, et al. Comparison of diagnostic criteria of tuberculous meningitis in human immunodeficiency virus-infected and uninfected children. *Pediatr Infect Dis J.* 2006;25:65–69.

54. Nourse PJ, Cotton MF, Bates WD. Renal manifestations in children co-infected with HIV and disseminated tuberculosis. *Pediatr Nephrol.* 2010;25:1759–1763.

55. Heller T, Wallrauch C, Brunetti E, Giordani MT. Changes of FASH ultrasound findings in TB-HIV patients during anti-tuberculosis treatment. *Int J Tuberc Lung Dis.* 2014;18:837–839.

56. Bosch-Marcet J, Serres-Creixams X, Zuasnabar-Cotro A, Codina-Puig X, Catala-Puigbo M, Simon-Riazuelo JL. Comparison of ultrasound with plain radiography and CT for the detection of mediastinal lymphadenopathy in children with tuberculosis. *Pediatr Radiol.* 2004;34:895–900.

57. ARROW Trial Team. Routine versus clinically driven laboratory monitoring and first-line antiretroviral therapy strategies in African children with HIV (ARROW): a 5-year open-label randomised factorial trial. *Lancet.* 2013;381:1391–1403.

58. Niemi M, Backman JT, Fromm MF, Neuvonen PJ, Kivisto KT. Pharmacokinetic interactions with rifampicin: clinical relevance. *Clin Pharmacokinet.* 2003;42:819–850.

59. Moultrie H, McIlleron H, Sawry S, et al. Pharmacokinetics and safety of rifabutin in young HIV-infected children receiving rifabutin and lopinavir/ritonavir. *J Antimicrob Chemother.* 2014;70:543–549.

60. Vernon A, Burman W, Benator D, Khan A, Bozeman L. Acquired rifamycin monoresistance in patients with HIV-related tuberculosis treated with once-weekly rifapentine and isoniazid. Tuberculosis Trials Consortium. *Lancet.* 1999;353:1843–1847.

61. Lawn SD, Meintjes G, McIlleron H, Harries AD, Wood R. Management of HIV-associated tuberculosis in resource-limited settings: a state-of-the-art review. *BMC Med.* 2013;11:253. doi:10.1186/1741-7015-11-253

62. Naidoo K, Baxter C, Abdool Karim SS. When to start antiretroviral therapy during tuberculosis treatment? *Curr Opin Infect Dis.* 2013;26:35–42.

63. Yotebieng M, Van Rie A, Moultrie H, et al. Effect on mortality and virological response of delaying antiretroviral therapy initiation in children receiving tuberculosis treatment. *AIDS.* 2010;24:1341–1349.

64. Bahr N, Boulware DR, Marais S, Scriven J, Wilkinson RJ, Meintjes G. Central nervous system immune reconstitution inflammatory syndrome. *Curr Infect Dis Rep.* 2013;15:583–593.

65. van Toorn R, Rabie H, Dramowski A, Schoeman JF. Neurological manifestations of TB-IRIS: a report of 4 children. *Eur J Paediatr Neurol.* 2012;16:676–682.

66. Torok ME, Yen NT, Chau TT, et al. Timing of initiation of antiretroviral therapy in human immunodeficiency virus (HIV)–associated tuberculous meningitis. *Clin Infect Dis.* 2011;52:1374–1383.

67. Link-Gelles R, Moultrie H, Sawry S, Murdoch D, Van Rie A. Tuberculosis immune reconstitution inflammatory syndrome in children initiating antiretroviral therapy for HIV infection: a systematic literature review. *Pediatr Infect Dis J.* 2014;33:499–503.

68. Orikiiriza J, Bakeera-Kitaka S, Boulware D, et al. Immune reconstitution inflammatory syndrome related mortality in HIV-infected children admitted after initiating ART in Uganda. 15th Conference on Retrovirology and Opportunistic Infection; 16–19 Feb 2010; San Francisco.

69. Boulware DR, Callens S, Pahwa S. Pediatric HIV immune reconstitution inflammatory syndrome. *Curr Clin HIV AIDS.* 2008;3:461–467.

70. Meintjes G, Rabie H, Wilkinson RJ, Cotton MF. Tuberculosis-associated immune reconstitution inflammatory syndrome and unmasking of tuberculosis by antiretroviral therapy. *Clin Chest Med.* 2009;30:797–810

71. Li N, Manji KP, Spiegelman D, et al. Incident tuberculosis and risk factors among HIV-infected children in Tanzania. *AIDS.* 2013;27:1273–1281.

72. Meintjes G, Lawn SD, Scano F, et al. Tuberculosis-associated immune reconstitution inflammatory syndrome: case definitions for use in resource-limited settings. *Lancet Infect Dis.* 2008;8:516–523.

73. Puthanakit T, Oberdorfer P, Akarathum N, Wannarit P, Sirisanthana T, Sirisanthana V. Immune reconstitution syndrome after highly active antiretroviral therapy in human immunodeficiency virus-infected Thai children. *Pediatr Infect Dis J.* 2006;25:53–58.

74. Violari A, Lindsey JC, Hughes MD, et al. Nevirapine versus ritonavir-boosted lopinavir for HIV-infected children. *New Engl J Med.* 2012;366:2380–2389.

75. Palumbo P, Lindsey J, Hughes MD, et al. Antiretroviral treatment for children with peripartum nevirapine exposure. *N Engl J Med.* 2010;363:1510–1520.

76. Ren Y, Nuttall JJ, Egbers C, et al. Effect of rifampicin on lopinavir pharmacokinetics in HIV-infected children with tuberculosis. *J Acquir Immune Defic Syndr.* 2008;47:566–569.

77. McIlleron H, Ren Y, Nuttall J, et al. Lopinavir exposure is insufficient in children given double doses of lopinavir/ritonavir during rifampicin-based treatment for tuberculosis. *Antivir Ther.* 2011;16:417–421.

78. Ren Y, Nuttall JJ, Egbers C, et al. High prevalence of subtherapeutic plasma concentrations of efavirenz in children. *J Acquir Immune Defic Syndr.* 2007;45:133–136.

79. McIlleron HM, Schomaker M, Ren Y, et al. Effects of rifampin-based antituberculosis therapy on plasma efavirenz concentrations in children vary by *CYP2B6* genotype. *AIDS.* 2013;27:1933–1940.

80. Oudijk JM, McIlleron H, Mulenga V, et al. Pharmacokinetics of nevirapine in HIV-infected children under 3 years on rifampicin-based antituberculosis treatment. *AIDS.* 2012;26:1523–1528

81. Fillekes Q, Mulenga V, Kabamba D, et al. Is nevirapine dose escalation appropriate in young, African, HIV-infected children? *AIDS.* 2013;27:2111–2115

82. Food and Drug Administration. Isentress; prescribing information. Version December, 2013. Available at https://http://www.merck.com/product/usa/pi_circulars/i/isentress/isentress_pi.pdf (accessed December 28, 2014).

83. Mayosi BM, Ntsekhe M, Bosch J, et al. Prednisolone and *Mycobacterium indicus pranii* in tuberculous pericarditis. *N Engl J Med.* 2014;371:1121–1130.

84. Schaaf HS, Cilliers K, Willemse M, Labadarios D, Kidd M, Donald PR. Nutritional status and its response to treatment of children, with and without HIV infection, hospitalized for the management of tuberculosis. *Paediatr Int Child Health*. 2012;32:74–81.

85. Rose PC, Hallbauer UM, Seddon JA, Hesseling AC, Schaaf HS. Linezolid-containing regimens for the treatment of drug-resistant tuberculosis in South African children. *Int J Tuberc Lung Dis*. 2012;16:1588–1593.

86. Seddon JA, Thee S, Jacobs K, Ebrahim A, Hesseling AC, Schaaf HS. Hearing loss in children treated for multidrug-resistant tuberculosis. *J Infect*. 2013;66(4):320–329. doi: 10.1016/j.jinf.2012.09.002

87. Frohoff C, Moodley M, Fairlie L, et al. Antiretroviral therapy outcomes in HIV-infected children after adjusting protease inhibitor dosing during tuberculosis treatment. *PloS One*. 2011;6:e17273. doi: 10.1371/journal.pone.0017273

88. Meyers T, Sawry S, Wong JY, et al. Virologic failure among children taking lopinavir/ritonavir-containing first-line antiretroviral therapy in South Africa. *Pediatr Infect Dis J*. 2014;34:175–179.

89. Reitz C, Coovadia A, Ko S, et al. Initial response to protease-inhibitor-based antiretroviral therapy among children less than 2 years of age in South Africa: effect of cotreatment for tuberculosis. *J Infect Dis*. 2010;201:1121–1131.

90. Walters E, Reichmuth K, Dramowski A, Marais BJ, Cotton MF, Rabie H. Antiretroviral regimens containing a single protease inhibitor increase risk of virologic failure in young HIV-infected children. *Pediatr Infect Dis J*. 2013;32:361–363.

91. van Zyl GU, Frenkel LM, Chung MH, Preiser W, Mellors JW, Nachega JB. Emerging antiretroviral drug resistance in sub-Saharan Africa. *AIDS*. 2014;28:2643–2648.

92. van Zyl GU, van der Merwe L, Claassen M, et al. Protease inhibitor resistance in South African children with virologic failure. *Pediatr Infect Dis J*. 2009;28:1125–1127.

15

ANTITUBERCULOSIS DRUGS IN CHILDREN

Helen McIlleron

HIGHLIGHTS OF THIS CHAPTER

- Children are likely to respond well to a drug regimen if given drug formulations and doses that achieve comparable pharmacokinetics to those in adults.
- Emerging pharmacokinetic data have suggested consistently that higher drug doses per kilogram of body weight are required in children than in adults.
- It is necessary to define the key pharmacokinetic measures associated with efficacy and toxicity in adults in order to optimize dosing in children based on pharmacokinetic targets.
- It is also necessary to evaluate the safety of drug regimens in children given doses achieving similar plasma exposures to adults.
- Extemporaneous preparations of antituberculosis drugs, especially the crushing of pills and creation of suspensions, typically have unknown bioavailability, their stability over time may not be adequately characterized, and potential toxicity of excipients is a concern.

TUBERCULOSIS DRUGS

Tuberculosis drugs are used for treatment of both tuberculosis infection and disease. This chapter outlines aspects of the pharmacology of the drugs relevant to their clinical applications in children.

Different Drugs Have Different Roles

A spectrum of mycobacterial phenotypes results from adaptation of *Mycobacterium tuberculosis* in response to its environment. A patient presenting with tuberculosis disease may harbor a variety of different mycobacterial subpopulations, defined by different rates of replication and metabolic states, with differing susceptibility to various drugs' mechanisms of action (Mitchison 2008). Rapidly dividing organisms, abundant in the aerobic environment of the lung cavities, are susceptible to drugs with good early bactericidal activity, like isoniazid. Drugs with sterilizing activity against the more slowly replicating and persisting organisms found in acidic and oxygen-restricted environments, like pyrazinamide and rifampicin, respectively, are key for effective regimens that will prevent relapse, and allow the design of shorter treatment regimens. Hence a variety of drugs with different roles are used against tuberculosis.

GENERAL PRINCIPLES

Treating Tuberculosis Infection

In an infected person without any symptoms or signs of disease, the mycobacterial burden is low and the risk of selecting organisms with drug-resistant mutations is insignificant even when only one drug is used. The World Health Organization (WHO) recommends giving six months of isoniazid for tuberculosis infected children at high risk of developing disease (WHO 2014). Addition of a drug with good sterilizing activity, however, allows shortening of the regimen. A three-month regimen of a rifamycin together with isoniazid is equally effective. The roles of shorter regimens with improved sterilizing activity are being further evaluated in children. The optimal approach to preventing tuberculosis disease in children exposed to or infected with a multidrug-resistant strain of *M. tuberculosis* (MDR-TB) requires further research; isoniazid and/or rifamycin-based preventive regimens are not likely to be effective (Sneag 2007).

Treating Tuberculosis Disease

Conversely, adults presenting with clinical evidence of pulmonary tuberculosis disease usually have a high bacterial load comprising metabolically diverse organisms. A multi-drug regimen is required to effect a cure. It should have excellent early bactericidal and sterilizing activities to achieve rapid reduction of the mycobacterial load and eradication of persisting mycobacterial populations, respectively. The regimen should include drugs able to penetrate in sufficient concentrations to the sites of infection—particularly the central nervous system in children—and should prevent the emergence of drug resistance through achieving sufficient concentrations of at least two effective drugs in the replicating mycobacterial populations. Although the mycobacterial burden in many children with tuberculosis disease is lower than in adults, these principles of treatment still apply.

Evidence for Antituberculosis Drug Use in Children

Few studies have been conducted to evaluate tuberculosis treatment regimens in children, especially infants and toddlers (Duke 2014). Hence, for many antituberculosis drugs, evidence to support dosing and suitable formulations is lacking. Generally the regimens and doses used in children have been extrapolated from those used in adults. Children are likely to respond well to a drug regimen if given drug formulations and doses that achieve comparable pharmacokinetics to those in adults (Burman 2008). However, although drug concentrations are influenced by changes in growth and development, confirmatory pharmacokinetic studies in children have been limited. Neonates and infants in whom the drug exposures are most difficult to predict have been most notably neglected. In response to emerging pharmacokinetic data suggesting that higher doses per kilogram of body weight are required in children compared to adults, the WHO recently increased the recommended doses of isoniazid, rifampicin, and pyrazinamide for children by 100%, 50%, and 40%, respectively (WHO 2014).

Pharmacokinetic and Safety Considerations in Children

That a higher dose per kilogram of body weight is required in children, who have a higher clearance per kilogram, is explained by allometric theory (Holford 2013). There is, however, a need for pharmacokinetic studies to confirm the optimal doses for children across the relevant ranges for age and weight. The nonlinear relationship between weight and drug clearance applies within the range of childhood weights. Moreover, immaturity of absorption and clearance processes, together with changes in body distribution, result in drug-specific differences in pharmacokinetics in children under two years of age. Emerging data support the theory that a single dose per kilogram of body weight is not appropriate across the range of childhood ages and weights, and will support further optimization of dosing recommendations in the future (Zvada 2014 abstr, Ramachandran 2013, Thee 2014a).

Pharmacokinetic data to support drug doses for children drug-resistant tuberculosis are particularly sparse.

More rapid absorption (which may occur when the drug is administered as a solution or a suspension instead of in a solid dosage form) and a relatively higher clearance, translate into a higher ratio for the peak drug concentration (C_{max}) to overall exposure (area under the concentration-time curve; AUC) in children compared to adults. Hence it is necessary to define the key pharmacokinetic measures associated with efficacy and toxicity in adults in order to optimize dosing in children based on these pharmacokinetic targets. The potential effects on antituberculosis drug exposures of factors such as HIV infection and malnutrition should also be evaluated in sufficiently representative and well-designed studies (Thee 2014 b, Ramachandran 2013). Pharmacogenetic factors predict drug exposures for isoniazid and rifampicin. The role of genotype in dose determination is a topic for future research. While the doses used in children should achieve the pharmacokinetic targets derived from studies in adults, the safety of those doses needs to be confirmed in children. This is especially needed for the second-line drugs for which there is only limited reported experience in children for extended periods. Confirmation of safety is particularly important in neonates and infants, who may be exposed to relatively high doses of excipients in liquid or extemporaneous formulations and as immaturity of their biochemical pathways, including those regulating drug disposition, may lead to unanticipated toxicity.

Different Drug Combinations, Doses, and Durations for Different Types of Tuberculosis

The optimal combinations of drugs, drug doses, and durations of treatment may vary according to the extent and site of infection and disease. For example, for children with non-severe paucibacillary tuberculosis, a shortened treatment period may be appropriate, while children with tuberculous meningitis may benefit from higher drug doses and the use of drugs with good penetration of the blood–brain barrier (Thwaites 2013, Ruslami 2013). The results of pediatric studies addressing some of these issues are eagerly awaited.

New Drugs for Tuberculosis

Several promising antituberculosis drugs are currently being developed. Bedaquiline and delamanid have received marketing authorization for adults. These new drugs offer the prospect of improved regimens for drug-susceptible and drug-resistant tuberculosis. There is growing recognition of the ethical imperative to include children in studies evaluating these drugs and regimens at an early stage, in order to provide the evidence needed for their safe and effective use in children as early as possible after licensing.

Formulations

A lack of suitable formulations is a considerable barrier to optimal treatment of children with tuberculosis. Appropriate investment in suitable formulations for infants and children is necessary to ensure correct dosing and to ensure that access to drugs is not delayed or denied. Ease of administration and acceptability are key considerations. Flexibility of the dose form is necessary to accommodate correct dosing by age and weight, and any specific dosing or drug combination requirements. Maintenance of an uninterrupted drug supply is essential, hence a sufficiently simplified formulary of products with good long-term stability is needed. Infants and young children cannot swallow solid dose forms, but liquid formulations are not suitable for most high-burden settings as they tend to be bulky, often need refrigeration, and have a short shelf life. Dispersible pediatric fixed-dose combinations of the first-line drugs are widely used; however, these do not easily accommodate the currently recommended doses (WHO 2014), as the ratio of rifampicin : isoniazid : pyrazinamide is different from that formerly used. The drugs for drug-resistant tuberculosis are frequently available only in adult formulations. For children they need to be divided and sometimes crushed; however, stability and absorption may be altered and accurate dosing is impossible (Weiner 2014, Pouplin 2014). Extemporaneous preparations typically have unknown bioavailability, their stability over time may not be adequately characterized, and potential toxicity of excipients is a concern. Moreover, large-volume doses or poorly palatable mixtures are difficult for children to tolerate and may be spat out. Little is known about dose preparation practices of caregivers, but there are concerns about the stability of rifampicin when it is mixed with isoniazid in the presence of water (a reaction that might be accelerated by ascorbic acid); the binding of drugs such as isoniazid, ethambutol, and fluoroquinolones to food constituents; and adsorption of rifampicin to certain plastics. In summary, there is an urgent need to invest in improved child-friendly antituberculosis drug formulations suited to high-burden settings, and they need to be widely available.

HIV-ASSOCIATED TUBERCULOSIS

Children with HIV infection should be started on antiretroviral treatment within eight weeks of starting tuberculosis treatment and, more urgently, within two weeks of starting tuberculosis treatment if the CD4+ T-cell count is below 50 cells/mL. Co-trimoxazole, pyridoxine supplementation, and nutritional support should also be provided. The combined treatments entail a high pill burden, the combined risks of drug side effects (Table 15.1), and the potential for drug–drug interactions (Table 15.2). Rifampicin and rifapentine are potent activators of the pregnane X receptor (PXR). PXR is a nuclear receptor that regulates the transcription of drug-metabolizing enzymes, including phase I enzymes such as cytochrome P450 (CYP) 2B6, 2B9, 2C8, 2C9, 3A4, and 3A7; phase II enzymes such as the glutathione- S- transferases, uridine diphosphate glucose (UDP) glucuronosyltransferases (UGTs), and sulphotransferases; and transporters such as P- glycoprotein, multidrug resistance protein 2, multidrug resistance- associated protein 2, and the organic anion transporter polypeptide (OATP)2. Hence the rifamycins reduce the concentrations of concomitantly administered drug substrates, including nonnucleoside reverse transcriptase inhibitors (NNRTIs) metabolized by CYP 2B6 and CYP 3A4, protease inhibitors (PIs) which are substrates of p-glycoprotein and CYP 3A4, and raltegavir, a UGT 1A1 substrate. Full induction of the activity of these enzymes and transporters takes several days to weeks, and their activity declines gradually after withdrawal of the activator. Ritonavir (and other peptide-mimetic PIs) also activates PXR, and efavirenz and nevirapine induce CYP 3A4 and 2B6 expression, largely via activation of the constitutive androstane receptor. On the other hand, ritonavir is a promiscuous mechanism-based inhibitor. It potently inhibits CYP 3A4 and p-glycoprotein. It is used in low doses to boost PI concentrations. Higher doses of ritonavir are used to counteract the effect of rifampicin on PI concentrations.

Antituberculosis drugs known to inhibit drug metabolizing enzymes include isoniazid (CYP 1A2, 2A6, 2C19, and 3A4), clarithromycin (P-glycoprotein and CYP 3A), ethambutol (CYP 1A2 and CYP2E1), and clofazamine (a weak CYP enzyme inhibitor). Inhibition reactions are rapid in onset and last hours to days, depending on the stability of the inhibitor and the target protein, and the strength of the bond between them. The currently recommended approaches (WHO 2013) for combining first-line tuberculosis treatment with antiretroviral regimens are based on studies performed in children on lower doses of rifampicin and isoniazid than those currently recommended, and should be confirmed for the current doses. Given the complex multidirectional nature of the drug interactions between the regimens, and differences between adult healthy volunteers and children with tuberculosis and HIV infection, studies in the relevant pediatric populations are important (Zhang 2013) and the findings should be confirmed in children receiving the recently revised antituberculosis drug doses. Among adults, HIV infection has been associated with reduced antituberculosis drug concentrations, although whether these findings are independent of nutritional and anthropomorphic effects is less clear (McIlleron 2006, Jeremiah 2014).

PHARMACOKINETICS, FORMULATIONS, AND GENERAL PHARMACOLOGICAL CHARACTERISTICS OF INDIVIDUAL ANTITUBERCULOSIS DRUGS

This section outlines basic information about the pharmacokinetics (Table 15.3), drug formulations (Table 15.4), and other general pharmacological information about antituberculosis drugs, including safety (Table 15.5) in children. These drugs are conventionally categorized in five groups: (1) the first-line oral drugs; (2) second-line injectable agents; (3) fluoroquinolones; (4) second-line oral bacteriostatic drugs; and (5) TB drugs with unclear efficacy or an unclear role that are used against drug-resistant tuberculosis.

Table 15.1. Shared side effects of antituberculosis drugs and antiretrovirals

SIDE EFFECT	ANTITUBERCULOSIS DRUGS	ANTIRETROVIRALS
Rash	Isoniazid, pyrazinamide, rifampicin, rifabutin, ethambutol, clofazamine, fluoroquinolones, cycloserine, terizidone PAS, ethionamide, aminoglycosides, capreomycin	Abacavir, nevirapine, efavirenz, stavudine, rarely: raltegravir
Hepatotoxicity	Isoniazid, ethionamide, protionamide, rifampicin, rifabutin, pyrazinamide, rarely: fluoroquinolones, PAS, cycloserine	Nevirapine, efavirenz, ritonavir and other protease inhibitors, nucleoside reverse transcriptase inhibitors, rarely: raltegravir
Neuropathy	Isoniazid, linezolid, ethionamide, protionamide, cycloserine, terizidone	Stavudine, didanosine, zalcitabine
Ophthalmological problems	Ethambutol, rifabutin, linezolid, ethionamide, protionamide	Didanosine
Central nervous system toxicity	Cycloserine, terizidone, ethionamide, protionamide, fluoroquinolones, isoniazid	Efavirenz, uncommonly: atazanavir
QT-interval prolongation	Fluoroquinolones (more marked with moxifloxacin), clarithromycin, clofazamine	Lopinavir, atazanavir,
Gastrointestinal disturbance	Ethionamide, protionamide, PAS, clofazamine, isoniazid, ethambutol, pyrazinamide, linezolid, clarithromycin, fluoroquinolones, rifampicin, rifabutin, isoniazid	Ritonavir, other protease inhibitors, didanosine, stavudine, nevirapine, raltegravir, others
Arthralgia	Pyrazinamide, ethambutol, fluoroquinolones, rifabutin	Raltegravir
Pancreatitis	Linezolid	Stavudine, didanosine, zalcitabine
Lactic acidosis	Linezolid	Stavudine, didanosine, zidovudine,
Renal impairment, electrolyte disturbance	Aminoglycosides, capreomycin, rarely: ethambutol	Tenofovir, rarely: raltegravir
Hematological abnormalities	Linezolid, rifabutin, rifampicin, isoniazid, fluoroquinolones, rarely: ethambutol, cycloserine, terizidone	Zidovudine, abacavir, trimethoprim/ sulphamethoxazole, rarely: raltegravir
Hypothyroidism	Ethionamide, protionamide, PAS	Stavudine
Dysglycemia	Ethionamide, protionamide, fluoroquinolones, isoniazid	Protease inhibitors
gynaecomastia hypersensitivity/ anaphylaxis	ethionamide, isoniazid fluoroquinolones	efavirenz, atazanavir, darunavir abacavir, tenofovir, atazanavir

PAS = p-aminosalicylic acid.

Table 15.2. Drug–drug interactions associated with the combination of rifampicin–based tuberculosis treatment* and antiretroviral regimens recommended for children with HIV-associated drug-sensitive TB (WHO 2013)

ART REGIMEN	COMMENTS	DRUG INTERACTION
EFV + 2 NRTIs	Recommended regimen for children 3 years and older, provided the child has no history of failure of an NNRTI-based regimen.	EFV is metabolized primarily by CYP 2B6, which is induced by rifampicin. Isoniazid inhibits the CYP 2A6-mediated accessory pathway. Model-based analyses show a modest reduction in EFV concentrations due to tuberculosis treatment among rapid metabolizers with a rapid NAT2 genotype. However, patients with a slow CYP 2B6 genotype have increased EFV concentrations during tuberculosis treatment, more marked in those with a slow NAT2 genotype. (McIleron 2013, Bertrand 2014)
NVP + 2 NRTIs	Recommended regimen for children younger than 3 years of age, provided the child has no history of failure of an NNRTI-based regimen. NVP should be commenced at full twice daily doses. There is a paucity of evidence supporting this approach in young children.	NVP is metabolized by both CYP 2B6 and CYP 3A4. Rifampicin potently induces both enzymes. Tuberculosis treatment reduces NVP concentrations in adults, in whom outcomes are acceptable. However, few studies report reductions of the magnitude reported in young children (Oudjik 2012). Toxicity concerns curtail increasing the dose.
LPV/r + additional ritonavir + 2 NRTIs	For children needing a PI-based regimen. The approach is not feasible in many settings, as ritonavir oral solution needs refrigeration and has a short shelf life. LPV/r and ritonavir oral solutions are poorly tolerated. Hepatotoxicity is a concern; children should be carefully monitored.	LPV is a substrate of CYP 3A4, p-glycoprotein, and OATP 1B1, which are induced by rifampicin and inhibited by ritonavir. LPV concentrations are profoundly reduced when standard doses of LPV/r are given with rifampicin. Adjusted doses of LPV and ritonavir are used to compensate. Super-boosting LPV with ritonavir to achieve a 1:1 ratio achieves adequate LPV concentrations in young children on tuberculosis treatment, while doubling the dose of LPV/r oral solution does not. In adults, twice the usual dose of LPV/r tablets is sufficient during tuberculosis treatment. This approach needs to be studied in children old enough to swallow LPV/r tablets.
Triple NRTI (ABC + 3TC + AZT)	Alternative regimen. Preferred regimen for children <3 years old if they are virologically suppressed on LPV/r-based ART when starting TB treatment. There is limited evidence to support this approach. There is concern that this is likely to be a weak regimen in children with a high viral load or failure of a prior ART regimen.	Major drug–drug interactions are avoided with this combination. Although metabolism of ABC and AZT (UGT substrates) may be induced rifampicin, the interaction is thought to be clinically insignificant.

*Rifampicin and isoniazid with pyrazinamide and ethambutol in the intensive phase.

ART = antiretroviral treatment; EFV = efavirenz; NRTI = nucleoside reverse transcriptase inhibitor; NNRTI = nonnucleoside reverse transcriptase inhibitor; CYP = cytochrome P450; NAT2 = N-acetyltransferase 2; NVP = nevirapine; LPV/r = ritonavir-boosted lopinavir; LPV = lopinavir; ABC = abacavir; 3TC = lamivudine; AZT = zidovudine; UGT = UDP glucuronosyltransferase.

Table 15.3. Selected pharmacokinetic measures for the antituberculosis drugs

DRUG	PROPOSED TARGET CONCENTRATION (MG/L)[a]	EXPECTED HALF-LIFE (H) IN ADULTS	PLASMA PROTEIN BINDING (%)	ESTIMATED RATIO (%) OF CSF TO PLASMA (THWAITES 2013)
Isoniazid	3–6	1.5/ 4[b]	<10	80–90
Rifampicin	8–24	2[c]	80–90	10–20
Rifapentine	C_{24} 5–14[d]	15	97–98	-
Rifabutin	0.45–0.9	30	70–85	-[e]
Pyrazinamide	20–60	9	±10	90–100
Ethambutol	2–6	3/10[f]	20–30	20–30
Amikacin	35–45	3	<10	10–20
Kanamycin	35–45	3	-	10–20
Capreomycin	35–45	-	-	-
Levofloxacin	8–13	9	24–38	70–80
Moxifloxacin	3–5	7	52	70–80
Ofloxacin	8[g]	9.5[g]	32	62 (Nau 2010)
Ethionamide	2–5	2	30	80–90
Cycloserine	20–35	7	-	80–90
p-aminosalicylic acid (PAS)	20–60	1	50–60	-
Clofazimine	0.5–2.0	11h/ 70 days[f]	-	-
Linezolid	12–26	5	10–30	40–70
Amoxicillin/ clavulanate	-	1.15	20	2 (Nau 2010)
Clarithromycin	2–7	5[h]	70–77	-

[a]C_{max}, or peak concentration, unless otherwise stated.
[b]In fast/slow acetylators, respectively.
[c]After multiple doses (auto-induced state).
[d]Concentration 24 h after 900 mg weekly dose in adults (Weiner 2014).
[e]Toxicity at high doses limits use for CNS infections.
[f]Biphasic elimination.
[g]Median in adults on 800 mg/day for MDR-TB (Chigutsa 2012); less effective than moxifloxacin 400 mg or high-dose levofloxacin.
[h]With 500 mg dose twice daily.

Isoniazid

The large population of rapidly dividing organisms present in lung cavities is highly susceptible to the action of isoniazid (Mitchison 2008). In patients on standard therapy, 90% of these organisms are eradicated within a few days. Isoniazid appears to have very little, if any, activity beyond the first few days, and may even be antagonistic to the sterilizing activity of pyrazinamide and rifampicin against persisting organisms (Almeida 2009, Chigutsa 2015). Hence, in most patients, its role after the first few days of therapy is largely as a companion drug to prevent the emergence of drug resistance. Isoniazid

Table 15.4. Antituberculosis drug doses and more widely used formulations

GROUP		USUAL DOSE (WHO 2014)	FORMULATIONS ON WHO'S PREQUALIFIED LIST, OR AVAILABLE FORMULATIONS (IN PARENTHESES AND *ITALICS*).
1	**First-line oral drugs**		
	Isoniazid (H)	7–15 mg/kg daily; maximum 300 mg/day[b,c,d]	FDCs[e] Tablets: 100, 300 mg
	Rifampicin (R)	10–20 mg/kg daily; maximum 600 mg/day[b,c]	FDCs[e] Capsules: 150, 300 mg
	Pyrazinamide (Z)	30–40 mg/kg daily[b]	FDCs[e] Tablets: 400, 500 mg tablet
	Ethambutol (E)	15–25 mg/kg daily[b]	FDCs[e] Tablets: 100, 400 mg
	Rifabutin	Not established[f]	(*capsule: 150 mg*)
2	**Injectable drugs**		
	Amikacin	15–22.5 mg/kg daily; maximum 1 g/day	Injection 500 mg/2ml
	Kanamycin	15–30 mg/kg daily; maximum 1 g/day	(*Injection 250 mg/ml - 2 mL, 4 mL; 50 mg/mL, 2 mL*)
	Capreomycin	15–30 mg/kg daily; maximum 1 g/day	Powder for injection 1g
3	**Fluoroquinolones**		
	Levofloxacin	7.5–10 mg/kg daily; maximum 750 mg/day	Tablets: 250, 500, 750 mg
	Moxifloxacin	7.5–10 mg/kg daily; maximum 400 mg/day	Tablets: 400 mg
	Ofloxacin	15–20 mg/kg daily in 1 or 2 doses; maximum 800 mg/day	Tablets: 200, 400 mg
4	**Second-line oral bacteriostatic drugs**		
	Ethionamide (or protionamide)	15–20 mg/kg twice daily; maximum 1 g/day	Tablets: 250 mg
	Cycloserine (or terizidone)	10–20 mg/kg/day in 1 or 2 doses; maximum 1g /day	Cycloserine capsules: 250 mg
	p-aminosalicylic acid (PAS)	150 mg/kg/day in 2 or 3 doses[g]; maximum 12 g/day	Powder (PAS-sodium) for oral solution 4 g; Delayed release granules 60% w/w
5[h]	**Drugs with unclear efficacy/role**		
	Clofazimine	In adults, 100 mg/day; higher doses not used for more than 3 months; *dose for children with tuberculosis not established.*[i]	(*Capsule: 50, 100 mg*)

Table 15.4. Continued

GROUP	USUAL DOSE (WHO 2014)	FORMULATIONS ON WHO'S PREQUALIFIED LIST, OR AVAILABLE FORMULATIONS (IN PARENTHESES AND *ITALICS*).
Linezolid	Adults: 10–12 mg/kg twice daily; *dose for children with tuberculosis not established.*	*(Tablets: 600 mg; Oral suspension: 20 mg/mL)*
Amoxicillin/clavulanate	Adults: 15 mg/kg amoxicillin, thrice daily; *dose for children with tuberculosis not established*	*(Tablets: 1000/62.5 mg; Powder for oral suspension liquid: 600/42.9 mg per 5mL)*
Clarithromycin	Adults: 7.5–15 mg/kg (maximum 500 mg) twice daily; *dose for children with tuberculosis not established.*	*(Tablets: 250, 500 mg; Oral suspension: 125 mg/5mL, 250 mg/5 mL)*

[a]Available at: http://apps.who.int/prequal/query/ProductRegistry.aspx?list=tb, last accessed 31 Dec. 2014.

[b]As children approach a body weight of 25 kg, adult dosing recommendations should be adopted.

[c]Daily doses are preferred; however, during the continuation phase of treatment, thrice-weekly regimens can be considered for HIV-uninfected children in settings with well-established directly-observed therapy (WHO 2014); 20–30 mg/kg/dose of isoniazid, 10–20 mg/kg (up to 600 mg) per dose.

[d]A high dose of H for children with low-level H resistance is not established; 16–20 mg/kg doses have been used in adults.

[e]The World Health Organization list of prequalified medicinal products includes the following FDCs: R/H/Z, 60/30/150 (dispersible tablet); R/H: 60/30 (dispersible tablet), 60/60 (dispersible tablet), 150/75 (tablet), 150/150 (tablet), 300/150 (capsule); R/H/Z/E: 150/75/400/275 (tablet); R/H/E: 150/75/275 (tablet); H/E: 150/400 (tablet).

[f]5–10 mg/kg daily doses are usually used for *M. avium* infections. Safe doses for children in conjunction with ritonavir-boosted protease inhibitors is not established.

[g]PAS doses are administered in an acidic medium (e.g., yoghurt or orange juice) for improved absorption.

[h]Thioacetazone (no longer widely available, and contraindicated in patients with HIV infection due to the high risk of life-threatening skin reactions). Carbapenems such as imipenem/cilastatin are used intravenously and are not feasible in most settings.

[i]1 mg/kg/day has been used in children; however, this is lower than the mg/kg dose in most adult patients. A dose of 3–5 mg/kg is recommended for adults under 33 kg (max 100 mg/d), but long-term doses at the top of this range may be associated with cardiotoxicity. There is a lack of suitable formulations for children; intermittent doses (2–3x/week) have been used.

[j]The recommended 600 mg twice daily dose in adults frequently causes side effects. Lower doses (300 mg twice daily, or once daily in adults) may be effective, and are less toxic. Dose reduction may be considered after an initial induction phase at the higher dose.

monotherapy for a duration of six or nine months is the most widely used regimen for the treatment of tuberculosis infection, although shorter regimens, including drugs with more potent sterilizing activity (rifamycins), are at least as effective.

Isoniazid is a prodrug requiring activation by mycobacterial catalase-peroxidase to act on its target enzyme, an NADH-dependent enoyl-acyl carrier protein reductase, which promotes cell wall synthesis. *M. tuberculosis* mutations in the *katG* and *inhA* genes, which encode the catalase-peroxidase and carrier protein reductase, respectively, are associated with isoniazid resistance. Patients infected with drug-resistant strains with a low level of isoniazid resistance (minimum inhibitory concentration >0.1 mg/L and <0.4 mg/L, which is associated with *inhA* promoter region mutations) may benefit from high doses of isoniazid. However, appropriate doses of isoniazid for children with low-level resistance have not yet been determined.

Oral isoniazid is rapidly absorbed when given in the fasted state. Food and antacids delay and further reduce absorption. Acetylation by N-acetyltransferase 2 (NAT2) is the primary metabolic pathway for isoniazid. Intestinal and hepatic NAT2 contribute to first-pass metabolism, while hepatic NAT2 is largely responsible for systemic clearance, before further metabolism and renal elimination. NAT2 is polymorphic, conferring a trimodal distribution of isoniazid plasma exposures, which

Table 15.5. Antituberculosis drugs, associated side effects, and measures to prevent and detect them

DRUG	SIDE EFFECTS	PREVENTION AND MONITORING
Isoniazid	Hepatitis (<0.1% of children on IPT; <1% with first-line regimen including rifampicin and pyrazinamide). Neurotoxicity (dose-related and more common in slow metabolizers): peripheral neuropathy, and rarely, ataxia, seizures, psychosis, optic neuritis. Rash, gastrointestinal intolerance, anemia (sideroblastic, hemolytic, or rarely, aplastic). Rarely, thrombocytopenia, neutropenia, interstitial nephritis, drug-induced lupus erythematosus.	Ensure correct dosing. Monitor clinically. Measure liver enzymes in children at increased risk of hepatitis. Provide pyridoxine supplementation to children with HIV, malnutrition, or on other drugs causing peripheral neuropathy.
Rifampicin	Hepatotoxicity, gastrointestinal intolerance, rash, pruritus, hypersensitivity (a rare flu-like syndrome with fever, urticaria, hemolysis, eosinophilia, thrombocytopenia, leucopenia, interstitial nephritis, acute tubular necrosis which is associated with intermittent high doses), drowsiness, headache, confusion. Induced glucocorticoid metabolism may precipitate adrenal insufficiency. Reduces the concentrations of many concomitantly administered drugs.	Monitor clinically and measure liver enzymes in children at increased risk of hepatitis (e.g., if on a protease inhibitor; underlying hepatic disease). Warn patients that rifampicin colors urine, tears, and other body fluids. Staining of soft contact lenses may occur. Consider drug-concentration monitoring of concomitantly administered drugs interacting with rifampicin.
Rifabutin	Dose-related and more frequent when administered with ritonavir or other enzyme inhibitors: rash, gastrointestinal intolerance, headache, neutropenia, thrombocytopenia, anemia, corneal opacities, and uveitis. Hepatotoxicity, hypersensitivity reactions. Drug–drug interactions with many other drugs.	Ensure correct dosing and monitor clinically. Perform regular liver function tests. Monitor the white blood cell and platelet counts. Patients should be warned to report any eye pain, redness, or loss of vision urgently. Rifabutin colors body fluids and may stain soft contact lenses. Gastrointestinal intolerance may be reduced by taking the drug with food. Consider rifabutin concentration monitoring, if available, especially if on concomitant protease inhibitors. Monitor concentrations of interacting drugs if indicated.
Pyrazinamide	Hepatotoxicity (more common at high doses), hyperuricemia and arthralgia, rashes, photosensitivity, gastrointestinal disturbance.	Ensure correct dosing, monitor clinically, and measure liver enzymes in children at increased risk of hepatitis.

Table 15.5. Continued

DRUG	SIDE EFFECTS	PREVENTION AND MONITORING
Ethambutol	Optic neuritis (dose-related), hyperuricemia with arthralgia, gastrointestinal disturbance, skin rashes, dizziness and confusion. Rarely, thrombocytopenia, renal toxicity.	Ensure correct dosing. Warn patients about potential for visual disturbances and that such symptoms should be reported without delay. Perform baseline and regular follow-up visual testing if it is possible.
Amikacin, kanamycin	Hearing loss related to dose and treatment duration (loss of high frequencies first), electrolyte imbalance (especially hypokalemia, hypomagnesemia), and renal impairment.	Ensure correct dosing. Perform regular audiology tests. Monitor serum creatinine and potassium regularly.
Capreomycin	Ototoxicity. Electrolyte imbalance (especially hypokalemia, hypomagnesemia) may be severe, and renal impairment is frequent.	Ensure correct dosing. Perform regular audiology tests. Monitor serum creatinine and potassium regularly.
Fluoroquinolones: levofloxacin, moxifloxacin, ofloxacin	Generally well tolerated. Gastrointestinal disturbance (rarely, pseudomembranous colitis). Headache, dizziness, restlessness, insomnia, drowsiness, depression, and rarely, hallucinations, seizures. QT prolongation (moxifloxacin > levofloxacin and ofloxacin). Hypersensitivity reactions including rashes, vasculitis, Stevens-Johnson syndrome, anaphylaxis. Raised liver enzymes, interstitial nephritis, blood dyscrasias, uveitis. Arthralgia and tendonitis (with increased risk of tendon rupture).	Monitor clinically. Advise patients of the risk of tendonitis, to avoid using the affected tendon if symptoms occur, and to report the symptoms as soon as possible. Use with caution in patients with risk factors for QT-prolongation (on other QT-prolonging agents, with electrolyte abnormalities, dysglycemia, cardiac abnormalities, hepatic failure).
Ethionamide, protionamide	Hepatitis, gastrointestinal disturbance (nausea and vomiting are common and may be severe), taste disturbance. Neurotoxicity (peripheral neuropathy responsive to pyridoxine, seizures, pellagra-like encephalopathy responsive to niacin, psychosis, anxiety, depression, optic neuritis). Endocrine effects include reversible hypothyroidism (increased risk with concomitant PAS), gynecomastia, hair loss, acne, impotence, menstrual irregularity.	Consider altering dose times to improve gastrointestinal tolerance. Monitor clinically and measure liver enzymes in children at increased risk of hepatitis. Monitor TSH and free T4 concentrations. Pyridoxine supplementation. Glycemic control may be affected in diabetics—monitor carefully.
Cycloserine, terizidone	Dose-related anxiety, depression, confusion, irritability, and psychosis are common. Headaches, vertigo, drowsiness, impaired speech, paresthesia, hyperreflexia, seizures, and coma may also occur. Dermatitis, photosensitivity, megaloblastic anemia, and heart failure have been reported.	Ensure correct dosing. Monitor clinically. Pyridoxine supplementation is recommended.

(continued)

Table 15.5. Continued

DRUG	SIDE EFFECTS	PREVENTION AND MONITORING
p-aminosalicylic acid (PAS)	Gastrointestinal intolerance (diarrhea, anorexia, bloating) Reversible hypothyroidism. Rarely, hepatotoxicity and coagulopathy.	Measure TSH and free T4 concentrations. Measure electrolytes if severe diarrhea.
Clofazimine	Pink or red discoloration of skin is almost universal. The conjunctiva, cornea, and body fluids may also be affected. Gastrointestinal intolerance is more frequent at higher doses. Photosensitivity, retinopathy, dry skin, pruritus, rash, ichthyosis are uncommon. Use of higher doses or concomitant QT-prolonging agents may be associated with QT-prolongation and *torsades de pointes*.	Monitor renal and hepatic function in patients with underlying kidney or liver impairment. Gastrointestinal symptoms may be reduced if drug taken with food.
Linezolid	Dose- and duration-dependent peripheral neuropathy, optic neuropathy, myelosuppression, lactic acidosis, and pancreatitis. Gastrointestinal disturbance (including diarrhea, nausea, vomiting, cramps, metallic taste), headache, fungal infections.	Monitor clinically for peripheral neuropathy and optic neuritis. Monitor full blood count regularly (weekly initially, then monthly). Avoid in patients taking serotonergic agents. Clinical monitoring and regular testing of full blood count and serum lactate. Consider pyridoxine supplementation. Consider dose reduction after initial induction period to prevent peripheral neuropathy and myelosuppression.

IPT = isoniazid preventive therapy; TSH = thyroid stimulating hormone; T4 = thyroxine.

varies by race and geographic region (Parkin 1997). NAT2 polymorphisms are the most important determinant of isoniazid exposures (with exposures 1.5- to 2.6-fold, and 1.9- to 4.6-fold, higher in children with a slow metabolizer genotype, compared to intermediate and rapid metabolizers, respectively [Zvada 2014, Kiser 2012, McIlleron 2009]) such that the range of exposures is very wide for any one dose across genotypes.

A minimum peak concentration of 3 mg/L is recommended for isoniazid (Alsultan 2014). While peak concentrations display enormous variability, the vast majority of children achieve a peak concentration greater than 3 mg/L when given doses in line with the currently recommended 7–15 mg/kg daily (Zvada 2014 abstr, Thee 2011, Kiser 2012). However, the proportion of children with a peak concentration under 3 mg/L may be greater when using currently available dispersible fixed-dose combinations (FDCs), possibly due to under dosing in some children or to formulation effects (Zvada 2014, Hiruy 2014, Zvada 2014 abstr). While the ratio of the peak concentration to the area under the concentration-time curve (AUC) is higher in children than in adults, both peak concentrations and AUC are considerably higher in children given 7–15 mg/kg doses than in adult populations receiving WHO-recommended doses in FDCs. Due to the effect of body size, lower body weight is associated with reduced plasma exposures for the same dose per kilogram; however, in infants this is counteracted by immature metabolic pathways (Zhu 2012, Zvada AAC 2014). The increase in clearance associated with increasing age is more pronounced in children with intermediate or rapid NAT2 genotypes (Zhu 2012). Notwithstanding, among low birthweight infants who underwent pharmacokinetic evaluation at an average of two weeks of age, infants with a slow NAT2 genotype had higher isoniazid exposures (Bekker 2014).

Isoniazid is generally well tolerated by children, but its safety alone and in combination therapy across age groups should be evaluated further in children, given the recently increased recommended dose. The vast majority of children who take isoniazid suffer no adverse effects. The most important side effects associated with isoniazid are peripheral neuropathy and hepatotoxicity. Concurrent rifampicin or certain other drugs and underlying liver disease increase the risk of hepatotoxicity. In children taking isoniazid alone, less than 0.1%, and under 1% of children on multidrug treatment regimens develop clinical evidence of hepatotoxicity, but 8% and 10%, respectively, have mildly elevated serum liver enzymes (Donald 2011). Patients with a slow acetylator genotype, HIV infection, or malnutrition are predisposed to develop peripheral neuropathy, which is caused by pyridoxine deficiency. Pyridoxine supplementation is used to prevent and to treat this dose-related toxicity. Relatively higher incidences of peripheral neuropathy (25%, grade 2 or higher) and alanine tranaminase (ALT) elevations (11%, elevations ≥5 times the upper limit of normal) have been reported among infants (3–24 months of age; 48% with HIV infection) on daily doses of 10–20 mg/kg isoniazid for treating tuberculosis infection (Kiser 2012).

Rifamycins

The rifamycins block transcription by binding to DNA-dependent RNA polymerase. The rifamycins have a relatively rapid onset of action allowing eradication of intermittently dividing or persistent mycobacteria, and a prolonged post-antibiotic effect (Mitchison 2008). The sterilizing activity of rifampicin underpins the contemporary six-month regimen for drug-susceptible tuberculosis. Recent studies suggest that patients with higher plasma concentrations of rifampicin have better bacteriological responses in sputum and improved long-term outcomes. Furthermore, they support a minimum target peak concentration of 8 mg/L, and suggest that rifampicin acts in synergy with pyrazinamide (Ramachandran 2013, Chigutsa 2015). Higher doses of rifampicin and rifapentine than those currently used are being evaluated for their potential to reduce the necessary duration of treatment.

Rifampicin or rifapentine, alone or in combination with isoniazid, provide shortened treatment regimens due to their improved sterilizing activity, but drug–drug interactions may limit their use in HIV-infected children. Rifapentine, which is highly protein-bound and has a much longer half-life (±15 hours) than rifampicin is currently licensed to treat tuberculosis infection in children over two years of age, in combination with isoniazid as a once-weekly regimen given for three months, but it is not licensed to treat tuberculosis disease in children under 12 years of age. There currently are no published pharmacokinetic data for rifapentine for children less than two years of age. Pediatric formulation development is underway.

The rifamycins interact with a wide range of concomitantly administered drugs, including key antiretrovirals (notably NNRTIs, PIs, and integrase inhibitors). This complicates the management of HIV-associated tuberculosis. Dose adjustments are necessary in some instances, and toxicity is a concern (Tables 15.1, 15.2,). In vitro evidence suggests that induction of mRNA by the rifamycins is dose-dependent (Williamson 2013), raising concern that the increased doses of rifampicin now recommended in children may lead to more extensive drug–drug interactions than previously recognized. The drug–drug interactions between rifampicin and rifapentine on one hand, and key antituberculosis drugs being evaluated in novel regimens on the other, including moxifloxacin, bedaquiline, delamanid, and pretonamid, limit their potential for inclusion in new combination regimens.

Rifabutin is a less potent enzyme inducer and an alternative rifamycin for patients needing protease inhibitor–based antiretroviral treatment. However, a safe and effective dose in combination with PIs has not been defined for children. A recent study evaluating the combination in young children was stopped due to the development of neutropenia (Moultrie 2014). Rifabutin may also have a role against drug-resistant strains of *M. tuberculosis*, with certain *rpoB* gene resistance mutations conferring rifampicin but not rifabutin resistance (Jamieson 2014). Rifabutin is available only in a 150 mg capsule, which is not suitable for young children.

Rifampicin concentrations are highly variable between and within individuals, even after adjustment for weight and sex, or lean body mass. Absorption of rifampicin varies considerably in rate and extent. Meals delay and modestly reduce absorption. Rifampicin undergoes intestinal and hepatic conversion to desacetyl rifampicin, its primary and active metabolite, by the microsomal enzyme arylacetamide deacetylase (AADAC) (Nakajima 2011). It is also a substrate of the efflux transporter P-glycoprotein and OATP 1B1 which mediates its entry into hepatocytes, and biliary excretion. Rifampicin undergoes autoinduction leading to a twofold increase in clearance, which is nearly complete after two weeks of daily doses. Genetic polymorphisms of *SLCO1B1* (the gene encoding OATP 1B1) have been associated with reduced rifampicin concentrations (Weiner 2010, Chigutsa 2011). Reduced concentrations have also been associated with low weight, low body mass index, male sex, diabetes, and HIV infection, which has been linked to substantially reduced rifampicin concentrations in some studies, but this has not been confirmed in children. Pharmacokinetic studies in children given the currently recommended 10–20 mg/kg daily (Zvada 2014 abst, Hiruy 2014, Zvada 2014) suggest that the median peak concentrations attained are similar to those in studies of adults with tuberculosis. Among infants, the exposure may increase disproportionately with the increase in dose (Thee 2011), as has been shown in adults (Chigutsa 2011). However, the optimal dose per kilogram of body weight appears to vary by age and weight; the AUC values are generally lower than those reported in adult patients; and peak concentrations in the majority of infants are below the 8 mg/L target.

Apart from gastrointestinal intolerance, rifampicin is generally well tolerated. Although it commonly causes mild transaminase elevations, overt hepatitis is rare, occurring more frequently in association with underlying hepatic disease or concomitant use of other drugs such as isoniazid and PIs. While the risk of mild to moderate transaminase elevations may increase with higher doses of rifampicin, the high doses currently being investigated in adults appear to be well tolerated in the short-term.

Pyrazinamide

Pyrazinamide is a prodrug that is converted by pyrazinamidase to pyrazinoic acid. Pyrazinoic acid requires an acid environment to diffuse passively into the mycobacterium where it causes acidification of the cell and membrane damage. It is excreted by an energy-dependent mycobacterial membrane pump; therefore, as bacterial metabolism decreases the intracellular concentration of pyrazoic acid increases. Hence it is uniquely active against nonreplicating bacilli, and also acts in synergy with other drugs inhibiting mycobacterial enzymes (Mitchison 2008). As part of a first-line regimen, higher doses augment sterilizing activity in synergy with rifampicin (Pasipanodya 2013, Chigutsa 2015). In conjunction with first-line drugs for drug-susceptible tuberculosis, it adds little activity after the first two months of treatment, probably because its activity is targeted to inflammatory lesions with a low pH, which resolve on an effective regimen. Pyrazinamide is also a key component of second-line regimens for drug-resistant tuberculosis (DR-TB), and is recommended for the duration of treatment (WHO 2011). Resistance to pyrazinamide (conferred by mutations in the *pncA* gene and also associated with pyrazinoic acid efflux pump efficiency), however, is common in MDR-TB strains (Louw 2008), and its role should be further evaluated in these settings. All strains of *Mycobacterium bovis* are resistant to pyrazinamide.

Pyrazinamide is reliably absorbed and widely distributed in the tissues. It is metabolized by multiple pathways, including xanthine oxidase, with only about 3% eliminated unchanged in the urine. Minor side effects of pyrazinamide are common. About 1% of adults experience hepatotoxicity on current doses less than 30 mg/kg, but higher doses have been associated with a substantially increased risk of hepatitis. Continued administration in spite of rising transaminase concentrations may lead to fulminant hepatitis. Pyrizinamide lowers the excretion of uric acid which can cause arthralgias and flares of gout; while children taking pyrazinamide have increased uric acid serum concentrations, symptoms are rare. Pyrazinamide also can cause mild to extreme pruritis which may necessitate discontinuation of the drug.

Ethambutol

Ethambutol inhibits cell wall synthesis. Its primary target is arabinosyl transferase, encoded by the *embA* and *embB* genes. Dose-related optic neuritis limits the use of bactericidal doses. At currently used doses (15–25 mg/kg in children), ethambutol is a relatively safe drug (WHO 2006) and prevents the emergence of resistance, but it does not contribute substantially to bactericidal activity. It is recommended during the two-month intensive phase for children with drug-susceptible tuberculosis, including severe forms of extrapulmonary disease such as osteoarticular tuberculosis, tuberculous meningitis, and for children living in high HIV-burden settings or where the prevalence of isoniazid resistance is high.

The rate and extent of ethambutol absorption are variable. Reduced absorption has been reported in HIV-infected adults (McIlleron 2006). It distributes well to many tissues, but penetration into cerebrospinal fluid is limited, and ethionamide is frequently used instead as the fourth drug for children with drug-susceptible tuberculous meningitis. Elimination is largely by excretion of unchanged drug in the urine, and the dosing interval should be lengthened in patients with moderate or severe renal impairment. Pharmacokinetic studies in children report lower exposures than those in adults for the same mg/kg doses (Zhu 2004, Graham 2006, Hiruy 2014). Ocular toxicity is the greatest concern; however, literature reviews report that ethambutol was stopped for possible ocular toxicity in only 0.05% of children receiving 15–30 mg/kg doses of ethambutol, compared to 1.9% for adults receiving 27.5 mg/kg/day, or less (WHO 2006, Ezer 2013). However, this side effect may be under-recognized as monitoring for the development of optic neuritis is difficult in young children. Vision should be monitored in older children using simple reading and color charts.

Injectable Agents

Aminoglycosides block ribosomal protein synthesis. They display dose-dependent killing of rapidly growing extracellular organisms and are also highly effective against slowly growing *in vitro* strains, but have reduced activity in acidic and intracellular environments. Together with the fluoroquinolones, they are the more potent drugs in standard regimens for MDR-TB (Falzon 2013). The requirement of parenteral administration, cumulative toxicity to the inner ear and nephron, and increasing resistance, limit the use of aminoglycosides. Daily intramuscular injections are painful, especially in wasted patients, and may contribute to poor clinic attendance as well as loss to follow-up. Administration can be given through an indwelling venous catheter but this modality is usually available only in the hospital, or outpatient setting in high resource environments. Hearing loss is reported in 15–20% of MDR-TB patients. Electrolyte imbalance and renal impairment can lead to serious complications and increase the need for patient monitoring. Amikacin or kanamycin is recommended as part of a 6–8-month intensive phase for MDR-TB treatment. Streptomycin is not recommended for MDR-TB due to high rates of resistance, as, until recently, it was commonly used along with other first-line agents in a retreatment regimen. Isolates developing resistance to streptomycin are usually susceptible to amikacin and kanamycin. Capreomycin is a cyclic polypeptide, but shares a similar mechanism of action, and side effects with the aminoglycosides. The renal complications are common (20–25%), can be severe, and they limit its use. There is little experience with capreomycin in children. The injectable agents should be used with caution in patients with renal disease, who should be carefully monitored. Dose-interval adjustments may be necessary.

Fluoroquinolones

Fluoroquinolones play a key role in the treatment of MDR-TB. Resistance to fluoroquinolones increases the risk of death, poor treatment outcomes, and relapse (Falzon 2013). In adults, ofloxacin has been widely replaced by moxifloxacin, a newer generation 8-methoxy fluoroquinolone, which, like gatifloxacin, has superior activity against *M. tuberculosis*. The fluoroquinolones target DNA gyrase and have exposure-related bactericidal activity best described by the ratio AUC/MIC. Higher doses of moxifloxacin have been proposed, especially for organisms with MICs ≥0.25 mg/L but still susceptible to ofloxacin by standard drug-susceptibility testing. However, dose-related toxicity (particularly QT-prolongation associated with the fatal arrhythmia *torsades de pointes*) is a concern, as there is little experience with prolonged use of the drug in high doses. High doses of levofloxacin (750–1000 mg daily) may be as effective for adults with MDR-TB as moxifloxacin 400 mg daily (Johnson 2006, Koh 2013). There is an urgent need for suitable regimens to prevent tuberculosis in contacts of MDR-TB cases, and a fluoroquinolone with good activity against *M. tuberculosis* is likely to be the key component of such regimens. Among a cohort of child contacts of MDR-TB cases, who were given ofloxacin together with ethambutol and isoniazid to prevent TB, the regimen was well tolerated, and few children developed disease (Seddon 2013). Recent observations suggest that moxifloxacin or levofloxacin, with or without ethambutol or ethionamide, provide excellent protection against the development of tuberculosis in adults and children who are contacts of cases with fluoroquinolone-susceptible MDR-TB (Bamrah 2014).

Regrettably, a lack of evidence to guide dosing, uncertainty about safety, and, most importantly, the absence of suitable formulations have limited the use of moxifloxacin and levofloxacin in children. The drugs are used off-label in children. The fluoroquinolones are generally absorbed well; however, they are chelated by di- and trivalent cations so they should not be given with food, medicines, or supplements containing, iron, magnesium, aluminum, calcium, or zinc. Moxifloxacin is a substrate of p-glycoprotein, and undergoes glucuronidation and sulphation in the liver. Ofloxacin and levofloxacin are eliminated largely in the urine. Recent reports suggest that the drugs are well tolerated by children as part of regimens to prevent or treat MDR-TB, but that higher doses than those currently recommended will be needed to match plasma drug exposures in adults (Thee 2014a, Thee 2014b, Watt 2012). The results of larger pharmacokinetic studies in children, and studies evaluating the effects of dose preparation (e.g., tablet crushing) on bioavailability, are eagerly awaited. Concerns about the musculoskeletal safety for fluoroquinolones arise from animal studies demonstrating dose- and duration-dependent cartilage injury in weight-bearing joints. Short-term use of fluoroquinolones in children seems to be relatively safe, and the limited evidence of longer term exposure is reassuring (Seddon 2013, Thee 2014a, Thee 2014b). However, safety should be carefully monitored, and pharmaco-epidemiological studies are warranted to document the risks of long-term use to prevent or treat TB in children.

Ethionamide and Protionamide (Also Called Prothionamide)

Ethionamide and protionamide (the propyl analogue of ethionamide) are thioamides that block mycolic acid synthesis and have weak bactericidal activity. The thioamides are more effective than cycloserine or p-aminosalicylic acid (PAS) against susceptible isolates. Resistance to ethionamide

is associated with *inhA* mutations which confer low-level isoniazid resistance. These patients may benefit from high doses of isoniazid instead of ethionamide. Ethionamide is widely used for the treatment of tuberculous meningitis in children in place of ethambutol, due to its superior penetration into the CSF. A recent study in children found that while there was wide variability in the pharmacokinetics of ethionamide, a 15–20 mg/kg dose resulted in systemic concentrations in the majority of older children similar to concentrations in adults on standard doses, but that younger children had lower exposures than older children for the same dose per kilogram of body weight (Thee 2011). A major limitation of the thioamides is their propensity to cause gastrointestinal side effects, particularly nausea and vomiting, although children appear to tolerate the drugs better than adults. Reversible thyroid function abnormalities are common in children treated with ethionamide, more so if they are treated with PAS concomitantly, or have HIV infection.

Cycloserine

Cycloserine and its analogue terizidone are broad-spectrum antibiotics with modest activity against *M. tuberculosis*. They inhibit cell wall synthesis and are bacteriostatic. Absorption of cycloserine is modestly decreased by food. The drug distributes well to most tissues, including the CSF. About 65% of the drug is excreted by kidneys unchanged. Dose-interval adjustments may be necessary in renal impairment. Dose-related CNS toxicity limits the use of cycloserine and terizidone. Inability to concentrate and lethargy are common. More serious side effects, including seizure, depression, psychosis, and suicidal ideation, usually occur with peak concentrations more than 35 mg/L, but also occur with lower drug exposures. Cycloserine is also implicated—among other antituberculosis drugs, antiretrovirals, alcohol use, HIV infection, diabetes, and nutritional deficiency—in the high incidence of peripheral neuropathy in MDR-TB patients (Conradie 2013), and pyridoxine should be given to children taking cycloserine.

Para-aminosalicylate (PAS)

PAS, a structural analogue of para-aminobenzoic acid, is a folate antagonist with bacteriostatic activity against *M. tuberculosis*. When PAS was used historically in combination with streptomycin and isoniazid, it could provide effective treatment, and it appears to reduce the incidence of drug resistance. A bulky dose is required. Absorption is variable, and increased doses may be required to achieve therapeutic concentrations. The granules should be kept in a refrigerator and taken with an acidic food (e.g., apple sauce or yoghurt) or beverage (e.g., orange, tomato, or apple juice). A sachet of the powder (PAS-sodium) is dissolved in 100 mL of boiled water and should be taken after a meal to reduce gastric irritation. The currently used PASER granules are aminosalicylic acid and best absorbed after a fat meal. Gastrointestinal intolerance (abdominal pain, vomiting, nausea, bloating, diarrhea, and soft stools) is common, although the symptoms improve over time and the delayed-release enteric coated granules are better tolerated. Skin hypersensitivity reactions, and adverse reactions relating to the nervous system (giddiness, vestibular syndrome) are frequent. Reversible hypothyroidism is common in children treated with PAS, especially if ethionamide is also being taken.

Clofazimine

Clofazamine is a riminophenazine with antimycobacterial activity and anti-inflammatory properties. It is licensed to treat leprosy. There is renewed interest in its role against drug-resistant tuberculosis following in vitro evidence of potent activity against hypoxic, nonreplicating M. tuberculosis, promising sterilizing activity in combination with other drugs in mice, and excellent results in observational studies of patients (Grosset 2013, Van Deun 2010, Gopal 2013). Absorption is slow and variable, and tissue distribution is high with a terminal half-life of 70 days. Tissue accumulation leads to red-black skin discoloration in almost all patients after prolonged use, and gastrointestinal side effects are common. Clofazimine should be used with caution in patients receiving other QT-interval-prolonging agents, with cardiac abnormalities, at risk of electrolyte imbalances, or with doses higher than 100 mg/day, due to the risk of torsades de pointes. It is currently used in the treatment of patients with extensive drug resistance.

Linezolid

Linezolid is an oxazolidinone antibiotic that is used off-label for tuberculosis. It inhibits protein synthesis by binding to 23S ribosomal RNA. Linezolid has bactericidal activity in vitro, and displays good efficacy as part of a regimen for MDR-TB with fluoroquinolone and/or injectable resistance. A recent meta-analysis confirmed that linezolid outperformed other group 5 agents in improving the possibility of a favorable treatment outcome in patients with pre-XDR and XDR-TB (Chang 2013). Its long-term use is limited by dose-related mitochondrial toxicity, which results in discontinuation of the drug in about a third of patients. Anemia, thrombocytopenia, peripheral neuropathy, and optic neuritis are common, while lactic acidosis and pancreatitis also occur, especially at doses higher than 600 mg per day. While the optimal dose for efficacy is not defined, reduced doses are better tolerated. Adults receiving 300 mg twice or even once daily (after an induction period at higher doses) have shown improved outcomes compared to patients not on linezolid. It has been used with success in children, although experience is limited, and careful monitoring for toxicity is necessary (Garcia-Prats 2014).

Other Group 5 Agents

Linezolid and clofazamine aside, the remaining group 5 agents should only be used in the therapeutically destitute. There is limited information about the efficacy of the beta-lactams against tuberculosis. They interfere with cell wall synthesis by binding to transpeptidases, which catalyze peptidoglycan cross-linking. Clavulanate ameliorates the effect of mycobacterial beta-lactamase. They may contribute bactericidal activity against rapidly dividing organisms, but nonreplicating organisms utilize alternative peptidoglycan cross-linking mechanisms conferring resistance to penicillins. Amoxicillin/clavulanate is widely used in children for other indications in whom diarrhea, gastrointestinal discomfort, and rashes are common side effects, and anaphylactic reactions occur in 0.01% of patients. Carbapenems appear to be active against such nonreplicating organisms, but their use is experimental, and intravenous administration is not feasible in most settings. Clarithromycin inhibits protein synthesis by binding to the 50S ribosomal subunit. Although it is active against nontuberculous mycobacteria, M. tuberculosis has intrinsic inducible resistance to clarithromycin, and its activity in a regimen for the treatment of tuberculosis is not clear, although it is attributed with anti-inflammatory properties. As a potent inhibitor of CYP 3A enzymes, it has wide potential for drug–drug interactions.

REFERENCES

1. Mitchison DA, Davies GR. Assessment of the efficacy of new anti-tuberculosis drugs. *Open Infect Dis J*. 2008 Dec;2:59–76.
2. WHO. *Guidance for National Tuberculosis Programmes on the Management of Tuberculosis in Children*. 2nd ed. Geneva: World Health Organization; 2014. WHO/HTM/TB/2014.03. Available at http://www.who.int/tb/publications/childtb_guidelines/en/; last accessed 6 Jan 2015.
3. Sneag DB, Schaaf HS, Cotton MF, Zar HJ. Failure of chemoprophylaxis with standard antituberculosis agents in child contacts of multidrug-resistant tuberculosis cases. *Pediatr Infect Dis J*. 2007 Dec;26(12):1142–1146.
4. Duke T, Fuller D. Randomised controlled trials in child health in developing countries: trends and lessons over 11 years. *Arch Dis Child*. 2014 Jul;99(7):615–620. Epub 2014 Mar 10. PubMed PMID: 24615625.
5. Burman WJ, Cotton MF, Gibb DM, et al. Ensuring the involvement of children in the evaluation of new tuberculosis treatment regimens. *PLoS Med*. 2008;5(8): e176. doi:10.1371/journal.pmed.0050176
6. Holford N, Heo YA, Anderson B. A pharmacokinetic standard for babies and adults. *J Pharm Sci*. 2013 Sep;102(9):2941–2952.
7. Zvada S, Prins M, Mulligan C, et al. *Pharmacokinetics of Rifampicin, Isoniazid and Pyrazinamide in Children on 2010 WHO/IUATLD Guideline Doses*. 7th International Workshop on Clinical Pharmacology of TB Drugs, 5 Sept. 2014, Washington, DC.
8. Ramachandran G, Hemanth Kumar AK, Bhavani PK, et al. Age, nutritional status and INH acetylator status affect pharmacokinetics of anti-tuberculosis drugs in children. *Int J Tuberc Lung Dis*. 2013 Jun;17(6):800–806.
9. Thee S, Garcia-Prats AJ, McIlleron HM, et al. Pharmacokinetics of ofloxacin and levofloxacin for prevention and treatment of multidrug-resistant tuberculosis in children. *Antimicrob Agents Chemother*. 2014;58(5):2948–2951.
10. Thee S, Garcia-Prats AJ, Draper HR, et al. Pharmacokinetics and safety of moxifloxacin in children with multidrug-resistant tuberculosis. *Clin Infect Dis*. 2014 Oct 30. pii: ciu868. [Epub ahead of print] PubMed PMID: 25362206.
11. Thwaites GE, van Toorn R, Schoeman J. Tuberculous meningitis: more questions, still too few answers. *Lancet Neurol*. 2013 Oct;12(10):999–1010.
12. Ruslami R, Ganiem AR, Dian S, et al. Intensified regimen containing rifampicin and moxifloxacin for tuberculous meningitis: an open-label, randomised controlled phase 2 trial. *Lancet Infect Dis*. 2013 Jan;13(1):27–35.
13. Weiner M, Savic RM, Mac Kenzie WR, et al., for the Tuberculosis Trials Consortium PREVENT TB Pharmacokinetic Group. Rifapentine pharmacokinetics and tolerability in children and adults treated once weekly with rifapentine and isoniazid for latent tuberculosis infection. *Pediatr Infect Dis*. 2014;3(2):132–145.
14. Pouplin T, Phuong PN, Toi PV, Nguyen Pouplin J, Farrar J. Isoniazid, pyrazinamide and rifampicin content variation in split fixed-dose combination tablets. *PLoS One*. 2014 Jul 8;9(7):e102047. doi: 10.1371/journal.pone.0102047
15. World Health Organization. *Consolidated Guidelines on the Use of Antiretroviral Drugs for Treating and Preventing HIV Infection. Recommendations for a Public Health Approach*. Geneva: World Health Organization; 2013.
16. McIlleron H, Wash P, Burger A, Norman J, Folb PI, Smith P. Determinants of rifampin, isoniazid, pyrazinamide, and ethambutol pharmacokinetics in a cohort of tuberculosis patients. *Antimicrob Agents Chemother*. 2006;50(4):1170–1177.
17. Jeremiah K, Denti P, Chigutsa E, et al. Nutritional supplementation increases rifampin exposure among tuberculosis patients coinfected with HIV. *Antimicrob Agents Chemother*. 2014;58(6):3468–3474.
18. Zhang C, Denti P, Decloedt EH, Ren Y, Karlsson MO, McIlleron H. Model-based evaluation of the pharmacokinetic differences between adults and children for lopinavir and ritonavir in combination with rifampicin. *Br J Clin Pharmacol*. 2013;76(5):741–751.
19. Almeida D, Nuermberger E, Tasneen R, et al. Paradoxical effect of isoniazid on the activity of rifampin-pyrazinamide combination in a mouse model of tuberculosis. *Antimicrob Agents Chemother*. 2009 Oct;53(10):4178–4184.
20. Chigutsa E, Pasipanodya JG, Visser ME, et al. The impact of non-linear interactions of pharmacokinetics and MICs on sputum bacillary kill rates as a marker of sterilizing effect in tuberculosis. *Antimicrob Agents Chemother*. 2015;1:38–45.
21. Parkin DP, Vandenplas S, Botha FJ, et al. Trimodality of isoniazid elimination: phenotype and genotype in patients with tuberculosis.

Am J Respir Crit Care Med. 1997 May;155(5):1717–1722.

22. Zvada SP, Denti P, Donald PR, et al. Population pharmacokinetics of rifampicin, pyrazinamide and isoniazid in children with tuberculosis: *in silico* evaluation of currently recommended doses. *J Antimicrob Chemother.* 2014;69(5):1339–1349.

23. Kiser JJ, Zhu R, D'Argenio DZ, et al. Isoniazid pharmacokinetics, pharmacodynamics, and dosing in South African infants. *Ther Drug Monit.* 2012 Aug;34(4):446–451.

24. McIlleron H, Willemse M, Werely CJ, et al. Isoniazid plasma concentrations in a cohort of South African children with tuberculosis: implications for international pediatric dosing guidelines. *Clin Infect Dis.* 2009;48(11):1547–1553.

25. Alsultan A, Peloquin CA. Therapeutic drug monitoring in the treatment of tuberculosis: an update. *Drugs.* 2014 Jun;74(8):839–854.

26. Thee S, Seddon JA, Donald PR, et al. Pharmacokinetics of isoniazid, rifampin, and pyrazinamide in children younger than two years of age with tuberculosis: evidence for implementation of revised World Health Organization recommendations. *Antimicrob Agents Chemother.* 2011 Dec;55(12):5560–5567.

27. Hiruy H, Rogers Z, Mbowane C, et al. Subtherapeutic concentrations of first-line anti-TB drugs in South African children treated according to current guidelines: the PHATISA study. *J Antimicrob Chemother.* 2015; 760:1115–1123.

28. Zhu R, Kiser JJ, Seifart HI, et al. The pharmacogenetics of NAT2 enzyme maturation in perinatally HIV exposed infants receiving isoniazid. *J Clin Pharmacol.* 2012 Apr;52(4):511–519.

29. Bekker A, Schaaf HS, Seifart HI, et al. Pharmacokinetics of isoniazid in low-birth-weight and premature infants. *Antimicrob Agents Chemother.* 2014;58(4):2229–2234.

30. Donald PR. Antituberculosis drug-induced hepatotoxicity in children. *Pediatr Rep.* 2011 Jun 16;3(2):e16. doi: 10.4081/pr.2011.e16

31. Williamson B, Dooley KE, Zhang Y, Back DJ, Owen A. Induction of influx and efflux transporters and cytochrome P450 3A4 in primary human hepatocytes by rifampin, rifabutin, and rifapentine. *Antimicrob Agents Chemother.* 2013;57(12):6366–6369.

32. Moultrie H, McIlleron H, Sawry S, et al. Pharmacokinetics and safety of rifabutin in young HIV-infected children receiving rifabutin and lopinavir/ritonavir. *J Antimicrob Chemother.* 2015; 70:543–549.

33. Jamieson FB, Guthrie JL, Neemuchwala A, Lastovetska O, Melano RG, Mehaffy C. Profiling of *rpoB* mutations and MICs for rifampin and rifabutin in *Mycobacterium tuberculosis. J Clin Microbiol.* 2014 Jun;52(6):2157–2162.

34. Nakajima A, Fukami T, Kobayashi Y, Watanabe A, Nakajima M, Yokoi T. Human arylacetamide deacetylase is responsible for deacetylation of rifamycins: rifampicin, rifabutin, and rifapentine. *Biochem Pharmacol.* 2011 Dec 1;82(11):1747–1756.

35. Weiner M, Peloquin C, Burman W, et al. Effects of tuberculosis, race, and human gene *SLCO1B1* polymorphisms on rifampin concentrations. *Antimicrob Agents Chemother.* 2010 Oct;54(10):4192–4200.

36. Chigutsa E, Visser ME, Swart EC, et al. The *SLCO1B1* rs4149032 polymorphism is highly prevalent in South Africans and is associated with reduced rifampin concentrations: dosing implications. *Antimicrob Agents Chemother.* 2011 Sep;55(9):4122–4127.

37. Pasipanodya JG, McIlleron H, Burger A, Wash PA, Smith P, Gumbo T. Serum drug concentrations predictive of pulmonary tuberculosis outcomes. *J Infect Dis.* 2013;208(9):1464–1473.

38. Louw GE, Warren RM, Donald PR, et al. Frequency and implications of pyrazinamide resistance in managing previously treated tuberculosis patients. *Int J Tuberc Lung Dis.* 2006 Jul;10(7):802–807.

39. World Health Organization. *Ethambutol Efficacy and Toxicity: Literature Review and Recommendations for Daily and Intermittent Dosage in Children.* Geneva: World Health Organization; 2006 (WHO/HTM/TB/2006.365).

40. Zhu M, Burman WJ, Starke JR, et al. Pharmacokinetics of ethambutol in children and adults with tuberculosis. *Int J Tuberc Lung Dis.* 2004 Nov;8(11):1360–1367.

41. Graham SM, Bell DJ, Nyirongo S, Hartkoorn R, Ward SA, Molyneux EM. Low levels of pyrazinamide and ethambutol in children with tuberculosis and impact of age, nutritional status, and human immunodeficiency virus infection. *Antimicrob Agents Chemother.* 2006 Feb;50(2):407–413.

42. Ezer N, Benedetti A, Darvish-Zargar M, Menzies D. Incidence of ethambutol-related visual impairment during treatment of active tuberculosis. *Int J Tuberc Lung Dis.* 2013 Apr;17(4):447–455.

43. Falzon D, Gandhi N, Migliori GB, et al.; Collaborative Group for Meta-Analysis of

Individual Patient Data in MDR-TB. Resistance to fluoroquinolones and second-line injectable drugs: impact on multidrug-resistant TB outcomes. *Eur Respir J.* 2013 Jul;42(1):156–168. doi: 10.1183/09031936.00134712. Epub 2012 Oct 25. PubMed PMID: 23100499.

44. Johnson JL, Hadad DJ, Boom WH, et al. Early and extended early bactericidal activity of levofloxacin, gatifloxacin and moxifloxacin in pulmonary tuberculosis. *Int J Tuberc Lung Dis.* 2006 Jun;10(6):605–612.

45. Koh WJ, Lee SH, Kang YA, et al. Comparison of levofloxacin versus moxifloxacin for multidrug-resistant tuberculosis. *Am J Respir Crit Care Med.* 2013 Oct 1;188(7):858–864.

46. Seddon JA, Hesseling AC, Finlayson H, et al. Preventive therapy for child contacts of multidrug-resistant tuberculosis: a prospective cohort study. *Clin Infect Dis.* 2013 Dec;57(12):1676–1684.

47. Bamrah S, Brostrom R, Dorina F, et al. Treatment for LTBI in contacts of MDR-TB patients, Federated States of Micronesia, 2009–2012. *Int J Tuberc Lung Dis.* 2014 Aug;18(8):912–918.

48. Watt KM, Massaro MM, Smith B, Cohen-Wolkowiez M, Benjamin DK Jr, Laughon MM. Pharmacokinetics of moxifloxacin in an infant with *Mycoplasma hominis* meningitis. *Pediatr Infect Dis J.* 2012 Feb;31(2):197–199.

49. Thee S, Seifart HI, Rosenkranz B, et al. Pharmacokinetics of ethionamide in children. *Antimicrob Agents Chemother.* 2011 Oct;55(10):4594–4600.

50. Thee S, Zöllner EW, Willemse M, Hesseling AC, Magdorf K, Schaaf HS. Abnormal thyroid function tests in children on ethionamide treatment. *Int J Tuberc Lung Dis.* 2011 Sep;15(9):1191–1193.

51. Conradie F, Mabiletsa T, Sefoka M, et al. Prevalence and incidence of symmetrical symptomatic peripheral neuropathy in patients with multidrug-resistant TB. *S Afr Med J.* 2013 Oct 11;104(1):24–26.

52. Grosset JH, Tyagi S, Almeida DV, et al. Assessment of clofazimine activity in a second-line regimen for tuberculosis in mice. *Am J Respir Crit Care Med.* 2013 Sep 1;188(5):608–612.

53. Van Deun A, Maug AK, Salim MA, et al. Short, highly effective, and inexpensive standardized treatment of multidrug-resistant tuberculosis. *Am J Respir Crit Care Med.* 2010 Sep 1;182(5):684–692. doi: 10.1164/rccm.201001-0077OC. Epub 2010 May 4. PubMed PMID: 20442432.

54. Gopal M, Padayatchi N, Metcalfe JZ, O'Donnell MR. Systematic review of clofazimine for the treatment of drug-resistant tuberculosis. *Int J Tuberc Lung Dis.* 2013 Aug;17(8):1001–1007.

55. Chang KC, Yew WW, Tam CM, Leung CC. WHO group 5 drugs and difficult multidrug-resistant tuberculosis: a systematic review with cohort analysis and meta-analysis. *Antimicrob Agents Chemother.* 2013 Sep;57(9):4097–4104.

56. Lee M, Lee J, Carroll MW, et al. Linezolid for treatment of chronic extensively drug-resistant tuberculosis. *N Engl J Med.* 2012 Oct 18;367(16):1508–1518. doi: 10.1056/NEJMoa1201964. PubMed PMID: 23075177; PubMed Central PMCID: PMC3814175.

57. Tang S, Yao L, Hao X, et al. Efficacy, safety and tolerability of linezolid for the treatment of XDR-TB: a study in China. *Eur Respir J.* 2015 Jan;45(1):161–170. doi: 10.1183/09031936.00035114. Epub 2014 Sep 18. PubMed PMID: 25234807.

58. Garcia-Prats AJ, Rose PC, Hesseling AC, Schaaf HS. Linezolid for the treatment of drug-resistant tuberculosis in children: a review and recommendations. *Tuberculosis (Edinb).* 2014 Mar;94(2):93–104.

59. Nau R, Sörgel F, Eiffert H. Penetration of drugs through the blood-cerebrospinal fluid/blood-brain barrier for treatment of central nervous system infections. *Clin Microbiol Rev.* 2010 Oct;23(4):858–883.

60. Chigutsa E, Meredith S, Wiesner L, et al. Population pharmacokinetics and pharmacodynamics of ofloxacin in South African patients with multidrug-resistant tuberculosis. *Antimicrob Agents Chemother.* 2012;56(7):3857–3863.

61. McIlleron HM, Schomaker M, Ren Y, et al. Effects of rifampin-based antituberculosis therapy on plasma efavirenz concentrations in children vary by *CYP2B6* genotype. *AIDS.* 2013;27(12):1933–1940

62. Bertrand J, Verstuyft C, Chou M, et al.; CAMELIA (ANRS 1295-CIPRA KH001) Study Group. Dependence of efavirenz-and rifampicin-isoniazid-based antituberculosis treatment drug–drug interaction on *CYP2B6* and *NAT2* genetic polymorphisms: ANRS 12154 Study in Cambodia. *J Infect Dis.* 2014 Feb 1;209(3):399–408.

63. Oudijk JM, McIlleron H, Mulenga V, et al. Pharmacokinetics of nevirapine in HIV-infected children under 3 years on rifampicin-based antituberculosis treatment. *AIDS.* 2012;26(12):1523–1528.

16

TREATMENT OF TUBERCULOSIS INFECTION IN CHILDREN

Amina Ahmed

HIGHLIGHTS OF THIS CHAPTER

- Isoniazid given daily for six to nine months (180–270 doses) is very effective in preventing tuberculosis disease in children, but completion rates are often below 50%.
- Isoniazid is effective when given twice weekly for nine months (78 doses) under directly observed therapy.
- Rifampin given daily for four months (120 doses) has higher completion rates than six to nine months of isoniazid; its efficacy is not well studied but has been high in the few published studies.
- Isoniazid and rifampin given together for three to four months (90–120 doses) is used widely in Europe and is very effective in children, with few adverse effects and high completion rates.
- The newest regimen is 12 once-weekly doses (12 doses) of isoniazid and rifapentine, a rifamycin with a long half-life. This regimen is safe in children and at least as effective as isoniazid taken daily for nine months (270 doses).
- A fluoroquinolone-based regimen should be used for children infected with an MDR strain of *M. tuberculosis*.

TUBERCULOSIS INFECTION is defined as the presence of *M. tuberculosis* in the absence of clinical or radiological evidence of tuberculosis disease. It is estimated that one-third of the global population, or 2 billion people, are infected with *M. tuberculosis*.[1] The lifetime risk of progression from infection to active and potentially infectious disease in otherwise healthy adults is 5–10%.[2] In children, the risk of progression to disease is substantially higher: 40% in infants under 12 months of age, 25% in children one to two years of age, and 10–15% in older children and adolescents.[3]

In developing countries with high tuberculosis incidence rates, elimination efforts are focused on the identification and treatment of persons with current disease. Active contact-tracing or screening of persons at high risk for tuberculosis infection or progression to disease are not priorities, given resource constraints. In industrialized nations with a low incidence of tuberculosis, priorities include both the treatment and the prevention of disease. For these countries, the identification and treatment of infected persons at highest risk for developing disease are essential components of national and local tuberculosis programs.

In the United States, the American Thoracic Society (ATS) and the Centers for Disease Control and Prevention (CDC) recommend a strategy of targeted testing of groups at high risk for tuberculosis infection and treatment of those who would most benefit from treatment. Children—especially those younger than age five years—who have been infected recently are at highest risk of rapid progression to disease, have more life-years to develop disease, and are most likely to benefit from treatment of infection, especially as antituberculosis drugs are well tolerated by these children. The United Kingdom and Canada follow a similar practice of targeted testing and treatment (Table 16.1). The World Health Organization (WHO) endorses these guidelines for high-income and upper-middle-income countries, but for resource-limited and other middle-income countries, treatment of tuberculosis infection is recommended only for persons living with HIV and for children younger than five years of age who either have tuberculosis infection documented by a test of infection or are recent close contacts of persons with infectious tuberculosis and have presumed infection.[7,8]

The concept of using a single drug to prevent tuberculosis disease began with Dr. Edith Lincoln, a pediatrician whose efforts to prevent progression of infection to tuberculous meningitis in young children at Bellevue Hospital in New York City led to the consideration of using isoniazid (INH) treatment for children recently exposed to infectious persons with tuberculosis:

> If these observations are substantiated, it may radically change the present indications for specific therapy in primary tuberculosis. The use of isoniazid will have to be considered for every child with active primary tuberculosis and probably also for children with known recent conversion of tuberculin tests even if chest roentgenograms are normal.[9]

The use of 6–12 months of daily INH treatment of tuberculosis infection in low-burden countries has contributed to significant declines in the incidence of tuberculosis disease. More recently, shorter regimens, including those with combinations of drugs, have been evaluated to overcome the low treatment-completion rates and perceived risk of toxicity associated with use of INH. In this chapter, regimens used for the treatment of tuberculosis infection studied since Dr. Lincoln's initial observations will be reviewed, with a focus on effectiveness and safety. Although the majority of data supporting the treatment of tuberculosis infection in children are derived from adult studies, evidence from pediatric trials will be highlighted to support the extrapolation of findings from adult studies to children. Challenges associated with treatment, such as adverse effects and adherence, will be discussed to provide guidance for choosing a regimen for the treatment of tuberculosis infection in children.

TREATMENT REGIMENS

Treatment of tuberculosis infection with INH was first formally recommended in the United States in 1965 for persons with previously untreated tuberculosis infection or recent tuberculin skin test (TST) conversion.[10] The recommendations were expanded in 1967 to include all children with a positive TST. INH monotherapy has been the mainstay of treatment for tuberculosis infection in the United States for over 40 years. However, treatment completion rates for six to nine months of INH taken daily are low, often below 50%, reducing the actual benefit of the regimen.[11] Shorter regimens that have been evaluated include three to four months of daily rifampin (RMP) monotherapy, three months of INH and RMP, and three months of once-weekly INH and rifapentine (RPT). These regimens have demonstrated equivalent efficacy and safety to standard treatment with INH, offering further options for the treatment of tuberculosis infection in children (Table 16.2).

Isoniazid

EFFICACY

Isoniazid (INH) monotherapy is the best-studied regimen for the treatment of tuberculosis infection. More than 20 randomized clinical trials were

Table 16.1. International guidelines for the treatment of tuberculosis infection in HIV-uninfected and HIV-infected infants, children and adolescents

SOURCE	AT-RISK PEDIATRIC POPULATION FOR WHOM TREATMENT IS RECOMMENDED	TREATMENT OPTIONS
Canadian Thoracic Society, Canada[4]	Infants, children, and adolescents with tuberculosis infection identified by targeted tuberculin testing and/or IGRA	*Standard regimen:* INH for 9 months *Alternative regimens:* INH for 6 months INH and RMP for 3–4 months INH and RPT for 3 months *HIV-infected:* INH for 9 months
National Institute for Health and Clinical Excellence, United Kingdom[5]	Infants, children, and adolescents with tuberculosis infection identified by tuberculin testing and, if indicated, IGRA	*Standard regimens:* INH and RMP for 3 months INH for 6 months *HIV-infected:* INH for 6 months
American Thoracic Society/Centers for Disease Control and Prevention, United States[6]	Infants, children and adolescents with tuberculosis infection identified by targeted tuberculin testing or IGRA	*Standard regimen:* INH for 9 months *Alternative regimen:* RMP for 6 months *HIV-infected:* INH for 9 months
World Health Organization: Resource-limited and middle-income countries[7]	Children <5 years of age who are contacts of persons with tuberculosis in whom tuberculosis disease has been excluded Children infected with HIV who are contacts of persons with tuberculosis, irrespective of age, in whom tuberculosis disease has been excluded	*Contacts:* INH for 6 months *HIV-infected:* INH for 6 months
World Health Organization: High-income or upper-middle-income countries[8]	Infants, children, and adolescents with tuberculosis infection identified by targeted tuberculin testing or IGRA	*Equivalent regimens:* INH for 6 months INH for 9 months INH and RPT for 3 months *Alternative regimens:* INH and RMP for 3 or 4 months RMP for 3 or 4 months

IGRA = interferon gamma release assay; INH = isoniazid; RMP = rifampin; RPT = rifapentine

Table 16.2. Recommended treatment regimens for tuberculosis infection in infants, children, and adolescents

REGIMEN	DRUG FORM(S)	DURATION	DOSAGE	INTERVAL	MINIMUM DOSES
Isoniazid (INH)	Tablets: 100 mg 300 mg Syrup: 10 mg/mL	9 months	10–20 mg/kg[a] Maximum dose: 300 mg	Daily	270
			20–40 mg/kg Maximum dose: 900 mg	Twice per week[b]	76
		6 months	10–15 mg/kg Maximum dose: 300 mg	Daily	180
			20–30 mg/kg Maximum dose: 900 mg	Twice per week	52
Rifampin (RMP)	Capsules: 150 mg 300 mg Syrup: Formulated	4 months[c]	10–20 mg/kg Maximum dose: 600 mg	Daily	120
INH and RMP	As above	3 or 4 months	INH: 10–15 mg/kg Maximum dose: 300 mg RMP: 10–20 mg/kg Maximum dose: 600 mg	Daily	90–120
INH and rifapentine[d] (RPT)	RPT tablets: 150 mg	3 months	INH: 15 mg/kg rounded to the nearest 50 mg or 100 mg Maximum dose: 900 mg RPT: 10.0–14.0 kg: 300 mg 14.1–25.0 kg: 450 mg 25.1–32.0kg: 600 mg 32.1–49.9 kg: 750 mg > 50 kg: 900 mg Maximum: 900 mg	Once per week	12

[a]The American Academy of Pediatrics recommends an INH dosage of 10–15 mg/kg for the daily regimen and 20–30 for the twice-weekly regimen.

[b]It is recommended that treatment with INH twice per week be administered by direct observation.

[c]The American Academy of Pediatrics currently recommends four months of RMP for the treatment of tuberculosis infection in infants, children, and adolescents when INH cannot be tolerated or if the child has had contact with a patient infected with an INH-resistant but RMP-susceptible organism.

[d]Recommended for children >2 years of age, administered as directly observed therapy.

conducted in the 1950s and 1960s by the United States Public Health Service (USPHS) and others in industrialized and developing countries. These studies compared 12 months of daily INH with placebo in more than 100,000 persons at risk for tuberculosis. Participants included children with primary tuberculosis, residents in psychiatric institutions, household contacts of previously diagnosed and newly diagnosed cases, residents of all ages in Alaskan communities, and patients with asymptomatic tuberculous lesions on chest radiographs. The efficacy of 12 months of INH, as measured by a decrease in incidence of tuberculosis among those treated, ranged from 25–92%.[6] Among those adherent with treatment regimens, the protective efficacy was approximately 90%.

In the only trial comparing durations of INH therapy, the International Union Against Tuberculosis (IUAT) found 3-, 6-, and 12-month regimens to be 21%, 65%, and 75% effective, respectively, for preventing tuberculosis among adult patients.[12] Among those who completed therapy, efficacy was significantly higher, at 30%, 69%, and 93%, respectively. Despite the superior efficacy of longer treatment, a cost-effectiveness analysis published in 1986 led to widespread adoption of the six-month daily INH regimen for the treatment of tuberculosis infection in the United States and most of the world.[13,14] A secondary analysis of randomized clinical trials later indicated maximal efficacy occurred with durations of daily INH of 9–12 months, with a plateau in efficacy between nine and ten months of therapy[15] (Figure 16.1). Although the nine-month duration was not studied directly until recently, the duration of INH treatment for adults in the United States has been nine months for many years.[6] The duration of INH treatment recommended by national organizations in some other countries is six to nine months (Table 16.1).

Data from randomized clinical trials evaluating INH for the treatment of tuberculosis infection in children are limited. Among children included in the early USPHS trials, INH therapy for tuberculosis infection appeared to be more effective than in adults, with several studies demonstrating a risk reduction for tuberculosis disease of 70–90%.[16,17] Hsu's observational studies of 1,882 children treated in Houston, Texas, with 12 months of INH demonstrated 99% protective efficacy in the setting of good adherence, with 75% completing the prescribed course, and 25% completing nine months.[18] Based on these observations, the regimen of choice recommended by the American Academy of Pediatrics (AAP) for the treatment of tuberculosis infection in children in the United States is nine months of daily INH.[19]

In resource-constrained areas, tuberculosis infection is usually only identified in the context of contact investigation following exposure of persons

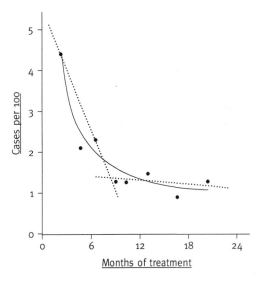

FIGURE 16.1   Tuberculosis case rates (%) in the Bethel Isoniazid Studies population, according to the number of months isoniazid was taken in the combined programs. Dots represent observed values; thin line, the calculated curve ($y = a + b/x$); and dotted lines, the calculated values based on the first four and last five observations ($y = a + bx$).

Reprinted by permission of the International Union against Tuberculosis and Lung Disease (*Int J Tuberc Lung Dis.* 1999;3:847–850).

to a case of contagious tuberculosis, and treatment is recommended only for those at highest risk for progression to disease. In these settings, the WHO recommends treatment only for children under five years of age who have either been identified as having tuberculosis infection or who have been exposed to a case of contagious tuberculosis and have presumed tuberculosis infection based on the absence of evidence of disease. The duration of treatment with INH recommended by the WHO for children is six months; the duration of treatment recommended by other international programs ranges from six to nine months, depending on the population being treated (Table 16.1).

EFFICACY IN HUMAN IMMUNODEFICIENCY VIRUS (HIV)-INFECTED PERSONS

The effectiveness of treating tuberculosis infection with 6–12 months of INH among HIV-infected persons has been demonstrated in multiple randomized clinical trials. Based on a recent Cochrane review of eight trials with 4,136 subjects, INH administered daily for six to nine months was 64% effective among

TST-positive persons living with HIV, compared with 14% among those that were TST-negative.[20] Although some of the trials included adolescents as young as 13 years of age, no trials of INH treatment have been conducted exclusively in adolescents or younger children with HIV infection. Based on the same rationale as that used for HIV-uninfected persons, and to ensure uniformity of recommendations, the ATS recommends nine months of INH for the treatment of tuberculosis infection in HIV-infected persons.[6] The AAP recommends the same duration for infants, children, and adolescents.[19] Outside of the United States, six to nine months of INH is recommended for the treatment for HIV-infected patients with tuberculosis infection, similar to the duration for HIV-uninfected patients (Table 16.1).

ISONIAZID PREVENTIVE THERAPY IN HIV-INFECTED PERSONS

Isoniazid preventive therapy (IPT) is the provision of INH to people at high risk of developing tuberculosis who do not necessarily have documented tuberculosis infection. Given the high risk of rapid progression to tuberculosis disease from infection among persons living with HIV, the WHO recommends IPT as part of a public health strategy to reduce the burden of tuberculosis in this population.[21] Because of operational challenges associated with implementation of testing for tuberculosis infection, a TST or an interferon-gamma release assay (IGRA) is not a requirement for giving IPT to adults or children living with HIV in resource-constrained settings, although it is acknowledged that the benefit of treatment of documented tuberculosis infection is likely to be higher.[20,21] The duration of IPT recommended strongly by the WHO for all patients living with HIV, determined by a comparison of trials using various durations of INH for the treatment of tuberculosis infection, is six months.[21] Based on evidence of the potential benefit of prolonged IPT for people living with HIV in settings of high tuberculosis prevalence and transmission,[22] the WHO also conditionally recommends 36 months of IPT as a surrogate for lifelong or continuous treatment in this population (Box 16.1). With evidence from several randomized controlled trials in adults demonstrating the value of giving IPT immediately after completion of treatment for tuberculosis disease,[23–25] the administration of six months of IPT after treatment of tuberculosis disease is also recommended for

adults; 36 months of secondary prophylaxis is conditionally recommended in settings of high rates of tuberculosis prevalence and transmission. Although it has been more than 15 years since the WHO first recommended IPT in persons living with HIV, the IPT strategy for these individuals remains controversial and has not been implemented in many high-burden countries due to resource constraints and the difficulty of excluding tuberculosis disease prior to initiating INH.[26]

The impact of IPT has been evaluated in children with contradictory results. Compared with placebo, INH administered for two years in HIV-infected children in South Africa was associated with a 54% reduction in all-cause mortality and a 72% reduction in the incidence of tuberculosis.[27] Among those with a negative TST, a 49% reduction in mortality and a 68% reduction in the incidence of tuberculosis were noted. In contrast, a multicenter African study found that there was no benefit of INH as pre-exposure prophylaxis compared with placebo in improving disease-free survival among HIV-infected infants treated for 96 weeks.[28] These infants had no known exposure to a tuberculosis source case, were identified in the first few months of life, and were given rapid access to antiretroviral therapy (ART) while being monitored for tuberculosis exposure and disease. Differences in outcomes of the two pediatric trials may be explained at least in part by differing study methodologies and the inclusion of older, more immunosuppressed and malnourished children in the earlier study.

The WHO recommends that all children living with HIV who are more than 12 months of age and who are unlikely to have tuberculosis disease based on available screening should receive six months of IPT as part of a comprehensive package of HIV care (Box 16.1). For children less than 12 months of age, only those who have been exposed to tuberculosis but do not have tuberculosis disease are eligible for IPT. There is no specific evidence to suggest that IPT extended beyond six months is of any benefit to children living with HIV. There is also no evidence supporting secondary prophylaxis in children after completion of treatment for tuberculosis disease, but administering six months of IPT is conditionally recommended in this situation.

SAFETY AND TOLERABILITY

INH is generally very well tolerated by children and adolescents. Potential toxicities associated with INH

Box 16.1 Recommendations for Intensified Tuberculosis (TB) Case-Finding and Isoniazid Preventive Therapy (IPT) for People Living with human immunodeficiency virus (HIV) in Resource-Constrained Settings with a High Tuberculosis Burden

1. Adults and adolescents living with HIV should be screened for tuberculosis disease with a clinical algorithm, and those who do not report any one of the symptoms of cough, fever, weight loss, or night sweats are unlikely to have active TB and should be offered IPT.
   Strong recommendation, moderate quality of evidence.[1]

2. Adults and adolescents living with HIV and screened with a clinical algorithm for TB, and who report any one of the symptoms of cough, fever, weight loss, or night sweats, may have tuberculosis disease and should be evaluated for tuberculosis and other diseases.
   Strong recommendation, moderate quality of evidence.

3. Adults and adolescents living with HIV who have an unknown or positive tuberculin skin test (TST) status and are unlikely to have tuberculosis disease should receive at least 6 months of IPT as part of a comprehensive package of HIV care. IPT should be given to such individuals irrespective of the degree of immunosuppression, and also to those taking antiretroviral therapy (ART), those who have previously been treated for tuberculosis and pregnant women.
   Strong recommendation, high quality of evidence.

4. Adults and adolescents living with HIV who have an unknown or positive TST status and who are unlikely to have tuberculosis disease should receive at least 36 months of IPT.[2] IPT should be given to such individuals irrespective of the degree of immunosuppression, and also to those on ART, those who have previously been treated for tuberculosis and pregnant women.
   Conditional recommendation, moderate quality of evidence.[3]

5. TST is not a requirement for initiating IPT in people living with HIV.
   Strong recommendation, moderate quality of evidence.

6. People living with HIV who have a positive TST benefit more from IPT; TST can be used where feasible to identify such individuals.
   Strong recommendation, high quality of evidence.

7. Providing IPT to people living with HIV does not increase the risk of developing isoniazid (INH)-resistant tuberculosis. Therefore, concerns regarding the development of INH resistance should not be a barrier to providing IPT.
   Strong recommendation, moderate quality of evidence.

8. Children living with HIV who do not have poor weight gain,[4] fever, or cough are unlikely to have tuberculosis disease.
   Strong recommendation, low quality of evidence.

9. Children living with HIV who have any one of the following symptoms—poor weight gain, fever, or cough, or who have a contact history with a tuberculosis case—may have tuberculosis and should be evaluated appropriately. If the evaluation shows no tuberculosis, such children should be offered IPT regardless of their age.
   Strong recommendation, low quality of evidence.

10. Children living with HIV who are more than 12 months of age and who are unlikely to have tuberculosis disease based on symptom-based screening, and have had no contact with a tuberculosis case should receive 6 months of IPT as part of a comprehensive package of HIV prevention and care services.
    Strong recommendation, moderate quality of evidence.

11. For children living with HIV who are less than 12 months of age, only those who have contact with a tuberculosis case and who are evaluated for tuberculosis should receive 6 months of IPT if their evaluation shows no tuberculosis disease.
   Strong recommendation, low quality of evidence.

12. All children living with HIV who have successfully completed treatment for tuberculosis disease should receive INH for an additional 6 months.
   Conditional recommendation, low quality of evidence.

---

include gastrointestinal disturbances, hepatotoxicity, and peripheral neuropathy. Discontinuation of treatment is generally related to hepatotoxicity, which may range from asymptomatic elevation of serum transaminases to, less commonly, clinical hepatitis.

The recognition of the potential hepatotoxicity of INH in the 1970s prompted several assessments of the risk of hepatitis. Although the studies differed in terms of populations, treatment regimens, and definitions of hepatotoxicity, the overall rate of INH-induced hepatitis in patients receiving up to 12 months of INH was estimated at less than 1%.[12,29-32] Age was defined as an important risk factor for INH hepatitis in these studies, with the highest rates of hepatotoxicity reported among those older than 50 years.[31] In the USPHS surveillance study of nearly 14,000 patients receiving INH monotherapy for tuberculosis infection in the 1970s, rates of probable INH hepatitis were 0.3% in those 20–34 years of age and as high as 4.6% among those older than 50 years.[29] The studies that included pediatric patients demonstrated that children and adolescents were at markedly decreased risk of hepatotoxicity compared with adults (Table 16.3).

Several studies have prospectively evaluated the rates of adverse effects associated with INH in children.[33-35] Again, the variable rates reported were probably due to differences in study design and definitions of hepatotoxicity. Among 2,250 infected children randomized to receive either INH (4–6 mg/kg) or placebo between 1955 and 1957, only 0.4% in the treatment arm developed nausea and emesis; serum transaminases were not monitored.[17] In Hsu's observational study of 1,882 children with tuberculosis infection treated with 6–20 mg/kg of INH for 12–18 months, clinical hepatitis was not reported, and only four cases of adverse events (rash, vomiting, diarrhea) were attributed to INH.[36] In a different pooled analysis of 965 children, 8% developed transient elevation of transaminases, but INH had to be discontinued only in 0.4%.[37] Of the 58 (1.3%) of 4,473 children undergoing treatment for tuberculosis infection who had transaminases measured for suspected hepatitis, only three had elevated values.

Chang recently reviewed 1,582 pediatric patients under 18 years of age treated with nine months of INH in California. Baseline laboratory values were assessed only in those at risk for hepatotoxicity, with biochemical monitoring only if the patient had signs or symptoms of hepatotoxicity; INH hepatotoxicity was defined by (1) alanine aminotransferase (ALT) >3 times upper limits of

Table 16.3. Prevalence of hepatotoxicity associated with isoniazid treatment for latent tuberculosis infection in children, adolescents, and adults

	SITE, YEARS	TOTAL NUMBER OF PATIENTS	RATE (%) OF HEPATITIS IN ADULTS	NUMBER OF CHILDREN (AGE)	RATE (%) OF HEPATITIS IN CHILDREN
Adult and pediatric studies	Multicenter, United States 1971–1972[29]	13,838	1.0	2,473 < 20 years	0.1
	Washington, 1989–1995[30]	11,141	0.1	1,468 <14 years	0
	California, 1999–2002[31]	3,788	0.3	1,277 < 14 years	0
Pediatric studies	California, 2005–2011[33]			1,582 < 18 years	0.8
	New York, 1978–1987[35]			564	0.18

Hepatitis was defined variably in the studies, based on measurement of serum transaminases with or without the presence of symptoms of hepatitis.

normal (ULN) and symptoms suggestive of hepatitis (nausea, vomiting, abdominal pain, jaundice or unexplained fatigue); or (2) ALT >5 times ULN without symptoms. INH hepatotoxicity was identified in 13 (0.8%) of 1,582 children who started INH, and 1.1% of the 1,235 who completed the nine-month regimen.[33] The more common symptoms included abdominal pain, anorexia, vomiting, and nausea. Although most patients who developed hepatotoxicity did so within six months of starting INH, in three, the hepatotoxicity was detected more than six months after the start of therapy. Elevations in aspartate aminotransferase (AST) and ALT were reversible in all children after discontinuation of therapy.

Despite the low risk of hepatitis in children, hepatic failure due to INH has been reported. In one study of 20 children with hepatic failure associated with INH treatment, ten children required liver transplantation, six children died before transplant, and only four children recovered without transplant.[38] In another report of two children who had severe adverse events from INH from 2004 to 2008, one child underwent liver transplant.[39] Clinical characteristics of children that predict mild or severe hepatotoxicity remain unknown, underscoring the importance of routine *clinical* monitoring (see "Monitoring During Treatment" below). Children receiving treatment for tuberculosis infection should be monitored at regular intervals for evidence of adverse effects, and families should be advised to stop the INH immediately if symptoms of possible hepatic toxicity are noted.

INTERMITTENT ISONIAZID ADMINISTRATION

Intermittent dosing regimens to treat tuberculosis infection allow the administration of a reduced number of doses, which enhances the feasibility of directly observed therapy (DOT) and thus improves adherence and completion of treatment. DOT is the term used to describe the observation of antituberculosis medication by a healthcare team member or, in resource-constrained settings, a community supporter. INH administered twice- or thrice-weekly at a higher dosage (Table 16.2) has been used extensively by tuberculosis-control programs to treat tuberculosis disease and infection in children. Given twice weekly, six months of INH resulted in significant reduction of disease compared with placebo in two trials in HIV-infected individuals.[40,41] In the only trial directly comparing intermittent with daily INH, six months of INH administered thrice weekly was somewhat less effective than INH administered daily for six months in HIV-infected children,[27] but the difference was insignificant.

Despite the potential advantages of intermittent dosing, there is concern that the higher dose required with less frequent dosing may result in increased rates of hepatotoxicity. A retrospective review of 441 children treated with INH (20–30 mg/kg) twice weekly by DOT demonstrated that the regimen was well tolerated.[42] Although 6.7% of the children developed some adverse effect, elevated transaminases were noted in only 0.4%, and no child had hepatic dysfunction. Based on these findings, the use of intermittent INH is an acceptable alternative to daily INH for the treatment of tuberculosis infection, especially in situations when DOT is preferred to assure success of treatment.

Rifampin

EFFICACY

A four-month regimen of rifampin (RMP) has been recommended by the ATS as an alternative regimen to nine months of INH for the treatment of LTBI in adults since 2000.[6] Although the recommendation was based on limited evidence, the regimen offers an option for patients intolerant of INH or those exposed to INH-resistant, RMP-susceptible tuberculosis.

The only randomized controlled trial evaluating RMP monotherapy compared six months of daily INH to three months of daily RMP, and three months of daily INH and RMP together, in adult males with silicosis in Hong Kong. At the five-year follow-up, all three regimens were significantly more efficacious than placebo, but not significantly different from each other.[43] Patients who received three months of RMP had the lowest rate of disease, with a protective efficacy of 63% in those who were adherent with treatment. Although the trial did not assess four months of RMP, the 10% rate of tuberculosis disease observed among subjects receiving three months of RMP was high enough for experts to conclude that four months would

be a more prudent duration than three months for the treatment of tuberculosis infection in this high-risk population. The four-month regimen is recommended conditionally (based on moderate evidence) by the Canadian Thoracic Society and is recommended as an alternative to INH by the WHO for the treatment of tuberculosis infection in high-income or middle–upper-income nations (Table 16.1).

Two smaller nonrandomized studies published prior to the 2000 ATS recommendations supported the use of RMP in the setting of infection with INH-resistant tuberculosis. Among homeless persons exposed to INH-resistant tuberculosis with TST conversion, none of the subjects treated with 6–12 months of RMP developed disease, compared with six of 71 (8.4 %) not treated and three of 38 (8%) treated with INH.[44] In the only trial involving children, no cases of tuberculosis disease were observed after two years of observation in 157 TST-positive high school students given six months of RMP after exposure to INH-resistant tuberculosis.[45]

There was minimal interest in the use of RMP for the treatment of tuberculosis infection prior to the 2000 ATS recommendations, probably due to the concern for potential development of resistance if used inadvertently in undiagnosed tuberculosis disease. Several programmatic assessments have since compared four months of RMP to nine months of INH. Although these assessments were not designed for analysis of efficacy, no differences were noted between the two regimens, suggesting a role for RMP as an alternative regimen even in the absence of INH resistance or intolerance.[46–48] A large international trial comparing four months of RMP with nine months of INH for the treatment of tuberculosis infection in children and adults is underway and should provide further evidence of the efficacy and tolerability of this regimen.

The AAP currently recommends four months of RMP for the treatment of tuberculosis infection in children and adolescents when INH is not tolerated or when the child is exposed to an INH-resistant RMP-susceptible source case.[19] The prior recommendation of a six-month duration of treatment was based on the single study of its effectiveness in children described above. The "children" were high-school students aged 15–23 years, with a mean age of 18 years, representing more of an adult population. There are no data favoring six months of treatment over four months in children, and the expected efficacy of four months in adults probably extrapolates to effectiveness in children.

EFFICACY IN HIV-INFECTED PERSONS

There are no studies of the efficacy of RMP monotherapy for the treatment of tuberculosis infection among HIV-infected persons. Tuberculosis disease is more difficult to exclude in HIV-infected persons, and the risk of acquired RMP resistance in persons with disease is high if monotherapy is given. For patients taking ART, drug interactions may prohibit the use of RMP. As a result, RMP monotherapy in this patient population is not recommended.

SAFETY AND TOLERABILITY

RMP administered for four months for the treatment of tuberculosis infection has proven to be a safe and well-tolerated regimen. In the Hong Kong study of adults with silicosis, the rate of adverse events was lowest for the three-month RMP regimen and similar to the rate with placebo.[43] None of the 165 patients developed hepatotoxicity, and transaminase levels were similar in the RMP and placebo groups. Menzies and colleagues, in a single-center randomized study comparing four months of RMP to nine months of INH, found adverse events resulted in permanent discontinuation of therapy for two (3%) patients taking RMP and eight (14%) patients taking INH; the three patients who developed hepatitis were all receiving INH.[46] In a much larger multinational open-label trial conducted by the same investigators, serious (grade 3 or 4) hepatotoxicity occurred in 16 (3.8%) of 422 recipients of INH versus three (0.7%) of 418 of those receiving RMP.[47] Rates of discontinuation due to drug-related adverse effects were lower for the RMP arm (3.8%) compared with the INH arm (5.7%).

Observational studies confirm the safety of RMP monotherapy, with rates of adverse events and rates of hepatotoxicity ranging from 0–0.4%.[48–50] When compared with nine months of INH, rates of discontinuation among those taking four months of RMP were equivalent or lower. Among homeless persons, seven (14%) of 49 subjects receiving 6–12 months of RMP developed adverse events, with no reports of hepatotoxicity despite high rates of alcoholism among the participants.[44] In 157 adolescents treated with six months of RMP, 18 (11.5%) interrupted therapy temporarily, and two (1.5%) discontinued treatment permanently; the rate of hepatotoxicity was low at 0.6%.[45] There are no currently published studies documenting the safety and tolerability of RMP used to treat tuberculosis infection in infants or young children.

Isoniazid and Rifampin

EFFICACY

A three-month course of daily INH and RMP has been recommended by the British Thoracic Society as an alternative to INH for the treatment of tuberculosis infection in adults and children since 1998.[51] At the time, the only data available from a randomized controlled trial in HIV-uninfected persons were in silicotic adults in Hong Kong. The efficacy among patients adherent with three months of INH and RMP was 41%, which was significantly higher than the placebo regimen, and not significantly different from an efficacy of 48% for six months of INH and 63% for three months of RMP.[43]

With an increase in interest in short-course regimens to improve adherence to therapy, additional studies have since evaluated three to four months of INH and RMP together for the treatment of tuberculosis infection. A meta-analysis published in 2005 identified five high-quality randomized controlled trials that demonstrated a three-month regimen of INH and RMP was equivalent in effectiveness and safety to a standard 6–12-month regimen of INH.[52] Including the Hong Kong trial, a total of 972 patients were treated with the two-drug regimen. Both HIV-infected and HIV-uninfected adults were enrolled at international sites; one of the Spanish studies included children. The only trial conducted exclusively in children compared four months of daily INH and RMP, to a nine-month course of INH and, in a separate period, to a shorter regimen of three months of INH and RMP in Greek children. New radiographic findings suggestive of tuberculosis disease were more common in children who received INH monotherapy than in those treated with four months of INH and RMP (24% versus 11.8 %, p = .001), suggesting superior efficacy of the RMP-containing regimens; the three- and four-month INH and RMP regimens were equally effective.[34] Children with radiographic changes were treated for tuberculosis disease, but none of the 850 children who were adherent to the prescribed regimens developed clinical disease.

The largest programmatic experience with the INH and RMP regimen comes from Blackburn, England, where, over the course of 23 years, Ormerod and colleagues treated children with sequentially declining durations of INH and RMP (9, 6, and then 3 months). The reduction in proportion of pediatric cases of tuberculosis observed after the introduction of this treatment in 1981 was maintained even with the shorter regimens.[53-55] Although not part of a controlled trial, the intervention proved highly successful in preventing tuberculosis disease and substantially encouraged the use of INH and RMP for the treatment of tuberculosis infection in children in the United Kingdom. Current recommendations from the National Institutes of Clinical Excellence in the United Kingdom continue to recommend three months of INH and RMP for the treatment of tuberculosis infection in HIV-uninfected children and adults.[5] Canada and the WHO endorse the regimen as an alternative to six to nine months of INH (Table 16.1).

EFFICACY IN HIV-INFECTED PERSONS

Several trials have evaluated INH and RMP for the treatment of tuberculosis infection in HIV-infected adults. Among 2,018 TST-positive Ugandan adults randomized to four treatment arms, the incidence of tuberculosis was significantly lower in the treatment groups than in the placebo group.[56] Daily self-administered INH and RMP was 60% effective in preventing disease. Although the reduced the risk of tuberculosis was substantial and similar to the 67% efficacy achieved with six months of INH, it narrowly missed the conservative level of statistical significance. In a more recent trial in South Africa, 1,148 TST-positive HIV-infected adults were randomized to treatment with 12 weeks of INH and RMP administered twice weekly by DOT, 12 weeks of INH and rifapentine (RPT) administered weekly by DOT, and, as a control arm, six months of INH self-administered daily. In the fourth treatment arm, termed "continuous," INH was administered daily for the duration of the study (mean 3.3. years, ≤6 years) to evaluate the efficacy of IPT in a setting of high tuberculosis transmission. No difference in progression to disease or death was noted among the four arms after three years of observation.[57] Three smaller Spanish trials have demonstrated that three months of INH and RMP is equivalent in efficacy to six or 12 months of INH in TST-positive and anergic HIV-infected adults.[58-60] No data are available for the effectiveness of the combination regimen in HIV-infected children or adolescents.

SAFETY AND TOLERABILITY

Despite the use of multiple drugs, a regimen of INH and RMP for the treatment of tuberculosis infection is as well tolerated as monotherapy. Adverse events, including hepatotoxicity, occur with similar or lower frequency in persons treated with three or four months of INH and RMP compared with those receiving 6–12 months of INH. The largest study conducted in HIV-uninfected persons found that eight (5%) of 167 silicotic Chinese adults receiving INH and RMP discontinued treatment due to adverse events, compared with eight (5%) of 173 who received six months of INH.[43] In the Greek pediatric trial described above, there were no serious adverse events noted among 926 children, and modification of treatment was not required in any patient.[34] Additional information from the programmatic Blackburn, England, experience demonstrated that none of the 334 children treated with INH and RMP between 1989 and 2004 required discontinuation of therapy due to adverse events.[55]

Among HIV-infected adults in Uganda, the drug discontinuation rate in subjects treated with INH and RMP was 2.3% (13 of 556), not significantly higher than the 0.6% discontinuation rate among those treated with six months of INH.[57] No patients developed serious adverse events, and, when measured, elevated liver enzymes were not found in any of the patients receiving the multidrug regimen. In the more recent study conducted in TST-positive HIV-infected South African adults, rates of serious adverse events were similar, at 5% or less for 329 patients treated with INH and RMP and 327 treated with six months of INH; rates of discontinuation were 3.8% in the INH and RMP arm and 2% in the INH arm.[58] Compared with standard treatment with INH, the combination regimen was found to be equally safe among HIV-uninfected and HIV-infected adults and children included in the meta-analysis of five studies evaluating INH and RMP, with 4.9% of 972 patients receiving the combination regimen requiring withdrawal from treatment, compared with 4.8 % of 954 treated with INH.[52] However, an important consideration for the use of this combined regimen in HIV-infected individuals is interaction between rifampin and ART.

Isoniazid and Rifapentine

EFFICACY

In 2011, the CDC recommended a combination of INH and RPT administered as 12 weekly doses via DOT as an equally effective alternative to nine months of daily INH for the treatment of tuberculosis infection in healthy patients ≥12 years of age.[61] The recommendations were largely based on the results of the PREVENT TB study of the Tuberculosis Trials Consortium.[62] A smaller trial from Brazil in largely HIV-uninfected adults previously demonstrated that the effectiveness of once-weekly, directly observed INH and RPT for three months was similar to that of two months of RMP and pyrazinamide (PZA) administered daily.[63] The PREVENT TB trial enrolled 7,731 subjects with tuberculosis infection from four low-incidence countries (Brazil, Canada, Spain, and the United States), including close contacts of cases of tuberculosis disease, recent TST converters, patients with radiographic evidence of healed tuberculosis, and HIV-infected persons not receiving ART. Participants were randomized to receive either 12 weeks of once-weekly, directly observed INH and RPT or nine months of daily self-administered INH and were followed for 33 months. The combination regimen proved to be as effective as standard treatment, with disease developing in seven of 3,986 (0.19%) subjects in the combination treatment group versus 15 of 3,745 (0.43%) subjects in the INH group. The recommendation for use of this regimen as an equal alternative to six months or nine months of INH was recently adopted by the WHO for middle- and upper-middle-income countries.[8] The Canadian Thoracic Society recommends it as an alternative regimen to be used with close monitoring.[4]

The PREVENT TB study was one of a few recent tuberculosis trials to enroll children. Ultimately, 1,058 children aged two to 17 were enrolled, 537 of them younger than 12 years of age. None of the 472 children randomized to 12 weeks of once-weekly, directly observed INH and RPT developed tuberculosis, compared with three (0.74%) of 365 randomized to nine months of INH.[64] Although safety analysis was the primary objective of the pediatric PREVENT TB study, the combination regimen proved to be as effective as standard therapy for the treatment of tuberculosis infection in children. It has been proposed that once-weekly DOT with INH and RPT for 12 weeks be considered an equal alternative to nine months of INH for children two years and older in future treatment guidelines. However, this regimen is not recommended for children under two years of age because of a lack of pharmacokinetic data for RPT in this age group.

EFFICACY IN HIV-INFECTED PERSONS

In the only study evaluating once-weekly INH and RPT in HIV-infected adults, Martinson and colleagues found no difference in the incidence of tuberculosis disease among 1,148 TST-positive South African adults randomized to one of four regimens for the treatment of tuberculosis infection: once-weekly INH and RPT, twice-weekly INH and RMP, both administered by DOT for 12 weeks; daily self-supervised INH for six months; or prolonged (continuous) daily INH.[57] Although the PREVENT TB study included 205 participants who were HIV-infected, there was no separate sub-analysis of the effectiveness of the regimen in this population.[62] However, due to the potential interactions of RPT with ART, the regimen is currently not recommended for HIV-infected individuals.

SAFETY AND TOLERABILITY

The data on the safety of INH and RPT are still accumulating, given the recent introduction of the regimen, but the regimen appears to be tolerated as well as standard therapy. The proportion of subjects over 12 years of age in the PREVENT TB trial with any adverse event was lower in the combination group than in the INH group, and there was no significant difference in the proportion of patients with grade 3 or 4 adverse effects.[62] However, those in the combination therapy group were more likely to have permanent drug discontinuation due to an adverse effect compared with the INH-only group (4.9% versus 3.7%, $p = 0.009$). The observation is probably due to the rate of hypersensitivity reactions observed in the group receiving INH and RPT compared with the group receiving INH (3.8% versus 0.5%, $p < 0.001$). Rates of hepatotoxicity attributable to the study drug were higher in the INH-only group (2.7% versus 0.4%, $p < 0.001$), as was the proportion of subjects who permanently discontinued the study drug because of hepatotoxicity (2.0% versus 0.3%). Monitoring for hypersensitivity reactions and other rare adverse effects will be important when combination treatment with INH and RPT is used in children. In the pediatric PREVENT TB study, 12 weeks of INH and RPT was well tolerated and safe among children two to 17 years of age.[64] Rates of discontinuation due to adverse events were similar for both arms (1.7% for INH and RPT versus 0.5% for INH, $p = 0.11$). Three (0.6%) of 539 children receiving combination therapy had a grade 3 adverse event compared with one (0.2%) of 493 for receiving INH alone (Table 16.4). Neither arm was associated with hepatotoxicity or any grade 4 adverse event, but several children receiving RPT had a mild hypersensitivity reaction.

Rifampin and Pyrazinamide

In early clinical trials evaluating RMP and PZA for the prevention of tuberculosis, two months of both drugs administered to HIV-infected adults was shown to be as effective and as safe as 6–12 months of INH.[65,66] Completion rates were significantly higher for the shorter regimen, and there were no significant differences in adverse events. Based on the promising trial results, the combination regimen was recommended for use in the United States in 2000.[6] However, when it was used widely in the general population, an unacceptably high rate of severe and fatal hepatotoxicity was recognized.[26,67–69] In a survey of state and city tuberculosis programs in the United States conducted by the CDC after initial

Table 16.4. Safety endpoints among children who received at least one dose of study medication in the PREVENT TB pediatric clinical trial (n = 1,032)

CHARACTERISTIC	PATIENTS, NO. (%)			
	ISONIAZID	RIFAPENTINE PLUS ISONIAZID	P-VALUE[a]	DIFFERENCE AND 95% CONFIDENCE INTERVAL[b]
	N = 493	N = 539		
AEs attributed to treatment:				
Grade 1 & 2	5 (1)	11 (2)	0.21	−1.0 (−2.5–0.5)
Grade 3	1 (0.2)	3 (0.6)	0.63	−0.4 (−1.1–0.4)
AEs not attributed to treatment:				
Grades 1 & 2	35 (7)	25 (5)	0.11	2.0 (−0.4–5.3)
Grade 3	5 (0.2)	3 (0.6)	0.49	0.4 (−0.6–1.5)
Grade 4	2 (0.4)	1 (0.2)	0.61	0.2 (−0.5–0.9)
Grades 3 & 4	7 (1)	4 (1)	0.37	0.7 (−0.6–2.0)
Grade 5 (Death)[c]	2 (0.4)	0 (0)	0.23	0.4 (−0.2–1.0)
Serious Adverse Events (SAE)[d]	7 (1.4)	0 (0)	0.01	1.0 (0.4–2.5)

Adapted with permission from Villarino ME, Scott NA, Weis SE, et al., for the International Maternal Pediatric and Adolescents AIDS Clinical Trials Group (IMPAACT), and the Tuberculosis Trials Consortium (TBTC). Treatment for preventing tuberculosis in children: a trial of a 3-month, 12-dose regimen of rifapentine and isoniazid. *JAMA Pediatr.* 2015;169:247–255.

AE = adverse event, NA = not available.

[a]p-value based on Fisher's exact test.

[b]95% CI for the differences in proportions using Wilson Score Interval method.

[c]Death #1: Malignant arrhythmia in a 16-year-old female in study day 201 of study treatment. Death #2: Gunshot injury in a 16-year-old year old male at study day 901 (approximately 657 days after the end of study treatment phase).

[d]Serious adverse events (SAE) include deaths on therapy or within 60 days of the last dose, life-threatening events, hospitalization, disability or permanent damage, and congenital anomaly/birth defect. For children ages 2–16: 6 had 1 SAE; 1 had >1 SAE. No SAE was attributed to treatment.

reports of severe hepatotoxicity, the rate of symptomatic hepatitis was 18.7 per 1,000 persons among 8,087 patients initiating treatment, with seven fatalities noted; the risk of hepatitis-associated death among persons receiving RMP and PZA was ten times higher than historic rates.[68] A subsequent report noted 50 cases of severe liver injury, including 12 deaths, attributable to RMP and PZA.[69] By 2003, the regimen was no longer recommended except in very limited circumstances.[70] However, for adults who initially receive four-drug therapy—including RMP and PZA—for suspected tuberculosis disease but are found to have only tuberculosis infection, having received the RMP and PZA for two months is considered adequate therapy.

In the only evaluation of the RMP and PZA regimen in children, two months of each drug was as well tolerated as six months of INH and four months of RMP in children in Poland, but, as with the earlier studies in HIV-infected individuals, the small sample size (143 children total) may have precluded the ability to detect toxicity.[71] Due to the observed hepatotoxicity in adults and the lack of efficacy data, RMP and PZA in combination was never recommended for the treatment of tuberculosis infection in children.

ADHERENCE

An important determinant of the effectiveness of treatment is acceptance and completion of the prescribed regimen. Approximately 50% of patients who start self-administered treatment for tuberculosis infection do not complete a six- or nine-month regimen of INH.[2,72] In a retrospective evaluation of clinics in the United States and Canada in 2002, approximately 17% of persons who were recommended for treatment of tuberculosis infection refused to accept it, and only 47% of those initiating therapy completed the full course.[72] Similarly, among 447 adult and pediatric contacts of tuberculosis cases identified at five health departments in the United States, a six-month course of INH was initiated in 89% but completed in only 51% of those initiating treatment.[73] The rate of completion among the 52 contacts under 15 years of age was only 63%, despite the use of DOT in a substantial portion of the children.

Rates of adherence with treatment in pediatric studies are variable and consistently suboptimal in both high- and low-burden countries. Early studies from the United States and Canada reported completion rates of 28–74% for treatment with six months of INH.[74–76] Treatment of recently immigrated children with tuberculosis infection identified by a school screening program in the United States reported a completion rate of 58%.[77] In South Africa, of 180 children younger than five years of age who were household contacts of acid-fast sputum smear-positive cases of tuberculosis, only 20% completed five months or more of self-administered INH, and 72% received fewer than two months.[78] Of the six children who developed tuberculosis, two had received no treatment, and four received fewer than two months. Higher rates of completion of 78% were achieved in Uganda under study conditions.[79]

Factors that contribute to lower rates of completion include drug-related adverse effects—perceived or actual—and prolonged duration of therapy. Among patients taking RMP for tuberculosis infection, the favorable tolerability and lower rates of adverse effects contribute to enhanced adherence.[46,47] Even more important for adherence than tolerability is the duration of treatment. Several studies have demonstrated that a shorter duration of treatment is a significant and independent predictor of increased adherence, with reported completion rates of 45–60% for nine months of daily INH, 69–78% for four months of daily RMP, and 75% for three months of daily INH and RMP.[11] Menzies and colleagues demonstrated in two randomized trials that completion rates of 78–91% achieved with four months of RMP were significantly higher than the 60–75% rates reported with nine months of INH.[46,47] Even with more complex regimens such as INH and RMP together, equivalent or higher completion rates appear to be achieved compared with longer treatment with INH monotherapy. The rate of completion in Greek children with tuberculosis infection treated with three or four months of INH and RMP was 78–90%, but only 66% of children in the nine-month INH arm completed treatment.[34] Completion rates of 70% were achieved in South African children receiving largely self-supervised treatment with three months of INH and RMP, compared with 28% completion among those treated with six months of INH.[80]

Additional barriers to completing therapy include individual patient or family characteristics, socioeconomic factors, the structure of health care services offered, the quality of the patient–physician relationship, and the social support of the family. Clinic-based factors such as hours of operation and availability of language and culturally competent services have been shown to affect adherence.[81] Treatment of tuberculosis infection of children relies on the parents or caregivers to administer drugs and monitor for adherence. Parents may lack understanding of the tuberculosis infection and need for treatment. Treatment usually requires multiple visits to a health care facility for monitoring and procurement of medication. Because tuberculosis infection is asymptomatic, parents often do not perceive any immediate benefit from treatment. It is important to engage caregivers and the child at the initial visit, educating them about the lifetime risk of development of disease and the benefit of treatment, whether the setting is in industrialized nations or in resource-limited settings with high burdens of tuberculosis.

Clinicians and program directors need to be aware of culturally influenced misconceptions about tuberculosis and tuberculosis infection that may impact acceptance or completion of treatment. In a hospital-based pediatric tuberculosis clinic in the United States serving a largely foreign-born population, parental refusal to start medication was noted in 54% of Eastern European children, none of whom completed treatment, and 80% of Asian children, of whom more than 50% did not complete treatment.[82] Not unexpectedly, parents from these regions often believed that the receipt of the Bacille Calmette-Guerin (BCG) vaccine accounted for positive tests of infection and that BCG would protect their children from the development of tuberculosis. Parents from high-burden countries where BCG vaccine is routinely administered frequently have been advised by family members or physicians in their native countries to refuse treatment for tuberculosis infection after moving to a locale where it is offered. It is important to explain why treatment of tuberculosis infection may not be offered routinely in their native country. Reinforcement of the education should be provided at subsequent monitoring visits to assure completion of therapy Additional strategies to enhance adherence include intensive case management, peer support, the use of lay health workers from the patient's social or cultural group, and the provision of incentives (e.g., gift cards or other rewards for children) and enablers (e.g., public transportation passes, food).

The intervention most likely to improve adherence for treatment of tuberculosis infection, especially in children, is DOT. While DOT is the standard of care in the United States for children with tuberculosis disease, it can also enhance treatment of tuberculosis infection in high-risk children.

In a study from Texas, the only variable positively associated with increased adherence among children completing treatment for tuberculosis infection was medication administration twice weekly by DOT through the public health department; children receiving treatment in this manner achieved 93% completion, whereas the completion rate for self- treatment with nine months of INH was only 49%.[83] Similarly, in South Africa, where treatment of tuberculosis infection is reserved for very young children with exposure to contagious cases of tuberculosis, overall adherence to self-treatment in one study was only 44%, but with direct supervision, either by a health care worker or a community supporter, 70% of these children completed treatment.[80] The benefit of DOT was clearly demonstrated in the recently completed PREVENT TB study comparing 12 weeks of INH and RPT administered by DOT compared with self-administered INH for nine months. Among 1,058 children aged 2–17 years, those randomized to the combination regimen given by DOT had a significantly higher rate of completion at 88%, compared with 80% of children receiving self-administered INH.[64]

Despite the advantages of DOT, it is often not feasible for treatment programs to utilize this technique due to the high cost of using staff for administration of the regimen. In industrialized countries, establishing school-based treatment programs or using school-based nurses to administer therapy may be a more cost-effective strategy. In two high school–based programs in New York City, significantly higher rates of treatment completion for tuberculosis infection were achieved in the adolescents receiving DOT (88%) compared with those receiving medications at home (50%).[84] Similarly, Sass et al.[85] reported significantly higher rates of completion among students receiving DOT (54%) compared with those receiving home treatment (26%). In resource-limited countries, the use of community workers for DOT can facilitate completion of therapy, especially when the person with tuberculosis disease in the household is receiving treatment via DOT.

ADMINISTRATION AND ADVERSE EFFECTS (TABLE 16.2)

Isoniazid

While the oral forms of INH are used almost exclusively, an intramuscular preparation is also available, administered at the same dosage as the oral formulations. When children are unable to swallow tablets, the pills can be crushed and mixed with a spoonful of soft food to mask the taste (e.g., applesauce, mashed bananas, pudding, yogurt). Some liquid preparations of INH contain sorbitol, which can cause gastric distress or diarrhea at higher dosages; use of tablets (crushed or whole) frequently results in resolution of symptoms. For infants, the tablet may be dissolved in a tablespoon of warm water and then mixed with a small amount of breast milk or formula. For optimal absorption, INH should be administered one hour before or two hours after meals. However, the drug may be taken with or shortly after a meal to avoid gastrointestinal upset.[86] No dosage adjustments are required in patients with renal insufficiency.

INH is very well tolerated by infants, children, and adolescents. The most important adverse effect is hepatotoxicity, which may manifest as asymptomatic or mildly symptomatic elevation of serum transaminases or symptomatic hepatitis. Mild, asymptomatic hepatic injury occurs in 10–20% of adults taking INH as manifested in elevations of transaminase serum concentrations (usually <100 IU/L). Virtually all cases are self-limited, and INH treatment can be continued with careful clinical and laboratory monitoring. Symptomatic INH hepatitis is less common, occurring in 0.1–0.5% of adults being treated with INH for tuberculosis infection.[87] Symptoms of INH hepatitis include anorexia, vomiting, abdominal pain, and unexplained malaise or fatigue. Patients may present with generalized influenza-like symptoms several weeks before the onset of jaundice, which is present in approximately 10% of affected adults and is less common in children.[33] Additional adverse effects associated with INH include gastrointestinal complaints (e.g., nausea, abdominal discomfort) and neurological symptoms (Table 16.5). Central nervous system side effects caused by INH include peripheral neuropathy and paresthesias and, less commonly, ataxia and seizures. Peripheral neuropathy occurs as a result of functional pyridoxine deficiency caused by INH-related antagonism of pyridoxine and interference with pyridoxine-dependent coenzymes.[88] Neurotoxicity can be prevented by pyridoxine supplementation. Peripheral neuropathy is rare in otherwise healthy children and adolescents, and pyridoxine is routinely recommended only for children with certain risk factors (Box 16.2).

Rifampin

An intravenous formulation of RMP is available for administration at the same dosages as the oral formulations. For children unable to swallow capsules, the medication can be compounded into a suspension. Alternatively, if the child's weight allows for rounding the dosage to use one or more capsules, the contents of the capsule can be mixed with small amounts of food to mask the bitter taste and prevent gastrointestinal upset. Absorption is improved if the drug is taken on an empty stomach. However, administration with small amounts of food may be warranted in children to avoid gastrointestinal upset. No dosage adjustments are required in patients with renal insufficiency. Although RMP may be used in patients with underlying hepatic dysfunction, no formal guidelines are available to guide dosing in this population.

Adverse reactions to rifamycins of clinical significance are uncommon in children and adolescents. The most common side effect associated with RMP is gastrointestinal upset, including nausea, vomiting, diarrhea, and anorexia (Table 16.5). Prior to initiation of treatment with RMP, it is important to caution families to anticipate these effects for the first week or two of treatment. Hepatotoxicity is infrequently associated with RMP and may range from hyperbilirubinemia without hepatocellular damage to elevations in transaminases.[89] Clinically significant hepatitis is rare but may be observed in patients with predisposing factors, including those receiving concomitant potentially hepatotoxic drugs such as INH.

RMP may cause dermatological reactions such as rash or pruritis, central nervous system effects such as headache, and, rarely, hypersensitivity reactions. Intermittent dosing of RMP, especially at dosages higher than 600 mg, may be associated with hematological effects (leukopenia, thrombocytopenia, or hemolytic anemia), an "influenza-like" syndrome (fever, chills, and malaise), or acute renal failure. These are hypersensitivity reactions presumed to be immune-mediated and are uncommon at recommended dosages. RMP is not recommended for intermittent therapy of tuberculosis infection, and the caregiver and patient should be cautioned against interruption of the daily treatment since rare renal hypersensitivity reactions have been reported when therapy was resumed. Temporary red-orange discoloration of urine, sweat, tears, and other body fluids is a normal and expected side effect; permanent discoloration of soft contact lenses may occur.

Table 16.5. Adverse reactions associated with medications used for the treatment of tuberculosis infection

DRUG	ADVERSE REACTIONS*	COMMENTS
Isoniazid	Rash Gastrointestinal distress Asymptomatic serum transaminase elevation Hepatitis Peripheral neuropathy Mild central nervous system effects	Peripheral neuropathy can be avoided by supplementation with pyridoxine.
Rifampin	Rash Gastrointestinal distress Asymptomatic serum transaminase elevation Hepatitis Influenza-like illness Thrombocytopenia Orange-colored body fluids Multiple drug interactions	Rifampin is contraindicated or should be used with caution in human immunodeficiency virus-infected patients taking protease inhibitors or non-nucleoside reverse transcriptase inhibitors. Permanent discoloration of contact lenses may occur.
Rifapentine	As above for rifampin Hypersensitivity reaction	As above for rifampin. Vigilance is recommended for mild (e.g., dizziness) and severe (e.g., hypotension) hypersensitivity reactions observed in the PREVENT TB trial.[62]

*See text for details.

Box 16.2 Characteristics of Infants, Children, and Adolescents for Whom Pyridoxine Supplementation Is Recommended During Treatment with Isoniazid for Tuberculosis Infection

Malnourished
On meat- and milk-deficient diet
Exclusively breastfed
Chronic liver disease
Renal failure
Pregnant or breastfeeding adolescents
Alcoholic
Symptomatic HIV infection
Seizure disorder

A recognized effect of rifamycins is induction of cytochrome P450 enzymes with resultant increased metabolism of a wide variety of drugs, including anticoagulants, oral contraceptives, anticonvulsants, antifungals (azoles), and certain antiretroviral drugs. Adolescents using oral contraceptives should be advised to use alternate forms of birth control while taking RMP. RMP is contraindicated in persons with HIV infection who are taking protease inhibitors (e.g., atazanavir, darunavir, fosamprenavir, saquinavir, or tipranavir) due to the potential of RMP to substantially reduce plasma concentrations and thereby the efficacy of the antiviral drugs. RMP should be taken with caution in HIV-infected patients receiving non-nucleoside reverse transcriptase inhibitors.

Rifapentine

RPT is a rifamycin derivative with a long half-life and greater potency against *M. tuberculosis* than

RMP. It was approved by the United States Food and Drug Administration in 2014 for the treatment of tuberculosis infection in combination with INH for patients two years and older. Currently, only the tablet formulation is available. Efforts are underway to develop a more child-friendly formulation. For children unable to swallow tablets, the pills can be crushed and mixed with a spoonful of soft food to mask the taste. In a pharmacokinetic analysis of RPT in 80 children (2–11 years) and 77 adults enrolled in the PREVENT TB trial, Weiner and colleagues found the geometric mean area under concentration time curve (AUC) to be higher for the children swallowing whole tablets compared with those receiving crushed tablets.[90] The geometric mean AUCs for both groups of children, however, were higher than that achieved in adults, and the higher weight-adjusted RPT doses were safe and effective in the clinical trial.

The toxicity profile of RPT is similar to that of RMP. Adverse effects associated with RPT are typically mild and confined to the gastrointestinal tract and hypersensitivity reactions. Gastrointestinal upset manifested as nausea, abdominal pain, and vomiting is uncommon. Elevations in serum liver enzymes have been reported. When given once weekly with INH for the treatment of tuberculosis infection in adults in the PREVENT TB trial, rare serious reactions, including hypotension and syncope, were observed.[62] Monitoring for these uncommon but severe adverse effects is important, as this new regimen is used in clinical practice. Symptoms of hypersensitivity include light headedness, dizziness, headache, nausea or vomiting, syncope, rash, or angioedema. As with RMP, RPT may produce an orange-red discoloration of body fluids and is a strong inducer of the cytochrome P450 system with multiple important and potentially prolonged drug interactions; it is not routinely recommended for patients receiving ART.

CHOOSING A REGIMEN

Recommendations for the treatment of tuberculosis infection in children have traditionally emphasized INH monotherapy, as this is the only regimen studied extensively in children. Outside of industrialized nations, INH remains the standard treatment for children due to its cost-effectiveness. The three other regimens—RMP monotherapy, INH and RMP, and INH and RPT—have been shown to have equivalent efficacy with similar or lower toxicity profiles in

adults. Although the data are more limited, existing evidence means that these regimens are likely to be effective for children and adolescents. Any of the four regimens can be considered for treatment of children and adults, with INH and RPT restricted to use in children older than two years of age. Preferred regimens according to international guidelines are outlined in Table 16.1.

Programs must consider resources for drug procurement, patient monitoring, and DOT when deciding which regimens can be offered to the patient. Healthcare providers must balance effectiveness of a regimen with rates of adverse events reported in trials while considering risk of progression to disease. It is important to consider the medical and social circumstances of the patient and family that may affect treatment. The choice of a regimen should be made with the patient's or parents' preferences in mind.

As the likelihood of completion is better, shorter duration regimens are generally preferred over those with longer duration by clinicians and recipients of treatment. Programs choosing shorter regimens must weigh the higher costs of drugs or DOT against the benefits of improved adherence. At the same time, DOT may lower acceptability of treatment by individuals receiving the treatment, either due to the time or cost for travel to receive DOT or the social stigma attached to DOT delivered at home or school.

PRETREATMENT EVALUATION AND MONITORING DURING TREATMENT

All patients with evidence of tuberculosis infection by history of close contact with a contagious patient (low-resource settings) or specific testing (high-resource settings) should undergo evaluation to the extent possible to make sure tuberculosis disease has not already developed. The decision to treat should take into account the individual's risk of developing tuberculosis disease and the risks of therapy. The risk–benefit ratio for initiating treatment of tuberculosis infection in children is more favorable than for adults because the risk of adverse effects is lower and the benefit is higher.

Pretreatment Evaluation

The management of a patient with tuberculosis should be coordinated through established programs at the health department, hospital, or community clinic, or through an institutional setting such as a school. The evaluation should be conducted in the family's primary language with the assistance of an interpreter, if needed. Once a child or adolescent has been identified as a candidate for treatment, medical evaluation should include a history, physical assessment, and family education. A medical history should be obtained to determine if the child has been treated previously for tuberculosis infection or disease and, if so, if the treatment was completed. Medical conditions that could complicate treatment or require more careful monitoring should be identified. A detailed listing of current medications should be obtained, with particular attention given to potential drug interactions. A physical examination is essential to exclude tuberculosis disease. Obtaining a chest radiograph is ideal but not usually obtained in low-resource settings if the child is asymptomatic and has a normal examination.

The pretreatment evaluation provides an opportunity for the provider to establish rapport with the patient and provide education to enhance adherence and minimize adverse outcomes. The difference between tuberculosis infection and disease and the benefits of treatment with reference to prevention of disease should be explained in plain, simple language. Options for treatment regimens should be reviewed and a regimen chosen based on available resources and provider and patient preferences. Potential adverse events associated with the chosen regimen should be reviewed, and the family should be educated about signs and symptoms of toxicity that warrant cessation of therapy and/or prompt medical evaluation. These include anorexia, nausea, vomiting, dark urine, jaundice, rash, persistent paresthesias of the hands and feet, unexplained fatigue or weakness, unexplained fever, abdominal tenderness (especially right upper quadrant discomfort), and easy bruising or bleeding (Table 16.6). Practitioners should consider implementation of a standardized history form to ensure that all elements of the pretreatment evaluation have been addressed.

Baseline laboratory testing is not routinely indicated for children and adolescents. Patients with a history of hepatic disorder or those receiving other potentially hepatotoxic drugs should undergo baseline measurements of AST, ALT, and bilirubin. Baseline testing should also be undertaken for patients with HIV infection, pregnant and immediately post-partum females, persons who drink alcohol regularly or may drink alcohol regularly (e.g., adolescents), and patients at risk for chronic liver disease (Table 16.6). Active hepatitis and liver disease are relative contraindications for the use of INH, RMP, and RPT. The risks and benefits of initiating INH for the treatment of tuberculosis infection in patients with abnormal baseline liver function (transaminases >3 times ULN) should be considered carefully. The risk of progression to disease should be weighed against the risk of potentiating liver dysfunction. If therapy is initiated, serum transaminases should be monitored carefully.[87]

Monitoring During Treatment

Clinical monitoring of patients being treated for tuberculosis infection should be conducted periodically by the tuberculosis program or provider. Periodic monitoring offers the opportunity to stress the importance of adherence and advise the family of signs and symptoms of toxicity. Families should be reminded to interrupt treatment and contact the provider upon onset of these symptoms or for unexplained illness during treatment. If no issues are noted, another month's supply of medications may be dispensed, with dosage adjusted for significant weight gain.

Adverse events related to any of the regimens used for the treatment of tuberculosis infection may occur any time during the course of treatment, underscoring the importance of routine monitoring throughout the treatment course. The most important factor in the management of INH-associated hepatotoxicity is early recognition and prompt discontinuation of INH. Severe effects are more likely in individuals continuing to take INH despite having symptoms of hepatotoxicity. The ATS recommends monthly clinical assessments for all patients being treated for tuberculosis infection. Patients should undergo a brief history and physical assessment to identify signs and symptoms of hepatitis or other adverse effects. Concomitant medications being received by the patient should be reviewed. Adolescents should be questioned about alcohol use and oral contraceptive use. As with the baseline evaluation, a standardized questionnaire may facilitate clinical monitoring.

Laboratory monitoring during treatment of tuberculosis infection is indicated for patients whose baseline liver function tests were abnormal, those with symptoms or signs of adverse events, and for persons at risk for hepatic disease (Table 16.6).

Table 16.6. Guidance for clinical monitoring of infants, children, and adolesecents during treatment of tuberculosis infection

	EVALUATION	COMMENTS
Pretreatment Evaluation	Medical history —Preexisting medical conditions —Concomitant medications	Risk factors for hepatotoxicity —HIV infection —Hepatic disorders —Regular alcohol use —Immediate post-partum period ($\leq$3 months after delivery) —Concomitant medications with potential hepatotoxicity
	Physical assessment —Signs of tuberculosis disease —Signs of underlying liver dysfunction Baseline laboratory assessment for those at risk for hepatotoxicity —ALT, serum bilirubin	
	Education —Review importance of treatment —Review importance of adherence —Review symptoms and signs of adverse events warranting cessation of treatment and medical evaluation	Symptoms of adverse events —Anorexia —Nausea, vomiting, abdominal pain —Unexplained fever —Dark urine —Jaundice —Rash, easy bruising or bleeding —Paresthesias —Unexplained fatigue or weakness
Periodic Monitoring (Monthly Recommended)	Interval history —Interim illnesses —Concomitant medications —Symptoms and signs of tuberculosis —Symptoms and signs of adverse events	For patients receiving INH and RPT, symptoms of hypersensitivity should be elicited in addition to symptoms of hepatotoxicity and hematological toxicity —Lightheadedness —Dizziness, syncope —Headache —Nausea/vomiting —Rash, angioedema
	Physical assessment —Weight of young infants and children —Signs of tuberculosis disease —Signs of adverse events	
	Periodic laboratory assessment —For those with abnormal baseline laboratory assessment —For those with symptoms or signs of adverse effects	Discontinue isoniazid if ALT >3 times the ULN with symptoms of hepatitis (nausea, vomiting, abdominal pain, jaundice, or unexplained fatigue) or 5 times the ULN in the absence of symptoms.
	Education —Review importance of treatment —Review importance of adherence —Review symptoms and signs warranting cessation of treatment and medical evaluation	

See text for details.

HIV= human immunodeficiency virus; ALT = alanine aminotransferase; ULN = upper limits of normal.

INH should be discontinued in patients with normal or unknown baseline liver function if monitoring demonstrates serum transaminase levels greater than three times the ULN, together with symptoms and/or jaundice.[87] For patients who are asymptomatic, INH should be discontinued if transaminase levels are more than five times the ULN. If serum transaminase levels increase rapidly but do not reach 3–5 times ULN, laboratory monitoring approximately every one to three weeks should continue.

SPECIAL CIRCUMSTANCES

Treatment of Household or Other Close Contacts of Recent Cases

In high-resource settings, children and adolescents who are recent household or close contacts of a person with suspected or proven infectious tuberculosis should undergo evaluation for tuberculosis infection or disease. Those with a positive TST or IGRA should be offered one of the recommended treatment regimens for tuberculosis infection, once disease has been excluded by history, physical examination, and a chest radiograph.

The tests for tuberculosis infection may not become positive until eight to ten weeks after the infection has actually occurred; as a result, children who have been exposed recently may be tested before enough time has elapsed for the test(s) to become positive. For children over five years of age and adolescents with an initially negative TST or IGRA result, repeat testing should be performed eight to ten weeks after the last exposure to the source case to be sure infection has not been established. If the repeat test is positive, treatment for tuberculosis infection should be initiated once disease is again excluded. However, young children—especially those younger than two years—and immunocompromised children can develop tuberculosis disease even before the repeat test can be performed. In exposed contacts younger than five years of age and immunosuppressed children who are at high risk of rapid progression to disease, treatment for tuberculosis infection should be initiated even when the child initially has a normal physical examination, chest radiograph, and a negative TST or IGRA result (so-called window prophylaxis). Experience with window prophylaxis is limited to INH monotherapy. Treatment is continued until testing can be repeated eight to ten weeks later. If the repeat TST or

IGRA result is negative, treatment can be discontinued. If the contact is immunosuppressed, or if tuberculosis infection cannot be excluded, a full course of treatment for tuberculosis infection should be completed. Some experts recommend completing treatment in young infants (i.e., <6 months of age) with significant exposure to a source case even with negative repeat testing, due to the high unreliability of negative TST or IGRA and high rate of progression from infection to disease in this age group.

In high-burden, low-resource settings, tests for tuberculosis infection and chest radiography are often unavailable. In these settings, children who are household contacts of a person recently diagnosed with tuberculosis disease should be examined and undergo symptom screening.[7] Children with an abnormal physical examination or symptoms compatible with tuberculosis should be referred to the local health facility for further evaluation; children less than five years of age without symptoms or physical findings should receive six months of INH. Although these recommendations have been made by WHO for over 30 years, they are not implemented in many high-burden settings. Studies are underway to determine the best methods to provide this potentially life-saving treatment.

Treatment of Tuberculosis Infection Caused by Multidrug-Resistant *M. Tuberculosis*

Multidrug-resistant tuberculosis (MDR-TB), defined as tuberculosis caused by *M. tuberculosis* resistant to at least INH and RIF, has become a major global public health issue. The prevalence of MDR tuberculosis is increasing, with reports of over 20% MDR-TB among new cases in some countries, and the transmission of MDR organisms to close contacts is common.[91] In three studies from South Africa, 5–12% of child contacts of MDR-TB developed disease, and 1–53% had tuberculosis infection.[92–94]

The rapid identification and treatment of patients with MDR-TB is essential to curing disease and interrupting further transmission. The management of adults and children in contact with these cases is less clear. Guidelines vary, as do expert opinion and published practice, but prospective studies on the effectiveness and safety of these regimens are lacking. One of the major concerns regarding the treatment of MDR-TB is toxicity. Second-line antituberculosis drugs considered for the treatment of tuberculosis infection due to MDR organisms are known to have lower safety and tolerability in children and adults than first-line drugs. Whereas the risk–benefit ratio of potentially toxic therapy is relatively clear for the treatment of disease, it is less clear when using it in children who are infected. If the regimen fails, and disease develops during treatment, there is a risk of further acquisition of resistance. Given these concerns, the treatment of contacts of cases with MDR-TB is sometimes deferred, and close clinical monitoring for disease is recommended instead. However, the implications of not providing adequate treatment to children infected with MDR strains are serious, given their high risk of developing disease.

Few studies have assessed treatment of child contacts of a case of MDR-TB, and there have been no randomized clinical trials. Of 41 children in Cape Town given a multidrug regimen tailored to the susceptibility pattern of the source case isolate, only two (5%) developed disease compared with 13 (20%) who were observed without treatment.[93] Most of the children were treated with PZA, ethambutol (EMB), and ethionamide (ETH), all administered by DOT. In New York City, 51 children with tuberculosis infection diagnosed after exposure to MDR-TB were treated with 2–7 drugs, most commonly a fluoroquinolone, cycloserine, and PZA for an average of ten months. Among those who were evaluable, eight (24%) had an adverse event, with gastrointestinal toxicity being the most common, although only two required discontinuation of therapy; no patients developed disease 2–10 years after treatment.[95] In a large prospective South African cohort of 186 children younger than five years of age treated with a three-drug regimen (ofloxacin, EMB, and high-dose INH) for six months, 3% developed a grade 3 adverse event, although half of these were caused by inadvertent overdosing of the fluoroquinolone.[96] The most common adverse events included gastrointestinal toxicity and dermatological reactions. After 12–24 months of follow up, six (3.2%) children had developed incident disease.[96] Most recently, adult and child contacts of MDR-TB in the Federated States of Micronesia were treated with a fluoroquinolone-based regimen tailored to source case drug-susceptibility testing (levofloxacin for those under 12 years of age, moxifloxacin for those over 12 years, with either EMB or ETH). Although 53% of the subjects reported at least one adverse effect, no serious adverse events were reported, and only 4% discontinued therapy related

to adverse effects.[91] Treatment was better tolerated by children than adults. Among 43 children under 18 years of age, only one discontinued treatment for hepatitis, which was attributed to hepatitis A infection. None of the children who were treated developed tuberculosis disease.

Based on these studies, fluoroquinolone-based treatment for child contacts to a case of MDR-TB is well tolerated and results in a low rate of incident disease. It is unclear if addition of a second drug adds to effectiveness. Until further evidence is available, consultation with an expert is recommended for the management of infants, children, and adolescents exposed to persons with MDR-TB. When possible, the selection of drugs for children and adolescents should be guided by drug susceptibility results of the isolate from the person to whom the patient was exposed. The optimal duration of therapy remains unclear, and DOT is recommended to enhance adherence and monitor for adverse effects. Given the unclear efficacy of any of the regimens proposed, children should be followed clinically for at least a year after completion of treatment to monitor for development of disease.

REFERENCES

1. World Health Organization. *Global Tuberculosis Control, Surveillance, Planning, Financing: 2010.* Report No.: WHO/HTM/TB/2006.362. World Health Organization 2010.
2. Lobue P, Menzies D. Treatment of latent tuberculosis infection: an update. *Respirology.* 2010;15:603–622.
3. Marais BJ, Gie RP, Schaaf HS, et al. The natural history of childhood intrathoracic tuberculosis: a critical review of literature from the pre-chemotherapy era. *Int J Tuberc Lung Dis.* 2004;8:392–402.
4. Menzies D, Alvarez GG, Khan K; Centre for Communicable Diseases and Infection Control; Public Health Agency of Canada and Canadian Lung Association. Chapter 6: Treatment of latent tuberculosis infection. In: *Canadian Tuberculosis Standards.* 7th ed. Ottawa: Public Health Agency of Canada and Canadian Lung Association; 2014.
5. National Institutes for Clinical Excellence. Tuberculosis: clinical diagnosis and management of tuberculosis, and measures for its prevention and control. Available at www.nice.org.uk/guidance/CG117, accessed January 17, 2015.

6. American Thoracic Society. Targeted tuberculin testing and treatment of latent tuberculosis infection. *Am J Respir Crit Care Med.* 2000;161:S221–S247.

7. World Health Organization. Recommendations for investigating contacts of persons with infectious tuberculosis in low- and middle-income countries. Report No.: WHO/HTM/TB/2012.9. Geneva: World Health Organization; 2012.

8. World Health Organization. Guidelines on the management of latent tuberculosis infection. Report No. WHO/HTM/TB/2015.01. Geneva: World Health Organization; 2015.

9. Lincoln EM. The effect of antimicrobial therapy on the prognosis of primary tuberculosis in children. *Am Rev Tuberc.* 1954;69:682–689.

10. American Thoracic Society. Preventive treatment in tuberculosis: a statement by the Committee on Therapy. *Am Rev Respir Dis.* 1965;91:297–298.

11. Horsburgh Jr CR, Rubin EJ. Latent tuberculosis infection in the United States. *N Engl J Med.* 2011;364:1441–1448.

12. International Union Against Tuberculosis Committee on Prophylaxis. Efficacy of various durations of isoniazid preventive therapy for tuberculosis: five years of follow-up in the IUAT trial. *Bull World Health Organ.* 1982;60:555–564.

13. Snider DE, Caras GJ, Koplan JP. Preventive therapy with isoniazid: cost-effectiveness of different durations of therapy. *JAMA.* 1986;255:1579–1583.

14. American Thoracic Society; Centers for Disease Control. Treatment of tuberculosis and tuberculosis infection in adults and children. *Am Rev Respir Dis.* 1986;134:355–363.

15. Comstock GQ. How much isoniazid is needed for prevention of tuberculosis among immunocompetent adults? *Int J Tuberc Lung Dis.* 1999;3:847–850.

16. Comstock GW, Hammes LM, Pio A. Isoniazid prophylaxis in Alaskan boarding school: a comparison of two doses. *Am Rev Respir Dis.* 1969;100:773–779.

17. Mount FW, Ferrebee SH. Preventive effects of isoniazid in the treatment of primary tuberculosis in children. *N Engl J Med.* 1961;265:713–721.

18. Hsu KH. Thirty years after isoniazid: its impact on tuberculosis in children and adolescents. *JAMA.* 1984;251:1283–1285.

19. American Academy of Pediatrics. Tuberculosis. In: Pickering LK, Baker CG, Kimberlin DW, et al., eds. *Red Book: 2012 Report of the Committee on Infectious Diseases.* 29th ed. Elk Grove Village, IL: American Academy of Pediatrics; 2012:736–759.

20. Akolo C, Adetifa I, Shepperd S, Volmink J. Treatment of latent tuberculosis infection in HIV infected persons. Review. *Cochrane Database Syst Rev.* 2010, Issue 1, Art. No.: CD000171.

21. World Health Organization. Guidelines for intensified tuberculosis case-finding and isoniazid preventive therapy for people living with HIV in resource-constrained settings. Geneva: World Health Organization; 2011. Available at www.who.int/hiv/topics/tb/en/index.html.

22. Samandari T, Agizew TB, Nyirenda S, et al. Six-month versus 36-month isoniazid preventive treatment for tuberculosis in adults with HIV infection in Botswana: a randomized, double-blind placebo-controlled trial. *Lancet.* 2011;377:1588–1598.

23. Perriens JH, St. Louis ME, Mukadi YB, et al. Pulmonary tuberculosis n HIV-infected patients in Zaire. A controlled trial of treatment for either 6 or 12 months. *N Engl J Med.* 1995;332:779–784.

24. Haller L, Sossouhounto R, Coulibaly IM, et al. Isoniazid plus sulfadoxine-pyrimethamine can reduce morbidity of HIV-positive patients treated for tuberculosis in Africa: a controlled clinical trial. *Chemotherapy.* 1999;45:452–465.

25. Fitzgerald DW, Desvarieux M, Severe P, et al. Effect of post-treatment isoniazid on prevention of recurrent tuberculosis in HIV-1-infected individuals: a randomized trial. *Lancet.* 2000;356:1470–1474.

26. Vernon A. Treatment of latent tuberculosis infection. *Semin Respir Crit Care Med.* 2013;34:67–86.

27. Zar HJ, Cotton MF, Strauss S, et al. Effect of isoniazid prophylaxis on mortality and incidence of tuberculosis in children with HIV: randomized controlled trial. *BMJ.* 2006;334:136–142.

28. Madhi SA, Nachman S, Violari A, et al. Primary isoniazid against tuberculosis in HIV-exposed children. *N Engl J Med.* 2011;365:21–31.

29. Kopanoff DE, Snider D, Caras G. Isoniazid related hepatitis: a U.S. Public Health Service cooperative surveillance study. *Am Rev Respir Dis.* 1979;117:991–1001.

30. Nolan CM, Goldberg S, Buskin S. Hepatotoxicity associated with isoniazid preventive therapy: a 7 year survey from a public health tuberculosis clinic. *JAMA.* 1999;281:1014–1018.

31. Lobue PA, Moser KS. Isoniazid- and rifampin-resistant tuberculosis in San Diego County, California, United States, 1993–2002. *Int J Tuberc Lung Dis.* 2005;9:501–506.

32. Fountain FF, Tolley E, Chrisman CR, Self TH. Isoniazid hepatotoxicity associated with

treatment of latent tuberculosis infection: a 7-year evaluation from a public health tuberculosis clinic. *Chest.* 2005;128:116–123.

33. Chang SH, Nahid P, Eitzman SR. Hepatotoxicity in children receiving isoniazid therapy for latent tuberculosis infection. *J Pediatr Infect Dis Soc.* 2014;3:221–227.

34. Spyridis NP, Spyridis PG, Gelesme A, et al. The effectiveness of a 9-month regimen of isoniazid alone versus 3- and 4-month regimens of isoniazid plus rifampin for treatment of latent tuberculosis infection in children: results of an 11-year randomized study. *Clin Infect Dis.* 2007;45:715–722.

35. Nakajo MM, Rao M, Steiner P. Incidence of hepatotoxicity in children receiving isoniazid chemoprophylaxis. *Pediatr Infect Dis J.* 1989;8:649–650.

36. Hsu KH. Isoniazid in the prevention and treatment of tuberculosis. A 20 year study of the effectiveness in children. *JAMA.* 1974;229:528–533.

37. Palusci VJ, O'Hare D, Lawrence RM. Hepatotoxicity and transaminase maeasurement during isoniazid chemoprophylaxis in children. *Pediatr Infect Dis J.* 1995;14;144–148.

38. Wu SS, Chao CS, Vargas JH, et al. Isoniazid-related hepatic failure in children: a survey of liver transplantation centers. *Transplantation.* 2007;84:173–179.

39. Centers for Disease Control and Prevention (CDC). Severe isoniazid-associated liver injuries among persons being treated for latent tuberculosis infection—United States, 2004–2008. *Morb Mortal Wkly Rep (MMWR).* 2010;59:224–229.

40. Halsey NA, Coberly JS, Desormeaux J, et al. Rifampin and pyrazinamide vs. isoniazid for prevention of tuberculosis in HIV-1 infected persons: an international randomized trial. *Lancet.* 1998;351:786–792.

41. Mwinga A, Hosp M, Godfrey-Faussett P, et al. Twice-weekly tuberculosis preventive therapy in HIV infection in Zambia. *AIDS.* 1998;12:2447–2457.

42. Cruz AT, Starke JR. Twice-weekly therapy for children with tuberculosis infection or exposure. *Int J Tuberc Lung Dis.* 2013; 17:169–174.

43. Hong Kong Chest Service Tuberculosis Research Centre MBMRC. A double-blind placebo-controlled clinical trial of three antituberculosis chemoprophylaxis regimens in patients with silicosis in Hong Kong. *Am Rev Respir Dis.* 1992;145:36–41.

44. Polesky A, Farber HW, Gottlieb DJ, et al. Rifampin preventive therapy for tuberculosis in Boston's homeless. *Am J Respir Crit Care Med.* 1996;154:1473–1477.

45. Villarino ME, Ridzon R, Weismuller PC, et al. Rifampin preventive therapy for tuberculosis infection: experience with 157 adolescents. *Am J Respir Crit Care Med.* 1997;155:1735–1738.

46. Menzies D, Dion MJ, Rabinovitch B, Mannix S, Brassard P, Schwartzman K. Treatment completion and costs of a randomized trial of rifampin for four months versus isoniazid for 9 months. *Am J Respir Crit Care Med.* 2004;170:445–449.

47. Menzies D, Long R, Trajman A, et al. Adverse events with four months rifampin or 9 months isoniazid therapy for latent tuberculosis infection: a randomized trial. *Ann Intern Med.* 2008;149:689–697.

48. Fountain FF, Tolley EA, Jacobs AR, Self TH. Rifampin hepatotoxicity associated with treatment of latent tuberculosis infection. *Am J Med Sci.* 2009;337:317–320.

49. Page KR, Sifakis F, Montes de Oca R, et al. Improved adherence and less toxicity with rifampin vs isoniazid for treatment of latent tuberculosis: a retrospective study. *Arch Intern Med.* 2006;166:1863–1870.

50. Lardizabal A, Passannante M, Kojakali F, Hayden C, Reichman LB. Enhancement of treatment completion for latent tuberculosis infection with four months of rifampin. *Chest.* 2006;130:1712–1717.

51. Joint Tuberculosis Committee of the British Thoracic Society. Chemotherapy and management of tuberculosis in the United Kingdom. *Thorax.* 1998;53:536–548.

52. Ena J, Valls V. Short course therapy with rifampin plus isoniazid, compared with standard therapy with isoniazid, for latent tuberculosis infection: a meta-analysis. *Clin Infect Dis.* 2005;40:670–676.

53. Ormerod LP. Reduced incidence of tuberculosis by prophylactic chemotherapy in subjects showing strong reactions to tuberculin testing. *Arch Dis Child.* 1987;62:1005–1008.

54. Ormerod LP. Rifampicin and isoniazid prophylactic chemotherapy for tuberculosis. *Arch Dis Child.* 1998;78:169–171.

55. Bright-Thomas R, Nandwani S, Smith J, Morris JA, Ormerod LP. Effectiveness of 3 months of rifampicin and isoniazid chemoprophylaxis for the treatment of latent tuberculosis infection in children. *Arch Dis Child.* 2010;95:600–602.

56. Whalen CC, Johnson JL, Okwera A, et al. A trial of three regimens to prevent tuberculosis

in Ugandan adults infected with the human immunodeficiency virus. *N Engl J Med*. 1997;337:801–808.

57. Martinson NA, Barnes GL, Moulton LH, et al. New regimens to prevent tuberculosis in adults with HIV infection. *N Engl J Med*. 2011;365:11–20.

58. Martinez-Alfaro E, Cuadra F, Solera J et al.; The GECMEI Group. Evaluation of 2 tuberculosis chemoprophylaxis regimens in patients infected with human immunodeficiency virus [in Spanish]. *Med Clin (Barc)*. 2000;115:161–165.

59. Rivero A, López-Cortés L, Castillo R, et al.; Grupo Andaluz para el estudio de las Enfermedades Infecciosas (GAEI). Randomized trial of three regimens to prevent tuberculosis in HIV-infected patients with anergy [in Spanish]. *Enferm Infecc Microbiol Clin*. 2003;21:287–292.

60. Rivero A, López-Cortés L, Castillo R, et al.; Grupo Andaluz para el estudio de las Enfermedades Infecciosas (GAEI). Randomized clinical trial investigating three chemoprophylaxis regimens for latent tuberculosis infection in HIV-infected patients [in Spanish]. *Enferm Infecc Microbiol Clin*. 2007;25:305–310.

61. Centers for Disease Control and Prevention. Recommendations for use of an isoniazid-rifapentine regimen with direct observation to treat latent *Mycobacterium tuberculosis* infection. *MMWR*. 2011;60:1650–1653.

62. Sterling TR, Villarino E, Borisov AS, et al., for the TB Trials Consortium PREVENT TB Study Team. Three months of rifapentine and isoniazid for latent tuberculosis infection. *N Engl J Med*. 2011;365:2155–2166.

63. Schechter M, Zajdenverg R, Falco G, et al. Weekly rifapentine/isoniazid or daily rifampin/ pyrazinamide for latent tuberculosis in household contacts. *Am J Respir Crit Care Med*. 2006;173:922–926.

64. Villarino ME, Scott NA, Weis SE, et al., for the International Maternal Pediatric and Adolescents AIDS Clinical Trials Group (IMPAACT), and the Tuberculosis Trials Consortium (TBTC). Treatment for preventing tuberculosis in children: a trial of a 3-month, 12-dose regimen of rifapentine and isoniazid. *JAMA Pediatr*. 2015;169:247–255.

65. Halsey NA, Coberly JS, Desormeaux J, et al. Rifampin and pyrazinamide vs. isoniazid for prevention of tuberculosis in HIV-1 infected persons: an international randomized trial. *Lancet*. 1998;351:786–792.

66. Gordin F, Chaisson RE, Matts JP, et al. Rifampin and pyrazinamide vs. isoniazid for prevention of tuberculosis in HIV-infected persons. *JAMA*. 2000;283:1445–1450.

67. Centers for Disease Control. Fatal and severe hepatitis associated with rifampin and pyrazinamide for the treatment of latent tuberculosis infection—New York and Georgia, 2000. *MMWR*. 2001;50:289–291.

68. McElroy PD, Ijaz K, Lambert LA, et al. National survey to measure rates of liver injury, hospitalization, and death associated with rifampin and pyrazinamide for latent tuberculosis infection. *Clin Infect Dis*. 2005;41 1125–1133.

69. Ijaz K, Jereb JA, Lambert LA, et al. Severe or fatal liver injury in 50 patients in the United States taking rifampin and pyrazinamide for latent tuberculosis infection. *Clin Infect Dis*. 2006;42:346–355.

70. American Thoracic Society and Centers for Disease Control and Prevention. Update: adverse event data and revised American Thoracic Society/CDC recommendations against the use of rifampin and pyrazinamide for the treatment of latent tuberculosis infection—United States, 2003. *MMWR*. 2003;52:735–739.

71. Magdorf K, Arizzi Rusche AF, Geiter LJ, O'Brien RJ, Wahn U. Short-course therapy for tuberculosis: a pilot study of rifampin-pyrazinamide regimens in children. *Am Rev Resp Dis*. 1991;143:A119.

72. Horsburgh Jr. CR, Goldberg S, Bethel J, et al.; and the Tuberculosis Epidemiologic Studies Consortium. Latent TB infection treatment acceptance and completion in the United States and Canada. *Chest*. 2010;137:401–409.

73. Reichler MR, Reves R, Bur S, et al. Treatment of latent tuberculosis infection in contacts of new tuberculosis cases in the United States. *South Med J*. 2002;95:414–420.

74. Yuan L, Richardson E, Kendall PRW. Evaluation of a tuberculosis screening program for high-risk students in Toronto schools. *Can Med Assoc J*. 1995;153:925–932.

75. Lobue PA, Moser KS. Use of isoniazid for latent tuberculosis infection in a public health clinic. *Am J Resp Crit Care Med*. 2003;168:443–447.

76. Bock NN, Metzger BS, Tapia JR, Blumberg HM. A tuberculin screening and isoniazid preventive therapy program in an inner-city population. *Am J Resp Crit Care Med*. 1999;159:295–300.

77. Brassard P, Steensma C, Cadieux L, Lands LC. Evaluation of a school-based tuberculosis-screening program and associate investigation targeting recently immigrated children in a low-burden country. *Pediatrics.* 2006;117:e148–e156.

78. Marais BJ, van Zyl S, Schaaf HS, van Aardt M, Gie RP, Beyers GN. Adherence to isoniazid preventive chemotherapy: a prospective community based study. *Arch Dis Child.* 2006;91:762–765.

79. Guwatudde D, Nakakeeto M, Jones-Lopez EC, et al. Tuberculosis in household contacts of infectious cases in Kampala, Uganda. *Am J Epidemiol.* 2003;158:887–898.

80. van Zyl S, Marais BJ, Hesseling AC, Gie RP, Beyers N, Schaaf HS. Adherence to anti-tuberculosis chemoprophylaxis and treatment in children. *Int J Tuberc Lung Dis.* 2006;10:13–18.

81. Colson PW, Franks J, Sondengam R, Hirsch-Moverman Y, El-Sadr W. Tuberculosis knowledge, attitudes and beliefs in foreign-born and US-born patients with latent tuberculosis infection. *J Immig Minor Health.* 2010;12:859–866.

82. Powell DA, Perkins L, Wang SH, Hunt G, Ryan-Wenger N. Completion of therapy for latent tuberculosis in children of different nationalities. *Ped Infect Dis J.* 2008;28:272–274.

83. Cruz AT, Starke JR. Increasing adherence for latent tuberculosis infection therapy with health department-administered therapy. *Pediatr Infect Dis J.* 2012;31:193–195.

84. Kohn MR, Arden MR, Vasilakis J, Shenker IR. Directly observed preventive therapy. Turning the tide against tuberculosis. *Arch Pediatr Adolesc Med.* 1996;150:727–729.

85. Sass P, Cooper K, Robertson V. School-based tuberculosis testing and treatment program: comparing directly observed preventive therapy with traditional preventive therapy. *J Public Health Manag Pract.* 1996;2:32–40.

86. Cruz AT, Ahmed A, Mandalakas AM, Starke JR. Treatment of latent tuberculosis infection in children. *J Pediatr Infectious Dis Soc.* 2014;2:248–258.

87. Saukkonen JJ, Cohn DL, Jasmer RM, et al.; American Thoracic Society Hepatotoxicity of Antituberculosis Therapy Subcommittee. An official ATS statement: hepatotoxicity of antituberculous therapy. *Am J Respir Crit Care Med.* 2006;174:935–952.

88. Kass JS, Shandera WX. Nervous system effects of antituberculosis therapy. *CNS Drugs.* 2010;24:655–667.

89. Package insert. Rifampin for injection, USP. Available at http://www.akorn.com/documents/catalog/sell_sheets/17478-151-42.pdf (accessed Dec. 27, 2014).

90. Weiner M, Savic RM, MacKenzie WR, et al. Rifapentine pharmacokinetics and tolerability in children and adults treated once weekly with rifapentine and isoniazid for latent tuberculosis infection. *J Ped Infect Dis Soc.* 2014;3:132–145.

91. Bamrah S, Brostrom R, Dorina F, et al. Treatment of LTBI in contacts of MDR-TB patients, Federated States of Micronesia, 2009–2012. *Int J Tuberc Lung Dis.* 2014;18:912–918.

92. Schaaf HS, Gie RP, Kennedy M, Beyers N, Hesseling PB, Donald PR. Evaluation of young children in contact with adult multidrug-resistant pulmonary tuberculosis: a 30-month follow-up. *Pediatrics.* 2002;109:765–771.

93. Schaaf HS, Van Rie A, Gie RP, et al. Transmission of multidrug-resistant pulmonary tuberculosis. *Pediatr Infect Dis J.* 2000;19:695–699.

94. Schaaf HS, Vermeulen HA, Gie RP, Beyers N, Donald PR. Evaluation of young children in household contact with adult multidrug-resistant pulmonary tuberculosis cases. *Pediatr Infect Dis J.* 1999;18:494–500.

95. Feja K, McNelley E, Tran CS, Burzynski J, Saiman L. Management of pediatric multidrug-resistant tuberculosis and latent tuberculosis infections in New York City from 1995–2003. *Pediatr Infect Dis J.* 2008;27:907–912.

96. Seddon JA, Hesseling AC, Finalyson H, et al. Preventive therapy for child contacts of multidrug-resistant tuberculosis: A prospective cohort study. *Clin Infect Dis.* 2013;57:1676–1684.

97. Fitzgerald DW et al. Effect of post-treatment isoniazid on prevention of recurrent tuberculosis in HIV-1 infected individuals: a randomized trial. *Lancet.* 2000;356:1470–1474.

17

MANAGEMENT OF DRUG-SUSCEPTIBLE TUBERCULOSIS IN CHILDREN

Soumya Swaminathan and N. Poorana Ganga Devi

HIGHLIGHTS OF THIS CHAPTER

- The main objectives of antituberculosis treatment are to cure the patient of the disease, minimize long-term sequelae, prevent relapse, prevent the development of drug resistance, and reduce transmission of the organism to others, and do all this with minimal toxicity.
- Drug regimens that are used currently in adults are effective for children; however, when any new drug or combination of drugs is introduced, it is critical that the safety, tolerability, and pharmacokinetics of the drug or regimen be studied in children of all ages.
- Children with suspected or confirmed pulmonary tuberculosis or tuberculosis lymphadenitis living in settings with a high HIV-prevalence infection and/or a high prevalence of isoniazid resistance (>4%), and/or children with extensive pulmonary disease, should be treated with a six-month regimen consisting of a four-drug regimen (INH, RMP, PZA, EMB) for two months followed by a two-drug regimen (INH and RMP) for four months.
- Children with suspected or confirmed tuberculous meningitis or osteoarticular tuberculosis should be treated with a 12-month regimen consisting of a four-drug regimen (INH, RMP, PZA, EMB) for two months, followed by a two-drug regimen (INH and RMP) for 10 months.
- Corticosteroids are often given together with antituberculosis treatment when post-inflammatory sequelae are likely to lead to obstructive complications, as in tuberculous meningitis, CNS tuberculomas, massively enlarged intrathoracic lymph nodes, pericardial effusion, and tuberculosis of the urinary tract.

PRINCIPLES OF TREATMENT IN CHILDREN

TREATMENT OF TUBERCULOSIS in children follows the same basic principles as in adults. A combination of drugs is used to achieve a bactericidal and sterilizing effect on the infection with *M. tuberculosis*. The main objectives of antituberculosis treatment are to cure the patient of the disease, minimize long-term sequelae, prevent relapse, and do this with minimal toxicity. Other goals of treatment are to prevent the development of drug resistance and reduce transmission of the organism to others. Both transmission and emergence of drug resistance are more likely when pulmonary disease is associated with high bacterial loads, a situation less likely for children than for adults. However, children with pulmonary disease can also transmit *M. tuberculosis* (especially if they have adult-type disease with cavitation and acid-fast sputum smear positivity), in which case the appropriate precautions must be taken. It is important to understand that treatment of tuberculosis benefits both the community as a whole and the individual patient. Thus, any public health program or private provider undertaking to treat a patient with tuberculosis is assuming a public health function that includes not only prescribing an appropriate regimen, but also ensuring adherence to the regimen until treatment is completed.

The tuberculosis treatment regimens we use today evolved after a series of clinical trials in adult tuberculosis patients conducted by the British Medical Research Council and others, which established the basic principles of treatment and tested various drug combinations given for varying periods of time.[1-5] These early trials and the microbiological studies that accompanied them demonstrated that different drugs had actions on different populations of the tubercle bacilli (actively replicating, intracellular, intermittently replicating, or dormant) and that monotherapy for tuberculosis disease invariably led to emergence of drug resistance. Starting from treatment regimens requiring 18–24 months' duration, the currently used modern short-course chemotherapy of six months, for which rifampin (RMP) and pyrazinamide (PZA) are essential, was developed.

Tuberculosis in young children is usually paucibacillary and involves the intrathoracic lymph nodes, but extrapulmonary disease is common, and the greatest risk of progression to disease after infection is in the first two years of life. Microbiological confirmation is often difficult, requiring multiple specimens other than sputum and is achieved in less than 30–50% of cases. The rates of primary drug resistance in most parts of the world are low (< 3%); however, the rates in children reflect adult drug resistance rates in a region and, therefore, culture and drug susceptibility testing must be carried out whenever possible.[6]

RECOMMENDED DOSAGES OF ANTITUBERCULOSIS DRUGS

Efficient killing of *M. tuberculosis* depends on peak drug levels (C_{max}) and area under the curve (AUC) and the ratio of C_{max}/MIC and AUC/MIC.[7] Almost every aspect of pharmacokinetics (absorption, distribution, metabolism, excretion) is subject to age-related differences (See also Chapter 15).[8] Previous dosing recommendations for children of various ages were extrapolated from adult studies, and mg/kg doses were calculated assuming that the metabolism of drugs in children would be similar to adults'. Pharmacokinetic studies evaluating whether these extrapolated doses achieved target blood levels in children were not done in the past.

Based on available evidence, the World Health Organization (WHO) revised treatment guidelines for children in 2010.[9] The dosages of the first-line antituberculosis medicines that should be used for the daily treatment of tuberculosis disease in children are listed in Table 17.1. These recommendations are independent of HIV status.

Age has a major influence on drug metabolism: a particular mg/kg dose of a drug when given to a child under five years of age generally achieves a lower serum concentration than when given to an older child or adult. Higher mg/kg dosages are therefore required in younger children to achieve levels that are considered to produce effective bactericidal or sterilizing activity.[10] For example, recent studies have shown that the bactericidal effect of RMP increases linearly with increasing dosage and concomitant C_{max}, suggesting that the previously used RMP dosage of 10 mg/kg for all children is suboptimal.[11] Under current guidelines for the dosing range for rifampin, a one-year-old child should be dosed at 20 mg/kg, an eight-year-old at 15 mg/kg, and a twelve-year-old at 10–12 mg/kg. In fact, the optimal dose of rifampin in children of various ages has not yet been firmly established. A safety, efficacy, pharmacokinetics, and early bactericidal

Table 17.1. Recommended daily doses of first-line antituberculosis drugs for children

ANTI-TB DRUG	DOSE AND RANGE (MG/KG BODY WEIGHT)	MAXIMUM DOSE (MG)
Isoniazid (INH)	10 (7–15)[a]	300
Rifampin (RMP)	15 (10–20)	600
Pyrazinamide (PZA)	35 (30–40)	-
Ethambutol (EMB)	20 (15–25)	-

[a]The higher end of the range for isoniazid dose applies to younger children; as the children grow older, the lower end of the dosing range becomes more appropriate.

Source: Rapid Advice: Treatment of Tuberculosis in Children. Geneva: World Health Organization; 2010. (WHO/HTM/TB/2010).

Remark: As children approach a body weight of 25 kg, clinicians can use adult dosing recommendations.

activity study in adults using rifampin at 20, 25, 30, and 35 mg/kg daily for two weeks demonstrated that all of these dosages were safe and well tolerated. Further, there was a nonlinear increase in exposure to rifampin without an apparent ceiling effect and a greater estimated fall in bacterial load in the higher dosing groups.[12] It is possible that even greater doses of rifampin in children would be more effective.

Other factors known to impact blood levels of antituberculosis drugs are nutritional status, pharmacogenetic differences, and HIV infection. Stunting has been shown to be associated with lower blood levels of pyrazinamide and rifampin.[13,14] Three acetylator genotypes (rapid, intermediate, and slow) result in two phenotypes (as rapid and intermediate behave similarly) of isoniazid metabolism, and peak levels and AUC of isoniazid are 40–50% lower in rapid acetylators. The proportion of slow and rapid acetylators varies between ethnic groups; the status of an individual can be checked either by genotyping the N-acetyltransferase gene or by an isoniazid excretion test.[15] Rapid acetylators may not respond as well when given drugs intermittently (twice-weekly or less). Similarly, polymorphisms in the *SLCO1* drug transporter gene have been shown to result in significantly lower rifampin exposure, and additional data are emerging from different parts of the world. In the African patient population with its high frequency of the *SLCO1B1* (rs4149032) polymorphism, peak rifampin levels were well below the acceptable range of 8–24 ug/ml[16] suggesting that higher dosages may be warranted. HIV infection has been shown to result in lower antituberculosis drug exposure both in adults and children; while the exact reason for this is not known, malabsorption due to other infections and HIV enteropathy are presumed to play a major role.[17]

Pharmacokinetic studies using the recently revised WHO dosages showed significantly higher blood levels in young children, including those under two years of age, compared to the previous doses.[9,11,18] Systematic review of the evidence also shows that the revised dosages have an excellent safety profile and are not associated with an increased risk of toxicity, including an increased risk of drug-induced hepatotoxicity due to isoniazid or pyrazinamide, or of optic neuritis due to ethambutol.[19,20] However, a recent study showed that drug concentrations of all first-line antituberculosis drugs were markedly below the target therapeutic concentrations in most South African children who received the revised WHO-recommended pediatric weight-based dosages.[21]

RECOMMENDED TREATMENT REGIMENS

Both the bacillary load and the type and anatomical site of disease may influence the effectiveness of treatment regimens. Treatment outcomes in children are generally good, even in young and immunocompromised children who are at higher risk of disease progression and disseminated disease, provided that treatment starts promptly. There is a low risk of adverse events associated with use of the recommended treatment regimens.

Antituberculosis treatment is divided into two phases: an intensive phase and a continuation phase. The purpose of the intensive phase is to rapidly eliminate the majority of organisms and to prevent the emergence of drug resistance. This phase uses a greater number of drugs than the continuation phase. The purpose of the continuation phase is to complete sterilization of the lesions by eliminating even the slowly growing and dormant organisms. Fewer drugs are generally used in this phase because the risk of acquiring drug resistance is low, as most of the organisms have already been eliminated.

WHO guidelines state that children with suspected or confirmed pulmonary tuberculosis or tuberculous peripheral lymphadenitis who live in settings with low HIV prevalence and low prevalence of isoniazid resistance, and children in any setting with low prevalence of isoniazid resistance who are known to be HIV-uninfected, can be treated with a six-month regimen consisting of a three-drug regimen of isoniazid (INH), rifampin (RMP), and pyrazinamide (PZA) for two months, followed by a two-drug (INH and RMP) regimen for four months at the specified dosages. Children with suspected or confirmed pulmonary tuberculosis or tuberculosis peripheral lymphadenitisliving in settings with a high HIV prevalence infection and/or a high prevalence of isoniazid resistance (>4%), and/or children with extensive pulmonary disease, should be treated with a six-month regimen consisting of a four-drug regimen (INH, RMP, PZA, and ethambutol [EMB]) for two months followed by a two-drug regimen (INH and RMP) for four months. In these settings, four drugs are preferred in order to reduce the risk of development and transmission of MDR-TB, and baseline isoniazid resistance is known to be the strongest risk factor for acquired rifampin resistance.[9,22,23]

Infants aged 0–3 months with suspected or confirmed pulmonary tuberculosis or tuberculous peripheral lymphadenitis should be promptly treated with standard treatment regimens described above. There are very limited data to inform drug dosages for neonates, who have certain characteristics—especially in the first week of life—that are likely to affect drug metabolism. Treatment may require dose adjustment to reconcile the effect of age and possible toxicity in young infants. The decision to adjust doses should be made by a clinician experienced in managing pediatric tuberculosis. If such expertise is not available, and tuberculosis disease has been either definitively diagnosed or is strongly suspected, treatment with the standard drug regimen should be considered.

During the continuation phase of treatment, twice- or thrice-weekly regimens can be considered for children known to be HIV-uninfected and living in settings with well-established directly-observed therapy (DOT). While there have been no clinical trials directly comparing daily and thrice-weekly treatment in children, a systematic review showed that twice-weekly therapy was less likely to achieve a cure than daily treatment.[24] However, a Cochrane review concluded that trials conducted to date are insufficient to support or refute the use of intermittent twice- or thrice-weekly, short-course treatment regimens in comparison to daily short-course treatment in children with tuberculosis.[25] Intermittent regimens may be an alternative in a non-HIV endemic setting, provided that each dose is directly observed, but should preferably not be used to treat children living in settings with high HIV prevalence (or with confirmed HIV infection) or children with extensive pulmonary tuberculosis or disseminated forms of disease such as miliary or meningeal tuberculosis.[10,23] A pharmacokinetic study in children treated with a thrice-weekly regimen in India found significantly lower peak rifampin levels in HIV-infected compared to HIV-uninfected patients, which was associated with worse treatment outcomes.[26] The 2010 WHO guidelines also advised that intermittent regimens not be used in HIV-infected patient populations. The guidelines further advised that streptomycin should not be used as part of first-line treatment regimens for children with most forms of tuberculosis.

Children with suspected or confirmed drug-susceptible tuberculous meningitis or osteo-articular tuberculosis should be treated with a 12-month regimen consisting of a four-drug regimen (INH, RMP, PZA, EMB) for two months, followed by a two-drug regimen (INH and RMP) for 10 months. The doses recommended for the treatment of tuberculous meningitis are the same as those described for pulmonary tuberculosis. A recently published Indonesian study showed that giving an initial regimen that included intravenous RMP at 13 mg/kg and moxifloxacin (400 mg or 800 mg), in addition to INH and PZA, halved six-month mortality due to tuberculous meningitis in adults, without significant toxicity.[27] A clinical trial (TBM Kids) to be initiated shortly will test this regimen in children.[28]

Table 17.2. Recommended treatment regimens for new cases of tuberculosis in children

TUBERCULOSIS DIAGNOSTIC CATEGORY	ANTITUBERCULOSIS DRUG REGIMENS*	
	INTENSIVE PHASE	CONTINUATION PHASE
Tuberculosis disease (except meningitis and osteoarticular tuberculosis) in HIV-uninfected children with low (≤4%) risk of INH resistance	2HRZ	4HR
Tuberculosis disease (except meningitis and osteoarticular tuberculosis) in children with HIV infection or with a high (>4%) risk of isoniazid resistance	2HRZE	4HR

*The standard code for antituberculosis treatment regimens uses an abbrevation for each drug: isoniazid (H), rifampin (R), pyrazinamide (Z), and ethambutol (E). A regimen consists of two phases—the initial and the continuation phase. The number at the front of each phase represents the duration of the phase in months.

Table 17.2 lists recommendations for treatment regimens made by various bodies, while Table 17.3 tabulates treatment outcomes from observational studies and clinical trials using a variety of short-course regimens. A review of national and international childhood tuberculosis treatment guidelines published to date indicates very little disagreement on recommended treatment regimens and modalities.[29] India is one of the last countries to switch over from thrice-weekly to daily treatment in the national program.[30]

OTHER MANAGEMENT ISSUES

Corticosteroids

Corticosteroids are often given together with antituberculosis treatment in the management of some forms of disease, especially those where post-inflammatory sequelae are likely to lead to obstructive complications (e.g., serosal surfaces and narrow passages). Examples are tuberculous meningitis, brain tuberculomas, massively enlarged mediastinal/paratracheal lymph nodes, pericardial effusion, and tuberculosis of the urinary bladder and ureters. The need for corticosteroids is less clear in some situations—e.g., massive pleural effusion, miliary, and intestinal tuberculosis—where their use is often based on clinical judgement. Most studies of corticosteroids in pulmonary and extrapulmonary tuberculosis have been conducted in adults and the results extrapolated to children (Table 17.4).

Corticosteroids have been shown to improve survival and reduce morbidity in tuberculous meningitis (TBM) and are recommended for all cases of tuberculous meningitis.[42] The mechanisms by which corticosteroids improve outcome in TBM are still not fully understood. A fascinating hypothesis recently suggested originates in a genetic hint. The gene *LTA4H* that encodes leukotriene A4 hydrolase determines the balance of pro-inflammatory and anti-inflammatory eicosanoids; in one study, corticosteroids reduced mortality only in TBM patients who were major allele homozygous for that gene, with a hyperinflammatory phenotype.[43] It could also explain why some patients get worse with corticosteroids—probably those with a hypoinflammatory genotype. In the future, it may be possible to target corticosteroid therapy (in meningitis as well as other forms of tuberculosis) only to those patients likely to benefit, based on genetic testing.[44]

Prednisone is used most frequently, in a dosage of 2 mg/kg daily, increased to 4 mg/kg daily in the case of the most seriously ill children, with a maximum dosage of 60 mg/day, for four weeks. The dose should then be gradually tapered over 1–2 weeks before stopping. Dexamethasone in an equivalent dose also is used commonly, especially for cases of TBM.

Pyridoxine Supplementation

Isoniazid may cause symptomatic pyridoxine deficiency, which presents as peripheral neuropathy

Table 17.3. Outcomes of tuberculosis treatment from clinical trials and observational studies in children treated with a variety of short-course regimens

S. NO.	AUTHOR[S], COUNTRY, PUBLICATION	DIAGNOSTIC CRITERIA	NO. OF CHILDREN	REGIMEN	RESULTS
1	Kabra, et al. India *Indian Pediatr.* 2004; 41:927–937.[31]	Clinical and radiological	459	2HRZE$_3$/4HR$_3$	365 (80%) completed the treatment. Of the 365, 302 (83%) were cured.
2	Al-Dossary, et al. USA *Pediatr Infect Dis J.* 2002;21:91–97.[32]	Clinical and radiological	175	0.5HRZ$_7$/ 1.5HRZ$_2$/4HR$_2$	81% treatment completion, 1 relapse
3	Water Naude, et al. S. Africa *Pediatr Infect Dis J.* 2000;19:405–410.[33]	Clinical and radiological	89 117	2HRZ$_2$/4HR$_2$ 6RHZ	Treatment outcome and adherence similar between regimens, 1 relapse
4	Ramachandran, et al. India *India J Tub.* 1998;45:83–87.[34]	Clinical, radiological, and bacteriological	68 69	2HRZ$_3$/4HR$_2$ 9HR	2% died, 0 failures, 3 relapses
5	Kumar, et al. India *Pediatr Infect Dis J.* 1990;9:802–806.[35]	Clinical and bacteriological	37 39	2HRZ$_2$/4HR$_2$ 2HRZ/4HR	2 non-tuberculosis deaths, 0 relapse
6	Biddulp, et al. New Guinea *Pediatr Infect Dis J.* 1990;9:794–801.[36]	Clinical and bacteriological	639	2SHRZ / 4HR$_2$2HRZ$_2$ /4HR$_2$	2% died, 1% relapse
7	Gocmen, et al. Turkey *Infection.* 1993;1(5):324–327.[37]	Clinical and radiological	130	0.5HRS$_7$/9HR$_2$ 0.5HR$_7$/9HR$_2$	1 relapse
8	Indumathi, et al. India *Indian Pediatr.* 2010;47(1):93–96.[38]	Clinical and radiological	65	2 EHRZ$_3$/4HR$_3$	95% cure rate

9	Bai, et al. India *Indian Pediatr.* 2002;39(5):458–462.[39]	Clinical and radiological	95	2HREZ$_7$/4HR$_7$	97% showed clinical improvement at the end of 1 month and 100% at the end of 2 months. Radiologically 22% showed complete clearance and 73% showed moderate clearance at the end of therapy
10	Abernathy United States Pediatrics. 1983;72(6):801–806.[40]	Clinical and radiological	50	1HR$_7$/8HR$_2$	Symptoms cleared in 1 to 2 months
11	Kansoy, et al. Turkey *Turkish J Med Sci.* 1996;26:41–43.[41]	Clinical and radiological	36	0.5SHR/8.5H2R$_2$	100 % cure rate

H = isoniazid, R = rifampin, P = pyrazinamide, E = ethambutol, S = streptomycin.
As an example, 2HRZE$_7$ means that the four drugs were given 7 days per week for 2 months.

Table 17.4. Studies related to the use of corticosteroids in various forms of tuberculosis

CONDITION	REFERENCE	RESULTS
Tuberculous meningitis (TBM)	Thwaites, et al. *N Engl J Med.* 2004;351:1741–1751.[45]	Adjunctive dexamethasone treatment improved survival in patients with TBM at nine months.
	Prasad, et al. *Cochrane Database Syst Rev.* 2008;1:CD002244.[46]	Corticosteroids reduced the risk of death by 22% (relative risk reduction) and improved disability-free survival by 22%.
	Prasad, et al. *Cochrane Database Syst Rev.* 2000;3:CD002244.[47]	Corticosteroids significantly reduced mortality among children with TBM.
Tuberculous pericarditis	Mayosi, et al. *Cochrane Database Syst Rev.* 2002;4:CD000526.[48]	Corticosteroids decreased the risk of all-cause mortality by 35% (relative risk reduction) in HIV-seronegative patients with tubercular pericarditis.
	Strang, et al. *QJM.* 2004; 97:525–535.[49]	The apparent clinical benefit of corticosteroids was maintained even 10 years after treatment.
Tuberculous pleural effusion	Lee, et al. *Chest.* 1988; 94:1256–1259.[50] Bang, et al. *Tuberc Respir Dis.* 1997;44–52[51]	Corticosteroids significantly decreased the duration of clinical symptoms, by 4.3 days
	Engel, et al. *Cochrane Database Syst Rev.* 2007;4:CD001876[52]	Corticosteroids significantly reduced the risk of pleural thickening, by 31%.
Peritoneal tuberculosis	Singh, et al. *N Engl J Med.* 1969;281:1091–1094.[53]	In 47 patients with peritoneal tuberculosis, a non-significant reduction in the development of late fibrotic complications (symptomatic intestinal obstruction) was found.
Miliary tuberculosis	Sun, et al. *Chin Med J.* 1981;94:309–314.[54]	In 55 patients with miliary tuberculosis, a statistically non-significant reduction in mortality was found.
Pulmonary tuberculosis	*Tubercle.* 1983;64–73[55]	In 530 sputum smear-positive patients, corticosteroids had no significant effect on radiological or bacteriological responses.
HIV co-infection with paradoxical tuberculosis-IRIS	Meintjes, et al. Proceedings of the 16th Conference on Retroviruses and Opportunistic Infections.[56]	In 109 patients, corticosteroids modestly improved the composite outcome of duration of hospital stay and outpatient therapeutic procedures (counted as one additional day of hospitalization).

(tingling or numbness, weakness, foot drop), particularly in severely malnourished children, breast-fed infants, pregnancy, and HIV-infected children on antiretroviral therapy (ART). Supplemental pyridoxine (5–10 mg/day) is recommended for children and adolescents in these categories being treated with INH for tuberculosis infection or disease.[57] Acute pyridoxine deficiency caused by an overdose of isoniazid—either accidental or in a suicide attempt—can cause generalized seizures that are difficult to control unless a large dose of pyridoxine is administered.

Nutritional Support

Severe malnutrition is associated with increased mortality in both children and adults with tuberculosis; hence, a child's nutritional status should be assessed before and regularly during treatment. Many children diagnosed with tuberculosis in developing countries have associated undernutrition (low weight for age) or stunting (low weight for height). Those who need treatment for severe acute malnutrition should be referred to the appropriate rehabilitation center, while all others require appropriate nutritional support and counseling. This includes early efforts to continue breastfeeding (until at least 24 months of age, when possible) and ensuring adequate nutrient intake on the basis of locally available and affordable foods. Additional energy is particularly important during the intensive phase of treatment and is best given through supplemental household foods, provided as part of a balanced and varied diet. Infants under six months of age with tuberculosis and malnutrition or growth failure require referral to a therapeutic feeding program. If this is not available or feasible, breastfeeding mothers should be given support to optimize breastfeeding. Nutritional supplementation often cannot be given directly to an infant under six months of age but can be provided for the lactating mother.[58–61]

Immune Reconstitution

Sometimes referred to as a paradoxical reaction, this temporary exacerbation of symptoms, signs, or radiographic manifestations of tuberculosis occurs a few days to weeks after beginning antituberculosis treatment. Although more common in children and adults with tuberculosis and HIV infection after they are started on both antituberculosis treatment and ART, it can happen in HIV-uninfected children, especially those with initially severe disease. It can simulate worsening local disease, with fever and increased size of peripheral or intrathoracic lymph nodes or tuberculomas, or can cause manifestations at previously uninvolved sites. Immune reconstitution can be brought about by improved nutritional status or by the antituberculosis treatment itself. When clinical deterioration due to immune reconstitution occurs after initiation of ART in immunosuppressed HIV-infected children with tuberculosis, it is known as the immune reconstitution inflammatory syndrome (IRIS). A rapidly rising CD4+ T-cell count, rapidly falling or undetectable viral load, high baseline CRP, IL-6, and IL-18 levels, and ruling out of other possibilities for clinical deterioration such as drug-resistant tuberculosis, all suggest the diagnosis of tuberculosis-related IRIS.[62] There have been no published randomized clinical trials for treatment of IRIS in children. However, anecdotal data and results from adult studies suggest that appropriate antituberculosis treatment should be continued and the addition of corticosteroids might be beneficial, especially in severe cases, when other anti-inflammatory drugs have not controlled the symptoms. The optimal dose and duration for corticosteroid therapy is unknown and usually is gauged by the clinical response.

Management of Common Adverse Effects

As is true with all medications, combination chemotherapy for tuberculosis is associated with a predictable incidence of adverse effects, some mild, and some serious (Table 17.5).

GASTROINTESTINAL: NAUSEA, VOMITING, POOR APPETITE, ABDOMINAL PAIN

Gastrointestinal reactions are common, particularly in the first few weeks of antituberculosis therapy. Many antituberculosis drugs can cause gastrointestinal upset, particularly INH.[63] In the presence of nausea, vomiting, or abdominal pain, serum aspartate aminotransferase (AST), alanine aminotransferase (ALT), and bilirubin should be measured. If the AST and ALT levels are less than three times the upper limit of normal, the symptoms are assumed

Table 17.5. First-line antituberculosis drugs: mechanisms of action, dosage, and adverse effects in children

FIRST-LINE DRUGS	MODE AND MECHANISM OF ACTION	MAIN TOXICITIES	DAILY DOSE MG/KG (RANGE); [MAXIMUM DAILY DOSE]
Isoniazid (INH)	Bactericidal: —Inhibits cell wall synthesis —Most potent early bactericidal activity offering the best protection to companion drugs —Contributes mainly by rapidly killing actively metabolizing extra-cellular bacilli, contributes to sterilization if given for a prolonged period	Hepatitis, peripheral neuropathy, psychosis (rare)	10 (7–15) [300 mg]
Rifampin (RMP)	Bactericidal and sterilizing: —Inhibits RNA synthesis —Contributes by killing extra-cellular and slower growing intracellular bacilli, important contribution to sterilization	Hepatitis; orange discoloration of secretions; drug–drug interactions because of hepatic enzyme induction	15 (10–20) [600 mg]
Pyrazinamide (PZA)	Sterilizing: —Disrupts energy metabolism —Contributes by specifically killing bacilli that persist within the acidic centers of caseating granulomas	Hepatitis; arthralgia; pruritis	35 (30–40) [2000 mg]
Ethambutol (EMB)	Bacteriostatic: —Inhibits cell wall synthesis —Contributes mainly by offering some additional protection against drug-resistant mutants	Visual disturbance (acuity, color vision)	20 (15–25) [1200 mg]
Streptomycin (SM)	Bactericidal-protein synthesis inhibitor: —Interacts directly with the small ribosomal subunit	Ototoxicity (hearing loss or vestibular dysfunction); renal toxicity	15 [1000 mg]

not to be due to hepatic toxicity. However, if the AST or ALT level is three or more times the upper limit of normal the symptoms should be assumed to represent hepatic toxicity (see below), and the patient should be evaluated appropriately.

The initial approach to gastrointestinal intolerance not associated with hepatic toxicity is to change the timing of drug administration and/or to administer the drugs with, or just after taking, small amounts of food. If patients are taking daily DOT, the timing of the drug administration should be altered, preferably to be closer to mealtime. Alternatively, food can be taken at the time of DOT administration (rifampin, however, should preferably be administered on an empty stomach due to interference by food in absorption). Patients receiving self-administered therapy can take the medications at bedtime. If gastrointestinal intolerance persists, it may be best for all medications to be taken half an hour after an anti-emetic is administered.

DRUG FEVER

Although drug fever caused by first-line antituberculosis drugs is rare in children, recurrence of fever in a patient who has been receiving therapy for several weeks should suggest drug fever, especially if the patient is showing clinical, microbiological, and radiographic improvement of the tuberculosis. It should be noted, however, that fever from tuberculosis may persist for as long as two months after ultimately successful therapy has been initiated.[64] Of course, children with tuberculosis may develop fever in association with community-acquired viral or bacterial infections. New onset of fever may also be a manifestation of a paradoxical reaction or IRIS, especially in patients with HIV infection. The clinical hallmark of drug fever is that the patient looks and feels well despite having a high fever (often greater than 39ºC). There is no specific pattern to the fever. Eosinophilia may or may not be present. The first step in management is to ensure that there is no superinfection or worsening of tuberculosis. If these potential causes are excluded, all antituberculosis drugs should be stopped. Drug-related fever usually will resolve within 24 hours. Patients with severe tuberculosis should be given at least three new drugs in the interim while it is being determined which drug is causing the fever. Once the fever has resolved, the initial drugs can be restarted sequentially to determine which drug caused the fever.

HEPATITIS

Three of the first-line antituberculosis drugs—INH, RMP, and PZA—can cause drug-induced liver injury (AST/ALT levels three or more times the upper limit of normal in the presence of symptoms, or five or more times the upper limit of normal in the absence of symptoms).[65] However, INH and PZA are more common causes of hepatotoxicity

than RMP. In the presence of nausea, vomiting, or abdominal pain, increases in the AST or ALT of greater than three times normal should be considered significant. In patients without specific symptoms, an AST or ALT level less than five times the upper limit of normal can be considered mild toxicity, an AST or ALT level 5–10 times normal defines moderate toxicity, and an AST or ALT level greater than 10 times normal is severe toxicity.[66] In addition to AST or ALT elevation, occasionally there are disproportionate increases in bilirubin and alkaline phosphatase; this pattern is more consistent with RMP hepatotoxicity. If there are clinical symptoms and/or the AST or ALT is more than five times upper limit of normal, INH, RMP, and PZA must be withheld, and a regimen of non-hepatotoxic drugs (usually ethambutol, a fluoroquinolone, and an injectable drug such as streptomycin or amikacin) is given. Liver tests should be checked at least weekly until the results return to normal. As soon as the serum liver enzymes are within the normal range, the original antituberculosis regimen can be reintroduced. There are a few ways of doing this: restart all drugs at full dose or with gradually increasing dosages together, or restart one at a time. Most clinicians prefer to reintroduce one drug at a time to help determine which drug caused the liver toxicity; if upon rechallenge of a specific drug the liver toxicity recurs, that drug usually needs to be eliminated from the regimen. However, according to the results of one adult trial, all three of the potentially hepatotoxic drugs can be reintroduced simultaneously at full dosage safely, especially for patients with bilateral extensive pulmonary tuberculosis, to halt disease transmission or to treat patients with life-threatening tuberculosis.[67]

MISCELLANEOUS ADVERSE EFFECTS

INH has rarely been associated with red cell aplasia, while RMP can cause thrombocytopenia. RMP and other rifamycins interfere with the metabolism of oral contraceptives, so an alternative form of birth control must be used while these medications are taken. Because rifamycins are excreted in tears, they can cause staining of contact lenses. PZA has been associated with both arthralgias and arthritis caused by increased uric acid levels; most children taking PZA have increased serum uric acid levels, but symptoms are much less common than in adults. PZA also can cause mild to severe pruritis, but this is more common in adolescents and adults. While EMB can cause optic neuritis, this is very rare in children taking the recommended doses; even in adults, EMB optic neuritis is often associated with underlying renal dysfunction that increases serum levels by slowing the excretion of the EMB.

Patient (Child)-Centered Care

Treatment of children with tuberculosis is most successful within a comprehensive framework that addresses both clinical and social issues of relevance to the patient and family. It is essential that treatment be tailored and supervision be based on each child's clinical and social circumstances; this is known as patient-centered care. It is strongly recommended that patient-centered care be the initial management strategy, regardless of the source of supervision. This strategy should always include an adherence plan based on the child's age and activities, and frequent communication between the family and patient and the health care team (doctor, nurse or social worker). This is important, as parents often have questions about the diet or dispensing of medicines after the initiation of treatment. It is extremely helpful to have an experienced person call the parent (or adolescent child) regularly for the first few weeks to troubleshoot as well as counsel and provide psychological support. Hence, tuberculosis treatment involves not just the prescribing physician and patient, but a whole team often consisting of a nurse, a counsellor or social worker, an outreach worker, a pharmacist, and a nutritionist.

Practicing child-centered care also allows the health care team to assess other household members. Reverse contact tracing—testing close contacts of children with suspected or confirmed tuberculosis disease—involves screening all adult and adolescent family members for any evidence of tuberculosis disease. The yields from these investigations are often substantial because the time between infection and development of disease in young children is often short, and the source of their infection is a family member who has not yet been identified or diagnosed.

Adherence Strategies

Due to the lack of availability of pediatric dosage forms for most antituberculosis medications, administration of the medications to young children is difficult and often involves the crushing of pills or opening of capsules. Many families need

and appreciate direct help with drug administration, especially at the beginning of treatment. Directly observed therapy (DOT) is a package of services designed to support a family through treatment. The central element of DOT involves providing the antituberculosis drugs directly to the patient and watching as he/she swallows the medications. Each patient's management plan should be individualized to incorporate measures that facilitate adherence to the drug regimen. In the case of children, such measures may include, for example, social service support and housing assistance for the family, treatment incentives and enablers (for parents), and coordination of tuberculosis services with those of other providers. Adherence to treatment in young children depends on the cooperation of their adult caregivers, usually a parent, and is generally excellent. Among adolescents, factors that interfere with adherence may include cultural and linguistic barriers to cooperation, lifestyle, homelessness, substance abuse, and a large number of other conditions and circumstances that, for the patient, are priorities that compete with taking treatment for tuberculosis.[68] Effective tuberculosis case management identifies and characterizes the terrain and determines an appropriate care plan based on each of the identified factors. Additional advantages of the patient-centered approach are that increasing communication with the patient and family provides opportunities for further education concerning tuberculosis and enables elicitation of additional information concerning contacts.

Treatment Response and Follow-up

The patient's clinical progress and the treatment plan must be reviewed periodically to evaluate the treatment response and to identify adherence problems. Ideally, each child should be assessed at least at the following intervals: two weeks after the start of treatment, at the end of the intensive phase, and every two months until completion of treatment (Table 17.6). The assessment should include, as a minimum: symptom assessment, assessment of treatment adherence, enquiry about any adverse events, and weight measurement. Dosages should be adjusted to take account of any weight gain. Adherence should be assessed by questioning the patient/caregiver and by reviewing the treatment card. A follow-up sputum (or other respiratory) sample for acid-fast smear microscopy/GeneXpertMTB/RIF and culture should be obtained at two months after the start of treatment

Table 17.6. Follow-up schedule for children on treatment for tuberculosis

Study visit	1	DECISION TREATMENT	Started on tuberculosis treatment			
			2	3	4	5
Time	0 Screening		2 wks	4 wks	8 wks	End of Rx
Symptom screening	Y		Y	Y	Y	Y
Tuberculosis risk factors and past medical history	Y					
Physical examination and anthropometry	Y		Y	Y	Y	Y
Tuberculin skin test (TST)	Y					
Chest radiograph, PA and lateral view	Y				Optional	Y
Symptoms, weight, and adherence check			Y	Y	Y	Y
Blood test for HIV	Y					
Respiratory specimen for acid-fast smear, culture, and DST	Y				Y (if positive initially)	Optional

from any child who was smear-, GeneXpert MTB/RIF-, or culture-positive at diagnosis. Follow-up chest radiographs are not routinely required in children who are improving symptomatically with treatment, particularly as many children will have a slow radiographic response to treatment. A five-year follow-up of children treated for tuberculosis with six-month regimens showed that 49% had an abnormal radiograph at the end of treatment, and 1.5% had some sequelae at five years, but no child had a relapse of tuberculosis.[69] In short, a normal chest radiograph is not a requirement to stop therapy. However, a chest radiograph is often taken at the end of treatment to document improvement and to provide a baseline for future assessments.

A child who is not responding to antituberculosis treatment should be referred for further assessment and management. This child may have drug-resistant tuberculosis, an unusual complication of pulmonary disease, a lung disease from another cause, or problems with treatment adherence. Malabsorption leading to low levels of antituberculosis drugs should also be considered, especially in HIV-infected and malnourished children, and therapeutic drug monitoring may have a role in this situation, although there are few published data for children.[70]

In addition, adherence monitoring by direct methods, such as the detection of drugs or drug metabolites in the patient's urine, or indirect methods such as pill counts or a medication monitor, should be a part of routine management, especially if the patient is not being given DOT. In one Indian study, treatment of tuberculosis in children was equally effective when given by an official DOT provider or a committed nongovernmental organization (NGO) worker.[71] Furthermore, family members, especially mothers, can be considered as primary DOT supporters, although true assessment of adherence is more difficult.[72]

Treatment Outcomes for Patients in Tuberculosis Control Program

Among the six WHO regions, the highest adult treatment success rates are in the Western Pacific Region (92%), the South-East Asia Region (88%),

Table 17.7. Programmatic treatment outcomes for drug-susceptible tuberculosis

OUTCOME	DEFINITION
Cured	A pulmonary tuberculosis patient with bacteriologically confirmed disease at the beginning of treatment who was acid-fast smear- or culture-negative in the last month of treatment and on at least one previous occasion.
Treatment completed	A tuberculosis patient who completed treatment without evidence of failure BUT with no record to show that sputum smear or culture results in the last month of treatment and on at least one previous occasion were negative, either because tests were not done or because results are unavailable.
Treatment failed	A tuberculosis patient whose sputum smear or culture is positive at month 5 or later during treatment.
Died	A tuberculosis patient who dies for any reason before starting or during the course of treatment.
Lost to follow-up	A tuberculosis patient who did not start treatment or whose treatment was interrupted for 2 consecutive months or more.
Not evaluated	A tuberculosis patient for whom no treatment outcome is assigned. This includes cases "transferred out" to another treatment unit, as well as cases for whom the treatment outcome is unknown to the reporting unit.
Treatment success	The sum of cured and treatment completed.

and the Eastern Mediterranean Region (87%). Of the 22 high-tuberculosis-burden countries, 15 reached or exceeded a treatment success rate of 85% among all new cases in 2012. The six countries that reported lower treatment success rates were Brazil (72%), the Russian Federation (69%, up from 65% in 2011), South Africa (77%), Thailand (81%), Uganda (77%, up from 73% in 2011), and Zimbabwe (81%).[73] Treatment outcomes in children in general are as good as or better than in adults, but are not specifically reported nor given high priority in most national tuberculosis program. This is because the focus of WHO and most national tuberculosis programs is to find and treat acid-fast sputum smear-positive, infectious patients. In children, the programmatic outcome reported most commonly is "treatment completed" (Table 17.7). As is obvious from the results tabulated in Table 17.3, cure rates in children are high and failure or relapse rates are low. Except in cases when there is a serious comorbid illness or extensive disease (usually due to delayed diagnosis) or problems with drug adherence, the majority of children with drug-susceptible tuberculosis should be cured.

FUTURE DIRECTIONS

There is an urgent need for rigorous, multicenter pharmacokinetic studies in children, combined with correlation with treatment outcomes, in order to determine optimal dosages of all first and second-line antituberculosis drugs. The efficacy of shorter (4 months) treatment regimens in children with uncomplicated pulmonary or lymph node tuberculosis is being tested (SHINE trial). Further, the role of higher dosages of RMP and use of fluoroquinolones in shortening treatment durations in children need to be explored. New antituberculosis drugs (bedaquiline, delamanid, and pretonamid) that have become available in the past few years need to be tested in children to establish their safety and optimal dosing. Hopefully, with newer drug combinations, it may be possible to cure most forms of tuberculosis in children in two months or less.

REFERENCES

1. East African/British Medical Research Councils. Controlled clinical trial of short-course (6-month) regimens of chemotherapy for

treatment of pulmonary tuberculosis. *Lancet.* 1972;i:1079–1085.

2. East African/British Medical Research Councils. Controlled clinical trial of four short-course (6-month) regimens of chemotherapy for treatment of pulmonary tuberculosis. Second report. *Lancet.* 1973;i:1331–1338.

3. East African/British Medical Research Councils. Controlled clinical trial of four short-course (6-month) regimens of chemotherapy for treatment of pulmonary tuberculosis. Third report. *Lancet.* 1974;237–240.

4. East African/British Medical Research Councils Study. Controlled clinical trial of four short-course (6-month) regimens of chemotherapy for treatment of pulmonary tuberculosis. Third report. *Lancet.* 1974;ii:1100–1106.

5. East African/British Medical Research Councils Study. Results at 5 years of a controlled comparison of a 6-month and a standard 18-month regimen of chemotherapy for pulmonary tuberculosis. *Am Rev Respir Dis.* 1977;ii:116:3–8.

6. Zignol M, Sismanidis C, Falzon D, Glaziou P, Dara M, Floyd K. Multidrug-resistant tuberculosis in children: evidence from global surveillance. *Eur Respir J.* 2013;42(3):701–707.

7. Peloquin CA. Antituberculosis Drugs: Pharmacokinetics. In Heifets L (Ed.), *Drug Susceptibility in the Chemotherapy of Mycobacterial Infections.* Boca Raton, FL: CRC Press; 1991:59–88.

8. Kearns GL, Abdel-Rahman SM, Alander SW, Blowey DL, Leeder JS, Kauffman RE. Developmental pharmacology-drug disposition, action, and therapy in infants and children. *N Engl J Med.* 2003;18;349(12):1157–1167.

9. WHO. Rapid advice: treatment of tuberculosis in children. Geneva: World Health Organization; 2010. (WHO/HTM/TB/2010) Available at http://whqlibdoc.who.int/publications/2010/9789241500449_eng.pdf. Accessed on 26 Feb. 2015.

10. Thee S, Seddon JA, Donald PR, et al. Pharmacokinetics of isoniazid, rifampin, and pyrazinamide in children younger than two years of age with tuberculosis: evidence for implementation of revised World Health Organization recommendations. *Antimicrob Agents Chemother.* 2011;55:5560–5567.

11. Donald PR, Maritz JS, Diacon AH. The pharmacokinetics and pharmacodynamics of rifampin in adults and children in relation to the dosage recommended for children. *Tuberculosis.* 2011;91:196–207.

12. Boeree MJ, Diacon AH, Dawson R, et al. A dose ranging trial to optimize the dose of rifampin in the treatment of tuberculosis. *Am J Respir Crit Care Med.* 2015 Feb 5. [Epub ahead of print.]

13. Graham SM, Bell DJ, Nyirongo S, Hartkoorn R, Ward SA, Molyneux EM. Low levels of pyrazinamide and ethambutol in children with tuberculosis and impact of age, nutritional status, and human immunodeficiency virus infection. *Antimicrob Agents Chemother.* 2006;50:407–413.

14. Ramachandran G, Hemanth Kumar AK, Bhavani PK, et al. Age, nutritional status and INH acetylator status affect pharmacokinetics of anti-tuberculosis drugs in children. *Int J Tuberc Lung Dis.* 2013;17(6):800–806.

15. Schaaf HS, Parkin DP, Seifart HI, et al. Acute paediatrics: isoniazid pharmacokinetics in children treated for respiratory tuberculosis. *Arch Dis Child.* 2005;90:614–618.

16. Gengiah TN, Botha JH, Soowamber D, Naidoo K, AbdoolKarim SS. Low rifampin concentrations in tuberculosis patients with HIV infection. *J Infect Dev Countries.* 2014;13;8(8):987–993.

17. Peloquin CA, MacPhee AA, Berning SE. Malabsorption of antimycobacterial medications. *N Engl J Med.* 1993;329(15):1122–1133.

18. McIlleron H, Willemse M, Werely CJ, et al. Isoniazid plasma concentrations in a cohort of South African children with tuberculosis: implications for international pediatric dosing guidelines. *Clin Infect Dis.* 2009;48(11):1547–1553.

19. Ethambutol efficacy and toxicity: literature review and recommendations for daily and intermittent dosage in children. Geneva: World Health Organization; 2006 (WHO/HTM/TB/2006.365). Available at http://www.stoptb.org/wg/dots_expansion/assets/documents/embreviewfinal070406.pdf, Accessed on 25 Feb. 2015.

20. Donald PR. Antituberculosis drug-induced hepatotoxicity in children. *Pediatr Rep.* 2011;3(2):e16.

21. Hiruy H, Rogers Z, Mbowane C, et al. Subtherapeutic concentrations of first-line anti-TB drugs in South African children treated according to current guidelines: the PHATISA study. *J Antimicrob Chemother.* 2014 Dec 11;pii:dku478. [Epub ahead of print.]

22. Treatment of tuberculosis: guidelines for national programmes. 4th ed. Geneva, World Health Organization, 2010 (WHO/HTM/TB/2009.420). Available at http://whqlibdoc.who.int/publications/2010/9789241547833_eng.pdf, accessed on 15 Feb. 2015.

23. Narendran G, Menon PA, Venkatesan P, et al. Acquired rifampin resistance in thrice-weekly TB therapy: impact of HIV and antiretroviral therapy. *Clin Infect Dis.* 2014;59(12):1798–1804.

24. Menon PR, Lodha R, Sivanandan S, Kabra SK. Intermittent or daily short course chemotherapy for tuberculosis in children: meta-analysis of randomized controlled trials. *Indian Pediatr.* 2010;47(1):67–73.

25. Bose A, Kalita S, Rose W, Tharyan P. Intermittent versus daily therapy for treating tuberculosis in children. *Cochrane Database Syst Rev.* 2014 Jan 28;1:CD007953. doi: 10.1002/14651858. CD007953.pub2

26. Ramachandran G, Kumar AK, Bhavani PK, et al. Pharmacokinetics of first-line antituberculosis drugs in HIV-infected children with tuberculosis treated with intermittent regimens in India. *Antimicrob Agents Chemother.* 2015;59(2):1162–1167.

27. Ruslami R, Ganiem AR, Dian S, et al. Intensified regimen containing rifampin and moxifloxacin for tuberculous meningitis: an open-label, randomised controlled phase 2 trial. *Lancet Infect Dis.* 2013;13(1):27–35.

28. Clinical trial titled "A Phase I/II Randomized, Open-Label Trial to Evaluate the Pharmacokinetics, Safety, and Treatment Outcomes of Multidrug Treatment Including High Dose Rifampin with or without Levofloxacin versus Standard Treatment for Pediatric Tuberculous Meningitis." The Eunice Kennedy Shriver National Institute of Child Health and Human Development (NICHD) (Protocol No:IRB00051196).

29. Berti E, Galli L, Venturini E, de Martini M, Chiappini E. Tuberculosis in childhood: a systematic review of national and international guidelines. *BMC Infect Dis.* 2014;14(Suppl 1):S3. doi: 10.1186/1471-2334-14-S1-S3

30. Standards for TB care in India (STCI World Health Organization, 2014). Available at http:// www.tbonline.info/media/uploads/docum ents/214586958-standards-for-tb-care-in-india-2014.pdf.,accessed 15 February, 2015.

31. Kabra SK, Lodha R, Seth V. Category-based treatment of tuberculosis in children. Brief reports. *Indian Pediatr.* 2004;41:927–937.

32. Al-Dossary FS, Ong LT, Correa AG, Starke JR. Treatment of childhood tuberculosis with a six month directly observed regimen of only two weeks of daily therapy. *Pediatr Infect Dis J.* 2002;21:91–97.

33. Te Water Naude JM, Donald PR, Hussey GD, et al. Twice-weekly vs. daily chemotherapy for childhood TB. *Pediatr Infect Dis J.* 2000;19:405–410.

34. Ramachandran P, Kripasankar AS, Duraipandian M. Short course chemotherapy for pulmonary tuberculosis in children. *Indian J Tuberc.* 1998;45:83–87.

35. Kumar L, Dhand R, Singhi PD, Rao KL, Katariya S. A randomised trial of fully intermittent and daily followed by intermittent short-course chemotherapy for childhood tuberculosis. *Pediatr Infect Dis J.* 1990;9:802–806.

36. Biddulph J. Short course chemotherapy for childhood tuberculosis. *Pediatr Infect Dis J.* 1990;9:794–801.

37. Göçmen A, Ozçelic U, Kiper N, et al. Short course intermittent chemotherapy in childhood tuberculosis. *Infection.* 1993;21:324–327.

38. Indumathi CK, Prasanna KK, Dinakar C, Shet A, Lewin S. Intermittent short course therapy for pediatric tuberculosis. *Indian Pediatr.* 2010;47(1):93–96.

39. Bai SS, Devi RL. Clinical spectrum of tuberculosis in BCG vaccinated children. *Indian Pediatr.* 2002;39(5):458–462.

40. Abernathy RS, Dutt AK, Stead WW, Moers DJ. Short-course chemotherapy for tuberculosis in children. *Pediatrics.* 1983;72(6):801–806.

41. Kansoy S, Kurtaþ N, Akþit S, Aksoylar S, Yaprak I, Çaðlayan S. Superiority of intermittent-short course chemotherapy in childhood pulmonary tuberculosis. *Turkish J Med Sci.* 1996;26:41–43.

42. Schoeman JF, Van Zyl LE, Laubscher JA, Donald PR. Effect of corticosteroids on intracranial pressure, computed tomographic findings, and clinical outcome in young children with tuberculous meningitis. *Pediatrics.* 1997;99:226–231.

43. Tobin DM, Roca FJ, Oh SF, et al. Host genotype-specific therapies can optimize the inflammatory response to mycobacterial infections. *Cell.* 2012;148:434–446.

44. Thwaites GE. Advances in the diagnosis and treatment of tuberculous meningitis. *Curr Opin Neurol.* 2013;26:295–300.

45. Thwaites GE, Nguyen DB, Nguyen HD, et al. Dexamethasone for the treatment of tuberculous meningitis in adolescents and adults. *N Engl J Med.* 2004;351:1741–1751.

46. Prasad K, Singh MB. Corticosteroids for managing tuberculous meningitis. *Cochrane Database Syst Rev.* 2008;1:CD002244.

47. Prasad K, Volmink J, Menon GR. Steroids for treating tuberculous meningitis. *Cochrane Database Syst Rev.* 2000;3:CD002244.

48. Mayosi BM. Interventions for treating tuberculous pericarditis. *Cochrane Database Syst Rev.* 2002;4:CD000526.

49. Strang JI, Nunn AJ, Johnson DA, Casbard A, Gibson DG, Girling DJ. Management of tuberculous constrictive pericarditis and tuberculous pericardial effusion in Transkei: results at 10 years follow-up. *QJM.* 2004;97:525–535.

50. Lee CH, Wang WJ, Lan RS, Tsai YH, Chiang YC. Corticosteroids in the treatment of tuberculous pleurisy: a double-blind, placebo-controlled, randomized study. *Chest.* 1988;94:1256–1259.

51. Bang JS, Kim MS, Kwak SM, Cho CH. Evaluation of steroid therapy in tuberculous pleurisy: a prospective, randomized study. *Tuberc Respir Dis.*1997;44:52–58.

52. Engel ME, Matchaba PT, Volmink J. Corticosteroids for tuberculous pleurisy. *Cochrane Database Syst Rev.* 2007;4:CD001876.

53. Singh MM, Bhargava AN, Jain KP. Tuberculous peritonitis: an evaluation of pathogenetic mechanisms, diagnostic procedures and therapeutic measures. *N Engl J Med.* 1969;281:1091–1094.

54. Sun TN, Yang JY, Zheng LY, Deng WW, Sui ZY. Chemotherapy and its combination with corticosteroids in acute miliary tuberculosis in adolescents and adults: analysis of 55 cases. *Chin Med J.* 1981;94:309–314.

55. Tuberculosis Research Centre. Study of chemotherapy regimens of 5 and 7 months' duration and the role of corticosteroids in the treatment of sputum-positive patients with pulmonary tuberculosis in South India. *Tubercle.*1983;64:73–91.

56. Meintjes G, Wilkinson R, Morroni C, et al. Randomised placebo-controlled trial of prednisone for the TB immune reconstitution inflammatory syndrome [Abstract 34]. In: Proceedings of the 16th Conference on Retroviruses and Opportunistic Infections; Feb. 8–11, 2009; Montreal, Canada. Available at http://retroconference.org/2009/Abstracts/34429.htm. Accessed 10 Feb. 2015.

57. Guidance for national tuberculosis programs on the management of tuberculosis in children. Geneva: World Health Organization; 2006 (WHO/HTM/TB/2006.371). Available at http://apps.who.int/medicinedocs/documents/s21535en/s21535en.pdf, accessed on 26 Feb. 2015.

58. Technical note: Supplementary foods for the management of moderate acute malnutrition in infants and children 6–59 months of age. Geneva: World Health Organization; 2012. Available at http://apps.who.int/iris/bitstream/10665/75836/1/9789241504423_eng.pdf, accessed on 26 Feb. 2015.

59. WHO child growth standards and the identification of severe acute malnutrition in infants and children. A joint statement by the World Health Organization and the United Nations Children's Fund. Geneva: World Health Organization and United Nations Children's Fund; 2009. Available at http://whqlibdoc.who.int/publications/2009/9789241598163_eng.pdf, accessed on 24 Feb. 2015.

60. The WHO Child Growth Standards. Geneva: World Health Organization; 2012; available at: http://www.who.int/childgrowth/standards/en/, accessed on 24 Feb. 2015.

61. Growth reference 5–19 years. Geneva: World Health Organization; 2012; available at: http://www.who.int/growthref/en/, accessed on 24 Feb. 2015.

62. Gopalan N, Andrade BB, Swaminathan S. Tuberculosis-immune reconstitution inflammatory syndrome in HIV: from pathogenesis to prediction. *Expert Rev Clin Immunol.* 2014;10(5):631–645.

63. Centers for Disease Control. Core curriculum on tuberculosis: what the clinician should know. 4th ed. Atlanta, GA: US Department of Health and Human Services, CDC, 2000. Available at http://www.cdc.gov/nchstp/tb/, accessed on 24 Feb. 2015.

64. Kiblawi SS, Jay SJ, Stonehill RB, Norton J. Fever response of patients on therapy for pulmonary tuberculosis. *Am Rev Respir Dis.* 1981;123:20–24.

65. Ormerod LP. Hepatotoxicity of antituberculosis drugs. *Thorax.* 1996;51:111–113.

66. World Health Organization Collaborating Center for International Drug Monitoring. Adverse drug reaction terminology (ART), 1979. Available at http://www.WHO-UMC.org (or email: info@WHO-UMC.org), accessed on 24 Feb. 2015.

67. Sharma SK, Singla R, Sarda P, et al. Safety of 3 different reintroduction regimens of antituberculosis drugs after development of antituberculosis treatment-induced hepatotoxicity. *Clin Infect Dis.* 2010;15;50(6):833–839.

68. Moss AR, Hahn JA, Tulsky JP, Daley CL, Small PM, Hopewell PC. Tuberculosis in the homeless: a prospective study. *Am J Respir Crit Care Med.* 2000;162:460–464.

69. Swaminathan S, Raghavan A, Duraipandian, et al. Short course chemotherapy for pediatric respiratory tuberculosis: 5 year report. *Int J Tuberc Lung Dis.* 2005;9(6):693–696.

70. Swaminathan S, Padmapriyadarsini C. Undernutrition and tuberculosis: Strongly linked, but ignored. *Natl Med J India.* 2014;27(3):125–127.

71. Singh M, Kumar L. A randomized controlled trial of directly observed treatment shortcourse (DOTS) for childhood tuberculosis by using an official DOTS provider and nongovernmental organizations. *Chest.* 2004;126(4_MeetingAbstracts):910S-a-910S.

72. Schoeman J, Malan G, van Toorn R, Springer P, Parker F, Booysen J. Home-based treatment of childhood neurotuberculosis. *J Trop Pediatr.* 2009;55(3):149–154.

73. WHO. Definitions and reporting framework for tuberculosis—2013 revision. WHO/HTM/TB/2013.2. Available at http://apps.who.int/iris/bitstream/10665/79199/1/9789241505345_eng.pdf, Accessed on 26 Feb. 2015.

18

MANAGEMENT OF DRUG-RESISTANT TUBERCULOSIS IN CHILDREN

James Seddon

HIGHLIGHTS OF THIS CHAPTER

- With currently available drugs and regimens, it is possible to achieve excellent outcomes for drug-resistant tuberculosis in children in a wide range of settings with varying resources.
- Children with drug-resistant tuberculosis (except for isolated isoniazid resistance) should be treated with at least 4 drugs and often more, with fluoroquinolones and injectable drugs often being the backbone of the initial regimen.
- The optimal length of therapy for the various forms of drug-resistant tuberculosis in children are unknown, but regimens lasting 12–24 months are commonly used.
- Children being treated for drug-resistant tuberculosis should be monitored closely to determine response to therapy, identify adverse events early, and promote adherence to treatment.
- Children tend to tolerate the second-line antituberculosis drugs better than adults with fewer interruptions in therapy.
- Whenever possible, treatment of drug-resistant tuberculosis should be given daily using directly observed therapy.

AT EVERY division of *Mycobacterium tuberculosis*, there is a small probability of a genetic mutation arising that will confer resistance to an antituberculosis medication. Therefore, at any time, within a large untreated population of *M. tuberculosis*, mycobacteria will exist that possess such mutations. Monotherapy with only one drug will give a selective advantage to these strains, allowing them to prosper, with drug-susceptible strains being killed.

Eventually, the entire population will possess that mutation and will be resistant to that medication. Isoniazid (INH) and rifampin (RMP) are the two most important medications used to treat *M. tuberculosis*, and the rate of spontaneous mutation to create resistance to isoniazid is 1 in 10^6 cell divisions and for rifampin, 1 in 10^8.[1] The use of an appropriate multidrug regimen should ensure that those mutant organisms resistant to one of the medications can be killed by one of the others in the regimen. A population of 10^{14} bacilli would be required to create the mathematical possibility of a mutation to both isoniazid and rifampin. Even in cavitary tuberculosis, with a high bacillary load, the number of organisms cannot reach this level.

For drug resistance to develop to a multidrug regimen, monotherapy must be given inadvertently. This occurs when serum levels are sub-therapeutic, treatment is intermittent or chaotic, or only some of the drugs in the regimen are taken. Resistance usually develops first to isoniazid, as this medication is the most bactericidal and therefore causes the greatest selective advantage. In addition, mutations to isoniazid occur more frequently than to rifampin. This leads to isoniazid mono-resistant *M. tuberculosis*. If rifampin is then given as monotherapy (or in combination with other medications given imperfectly), resistance to rifampin will develop. Resistance to only rifampin was rare prior to the HIV epidemic. However, and for reasons that are still not entirely clear, it is now seen more frequently, especially in persons living with HIV.[2,3] Once resistant to isoniazid and rifampin, *M. tuberculosis* is termed multidrug-resistant (MDR).[4] If resistance additionally develops to one of the injectable medications used to treat tuberculosis (an aminoglycoside or a polypeptide) as well as to a fluoroquinolone, it is said to be extensively drug-resistant (XDR).[5] Definitions used in pediatric drug-resistant tuberculosis (DR-TB) are shown in Table 18.1.

Drug resistance can be acquired as described above, through sequential, selective pressure in the face of inadequate therapy, when a previously drug-susceptible organism develops resistance within one human host. Alternatively, resistance can be transmitted when mycobacteria, already resistant, are transmitted to a new host. Additionally, a combination of the two can occur when one individual is infected with a mycobacterium already resistant to one or more medications and then in the face of inadequate treatment develops resistance to further antibiotics. It is unclear what proportion of drug resistance in tuberculosis is transmitted and what is acquired. Children usually have transmitted resistance as their disease is normally paucibacillary, making acquired resistance less likely.

The management of any child with tuberculosis disease can be challenging due to the problems of diagnosis, making sure that the appropriate drugs are prescribed and consumed at appropriate doses, difficulties in monitoring the response to treatment,

and managing the adverse effects of the medications. All of these challenges are compounded when treating a child with DR-TB.

The World Health Organization (WHO) estimated that in 2013 there were 480,000 incident cases of MDR-TB globally,[6] and in many high-burden settings, children compose up to 20% of the tuberculosis caseload.[7,8] A recent modeling exercise estimated that 32,000 children developed MDR-TB in 2010,[9] and of these, the vast majority were never diagnosed with MDR-TB and fewer still were started on therapy. For those treated appropriately with a regimen tailored to the drug susceptibility test (DST) pattern of the infecting organism, treatment outcomes are generally very good.[10] Currently this is carried out only in certain areas by a small number of specialists. However, with the rollout of genotypic tests for diagnosing MDR-TB (both the line probe assays [LPA][11] and the GeneXpert MTB/RIF assay [Cepheid][12] have been endorsed by WHO), and as national programs become more committed to treating children with tuberculosis, more pediatric MDR-TB cases will be diagnosed and will require treatment. Furthermore, many more adults with MDR-TB will be identified who are in close contact with children, necessitating consideration of treatment for MDR-TB infection in the contacts.

Few studies have looked at the management of MDR-TB in children, and the presentation, treatment, and outcomes are poorly described. Pediatric treatment guidelines are often based on adult studies, but this is not always appropriate, as children have a different disease spectrum. They usually have paucibacillary disease, a greater frequency of intra- and extra-thoracic lymph node disease, higher rates of extrapulmonary tuberculosis (EPTB), and more often present with severe forms of disease such as miliary tuberculosis or tuberculous meningitis. In addition, the diagnosis is more often presumptive and less frequently confirmed with acid-fast smear or culture. Children generally metabolize drugs in a different way than adults do, and they have a different spectrum of adverse effects and psychosocial needs.

This chapter reviews the management of a child with MDR-TB disease, including when to start treatment, the design of regimens, the use of concomitant medications, the interplay with human immunodeficiency virus (HIV), the monitoring of response to treatment, the management of adverse effects, and infection control. It will also discuss the management of well children exposed to MDR-TB.

Table 18.1. Definitions for use in pediatric drug-resistant tuberculosis

		DEFINITION
Drug resistance	Drug-resistant tuberculosis (DR-TB)	Resistant to any antituberculosis drug
	Mono-resistant tuberculosis	Resistance to one antituberculosis drug
	Poly-resistant tuberculosis	Resistance to two or more antituberculosis drugs other than to both rifampin and isoniazid
	Multidrug-resistant tuberculosis (MDR-TB)	Resistant to rifampin and isoniazid
	Pre-extensively drug-resistant tuberculosis	MDR-TB with resistance to either a fluoroquinolone or an injectable second-line antituberculosis drug, but not both
	Extensively drug-resistant tuberculosis (XDR-TB)	MDR-TB with resistance to both a fluoroquinolone and an injectable second-line antituberculosis drug
Episodes and treatment	Previous tuberculosis episode	Treatment taken for at least one month, after which there was a reported symptom-free period of ≥6 months before the start of the current DR-TB episode[139]
	DR-TB episode	If DR-TB is subsequently confirmed, the episode begins when the child is first documented to have presented to the health care system, when the specimen was obtained that eventually confirmed DR-TB, or when the child began antituberculosis treatment
	Previous tuberculosis treatment	Any antituberculosis treatment prior to the initiation of DR-TB treatment for more than one month
Reason for treatment	Confirmed DR-TB	Isolation of *M. tuberculosis* from the child with genotypic or phenotypic demonstration of resistance
	Presumed DR-TB due to contact	DR-TB treatment started on the basis of symptoms, signs, radiology, and/or immunology consistent with tuberculosis, together with a close, infectious source case with confirmed DR-TB or with risk factors for DR-TB
	Presumed DR-TB due to treatment failure	DR-TB treatment started on the basis of a clinical or radiological deterioration on effective, well-adhered-to, first-line therapy, with the exclusion of other possible diagnoses or explanations

(continued)

Table 18.1. Continued

		DEFINITION
Outcome	Cure	Completion of treatment, clinical and radiological improvement, and three or more negative sputum cultures
	Probable cure	Completion of treatment with clinical and radiological improvement
	Treatment completed	Completion of prescribed treatment
	Default	Treatment interruption for two or more months
	Died	Death for any reason while on treatment
	Treatment failure	Ongoing sputum culture positivity or clinical or radiological deterioration after six months of an effective, well-adhered-to therapy
	Transferred out	Transfer to another reporting region for ongoing care

STUDIES OF PEDIATRIC DR-TB TREATMENT AND INTERNATIONAL GUIDELINES

A systematic review and meta-analysis published in 2012 identified only eight studies reporting the treatment of MDR-TB in 315 children.[10] Successful outcomes were seen in 82% of children, compared to 62% in adults.[13,14] It is difficult to draw too many firm conclusions from such small numbers, but it does appear that if children are identified, diagnosed, and treated with appropriate therapy, outcomes are very good. However, these individualized approaches require high levels of expertise from the clinicians who manage these children; the treatment is long (often for longer than 18 months) and is associated with significant adverse events; a quarter of children treated with injectable drugs experience some degree of permanent hearing loss;[15] and over half of children given ethionamide develop reversible thyroid dysfunction.[16,17]

Since this systematic review, however, there has been a large number of cases, case series, and studies published that have described the treatment of MDR-TB in children[18–36] (Table 18.2). An individual patient systematic review and meta-analysis is underway, commissioned by WHO, to inform treatment recommendations. In one study of confirmed and presumed MDR-TB, children were classified as having had severe and non-severe disease,[36] based on established criteria.[37] The children with non-severe disease were younger, better nourished, less likely to have HIV infection, less likely to have microbiologically confirmed disease, and less likely to have sputum acid-fast smear-positive tuberculosis. They were more commonly treated as outpatients, were less likely to receive an injectable medication, and were given shorter total durations of medication (median 12 months vs. 18 months in the severe cases). Although not a trial, this does suggest that for more limited disease it may be possible to give shorter durations of therapy and even omit the injectable medication altogether. It is clear that shorter and safer regimens are required.

Guidelines to treat MDR-TB in children are lacking, and those that exist are rarely evidence-based. Often treatment recommendations are extrapolated from adult guidelines, but as children frequently have more limited disease, the long treatment courses may not always be necessary. The WHO,[38–40] South African Department of Health,[41] American Academy of Pediatrics,[42] Francis Curry TB Center,[43] and Partners in Health[44,45] have produced guidelines that give some direction to pediatric MDR-TB management. More recently the Sentinel Project on Pediatric Drug-Resistant Tuberculosis[46] has developed a field guide specifically for childhood DR-TB.[47] The Sentinel Project is a global partnership that aims to develop and deploy evidence-based strategies to prevent child deaths from DR-TB.

Table 18.2. Studies describing drug-resistant tuberculosis treatment in children

FIRST AUTHOR	YEAR OF STUDY	LOCATION	NUMBER OF CHILDREN INCLUDED	NUMBER CULTURE-CONFIRMED	TREATMENT SUCCESS (%)	ADVERSE EVENTS
Chauny[30]	2005–2011	Paris, France	3	3	3 (100)	2
Drobac[118]	1999–2003	Lima, Peru	38	28	36 (95)	16
Esposito[18]	2012	Milan, Italy	1	1	1 (100)	0
Esposito[76]	2013	Milan, Italy	1	1	1 (100)	0
Fairlie[140]	2008	Johannesburg, South Africa	13	13	7 (54)	2
Feja[141]	1995–2003	New York, USA	20	6	16 (80)	4
Garazzino[29]	2007–2012	Turin, Italy	8	5	7 (88)	2
Gegia[20]	2009–2011	Georgia	45	41	27/35 (77)	NS
Granich[142]	1994–2003	California, USA	10	NS	9 (90)	NS
Isaakidis[31]	2007–2013	Mumbai, India	11	11	4 (36)	8/8
Katragkou[19]	2010–2011	Thessaloniki, Greece	2	2	1 (50)	2
Kjöllerström[84]	2011*	Lisbon, Portugal	4	4	4 (100)	3
Lapphra[22]	2008–2011	Bangkok, Thailand	33	18	18 (55)	NS
Leimane[143]	1998–2006	Latvia	76	NS	70 (92)	26
Mendez Echevarria[144]	1994–2005	Madrid, Spain	8	5	8 (100)	4
Mignone[33]	2006–2010	Italy	22	17	21 (95)	4
Padayatchi[145]	1992–2003	Durban, South Africa	8	8	1 (13)	NS
Pinon[85]	2010*	Turin, Italy	2	NS	1 (50)	0
Rodrigues[35]	2013*	Lisbon, Portugal	2	2	2 (100)	2
Rose[23]	2007–2012	Cape Town, South Africa	7	7	4/4 (100)	3
Santiago[34]	2005–2010	Madrid, Spain	24	24	NS	NS

(continued)

Table 18.2. Continued

FIRST AUTHOR	YEAR OF STUDY	LOCATION	NUMBER OF CHILDREN INCLUDED	NUMBER CULTURE-CONFIRMED	TREATMENT SUCCESS (%)	ADVERSE EVENTS
Satti[24]	2007–2011	Lesotho	19	5	15/17 (88)	18
Schaaf[17]	1998–2001	Cape Town, South Africa	39	39	21 (54)	20
Schluger[146]	1983–1993	New York, USA	2	2	2 (100)	NS
Seddon[147]	2003–2008	Cape Town, South Africa	111	111	88 (79)	NS
Seddon[36]	2009–2010	Cape Town, South Africa	149	59	137 (92)	32
Shah[26]	2003–2005	Mumbai, India	4	4	3 (75)	NS
Shah[28]	2012*	Mumbai, India	1	1	1 (100)	NS
Shah[25]	2012*	Mumbai, India	3	3	2 (67)	1
Suessmuth[148]	2005	Hanover, Germany	1	1	1 (100)	NS
Uppuluri[32]	2014*	Mumbai, India	1	1	1 (100)	NS
Williams[21]	2006–2010	United Kingdom	17	17	14 (82)	6

*Year of publication, as year of study unclear.
NS = not stated

MOLECULAR ASPECTS OF DRUG-RESISTANT TUBERCULOSIS

Traditionally, DST is determined by phenotypic methods whereby bacilli are grown in the presence of an antibiotic. If more than a certain percentage (usually 1% or more) of bacilli grow in comparison to a control without antibiotic, the bacilli are classified as resistant. More recently, polymerase chain reaction (PCR) tests have been developed to identify genetic mutations that are commonly associated with antibiotic resistance. The great majority (>95%) of rifampin-resistant strains possess mutations in the *rpoB* gene. Most, but not all, strains that are resistant to isoniazid possess mutations in either the *inhA* promoter region or the *katG* gene. *KatG* mutations are associated with complete resistance, but resistance due to *inhA* mutations can often be overcome by giving isoniazid at a higher dose (15–20 mg/kg).[48] Co-resistance occurs between isoniazid and ethionamide, however, and if an *inhA* mutation is present, ethionamide is unlikely to be of use.[49] Mutations in the *ethA* gene also usually cause resistance to ethionamide. Mutations in the *embB* gene commonly confer resistance to ethambutol, and those in the *pncA* gene to pyrazinamide. Resistance to the fluoroquinolones is usually coded for on the *gyrA* gene, but the situation is complex, and there is some evidence that for later-generation drugs (levofloxacin and moxifloxacin), multiple mutations are required to confer complete resistance. This may imply that if an isolate is resistant to ofloxacin, later-generation fluoroquinolones may still be effective.[50] Resistance to the injectables is also complex, with variable and unclear cross-resistance. Cross-resistance between amikacin or kanamycin is common,[51] and there is evidence that if a strain is resistant to an aminoglycoside it will already be resistant to capreomycin.[52,53] The converse is not necessarily true, however.

STARTING TREATMENT FOR DRUG-RESISTANT TUBERCULOSIS IN CHILDREN

The diagnosis of MDR-TB in children is either confirmed or presumed (Figure 18.1). Confirmed disease occurs when *M. tuberculosis* is isolated from the child and is demonstrated to grow in the presence of isoniazid and rifampin (phenotypic resistance)

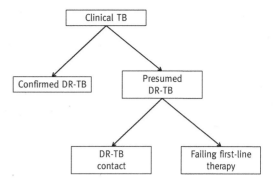

FIGURE 18.1 A brief algorithm for suspecting drug-resistant tuberculosis.

or to contain genes that are frequently associated with resistance to both these drugs (genotypic resistance). A diagnosis of presumed MDR-TB should be considered when the child is diagnosed with tuberculosis on the basis of symptoms, signs, and radiology, in combination with risk factors that might imply drug resistance. Such risk factors include the child being treated previously for tuberculosis or being in contact with a contagious source case that is known to have MDR-TB or who has died, failed treatment, or defaulted. In addition, if a child being treated for tuberculosis with first-line medications is failing treatment in spite of a well-adhered-to regimen, it may be appropriate, in certain circumstances, to also treat for MDR-TB. When presented with a child with symptoms suggestive of pulmonary tuberculosis (PTB) and a chest radiograph (CR) that could be consistent with either tuberculosis or bacterial pneumonia, it is appropriate to give a trial of antibiotics and review the child in a few weeks (Figure 18.2). It must be noted that when undertaking this approach, amoxicillin-clavulanic acid, the fluoroquinolones, and the macrolides clarithromycin and azithromycin have activity against *M. tuberculosis* and should not be used in this capacity, as treatment response may falsely reassure the clinician that the child does not have PTB. The treatment of tuberculous meningitis and miliary tuberculosis are medical emergencies, however, and as delay in starting appropriate therapy is associated with poor outcome,[54,55] and as median time to death is 19.5 days if untreated,[56] MDR-TB treatment should be commenced as soon as the diagnosis is suspected.

If the child is diagnosed with presumed MDR-TB, extensive efforts should be made to confirm the diagnosis with multiple samples. Dependent on the child's age, attempts should be

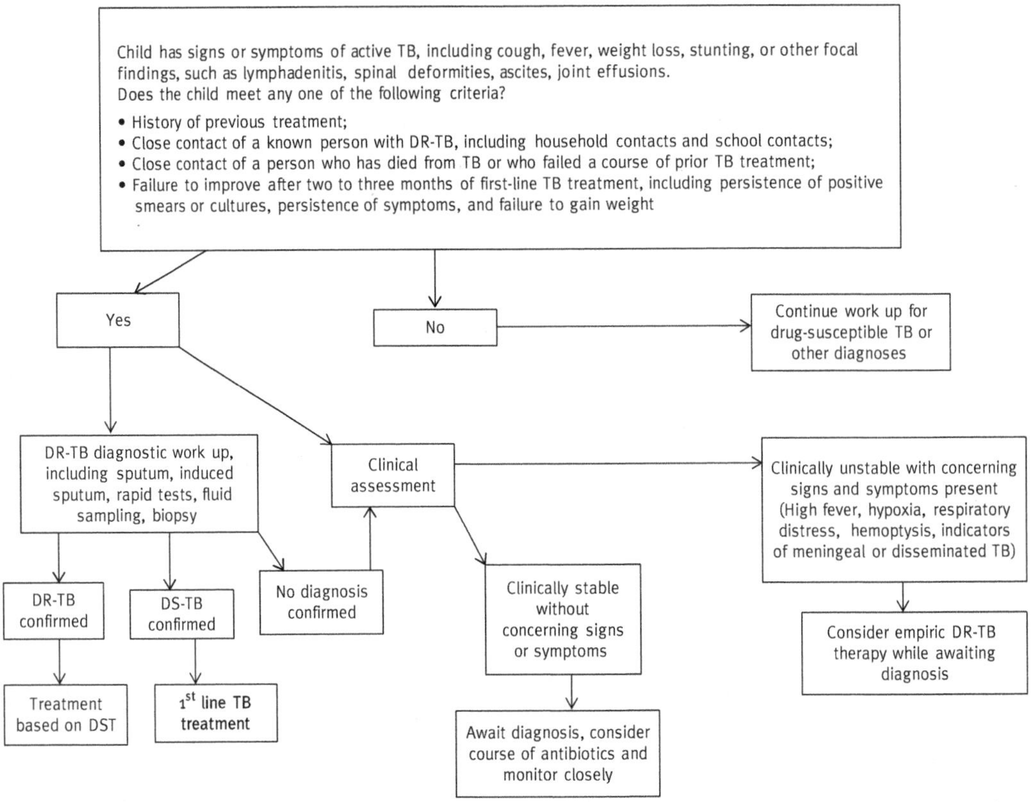

FIGURE 18.2   A more extensive algoritm for the avaluation of a child for suspected drug-resistant tuberculosis.

Figure reproduced courtesy of The Sentinel Project.[47]

made to obtain sputum samples, gastric aspirates, induced sputum samples, lymph node biopsy, or tissue biopsy. Although invasive, giving a general anesthetic to the child in order to perform bronchoalveolar lavage, bronchoscopic biopsy, or open lung biopsy may well be in the child's best interest, as confirming the diagnosis of tuberculosis and the organisms' drug susceptibility will allow appropriate treatment, increasing probability of success and minimizing adverse effects. All samples confirmed as MDR should be sent automatically for full second-line DST testing to determine susceptibility to at least the injectables, the fluoroquinolones and ethionamide.

CONSTRUCTING A DRUG-RESISTANT TUBERCULOSIS REGIMEN FOR CHILDREN

WHO has placed the drugs used in the treatment of DR-TB into five groups, summarized in Table 18.3.[39] Group 1 drugs are considered first-line, with the remainder second-line. Few of the second-line drugs are produced in pediatric formulations, and the pharmacokinetics of most are incompletely studied in young children. This means that tablets must be broken or cut, potentially leading to inaccurate dosages, which may lead to blood concentrations that are sub-therapeutic or toxic. The taste of the medications is often unpalatable, and several of the drugs can cause vomiting and diarrhea, which may affect the amount absorbed. The daily pill burden can be vast, as the child may require multiple medications, ART, other antibiotics, as well as supplements for vitamins and calories. (Figure 18.3 shows the daily number of tablets for a child with MDR-TB and HIV. A programmatic dosing table has been designed by the Sentinel Project and is demonstrated in Figure 18.4.) The number of tablets can be divided and spread over the course of the day; they can be mixed with different foods or drinks; and, in some situations, nasogastric or

Table 18.3. The drugs used to treat tuberculosis in children

GROUP	GROUP NAME	DRUGS	DOSAGE*	ADVERSE EVENTS
1	First-line oral agents	Isoniazid	10–15	Hepatitis, peripheral neuropathy
		Rifampin	10–20	Hepatitis, discoloration of secretions
		Ethambutol	15–25 (DR-TB: 20–25)	Optic neuritis
		Pyrazinamide	30–40	Hepatitis, arthritis
2	Injectable agents	Kanamycin	15–30	Ototoxicity, nephrotoxicity
		Amikacin	15–22.5	As above
		Capreomycin	15–30	As above
		Streptomycin	15–20	As above
3	Fluoro-quinolones	Ofloxacin	15–20	Sleep disturbance, gastrointestinal disturbance, arthritis, peripheral neuropathy
		Ciprofloxacin	20 twice daily	As above
		Levofloxacin	7.5–10**	As above
		Moxifloxacin	7.5–10	As above but including prolonged QT syndrome
4	Oral bacteriostatic second-line agents	Ethionamide	15–20	Gastrointestinal disturbance, metallic taste, hypothyroidism
		Prothionamide	15–20	As above
		Cycloserine	15–20	Neurological and psychological effects
		Terizidone	15–20	As above
		Para-aminosalicylic acid	150	Gastrointestinal intolerance, hypothyroidism, hepatitis
5	Agents with unclear efficacy/role	Clofazimine	3–5	Skin discoloration, xerosis, abdominal pain
		Linezolid	10**	Diarrhea, headache, nausea, myelosuppression, neurotoxicity, lactic acidosis, pancreatitis, and optic neuropathy
		Amoxicillin-clavulanic acid	10–15 (amoxicillin component) three times a day	Gastrointestinal intolerance, hypersensitivity reactions, seizures, liver and renal dysfunction
		Imipenem/cilastatin		As above

(continued)

Table 18.3. Continued

GROUP	GROUP NAME	DRUGS	DOSAGE*	ADVERSE EVENTS
		Thiacetazone	2.5	Stevens Johnson Syndrome in HIV-infected patients, gastrointestinal intolerance, hepatitis, skin reactions
		High dose isoniazid	15–20	Hepatitis, peripheral neuropathy, neurological and psychological effects
		Clarithromycin	7.5–15 b.i.d.	Gastrointestinal intolerance, rash, hepatitis, prolonged QT syndrome, ventricular arrhythmias
		Bedaquiline	Unknown	Possible QTc prolongation
		Delamanid	Unknown	Possible QTc prolongation

*Daily unless otherwise specified.
**Twice daily for <5 years.

percutaneous endoscopic gastrostomy feeding may be appropriate. The efficacy of these practical suggestions has little evidence base, however, and few studies have assessed drug absorption with differing foods. Dividing the doses can make directly observed therapy (DOT) challenging, but healthcare staff must work with the child and family to find the best ways of managing this.

When designing a regimen to treat children with MDR-TB, the target should be to use at least four,

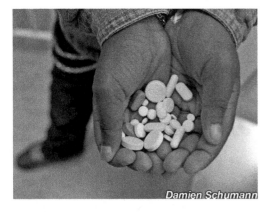

FIGURE 18.3   The volume of pills that may be required for a child being treated for MDR-TB.

Photograph courtesy of The Desmond Tutu TB Centre. Taken by Damien Schumann.

but preferably five drugs, which are likely to have activity against the infecting organism (Figure 18.5). Decisions on which drugs to include in a DR-TB treatment regimen should be guided by the DST of the child's isolate. If this is not available, it should be guided by the DST pattern of the presumed source case. If treatment is given for failure of a first-line regimen, the child should be assumed to have tuberculosis that is resistant to rifampin and isoniazid. In all situations, the previous treatment history of the child and source case should be considered, as drugs previously used by either may no longer be effective.

As they are the most potent drugs with the fewest adverse effects, any first-line drugs (group 1) to which the organism is still susceptible should be used. As DST to pyrazinamide is difficult to perform and the phenotypic DST to ethambutol is unreliable, these drugs should not be assumed to be effective if they have been used for longer than a month prior to the diagnosis of MDR-TB, even if DST indicates susceptibility. Although a high proportion of MDR isolates are already resistant to ethambutol and pyrazinamide,[57,58] pyrazinamide is frequently included in MDR-TB treatment regimens. This is due to its unique mechanism of action, its tolerability, and its synergistic relationship with other drugs. The treatment history of the child and the likely source case should be considered and drugs avoided if they have been used previously as inadvertent

MDR-TB Weight-Based Dosing Chart for Children

Group 1: Oral first-line anti-TB drugs / Group 3: Fluoroquinolones / Group 4: Oral bacteriostatis agents

Wt (kg)	Ethambutol (15–25 mg/kg)		Pyrazinamide (30–40 mg/kg)	Levofloxacin (15–20 mg/kg)		Moxifloxacin (7.5–10 mg/kg)		Ofloxacin (15–20 mg/kg)	Cycloserine/Terizidone (15–20 mg/kg)		PAS (150–200 mg/kg) Daily	PAS Twice Daily	Prothionamide/Ethionamide (15–20 mg/kg)
Available Formulations	100 mg tablet	Suspend 400 mg tab in 8 mL of water for a 50 mg/mL suspension	400 mg tablet / 500 mg tablet	250 mg tablet	25 mg/mL suspension	400 mg tablet	20 mg/mL suspension	200 mg tablet	250 mg capsule	1 capsule in 10 mL water			250 mg tablet
<3	Consult with a clinician experienced in paediatric MDR-TB prescribing for neonates (<28 days of age) and infants weighing <3 kg												
3–3.9	1 tab	2 mL	0.25 tab	0.25 tab	2.5 mL		1.5 mL	not recommended	0.25 cap	2.5 mL	500 mg	250 mg	0.25 tab
4–4.9	1 tab	2 mL	0.25 tab	0.25 tab	2.5 mL		2 mL	0.5 tab	0.25 cap	2.5 mL	500 mg	250 mg	0.25 tab
5–5.9	2 tabs	4 mL	0.5 tab	0.5 tab	5.0 mL		2.5 mL	0.5 tab	0.5 cap	5 mL	500 mg	250 mg	0.5 tab
6–6.9	2 tabs	4 mL	0.5 tab	0.5 tab	5.0 mL		2.5 mL	0.5 tab	0.5 cap	5 mL	1000 mg	500 mg	0.5 tab
7–7.9	2 tabs	4 mL	0.5 tab	0.5 tab	5.0 mL		2.5 mL	0.5 tab	0.5 cap	5 mL	1000 mg	500 mg	0.5 tab
8–8.9	2 tabs	4 mL	0.5 tab	0.5 tab	5.0 mL		2.5 mL	0.5 tab	0.5 cap	5 mL	1000 mg	500 mg	0.5 tab
9–9.9	3 tabs	6 mL	1 tab	0.75 tab	7.5 mL		5 mL	1 tab	0.75 cap	7.5 mL	1500 mg	750 mg	0.75 tab
10–10.9	3 tabs	6 mL	1 tab	0.75 tab	7.5 mL		5 mL	1 tab	0.75 cap	7.5 mL	1500 mg	750 mg	0.75 tab
11–11.9	3 tabs	6 mL	1 tab	0.75 tab	7.5 mL		5 mL	1 tab	0.75 cap	7.5 mL	1500 mg	750 mg	0.75 tab
12–12.9	3 tabs	6 mL	1 tab	1 tab	10 mL		5 mL	1 tab	1 cap	10 mL	2000 mg	1000 mg	1 tab
13–13.9	4 tabs	8 mL	1 tab	1 tab	10 mL		5 mL	1 tab	1 cap	10 mL	2000 mg	1000 mg	1 tab
14–14.9	4 tabs	8 mL	1 tab	1 tab	10 mL		5 mL	1 tab	1 cap	10 mL	2000 mg	1000 mg	1 tab
15–15.9	4 tabs	8 mL	1.5 tabs	1 tab	10 mL	0.5 tab	7.5 mL	1 tab	1 cap	10 mL	2500 mg	1250 mg	1 tab
16–16.9	4 tabs	8 mL	1.5 tabs	1 tab	10 mL	0.5 tab	7.5 mL	1 tab	1 cap	10 mL	2500 mg	1250 mg	1 tab
17–17.9	5 tabs	10 mL	1.5 tabs	1.5 tabs	15 mL	0.5 tab	7.5 mL	1.5 tabs	1.5 caps	15 mL	2500 mg	1250 mg	1.5 tabs
18–18.9	5 tabs	10 mL	1.5 tabs	1.5 tabs	15 mL	0.5 tab	7.5 mL	1.5 tabs	1.5 caps	15 mL	3000 mg	1500 mg	1.5 tabs
19–19.9	5 tabs	10 mL	1.5 tabs	1.5 tabs	15 mL	0.5 tab	7.5 mL	1.5 tabs	1.5 caps	15 mL	3000 mg	1500 mg	1.5 tabs
20–20.9	5 tabs	10 mL	1.5 tabs	1.5 tabs	15 mL	0.5 tab	7.5 mL	1.5 tabs	1.5 caps	15 mL	3000 mg	1500 mg	1.5 tabs
21–21.9	5 tabs	10 mL	2 tabs	1.5 tabs	15 mL	0.5 tab	10 mL	2 tabs	1.5 caps	15 mL	4000 mg	2000 mg	1.5 tabs
22–22.9	5 tabs	10 mL	2 tabs	1.5 tabs	15 mL	0.5 tab	10 mL	2 tabs	1.5 caps	15 mL	4000 mg	2000 mg	1.5 tabs
23–23.9	5 tabs	10 mL	2 tabs	1.5 tabs	15 mL	0.5 tab	10 mL	2 tabs	1.5 caps	15 mL	4000 mg	2000 mg	1.5 tabs
24–24.9	5 tabs	10 mL	2 tabs	2 tabs	20 mL	0.5 tab	10 mL	2 tabs	2 caps	20 mL	5000 mg	2500 mg	2 tabs
25–25.9	5 tabs	10 mL	2.5 tabs	2 tabs	20 mL	0.5 tab	12.5 mL	2.5 tabs	2 caps	20 mL	5000 mg	2500 mg	2 tabs
26–26.9	5 tabs	10 mL	2.5 tabs	2 tabs	20 mL	0.5 tab	12.5 mL	2.5 tabs	2 caps	20 mL	5000 mg	2500 mg	2 tabs
27–27.9	5 tabs	10 mL	2.5 tabs	2 tabs	20 mL	0.5 tab	12.5 mL	2.5 tabs	2 caps	20 mL	6000 mg	3000 mg	2 tabs
28–28.9	5 tabs	10 mL	2.5 tabs	2 tabs	20 mL	0.5 tab	12.5 mL	2.5 tabs	2 caps	20 mL	6000 mg	3000 mg	2 tabs
29–29.9	5 tabs	10 mL	2.5 tabs	2 tabs	20 mL	0.5 tab	12.5 mL	2.5 tabs	2 caps	20 mL	6000 mg	3000 mg	2 tabs

Group 2

	Streptomycin	Amikacin	Kanamycin	Capreomycin
Daily Dose	20–40 mg/kg once daily	15–20 mg/kg once daily	15–20 mg/kg once daily	15–20 mg/kg once daily
Maximum Daily Dose	1000 mg	1000 mg	1000 mg	1000 mg

Group 5

	Clofazimine (CFZ)	Amoxicillin-clavulanate (AMX-CLV)	Meropenem (MPN)	Linezolid (LZD)	Clarithromycin (CLR)
Daily Dose	2–3 mg/kg once daily. If the child is <25kg give 100mg every second day	80 mg/kg in two divided doses based on the amoxicillin component	20–40 mg/kg IV every 8 hours	10 mg/kg dose twice daily for children <10 years of age; 300 mg daily for children >10 years of age (also give vitamin B6)	7.5 mg/kg twice daily
Maximum Daily Dose	200 mg	4000 mg amoxicillin and 500 mg clavulanate	6000 mg	600 mg	1000 mg

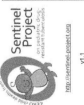

Sentinel Project on paediatric drug-resistant tuberculosis

ZERO child deaths from DR-TB

http://sentinel-project.org

v1.1

FIGURE 18.4 A dosing table based on weight that is commonly used for drugs included in regimens for treating MDR-TB in children.

Figure reproduced and adapted courtesy of The Sentinel Project.[47]

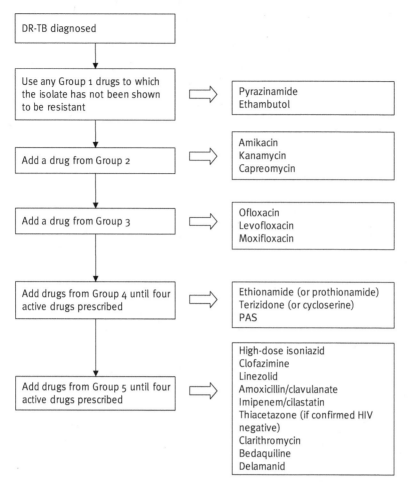

FIGURE 18.5   The grouping of drugs used to treat MDR-TB.

monotherapy. Even though the organism is resistant to isoniazid, it is sometimes used at a high dose in cases of low-level resistance.[59] With increasing use of genotypic diagnostics, clinicians will need to become familiar with the implications of different mutations. For children with confirmed MDR-TB, or those with a clear MDR-TB source case, there is no role for rifampin. However, if the child is either failing first-line therapy or there are multiple source cases, it may be appropriate to include rifampin due to its potency. However, the drug–drug interactions seen with rifampin must be considered, especially in persons living with HIV, and there is some evidence that the fluoroquinolones are less effective in rifampin-containing regimens.[60,61]

The next step is to add an injectable drug from group 2 which includes aminoglycosides (amikacin and kanamycin) and polypeptides (capreomycin). Normally, an aminoglycoside is used to treat MDR-TB, with capreomycin reserved for the treatment of XDR-TB. A fluoroquinolone should then be added from group 3. The later-generation drugs (moxifloxacin and levofloxacin) are more effective than earlier-generation drugs (ofloxacin) in vitro.[62–64] Additional drugs from group 4 should then be added. Either ethionamide or prothionamide should be used (if no inhA mutation is documented), as their metabolic pathways are similar and cross-resistance is total. The same is true for cycloserine and terizidone, and only one of these two drugs should be used. Para-aminosalicylic acid (PAS) can be added if there are not sufficient effective drugs at this stage, but due to gastrointestinal intolerance, the other drugs from group 4 are usually used in preference. Finally, agents from group 5 can be added if required. Drugs from this group are described as having relatively weak or uncertain activity against M. tuberculosis.[39,40] However, both clofazimine and linezolid have, in recent studies, demonstrated promising efficacy and should be considered useful drug options.[65,66] Two newly licensed drugs, bedaquiline and delamanid, appear to have good efficacy against *M. tuberculosis* and may in the future have a more prominent role in the treatment of pediatric MDR-TB. Pharmacokinetic and safety data are limited in children, and appropriate formulations have yet to be developed. These drugs are discussed in more detail later in this chapter, but currently their role and place in the treatment of MDR-TB in children is unclear.

The decision on number of drugs and treatment duration depends on both the extent of disease and the degree of drug resistance, as well as penetration to different body sites and treatment response.

For children with cavitary pulmonary or widespread disease, with resistance to only rifampin and isoniazid, treatment should continue for 18 months from the time of sampling of the first negative culture (assuming that there are no further positive cultures and the child is responding well clinically and radiologically). Treatment should include an injectable agent for the first four to six months; this should be given daily (5 or 7 times per week) until better evidence emerges regarding the efficacy, and reduced toxicity, of thrice-weekly treatment. WHO has recently recommended that injectables should be given for eight months, as longer durations are associated with better outcomes in adults;[38] this is rarely required in children, however. For children with limited, paucibacillary disease, such as isolated intra- or extra-thoracic lymph node involvement and with susceptibility to the second-line drugs, it may be possible to treat the child for 12–15 months in total, depending on the response. It may be possible in such situations to give a shorter duration of the injectable medication or omit the injectable medication altogether and treat only with oral drugs. Evidence for such shorter regimens is lacking, however, and more research is required. If the isolate is XDR or pre-XDR, treatment must rely on less effective drugs, and in this context, more drugs must be used and the treatment given for a minimum of 24 months in total. The choice of drugs will also be determined by the medications available. In the treatment of XDR-TB, consideration should be given to the inclusion of streptomycin, as cross-resistance between second-line injectables is incomplete. Follow-up should continue after the child has completed treatment, to monitor the possibility of relapse. The majority of relapses, if they are to occur, will present in the 12 months

following the end of therapy, and all children should be followed up for at least a year after treatment finishes.

INH mono-resistance can be treated for 9–12 months with rifampin, pyrazinamide, and ethambutol. In cases with additional known or suspected resistance to pyrazinamide or ethambutol, or in cases of extensive disease, a fluoroquinolone can be added along with either high-dose isoniazid or ethionamide, depending on the specific isoniazid mutation. Children with rifampin mono-resistant (RMR) isolates can be treated with isoniazid, pyrazinamide, ethambutol, and a fluoroquinolone for 12–15 months. In cases of additional resistance to pyrazinamide or ethambutol or for extensive disease, an injectable agent can be employed for the first few months, ethionamide can be added, and treatment extended to 18 months. If genotypic tests are employed to perform DST, most national programs advise treating RMR-TB with an MDR-TB regimen in case the child has MDR-TB caused by a mutation other than in the *inhA* promoter region or in the *katG* gene.

In addition to the antituberculosis drugs, children should be given pyridoxine if they are HIV-infected, malnourished, breastfed, or are being given terizidone or cycloserine. There is an argument for putting all children being treated for MDR-TB on multivitamin supplements. Careful consideration should be given to their nutritional requirements, as these children have often been in a catabolic state prior to the diagnosis of MDR-TB and the start of appropriate therapy. Remembering that the old name for tuberculosis was "consumption," note that they may also have high caloric requirements due to the ongoing tissue damage, repair, and inflammation.

Other adjunctive treatments include surgery and bronchoscopy. Both interventions may be employed to assist in making a tissue diagnosis, which is vital in providing appropriate therapy. In addition, in certain circumstances, both may play a therapeutic role. In cases of extensive resistance, where the disease is localized to one anatomical lobe or part of the lung, resection may still have a place. If there is extensive destruction and fibrosis, it is very difficult for the drugs to penetrate into the lesion. In cases of intrathoracic lymph node disease, with external pressure on the airways leading to compression and respiratory compromise, assessment by bronchoscopy is vital. Enucleation of the nodes may be required either bronchoscopically or surgically, both to relieve the pressure on the airway and also to de-bulk the lymph node lesion.

NEW AND RETOOLED ANTITUBERCULOSIS DRUGS IN CHILDREN

Until recently, no new antituberculosis drug classes had been developed for over 40 years.[67] However, in the last decade, the drug research and development pipeline has become much more promising.[68] Not only have a number of entirely new chemical entities been discovered and are proceeding through the stages of drug evaluation, but a number of older drugs are being retooled and used in different ways, in different combinations, or at different dosages.

Two new drugs are at an advanced stage of clinical evaluation: bedaquiline (BDQ) and delamanid (DLM). Bedaquiline is a diarylquinoline that acts by inhibiting intracellular ATP synthase. It has a very long half-life and is effective against actively replicating as well as dormant bacilli. In clinical trials, it has been shown to reduce the time to culture conversion in adults with pulmonary MDR-TB, as well as increasing the proportion who culture-convert.[69] Bedaquiline has been approved recently by the U.S. Federal Drug Administration (FDA) for use in MDR-TB and has been given an interim recommendation by WHO.[70] Although it has not been licensed for use in children, bioequivalence studies of two pediatric formulations (granules and water-dispersible tablets) have been conducted,[71] and pharmacokinetic studies are planned in older children. The CDC advises that on a case-by-case basis bedaquiline might be considered in children when "an effective treatment regimen cannot otherwise be provided."[72] Delamanid is a nitroimidazole (like metronidazole) and acts predominantly on mycolic acid synthesis to stop cell wall production. It has been shown to increase culture conversion and also to improve outcome in adult studies.[73,74] It has been approved by the European Medicines Agency (EMA) and has also been given an interim recommendation by WHO. Pediatric formulations have been developed, and pharmacokinetic and safety studies are underway in children.[75] A single case report describes the successful use of delamanid in a 12-year-old boy who was failing treatment and was infected with a highly resistant organism.[76]

A number of antibiotics traditionally used for the treatment of other infections have also been investigated recently.[77-81] Linezolid has gained much attention following a trial published in 2012, which showed the drug to be highly effective in adult patients with XDR-TB who were failing therapy.[82] Almost all the adults developed side effects to some degree, however, some severe, necessitating cessation of therapy. Linezolid in children seems as effective as in adults, but without the high proportion who develop serious adverse events.[23,83-85] The evidence base is increasing, but experience remains limited. Clofazimine, traditionally an anti-leprosy drug, has also received a great deal of interest recently, mainly due to its central role in the Bangladesh regimen, which will be discussed later.[66] Although there are few reports of children being treated for tuberculosis with clofazimine, there is good experience of using the drug in children with leprosy. Apart from reversible skin discoloration, it appears to be well tolerated.[86] Thioridazine (an antipsychotic), paramomycin (an aminoglycoside), clarithromycin, meropenem, and doxycycline have all been reevaluated recently and have been used when few other drugs are available. Their role in future tuberculosis treatment regimens for children is still unclear.

NEW REGIMENS FOR THE TREATMENT OF TUBERCULOSIS IN CHILDREN

Early in the development of antituberculosis treatment regimens, it was discovered that multidrug regimens were required to effectively prevent the development of resistance.[87] Therefore, in addition to the developments in individual drugs, it is also important to consider the development of regimens. Novel regimens have recently been identified by using contrasting mechanisms.

In 2010, a seminal article was published describing an observational study conducted in Bangladesh.[66] Sequential cohorts of adults with MDR-TB were given different treatment regimens, each differing from the previous by the substitution or addition of one drug. The final cohort was given a nine-month regimen, consisting of kanamycin, clofazimine, gatifloxacin, ethambutol, isoniazid, pyrazinamide, and prothionamide for four months, followed by gatifloxacin, ethambutol, pyrazinamide, and clofazimine for five months. Eighty-eight percent of these patients had a favorable outcome (cured or treatment completed), compared to substantially poorer outcomes for the five previous cohorts who had been given longer regimens (typically 15 months) with drugs including an earlier-generation fluoroquinolone (ofloxacin) and without clofazimine. This study has generated much interest and has led to a number of trials and observational cohorts which seek to further evaluate this nine-month regimen for MDR-TB. One such study, the STREAM trial, is a randomized, non-inferiority trial that compares a similar nine-month regimen to the standard WHO-recommended regimen. It should complete by the end of 2016.[88] *If a drug or regimen has been shown effective in adults, it can be assumed it is effective in children if the pharmacokinetic exposure is similar.* Although all of the individual drugs with in the "Bangladesh regimen" are available for children in some form and are used either to treat tuberculosis already or are used for other indications, no children have been included in these studies. However, consideration should be given to treating children with MDR-TB using this shortened regimen if the STREAM trial shows it to be effective in adults.

A new way of identifying potentially effective regimens is to first carry out murine studies of different drug combinations, based on knowledge of the efficacy of individual agents, to identify combinations that offer synergy. The most promising combinations then advance to early bactericidal activity (EBA) studies, and the best of these then move into longer clinical studies of efficacy and toxicity. This is the route that has taken place to identify the promising combination of pyrazinamide, moxifloxacin, and Pa-824. Initial mouse studies demonstrated that Pa-824 and pyrazinamide worked well together,[89] as did bedaquiline and pyrazinamide.[90] EBA studies identified the combination of pyrazinamide, moxifloxacin, and Pa-824 as the most promising regimen,[91] and this is now being explored in multiple larger studies.[92]

INTERACTION WITH OTHER MEDICAL CONDITIONS

Comorbid medical conditions can increase the risk of tuberculosis disease and affect treatment outcomes. Examples include HIV infection,[93] diabetes,[94] and malnutrition.[95] HIV-infected children are at significantly higher risk of developing tuberculosis than those who are HIV-uninfected,[93] and rates of HIV infection in cohorts of children with MDR-TB are as high as 40%. Adults with diabetes are at increased risk,[94] and children with malnutrition are more vulnerable to the progression of tuberculosis infection.[95] In most regimens used to treat MDR-TB, the drug most likely to cause drug–drug interaction, rifampin, is not used, so the potential for altering the metabolism of other drugs is reduced. However, a number of the antiretroviral therapy (ART) medications alter the blood concentrations of the antituberculosis drugs, and vice versa.[96]

Important practical considerations in the co-treatment of tuberculosis and HIV infection include the timing of initiation of ART, immune reconstitution inflammatory syndrome (IRIS), and drug–drug interactions,[96] together with overlapping toxicities of ART and tuberculosis therapy.[97] If a child with suspected MDR-TB disease is known to have HIV infection and is being treated with ART, MDR-TB treatment should be commenced and adverse effects monitored. In children with tuberculosis who have never been tested or not tested recently, an HIV test is mandatory, following informed consent from the parent, legal guardian, or the child if old enough to assent. For those found to be HIV-infected, MDR-TB is an indication to start ART as soon as is possible.[39,41,98] In practice, it is usually prudent to start the antituberculosis therapy and then wait for a week or two to allow the worst of the initial antituberculosis drug adverse effects to subside before starting ART. This will decrease the likelihood of adverse drug reactions, while allowing rapid initiation of immuno-restorative therapy (Figure 18.6). The management of tuberculous meningitis in this situation is complex, as some studies in adults demonstrate worse outcomes when ART is started early.[99] This field requires further investigation, particularly in children. IRIS occurs within the first few weeks of ART when a resurgent immune system begins to react to *M. tuberculosis* antigens. IRIS can be divided into paradoxical and unmasking IRIS.[100–102] Paradoxical IRIS occurs when a child on antituberculosis treatment becomes worse following the initiation of ART. Unmasking IRIS, however, must be considered in any HIV-infected child with a risk of tuberculosis infection, including MDR-TB, following initiation of ART. The role of corticosteroids is still inconclusive, but they may give some protection in certain situations.[103] Differentiating IRIS from treatment failure can be challenging, but decreasing HIV viral load and improving CD4+ T-cell count should point to IRIS. Few data exist on the interactions between ART and second-line antituberculosis therapy, but, in general, stavudine

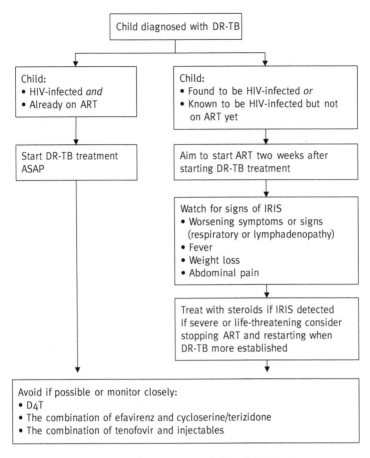

```
                    ┌─────────────────────────────┐
                    │  Child diagnosed with DR-TB │
                    └─────────────────────────────┘
```

Child:
• HIV-infected *and*
• Already on ART

Child:
• Found to be HIV-infected *or*
• Known to be HIV-infected but not
  on ART yet

Start DR-TB treatment
ASAP

Aim to start ART two weeks after
starting DR-TB treatment

Watch for signs of IRIS
• Worsening symptoms or signs
  (respiratory or lymphadenopathy)
• Fever
• Weight loss
• Abdominal pain

Treat with steroids if IRIS detected
If severe or life-threatening consider
stopping ART and restarting when
DR-TB more established

Avoid if possible or monitor closely:
• D4T
• The combination of efavirenz and cycloserine/terizidone
• The combination of tenofovir and injectables

FIGURE 18.6   Approach to the treatment of MDT-TB in a child with HIV infection.

Figure reproduced courtesy of The Sentinel Project.[47]

should be avoided, and concomitant use of tenofo-vir and an injectable requires weekly testing of renal function and electrolytes. HIV-infected children frequently have chronic diarrhea, which may affect the absorption of both the first- and second-line antituberculosis drugs as well as ART medications.[104]

For children with DR-TB and diabetes, more frequent glucose monitoring may be indicated, as both tuberculosis disease and some antituberculosis drugs (ethionamide, PAS, and fluoroquinolones) can disrupt glycemic control. Malnourished children should be treated according to UNICEF protocols, and malnutrition should be prevented by the provision of nutritional support to children and their families. This should ideally avoid the use of specific vitamin supplements, which can add more pills to an already overburdened child, and rather focus on ingestion of vitamins along with calories in the terms of vitamin- and protein-rich foods, such a leafy greens, eggs, peanuts, and legumes.

MONITORING CHILDREN ON DRUG-RESISTANT TUBERCULOSIS TREATMENT

Children should be monitored for three reasons: to determine response to therapy; to identify adverse events early; and to promote adherence to treatment. Directly observed therapy (DOT) is a key component of successful treatment, and the use of community health workers (CHW) or DOT supporters can be invaluable for promoting adherence and identifying adverse events early. DOT should be a comprehensive package of support and assistance, rather than a paternalistic observation of ingestion. Although young children, in effect, always receive their treatment under DOT, in a programmatic sense DOT implies treatment given under the supervision of someone outside the family. A suggested monitoring schedule, which should be adapted to local conditions and resources, is demonstrated in Table 18.4.

Table 18.4. A proposed monitoring schedule to determine response and detect adverse events when treating drug-resistant tuberculosis in children

ALL CHILDREN	BASELINE	\ 1	\ 2	\ 3	\ 4	\ 5	\ 6	\ 9	12	15	18	ONGOING
						MONTH						
HIV status	•											
Toxicity (symptoms, signs)	•	•	•	•	•	•	•	•	•	•	•	•
Height and weight	•	•	•	•	•	•	•	•	•	•	•	•
Audiology[1]	•	•	•	•	•	•	•					
Color vision testing[2]	•	•	•	•	•	•	•	•	•	•	•	•
CXR[3]	•					•					•	
TB culture and DST[4]	•	•	•	•	•	•	•					
Creatinine and potassium[1]	•	•	•	•	•	•	•					
TSH, T$_4$[5]	•	•				•		•				
Hematology (FBC, diff)[6]	•	•	•		•		•	•	•	•	•	•
ECG[7]	•	•	•		•		•	•	•	•	•	•
HIV-infected												
LFTs, Cholesterol	•						•			•		
CD4 count and viral load	•						•		•			•

Figure reproduced courtesy of The Sentinel Project.[47]

[1] Monthly whilst on an injectable, and at six months following termination of injectable.

[2] If on ethambutol.

[3] If any pulmonary involvement or at any point if clinically indicated. To be repeated at the end of treatment.

[4] Monthly if old enough to expectorate. If unable to expectorate and initially smear- or culture-positive, monthly until culture-converted, then thrice monthly. If initially smear- and culture-negative, to perform if clinically indicated.

[5] If on ethionamide, prothionamide, or PAS.

[6] If on linezolid or HIV-infected.

[7] If on bedaquiline or delamanid.

Response to therapy includes clinical, microbiological, and radiological monitoring. Children should be clinically assessed on a regular basis to identify symptoms or signs that might signal lack of response; activity levels, respiratory function, and neurological development. Height and weight should be measured monthly and plotted on an appropriate percentile chart. For children with pulmonary disease, respiratory samples should be collected. For older children, able to expectorate, the adult schedule should be followed with monthly sampling. For younger children, with an initial positive acid-fast smear or culture result, samples initially should be taken monthly. After culture conversion to negative, sampling should be carried out every two to three months. For those with negative acid-fast smear and culture samples at treatment initiation, samples should be obtained if the clinical or radiological situation deteriorates. All samples should be sent for culture and DST, in addition to acid-fast smear microscopy. Finally, children with pulmonary disease should have a chest radiograph at three and six months of treatment and at any time if clinically indicated. It is also useful to have a chest radiograph at the end of therapy to provide a baseline for follow-up. Although chest radiographic improvement is an important indicator of successful treatment response, complete resolution may not occur, and a normal chest radiograph is not required to complete therapy.

Children should be assessed clinically for adverse effects on a regular basis and investigated if signs or symptoms are present. Prior to the start of treatment, children should have a baseline assessment of thyroid function and renal function and have audiological and vision examinations. Both ethionamide and PAS may cause hypothyroidism,[16,17,105–108] and thyroid function should be checked at least every two months while either of these drugs is taken. The injectable drugs can cause renal impairment and hearing loss.[109–112] Renal function should be determined every two months and hearing every month. If circumstances allow, hearing should be tested more frequently. The testing of hearing is age-dependent, and for those older than five years with normal neuro-development, pure tone audiometry (PTA) is the best assessment. Otoacoustic emissions can be used to test the hearing in younger children, but visual testing is challenging for this age group. Children being given ethambutol who are able to cooperate with color-vision testing should be assessed monthly, using an appropriate Ishihara or Snellen chart. This is usually possible from the age of five years. Clinicians should, however, be reassured that ocular toxicity is very rare when ethambutol is given at the recommended dosage.[113] A full blood count should be undertaken monthly if the child is receiving linezolid. There is no need to monitor full blood count or liver function routinely. Transient elevations in transaminase levels are common at the start of antituberculosis therapy and are rarely associated with significant adverse effects.[114] Drugs to alleviate adverse events should be provided free of charge, as adherence may be compromised if the family has to pay. The management of adverse events is described in Table 18.5. If the child has other medical conditions such as HIV or diabetes, however, other regular blood tests may be required.

PROMOTING ADHERENCE FOR TREATMENT OF DR-TB

As with the treatment of drug-susceptible tuberculosis in children, adherence to treatment is critical but even more difficult for children with MDR- or XDR-TB. Children on treatment for MDR-TB must take multiple medications, vitamin and calorie supplements, and if HIV-infected, ART drugs every day for at least a year. A number of the drugs are highly unpalatable and can cause profound nausea, vomiting, and diarrhea. It is not surprising that adherence can be challenging. Usually during the initial, intensive phase, when an injectable medication is given, the child is either in a hospital or in regular contact with the health services. Treatment during this phase should be under DOT. It is during this phase that the worst of the adverse effects are likely to occur, and at this point the child has not become familiar with the daily routine of pill-taking. It is also during this phase that adherence is most important as, with the highest bacillary load, the organisms are at the greatest probability of developing further resistance if adherence lapses. The daily injections can be particularly distressing for children. Usually they are given into the muscle, but if resources permit, intravenous administration is less painful. The use of local anesthetic mixed with the antibiotic, as well as hot compresses and varying the site of injection, can help.

For the continuation phase, DOT is desirable but not always practical. It should be made as easy as possible for the child to have the medications under DOT, with consideration given to allowing

Table 18.5. The management of adverse events in the treatment of drug-resistant tuberculosis in children

	LIKELY CULPRIT DRUGS	IDENTIFICATION	MANAGEMENT
Hepato-toxicity	INH; PZA; RIF; ETH; PAS; CTZ; TZD	Tender liver, visible jaundice	Stop all drugs Wait for liver function to return to normal Reintroduce drugs one-by-one sequentially, every two days with monitoring of liver function before introducing the next drug
Visual problems	EMB, INH	Regular testing with Ishihara Chart	Stop EMB or substitute for alternative drug
Hearing problems	AMK; Km; CAP	Identified through audiometry or problems in communication	Consider stopping the injectable drug, substituting for an alternative drug, reducing dose, or increasing dose interval
Thyroid dysfunction	ETH; PAS	Regular blood testing, clinical hypothyroidism, or goiter	Consider thyroxine supplementation (0.05 mg daily) if (a) clinical hypothyroidism or (b) raised TSH and decreased fT4 If raised TSH and normal fT4, repeat test in one month
Renal impairment	AMK; Km; CAP	Regular blood testing, symptoms of high potassium	If creatinine rises or potassium is elevated, stop injectable, substitute for alternative drug, dose three times a week, or reduce dose
Severe rash (SJS)	Any drug	Severe rash, peeling mucus membranes, child unwell	Stop all drugs Wait until clinical condition has improved Reintroduce drugs one-by-one sequentially, every two days, monitoring clinically
Nausea and vomiting	ETH; EMB; PAS	Clinically	Consider anti-emetics Consider separating the dosing of ETH from the other drugs by giving it in the evening Consider reducing the dose of ETH and building the dose up to full dose over two weeks
Diarrhea	PAS	Clinically	Split dose of granules to give small doses throughout day Reduce dose Consider loperamide
Peripheral neuropathy	INH	Clinically	Give or increase pyridoxine If persistent or severe, stop INH

(continued)

Table 18.5. Continued

	LIKELY CULPRIT DRUGS	IDENTIFICATION	MANAGEMENT
Neuro-psychiatric problems	INH; OFL; LEV; MOX; TZD; CLS	Seizures, headache, behavior changes, sleep disturbances	Verify correct dosing Stop likely culprit drug If symptoms persist, reintroduce and stop next most likely drug If symptoms severe or persistent, stop all likely drugs or reduce dose
Joint problems	PZA; OFL; LEV; MOX	Clinically	Verify correct dosing Consider reducing dose/stopping possible culprit drug Consider trial of allopurinol
Painful injection sites	AMK; Km; CAP	Clinically	Add local anesthetic to drug in equal volumes Vary site of injection on a daily basis If severe, consider splitting dose and giving half into two different sites

this to happen in school or with a nearby clinic.[115] Long waiting times, unsympathetic staff, and stigmatization at health facilities can deter attendance. During this phase, if the child is old enough to understand, it is important to invest time and effort in educating children about the disease and allowing them to take responsibility for their illness and their treatment. If the child is not old enough, the parents must be prepared appropriately. The child and family should be warned about the possibility of all adverse effects and what to do if they occur. These adverse effects should be managed aggressively, and early and anti-emetic medications can be very useful. Creative mechanisms should be employed to encourage adherence, with reward systems appropriate to the child's age. Mobile telephone technology, lay DOT support workers, or decentralized care in the community may all play a role.[115,116] Parents and medical staff also need to be creative about how the medications are delivered—whether as tablets or ground up and mixed with strong-tasting foods such as yogurts, fruit juices, jams, or sauces.

MANAGING ADVERSE EVENTS

Most antituberculosis drugs can cause rash and gastrointestinal upset, but in most instances these resolve without treatment and without compromising therapy. Stevens Johnson–like reactions, however, necessitate immediate cessation of all drugs (including all antituberculosis and HIV medications) until the symptoms have resolved. Sequential reintroduction can then occur. In this situation, it is best to restart the antituberculosis medications one by one every two to three days and monitor response. If the child was on ART medications, once tuberculosis treatment is reestablished, all ART medications should be restarted at the same time. Once antituberculosis and ART drugs are established, other agents can be added. Co-trimoxazole is an important, but rare, cause of severe skin reactions. Gastrointestinal upset is most pronounced with ethionamide and PAS: ethionamide generally causing nausea and vomiting, and PAS, diarrhea. If nausea and vomiting compromise drug delivery, it may be prudent to start ethionamide initially with a half dose and give it in the evening, separately from the other medications. Antiemetics can also be used. After a week, the other half of the dose can be given in the morning. After a further week, the full dose can be given in the evening, and eventually the full dose can be given with the other medications in the morning. PAS is usually given twice a day, but if diarrhea is severe, the dosage can be reduced or the drug given in smaller quantities more frequently.

If diarrhea is profuse, regular monitoring of hydration status and serum potassium is necessary.

If either color vision or hearing are found to be deteriorating, strong consideration should be given to stopping the ethambutol (vision) or injectable medication (hearing). If necessary, further drugs from group 4 or 5 can be substituted. As this is a drug substitution within a functional regimen, it is not considered to be the addition of a single drug to a failing regimen. If the thyroid stimulating hormone (TSH) is elevated and the free T4 is low, then consideration should be given to starting thyroxine substitution at an initial dose of 0.05 mg daily. Peripheral neuropathy can be treated by either increasing the dose of pyridoxine or reducing the dose of isoniazid. If it persists, the isoniazid should be stopped. However, peripheral neuropathy associated with linezolid usually necessitates stopping the drug. Determining the cause of neuropsychiatric adverse events can be complicated. Isoniazid can cause behavioral changes and psychosis, and the fluoroquinolones can cause headache and hallucinations and can affect sleep. Terizidone and cycloserine can cause seizures, behavioral changes, hallucinations, and psychosis. In addition, if the child is on efavirenz as part of ART, that drug may be responsible. As a first step, it is important to verify that the child has been prescribed and is receiving the correct dose, as over-dosages can be associated with adverse effects. The next step is to reduce the dosage of the drug felt most likely to be responsible and to monitor the effect. If this does not help, then the drug should be stopped. If there is no resolution, the drug should be reintroduced and the next most likely drug reduced in dose and then, if necessary, stopped. Joint problems can be caused by pyrazinamide and the fluoroquinolones, and management options include reducing or stopping one or both of these drugs or adding allopurinol (if PZA is the likely cause). Clinical hepatitis (tender liver, visible jaundice) necessitates immediate cessation of all hepatotoxic drugs. These include rifampin, isoniazid, pyrazinamide, ethionamide, PAS, beta-lactams, macrolides, and thiacetazone. Treatment should continue with the remaining drugs and consideration given to starting any other available medications that are not hepatotoxic. The hepatotoxic drugs can be reintroduced one by one every two days, but given that the child is on treatment for MDR-TB, the relative merits of reintroducing isoniazid, rifampin, and pyrazinamide should be considered.

INFECTION CONTROL

Children traditionally have been considered to pose a low infection-control risk as they generally have paucibacillary disease and limited tussive force. However, as the diagnosis of DR-TB is frequently delayed in children,[117-119] those with DR-TB tend to be older than those with drug-susceptible disease[120,121] and have more severe pathology; in a recent cohort of pediatric culture-confirmed MDR-TB cases, over 60% were sputum smear-positive.[122] Infection control should form a vital part of any management strategy for children with DR-TB.

Children should be considered a significant infection risk if they have sputum acid-fast smear-positive disease and a moderate risk while they still have sputum culture-positive disease. While acid-fast smear-positive, they should sleep in a room separate from others and while inside should wear a mask. Masks for patients need to limit the spread of aerosolized bacilli, and, for this purpose, simple surgical masks suffice. This is challenging to enforce in young children. Those who are culture-positive should not sleep in the same room as other vulnerable children, such as those who are HIV-infected or the very young. Children should be encouraged to spend as much of their time outside as possible. When outside, it is reasonable to allow children to play and eat without a mask. Where it is not possible to spend long periods of time outside, windows should be kept open, passive air-extraction systems put in place, and areas with sufficient resources should consider active airflow management systems. Those without pulmonary disease are unlikely to pose an infection risk unless there is pus discharging from an uncovered body site.

Staff should protect themselves when interacting with potentially contagious children. If the child is sputum acid-fast smear-positive, staff should wear a fit-tested respirator mask to prevent the inhalation of infectious aerosolized droplets. Respiratory protective devices with a filter efficiency of 95% or greater (e.g., N95, N99, N100) should be used.

MULTIDISCIPLINARY CARE

Multidisciplinary care is a cornerstone of the successful management of children with DR-TB. In addition, the child and caregiver should be engaged as active members of the health care team. In settings with good healthcare resources, input from pharmacists can be invaluable in providing appropriate medications, formulations, and advice concerning interactions and pharmacokinetics. Support from a dietician, where possible, is important in monitoring and planning calorie intake and the correct balance of nutrients, vitamins, and minerals. Where they exist, physiotherapy and occupational therapy are beneficial, not only for those with neurodevelopment involvement but also for those with respiratory and musculoskeletal deficits. Social services should assess home circumstances and support the caregiver to look after a child who may have complex medical needs and must take multiple medications. They must also assist the family in securing any insurance, funding, or grants that they are eligible for to assist in the process of home-based care. In cases of neglect, abuse, or drug and alcohol use, child placement with alternative caregivers may be necessary. Early involvement is vital. Ongoing education is important, and when they are no longer contagious, children should be encouraged to return to school.

Children are treated for long durations in hospital, so structured daytime activities are important. For younger children, play specialists can structure development-promoting activities; and for older children, hospital schools with dedicated teaching staff make sure that children do not miss out on too much of their education while inpatients.

DRUG-RESISTANT TUBERCULOSIS DEFINITIONS IN CHILDREN

From clinical, programmatic, and academic perspectives, it is important to define treatment characteristics and outcome in a standardized manner. It is important to define and record if the child has been previously treated and what that treatment was, and also to determine if the child has previously experienced a tuberculosis disease episode. For the current episode, the reason for treatment initiation is important, as is the site of disease. A list of suggested definitions is shown in Table 18.1.

The definition of "cure" for adults with MDR-TB is completion of treatment with five negative cultures in the final 12 months of treatment.[123] For children with drug-susceptible tuberculosis, cure is defined as being sputum culture or acid-fast smear-negative in the last month of treatment and on at least one previous occasion.[124,125] Both of these definitions seem inappropriate for children with MDR-TB, so it is likely that a compromise is necessary. A more

appropriate definition is three consecutive negative respiratory cultures obtained at least one month apart, with no positive cultures after the first negative result, in the presence of treatment completion.[122] A significant proportion of children treated for MDR-TB either will not have confirmed MDR-TB or will not have an initial sputum sample (EPTB). For these children, it is important that the category of treatment completed include components of clinical and radiological resolution in the context of completion of the prescribed treatment course. Weight gain should form part of this assessment. Treatment failure should include a poor clinical or radiological response, or microbiology that persists in being culture or acid-fast smear positive. Default will include those children who either did not take or were not given their treatment for longer than two months. Death is from any cause on MDR-TB treatment.

TREATMENT OF DR-TB INFECTION

The correct management of children exposed to DR-TB is unclear,[126] with a limited evidence base to support policy,[127,128] and variable international guidelines.[129] The British National Institute for Health and Clinical Excellence advises follow-up with no medical treatment,[130] as does the WHO.[40] The US Centers for Disease Control and Prevention, the American Thoracic Society, the American Academy of Pediatrics, and the Infectious Diseases Society of America advise giving two drugs to which the source case's strain is susceptible.[131] The European Centre for Disease Prevention and Control suggests that either treatment or close follow-up are legitimate options.[132] A possible approach is shown in Figure 18.7.

Only a few studies have assessed treatment of MDR-TB child contacts. In Israel, 476 adult and child contacts of 78 pulmonary MDR-TB patients were evaluated. Twelve were given a therapy regimen tailored to the known DST results, 71 were given isoniazid, 6 were given other treatments, and 387 were not given any treatment. No contacts developed tuberculosis disease.[133] In Cape Town, from 1994–2000, 103 child contacts of 73 MDR-TB source cases were identified and followed up. Two (5%) of the 41 children who received tailored treatment developed tuberculosis disease, opposed to 13 (20%) out of the 64 children who were not given any treatment.[134] In a retrospective study in Brazil,

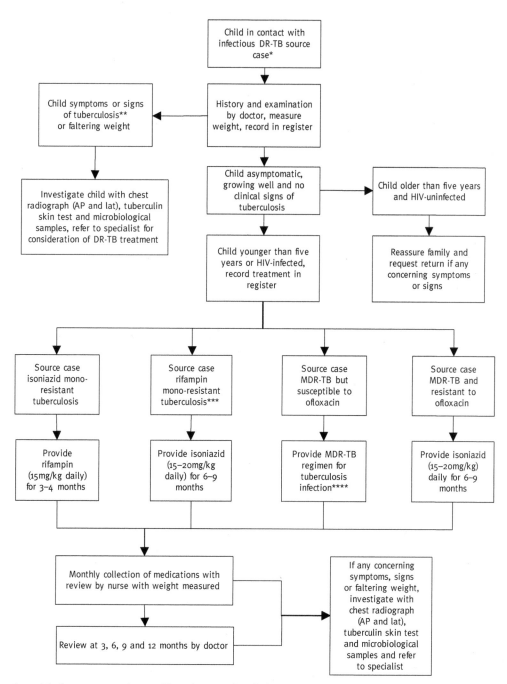

*   Infectious–smear or culture positive pulmonary tuberculosis
**   Cough, reduced playfulness, fever, lethargy, abnormal bones or joints
***   If diagnosed by GeneXpert, consider MDR until confirmation by line probe assay
****   A number of preventive therapy options have been proposed. One option might include: isoniazid (15-20mg/kg daily), ethambutol (20–25mg/kg daily) and ofloxacin (15–20mg/kg daily) for six months

FIGURE 18.7   An algorithm for assessing a child for treatment of drug-resistant tuberculosis infection after contact with a source case.

Figure reproduced courtesy of The Sentinel Project (reference 47).

218 contacts of 64 MDR-TB source cases were given isoniazid, while the remainder were observed without treatment. The rate of subsequent tuberculosis was similar in the group given isoniazid (1.2 per 1,000-person-months of contact) compared to the group that was not (1.7 per 1,000-person-months of contact; $p = 0.47$). In two outbreaks in Chuuk, Federated States of Micronesia, 5 MDR-TB source cases were identified. Of 232 contacts identified, 119 were offered treatment, of whom 104 initiated a fluoroquinolone-based regimen. None of those who started treatment developed tuberculosis disease, compared with 3 of the 15 who did not take treatment.[135-137]

A recent prospective study from Cape Town recruited 186 children who had been exposed to adult source cases with MDR-TB. All were offered three-drug treatment with ofloxacin, ethambutol, and high-dose isoniazid. Six children developed tuberculosis disease, and one infant died. Factors associated with poor outcome were age less than 12 months, HIV infection, and poor adherence.[138] Several randomized, double-blind, placebo-controlled trials are planned to evaluate levofloxacin as a single agent for the prevention of tuberculosis in MDR-TB contacts. However, in the meantime, these observational studies suggest that providing treatment may be effective in stopping the progression from infection to disease in children.

CONCLUSION

Treating children with DR-TB is perceived to be challenging. However, it is possible to achieve excellent outcomes in a wide range of settings with varying resources. The child and family should be actively engaged in the treatment process and supported by the healthcare team. They should be treated with at least four drugs likely to be effective, and the child should be monitored carefully for adverse events and response to treatment. More children will be diagnosed with MDR-TB in the future, and clinicians must be well prepared in order to treat them.

REFERENCES

1. Zhang Y, Yew WW. Mechanisms of drug resistance in *Mycobacterium tuberculosis*. *Int J Tuberc Lung Dis.* 2009;13(11):1320–1330.
2. Dramowski A, Morsheimer MM, Jordaan AM, Victor TC, Donald PR, Schaaf HS. Rifampin-monoresistant *Mycobacterium tuberculosis* disease among children in Cape Town, South Africa. *Int J Tuberc Lung Dis.* 2012;16(1):76–81.
3. Mukinda FK, Theron D, van der Spuy GD, et al. Rise in rifampin-monoresistant tuberculosis in Western Cape, South Africa. *Int J Tuberc Lung Dis.* 2012;16(2):196–202.
4. Pablos-Mendez A, Raviglione MC, Laszlo A, et al. Global surveillance for antituberculosis-drug resistance, 1994–1997. World Health Organization–International Union against Tuberculosis and Lung Disease Working Group on Anti-Tuberculosis Drug Resistance Surveillance. *N Engl J Med.* 1998;338(23):1641–1649.
5. Mitnick CD, Shin SS, Seung KJ, et al. Comprehensive treatment of extensively drug-resistant tuberculosis. *N Engl J Med.* 2008;359(6):563–574.
6. World Health Organization, Geneva, Switzerland. Global Tuberculosis Report. 2014.
7. van Rie A, Beyers N, Gie RP, Kunneke M, Zietsman L, Donald PR. Childhood tuberculosis in an urban population in South Africa: burden and risk factor. *Arch Dis Child.* 1999;80(5):433–437.
8. Dodd PJ, Gardiner E, Coghlan R, Seddon JA. Burden of childhood tuberculosis in 22 high-burden countries: a mathematical modelling study. *Lancet Global Health.* 2014;2(8):e453–e459.
9. Jenkins HE, Tolman AW, Yuen CM, et al. Incidence of multidrug-resistant tuberculosis disease in children: systematic review and global estimates. *Lancet.* 2014;383(9928):1572–1579.
10. Ettehad D, Schaaf HS, Seddon JA, Cooke GS, Ford N. Treatment outcomes for children with multidrug-resistant tuberculosis: a systematic review and meta-analysis. *Lancet Infect Dis.* 2012;12(6):449–456.
11. World Health Organization, Geneva, Switzerland. Molecular Line Probe Assays for the rapid screening of patients at risk of multidrug-resistant tuberculosis (MDR-TB). Policy statement, 2008. Available at: http://www.who.int/tb/features_archive/policy_statement.pdf (accessed August 2012).
12. World Health Organization, Geneva, Switzerland. Roadmap for rolling out Xpert MTB/RIF for rapid diagnosis of TB and MDR-TB. 2010. Available at: http://www.who.int/tb/laboratory/roadmap_xpert_mtb_rif.pdf (accessed August 2012).
13. Orenstein EW, Basu S, Shah NS, et al. Treatment outcomes among patients with

multidrug-resistant tuberculosis: systematic review and meta-analysis. *Lancet Infect Dis.* 2009;9(3):153–161.

14. Johnston JC, Shahidi NC, Sadatsafavi M, Fitzgerald JM. Treatment outcomes of multidrug-resistant tuberculosis: a systematic review and meta-analysis. *PLoS One.* 2009;4(9):e6914.

15. Seddon JA, Thee S, Jacobs K, Ebrahim A, Hesseling AC, Schaaf HS. Hearing loss in children treated for multidrug-resistant tuberculosis. *J Infect.* 2013;66(4):320–329.

16. Thee S, Zollner EW, Willemse M, C. HA, Magdorf K, Schaaf HS. Abnormal thyroid function tests in children on ethionamide treatment (short communication). *Int J Tuberc Lung Dis.* 2011;15(9):1191–1193.

17. Hallbauer UM, Schaaf HS. Ethionamide-induced hypothyroidism in children. *South Afr J Epidemiol Infect.* 2011;26(3):161–163.

18. Esposito S, Bosis S, Canazza L, Tenconi R, Torricelli M, Principi N. Peritoneal tuberculosis due to multidrug-resistant *Mycobacterium tuberculosis. Pediatr Int (Japan).* 2013;55(2):e20–e22.

19. Katragkou A, Antachopoulos C, Hatziagorou E, Sdougka M, Roilides E, Tsanakas J. Drug-resistant tuberculosis in two children in Greece: report of the first extensively drug-resistant case. *Eur J Pediatr.* 2013;172(4):563–567.

20. Gegia M, Jenkins HE, Kalandadze I, Furin J. Outcomes of children treated for tuberculosis with second-line medications in Georgia, 2009–2011. *Int J Tuberc Lung Dis.* 2013;17(5):624–629.

21. Williams B, Ramroop S, Shah P, et al. Multidrug-resistant tuberculosis in UK children: presentation, management and outcome. *Eur Respir J.* 2013;41(6):1456–1458.

22. Lapphra K, Sutthipong C, Foongladda S, et al. Drug-resistant tuberculosis in children in Thailand. *Int J Tuberc Lung Dis.* 2013;17(10):1279–1284.

23. Rose PC, Hallbauer UM, Seddon JA, Hesseling AC, Schaaf HS. Linezolid-containing regimens for the treatment of drug-resistant tuberculosis in South African children. *Int J Tuberc Lung Dis.* 2012;16(12):1588–1593.

24. Satti H, McLaughlin MM, Omotayo DB, et al. Outcomes of comprehensive care for children empirically treated for multidrug-resistant tuberculosis in a setting of high HIV prevalence. *PLoS One.* 2012;7(5):e37114.

25. Shah I, Rahangdale A. Partial extensively drug resistant (XDR) tuberculosis in children. *Indian Pediatr.* 2011;48(12):977–979.

26. Shah I. Multidrug-resistant tuberculosis in children from 2003 to 2005: a brief report. *Indian J Med Microbiol.* 2012;30(2):208–211.

27. Shah I, Chilkar S. Clinical profile of drug resistant tuberculosis in children. *Indian Pediatr.* 2012;49(9):741–744.

28. Shah I, Mohanty S. Multidrug-resistant tuberculosis in an HIV-infected girl. *Natl Med J India.* 2012;25(4):210–211.

29. Garazzino S, Scolfaro C, Raffaldi I, Barbui AM, Luccoli L, Tovo PA. Moxifloxacin for the treatment of pulmonary tuberculosis in children: a single center experience. *Pediatr Pulmonol.* 2014;49(4):372–376.

30. Chauny JV, Lorrot M, Prot-Labarthe S, et al. Treatment of tuberculosis with levofloxacin or moxifloxacin: report of 6 pediatric cases. *Pediatr Infect Dis J.* 2012;31(12):1309–1311.

31. Isaakidis P, Paryani R, Khan S, et al. Poor outcomes in a cohort of HIV-infected adolescents undergoing treatment for multidrug-resistant tuberculosis in Mumbai, India. *PLoS One.* 2013;8(7):e68869.

32. Uppuluri R, Shah I. Partial extensively drug-resistant tuberculosis in an HIV-infected child: a case report and review of literature. *J Int Assoc Provid AIDS Care.* 2014;13(2):117–119.

33. Mignone F, Codecasa LR, Scolfaro C, et al. The spread of drug-resistant tuberculosis in children: an Italian case series. *Epidemiol Infect.* 2013:1–8.

34. Santiago B, Baquero-Artigao F, Mejias A, Blazquez D, Jimenez MS, Mellado-Pena MJ. Pediatric drug-resistant tuberculosis in Madrid: family matters. *Pediatr Infect Dis J.* 2014;33(4):345–350.

35. Rodrigues M, Brito M, Villar M, Correia P. Treatment of multidrug-resistant and extensively drug-resistant tuberculosis in adolescent patients. *Pediatr Infect Dis J.* 2014;33(6):657–659.

36. Seddon JA, Hesseling AC, Godfrey-Faussett P, Schaaf HS. High treatment success in children treated for multidrug-resistant tuberculosis: an observational cohort study. *Thorax.* 2014;69(5):458–464.

37. Wiseman CA, Gie RP, Starke JR, et al. A proposed comprehensive classification of tuberculosis disease severity in children. *Pediatr Infect Dis J.* 2012;31(4):347–352.

38. World Health Organization, Geneva, Switzerland. Guidelines for the programmatic management of

drug-resistant tuberculosis. 2011 update. WHO/HTM/TB/2011.6.

39. World Health Organization, Geneva, Switzerland. Guidelines for the programmatic management of drug-resistant tuberculosis—Emergency update, 2008. WHO/HTM/TB/2008.402. Available at: http://whqlibdoc.who.int/publications/2008/9789241547581_eng.pdf (accessed July 2013).

40. World Health Organization, Geneva, Switzerland. Guidance for national tuberculosis programme on the management of tuberculosis in children. 2nd ed., 2014. Available at: http://apps.who.int/iris/bitstream/10665/112360/1/9789241548748_eng.pdf?ua=1 (accessed 29 May 2014).

41. Department of Health, Republic of South Africa. Management of drug-resistant tuberculosis. Policy guidelines. Cape Town, South Africa, 2010.

42. American Academy of Pediatrics. Tuberculosis. In: Pickering LK, ed. *Red Book: Report of the Committee on Infectious Diseases*. 28th ed. Elk Grove Village, IL: American Academy of Pediatrics; 2009:680–701.

43. Francis J Curry National Tuberculosis Center. Drug-resistant tuberculosis: a survival guide for clinicians. 2nd ed., 2008. Available at: http://www.currytbcenter.ucsf.edu/drtb/docs/MDRTB_book_2011.pdf (accessed July 2013).

44. Partners in Health. The Partners in Health guide to the medical management of multidrug-resistant tuberculosis; 2003. Available at: http://parthealth.3cdn.net/7b69fbe8784f6c73c9_cwm6v2gyk.pdf (accessed July 2013).

45. Partners in Health, Harvard Medical School, Bill & Melinda Gates Foundation. A DOTS-Plus handbook—guide to the community-based treatment of MDR TB. Boston, MA: Harvard Medical School, 2004.

46. The Sentinel Project on Pediatric Drug-Resistant Tuberculosis. Available at: www.sentinel-project.org (accessed November 2012).

47. The Sentinel Project for Pediatric Drug-Resistant Tuberculosis. Management of multidrug-resistant tuberculosis in children: a field guide. 2012. Available at: http://sentinelproject.files.wordpress.com/2012/11/sentinel_project_field_guide_2012.pdf (accessed 6 June 2014).

48. Schaaf HS, Victor TC, Engelke E, et al. Minimal inhibitory concentration of isoniazid in isoniazid-resistant *Mycobacterium tuberculosis* isolates from children. *Eur J Clin Microbiol Infect Dis*. 2007;26(3):203–205.

49. Muller B, Streicher EM, Hoek KG, et al. inhA promoter mutations: a gateway to extensively drug-resistant tuberculosis in South Africa? *Int J Tuberc Lung Dis*. 2011;15(3):344–351.

50. Kam KM, Yip CW, Cheung TL, Tang HS, Leung OC, Chan MY. Stepwise decrease in moxifloxacin susceptibility amongst clinical isolates of multidrug-resistant *Mycobacterium tuberculosis*: correlation with ofloxacin susceptibility. *Microb Drug Resist*. 2006;12(1):7–11.

51. Allen BW, Mitchison DA, Chan YC, Yew WW, Allan WG, Girling DJ. Amikacin in the treatment of pulmonary tuberculosis. *Tubercle*. 1983;64(2):111–118.

52. Caminero JA, Sotgiu G, Zumla A, Migliori GB. Best drug treatment for multidrug-resistant and extensively drug-resistant tuberculosis. *Lancet Infect Dis*. 2010;10(9):621–629.

53. Maus CE, Plikaytis BB, Shinnick TM. Molecular analysis of cross-resistance to capreomycin, kanamycin, amikacin, and viomycin in *Mycobacterium tuberculosis*. *Antimicrob Agents Chemother*. 2005;49(8):3192–3197.

54. Donald PR, Schoeman JF. Tuberculous meningitis. *N Engl J Med*. 2004;351(17):1719–1720.

55. van Well GT, Paes BF, Terwee CB, et al. Twenty years of pediatric tuberculous meningitis: a retrospective cohort study in the Western Cape of South Africa. *Pediatrics*. 2009;123(1):e1–e8.

56. Lincoln EM. Tuberculous meningitis in children; with special reference to serous meningitis; tuberculous meningitis. *Am Rev Tuberc*. 1947;56(2):75–94.

57. Mphahlele M, Syre H, Valvatne H, et al. Pyrazinamide resistance among South African multidrug-resistant *Mycobacterium tuberculosis* isolates. *J Clin Microbiol*. 2008;46(10):3459–3464.

58. Hoek KG, Schaaf HS, Gey van Pittius NC, van Helden PD, Warren RM. Resistance to pyrazinamide and ethambutol compromises MDR/XDR-TB treatment. *S Afr Med J*. 2009;99(11):785–787.

59. Schaaf HS, Victor TC, Venter A, et al. Ethionamide cross- and co-resistance in children with isoniazid-resistant tuberculosis. *Int J Tuberc Lung Dis*. 2009;13(11):1355–1359.

60. Louw GE, Warren RM, Gey van Pittius NC, et al. Rifampin reduces susceptibility to ofloxacin in rifampin-resistant *Mycobacterium tuberculosis* through efflux. *Am J Respir Crit Care Med*. 2011;184(2):269–276.

61. Weiner M, Burman W, Luo CC, et al. Effects of rifampin and multidrug resistance gene polymorphism on concentrations of

moxifloxacin. *Antimicrob Agents Chemother.* 2007;51(8):2861–2866.

62. Hu Y, Coates AR, Mitchison DA. Sterilizing activities of fluoroquinolones against rifampin-tolerant populations of *Mycobacterium tuberculosis. Antimicrob Agents Chemother.* 2003;47(2):653–657.

63. Global Alliance for TB Drug Development. Handbook of Anti-Tuberculosis Agents. *Tuberculosis (Edinb).* 2008;88(2):85–170.

64. Rodriguez JC, Cebrian L, Lopez M, Ruiz M, Jimenez I, Royo G. Mutant prevention concentration: comparison of fluoroquinolones and linezolid with *Mycobacterium tuberculosis. J Antimicrob Chemother.* 2004;53(3):441–444.

65. Cox H, Ford N. Linezolid for the treatment of complicated drug-resistant tuberculosis: a systematic review and meta-analysis [Review article]. *Int J Tuberc Lung Dis.* 2012; 16(4):447–454.

66. Van Deun A, Maug AK, Salim MA, et al. Short, highly effective, and inexpensive standardized treatment of multidrug-resistant tuberculosis. *Am J Respir Crit Care Med.* 2010;182(5):684–692.

67. Zumla A, Nahid P, Cole ST. Advances in the development of new tuberculosis drugs and treatment regimens. *Nat Rev Drug Discov.* 2013;12(5):388–404.

68. Working Group on New TB Drugs. Drug pipeline. Available at: http://www.newtbdrugs. org/pipeline.php, 2015 (accessed 6 June 2015).

69. Diacon AH, Pym A, Grobusch M, et al. The diarylquinoline TMC207 for multidrug-resistant tuberculosis. *N Engl J Med.* 2009;360(23):2397–2405.

70. World Health Organization, Geneva, Switzerland. The use of bedaquiline in the treatment of multidrug-resistant tuberculosis: Interim policy guidance (WHO/HTM/TB/2013.6), 2013. Available at: http://apps.who.int/iris/ bitstream/10665/84879/1/9789241505482_ eng.pdf?ua=1 (accessed 6 June 2014).

71. Clinicaltrials.gov. A study to assess the relative bioavailability of TMC207 following single-dose administrations of two pediatric formulations in healthy adult participants. Available at: http:// clinicaltrials.gov/ct2/show/record/NCT018033 73?term=bedaquiline&rank=6, 2014 (accessed 6 June 2014).

72. Provisional CDC guidelines for the use and safety monitoring of bedaquiline fumarate (Sirturo) for the treatment of multidrug-resistant tuberculosis. *MMWR Recomm Rep.* 2013;62(RR-09):1–12.

73. Skripconoka V, Danilovits M, Pehme L, et al. Delamanid improves outcomes and reduces mortality in multidrug-resistant tuberculosis. *Eur Respir J.* 2013;41(6):1393–1400.

74. Gler MT, Skripconoka V, Sanchez-Garavito E, et al. Delamanid for multidrug-resistant pulmonary tuberculosis. *N Engl J Med.* 2012;366(23):2151–2160.

75. ClinicalTrials.gov. Pharmacokinetic and safety trial to determine the appropriate dose for pediatric patients with multidrug resistant tuberculosis. Available at: http://clinicaltrials. gov/ct2/show/record/NCT01856634, 2014 (accessed 6 June 2014).

76. Esposito S, D'Ambrosio L, Tadolini M, et al. ERS/ WHO Tuberculosis Consilium assistance with extensively drug-resistant tuberculosis management in a child: case study of compassionate delamanid use. *Eur Respir J.* 2014 44(3):811–815.

77. Alsaad N, Wilffert B, van Altena R, et al. Potential antimicrobial agents for the treatment of multidrug-resistant tuberculosis. *Eur Respir J.* 2014;43(3):884–897.

78. Zumla AI, Gillespie SH, Hoelscher M, et al. New antituberculosis drugs, regimens, and adjunct therapies: needs, advances, and future prospects. *Lancet Infect Dis.* 2014;14(4):327–340.

79. Kaufmann SH, Lange C, Rao M, et al. Progress in tuberculosis vaccine development and host-directed therapies—a state of the art review. *Lancet Respir Med.* 2014;2(4):301–320.

80. Dooley KE, Obuku EA, Durakovic N, et al. World Health Organization group 5 drugs for the treatment of drug-resistant tuberculosis: unclear efficacy or untapped potential? *J Infect Dis.* 2013;207(9):1352–1358.

81. Dooley KE, Mitnick C, Degroote MA, et al. Old drugs, new purpose: Retooling existing drugs for optimized treatment of resistant tuberculosis. *Clin Infect Dis.* 2012;55(4):572–581.

82. Lee M, Lee J, Carroll MW, et al. Linezolid for treatment of chronic extensively drug-resistant tuberculosis. *N Engl J Med.* 2012;367(16):1508–1518.

83. Garcia-Prats AJ, Rose PC, Hesseling AC, Schaaf HS. Linezolid for the treatment of drug-resistant tuberculosis in children: a review and recommendations. *Tuberculosis (Edinb).* 2014;94(2):93–104.

84. Kjollerstrom P, Brito MJ, Gouveia C, Ferreira G, Varandas L. Linezolid in the treatment of multidrug-resistant/extensively drug-resistant tuberculosis in paediatric patients: experience of a paediatric infectious diseases unit. *Scand J Infect Dis.* 2011;43(6–7):556–559.

85. Pinon M, Scolfaro C, Bignamini E, et al. Two pediatric cases of multidrug-resistant tuberculosis treated with linezolid and moxifloxacin. *Pediatrics*. 2010;126(5):e1253–e1256.

86. Kroger A, Pannikar V, Htoon MT, et al. International open trial of uniform multi-drug therapy regimen for 6 months for all types of leprosy patients: rationale, design and preliminary results. *Trop Med Int Health*. 2008;13(5):594–602.

87. Iseman MD. Tuberculosis therapy: past, present and future. *Eur Respir J (Suppl)*. 2002;36:87s–94s.

88. ClinicalTrials.gov. The evaluation of a standardised treatment regimen of anti-tuberculosis drugs for patients with multi-drug-resistant tuberculosis (MDR-TB): STREAM. Available at: http://www.controlled-trials.com/ISRCTN78372190/STREAM, 2014 (accessed 9 June 2014).

89. Tasneen R, Tyagi S, Williams K, Grosset J, Nuermberger E. Enhanced bactericidal activity of rifampin and/or pyrazinamide when combined with PA-824 in a murine model of tuberculosis. *Antimicrob Agents Chemother*. 2008;52(10):3664–3668.

90. Ibrahim M, Andries K, Lounis N, et al. Synergistic activity of R207910 combined with pyrazinamide against murine tuberculosis. *Antimicrob Agents Chemother*. 2007;51(3):1011–1015.

91. Diacon AH, Dawson R, von Groote-Bidlingmaier F, et al. 14-day bactericidal activity of PA-824, bedaquiline, pyrazinamide, and moxifloxacin combinations: a randomised trial. *Lancet*. 2012;380(9846):986–993.

92. Bagcchi S. Novel drug combination for tuberculosis to be tested across 50 sites. *BMJ*. 2014;348:g3535.

93. Hesseling AC, Cotton MF, Jennings T, et al. High incidence of tuberculosis among HIV-infected infants: evidence from a South African population-based study highlights the need for improved tuberculosis control strategies. *Clin Infect Dis*. 2009;48(1):108–114.

94. Webb EA, Hesseling AC, Schaaf HS, et al. High prevalence of *Mycobacterium tuberculosis* infection and disease in children and adolescents with type 1 diabetes mellitus. *Int J Tuberc Lung Dis*. 2009;13(7):868–874.

95. Singh M, Mynak ML, Kumar L, Mathew JL, Jindal SK. Prevalence and risk factors for transmission of infection among children in household contact with adults having pulmonary tuberculosis. *Arch Dis Child*. 2005;90(6):624–628.

96. Coyne KM, Pozniak AL, Lamorde M, Boffito M. Pharmacology of second-line antituberculosis drugs and potential for interactions with antiretroviral agents. *AIDS*. 2009;23(4):437–446.

97. Seddon JA, Hesseling AC, Marais BJ, et al. Paediatric use of second-line anti-tuberculosis agents: a review. *Tuberculosis (Edinb)*. 2012;92(1):9–17.

98. World Health Organization, Geneva, Switzerland. Antiretroviral therapy for HIV infection in infants and children: towards universal access. Recommendations for a public health approach. 2010 revision.

99. Torok ME, Yen NT, Chau TT, et al. Timing of initiation of antiretroviral therapy in human immunodeficiency virus (HIV)-associated tuberculous meningitis. *Clin Infect Dis*. 2011;52(11):1374–1383.

100. International Network of the Study of HIV-Associated IRIS. Case definition: consensus criteria for diagnosis of paediatric TB IRIS. 2008. Available at http://www.inshi.umn.edu/definitions/Peds_TB_IRIS/home.html (accessed on 29 May 2011).

101. Boulware DR, Callens S, Pahwa S. Pediatric HIV immune reconstitution inflammatory syndrome. *Curr Opin HIV AIDS*. 2008;3(4):461–467.

102. Zampoli M, Kilborn T, Eley B. Tuberculosis during early antiretroviral-induced immune reconstitution in HIV-infected children. *Int J Tuberc Lung Dis*. 2007;11(4):417–423.

103. Muller M, Wandel S, Colebunders R, Attia S, Furrer H, Egger M. Immune reconstitution inflammatory syndrome in patients starting antiretroviral therapy for HIV infection: a systematic review and meta-analysis. *Lancet Infect Dis*. 2010;10(4):251–261.

104. Peloquin CA, Berning SE, Huitt GA, Iseman MD. AIDS and TB drug absorption. *Int J Tuberc Lung Dis*. 1999;3(12):1143–1144.

105. McDonnell ME, Braverman LE, Bernardo J. Hypothyroidism due to ethionamide. *N Engl J Med*. 2005;352(26):2757–2759.

106. Soumakis SA, Berg D, Harris HW. Hypothyroidism in a patient receiving treatment for multidrug-resistant tuberculosis. *Clin Infect Dis*. 1998;27(4):910–911.

107. Moulding T, Fraser R. Hypothyroidism related to ethionamide. *Am Rev Respir Dis*. 1970;101(1):90–94.

108. Davies HT, Galbraith HJ. Goitre and hypothyroidism developing during treatment with P.A.S. *Br Med J.* 1953;1(4822):1261.

109. Selimoglu E. Aminoglycoside-induced ototoxicity. *Curr Pharm Des.* 2007;13(1):119–126.

110. Duggal P, Sarkar M. Audiologic monitoring of multi-drug resistant tuberculosis patients on aminoglycoside treatment with long term follow-up. *BMC Ear Nose Throat Disord.* 2007;7:5.

111. Peloquin CA, Berning SE, Nitta AT, et al. Aminoglycoside toxicity: daily versus thrice-weekly dosing for treatment of mycobacterial diseases. *Clin Infect Dis.* 2004;38(11):1538–1544.

112. de Jager P, van Altena R. Hearing loss and nephrotoxicity in long-term aminoglycoside treatment in patients with tuberculosis. *Int J Tuberc Lung Dis.* 2002;6(7):622–627.

113. Donald PR, Maher D, Maritz JS, Qazi S. Ethambutol dosage for the treatment of children: literature review and recommendations. *Int J Tuberc Lung Dis.* 2006;10(12):1318–1330.

114. Frydenberg AR, Graham SM. Toxicity of first-line drugs for treatment of tuberculosis in children: review. *Trop Med Int Health.* 2009;14(11):1329–1337.

115. Barker RD, Millard FJ, Nthangeni ME. Unpaid community volunteers—effective providers of directly observed therapy (DOT) in rural South Africa. *S Afr Med J.* 2002;92(4):291–294.

116. Economist. Taken your medicine? *The Economist Technology Quarterly (June 6th).* 2009:7–8.

117. Schaaf HS, Shean K, Donald PR. Culture-confirmed multidrug-resistant tuberculosis: diagnostic delay, clinical features, and outcome. *Arch Dis Child.* 2003;88(12):1106–1111.

118. Drobac PC, Mukherjee JS, Joseph JK, et al. Community-based therapy for children with multidrug-resistant tuberculosis. *Pediatrics.* 2006;117(6):2022–2029.

119. Ettehad D, Schaaf HS, Seddon JA, Cooke G, Ford N. Treatment outcomes for children with multidrug-resistant tuberculosis: a systematic review and meta-analysis. *Lancet Infect Dis (in press).* 2012.

120. Schaaf HS, Marais BJ, Hesseling AC, Brittle W, Donald PR. Surveillance of antituberculosis drug resistance among children from the Western Cape Province of South Africa—an upward trend. *Am J Public Health.* 2009;99(8):1486–1490.

121. Schaaf HS, Marais BJ, Hesseling AC, Gie RP, Beyers N, Donald PR. Childhood drug-resistant tuberculosis in the Western Cape Province of South Africa. *Acta Paediatr.* 2006;95(5):523–528.

122. Seddon JA, Hesseling AC, Willemse M, Donald PR, Schaaf HS. Culture-confirmed multidrug-resistant tuberculosis in children: clinical features, treatment, and outcome. *Clin Infect Dis.* 2012;54(2):157–166.

123. World Health Organisation, Geneva, Switzerland. Guidelines for the programmatic management of drug-resistant tuberculosis—Emergency update; 2008. WHO/HTM/TB/2008.402.

124. World Health Organisation, Geneva, Switzerland. Guidelines for National Tuberculosis Programmes on the management of tuberculosis in children; 2006. WHO/HTM/TB/2006.371, WHO/FCH/CAH/2006.7.

125. Franck C, Seddon JA, Hesseling AC, Schaaf HS, Skinner D, Reynolds L. Assessing the impact of multidrug-resistant tuberculosis in children: an exploratory qualitative study. *BMC Infect Dis.* 2014;14(1):426.

126. Seddon JA, Godfrey-Faussett P, Hesseling AC, Gie RP, Beyers N, Schaaf HS. Management of children exposed to multidrug-resistant *Mycobacterium tuberculosis. Lancet Infect Dis.* 2012;12(6):469–479.

127. van der Werf MJ, Langendam MW, Sandgren A, Manissero D. Lack of evidence to support policy development for management of contacts of multidrug-resistant tuberculosis patients: two systematic reviews. *Int J Tuberc Lung Dis.* 2012;16(3):288–296.

128. Fraser A, Paul M, Attamna A, Leibovici L. Drugs for preventing tuberculosis in people at risk of multiple-drug-resistant pulmonary tuberculosis. *Cochrane Database Syst Rev.* 2006(2):CD005435.

129. van der Werf MJ, Sandgren A, Manissero D. Management of contacts of multidrug-resistant tuberculosis patients in the European Union and European Economic Area. *Int J Tuberc Lung Dis.* 2012;16(3):426.

130. National Institute for Health and Clinical Excellence. Tuberculosis. Clinical diagnosis and management of tuberculosis, and measures for its prevention and control; 2011. Available at: http://www.nice.org.uk/nicemedia/live/13422/53642/53642.pdf (accessed July 2013). NICE clinical guideline 117.

131. Centers for Disease Control, Atlanta, Georgia. Management of persons exposed

to multidrug-resistant tuberculosis. *MMWR Recomm Rep.* 1992;41(RR-11):61–71.

132. European Centre for Disease Prevention and Control. Management of contacts of MDR TB and XDR TB patients; 2012. Available at: http://ecdc.europa.eu/en/publications/Publications/201203-Guidance-MDR-TB-contacts.pdf (accessed July 2013).

133. Attamna A, Chemtob D, Attamna S, et al. Risk of tuberculosis in close contacts of patients with multidrug resistant tuberculosis: A nationwide cohort. *Thorax.* 2009;64(3):271.

134. Schaaf HS, Gie RP, Kennedy M, Beyers N, Hesseling PB, Donald PR. Evaluation of young children in contact with adult multidrug-resistant pulmonary tuberculosis: a 30-month follow-up. *Pediatrics.* 2002;109(5):765–771.

135. Bamrah S, Brostrom R, Dorina F, et al. Treatment for LTBI in contacts of MDR-TB patients, Federated States of Micronesia, 2009–2012. *Int J Tuberc Lung Dis.* 2014;18(8):912–918.

136. Brostrom R, Fred D, Heetderks A, et al. Islands of hope: building local capacity to manage an outbreak of multidrug-resistant tuberculosis in the Pacific. *Am J Public Health.* 2011;101(1):14–18.

137. Fred D, Desai M, Song R, et al. Multi-drug resistant tuberculosis in Chuuk State Federated States of Micronesia, 2008–2009. *Pacific Health Dialog.* 2010;16(1):123–127.

138. Seddon JA, Hesseling AC, Finlayson H, et al. Preventive therapy for child contacts of multidrug-resistant tuberculosis: a prospective cohort study. *Clin Infect Dis.* 2013;57(12):1676–1684.

139. Schaaf HS, Krook S, Hollemans DW, Warren RM, Donald PR, Hesseling AC. Recurrent culture-confirmed tuberculosis in human immunodeficiency virus-infected children. *Pediatr Infect Dis J.* 2005;24(8):685–691.

140. Fairlie L, Beylis NC, Reubenson G, Moore DP, Madhi SA. High prevalence of childhood multi-drug resistant tuberculosis in Johannesburg, South Africa: a cross sectional study. *BMC Infect Dis.* 2011;11:28.

141. Feja K, McNelley E, Tran CS, Burzynski J, Saiman L. Management of pediatric multidrug-resistant tuberculosis and latent tuberculosis infections in New York City from 1995 to 2003. *Pediatr Infect Dis J.* 2008;27(10):907–912.

142. Granich RM, Oh P, Lewis B, Porco TC, Flood J. Multidrug resistance among persons with tuberculosis in California, 1994–2003. *JAMA.* 2005;293(22):2732–2739.

143. Leimane V, Ozere I. Challenges of managing a child with MDR-TB: 41st World Conference on Lung Health of the International Union Against Tuberculosis and Lung Disease (The Union), Cancun, Mexico, 3–7 December, 2009.

144. Mendez Echevarria A, Baquero Artigao F, Garcia Miguel MJ, et al. Multidrug-resistant tuberculosis in the pediatric age group. *Anales de Pediatria.* 2007;67(3):206–211.

145. Padayatchi N, Bamber S, Dawood H, Bobat R. Multidrug-resistant tuberculous meningitis in children in Durban, South Africa. *Pediatr Infect Dis J.* 2006;25(2):147–150.

146. Schluger NW, Lawrence RM, McGuiness G, Park M, Rom WN. Multidrug-resistant tuberculosis in children: two cases and a review of the literature. *Pediatr Pulmonol.* 1996;21(2):138–142.

147. Seddon JA, Hesseling AC, Willemse M, Donald PR, Schaaf HS. Culture-confirmed multidrug-resistant tuberculosis in children: clinical features, treatment, and outcome. *Clin Infect Dis.* 2012;54(2):157–166.

148. Suessmuth S, Bange FC, Gappa M. Multidrug resistant tuberculosis in a 6 year old child. *Paediatr Respir Rev.* 2007;8(3):265–268.

19

BACILLE CALMETTE–GUÉRIN VACCINES

Kim Connelly Smith, Ian M. Orme, and Jeffrey R. Starke

HIGHLIGHTS OF THIS CHAPTER

- Bacille Calmette–Guérin vaccination has worked well in some situations but poorly in others. Because only a small fraction of the cases in the general population of contagious, smear-positive adult pulmonary tuberculosis are potentially preventable by BCG vaccination, BCG has had little effect on the ultimate control of tuberculosis.
- Meta-analysis of published studies of BCG vaccination calculate that the overall protective efficacy against all forms of tuberculosis for those vaccinated at birth or during infancy was 50% on average, and protection against death was 65%, meningitis 64%, and disseminated tuberculosis 78%.
- Localized adverse effects (adenopathy, drainage at the injection site) are common after BCG vaccination, but serious long-term complications are rare, except in severely immunocompromised children.
- Currently, the World Health Organization considers HIV infection a contraindication for BCG vaccination and recommends delay of immunization in HIV-exposed infants until HIV infection has been ruled out. In reality, the lack of available HIV serodiagnosis or antigen detection in many regions of the world means that, in some areas, large numbers of HIV-infected infants and children are still receiving BCG vaccines.

THE BACILLE Calmette–Guérin (BCG) vaccines have been given to over 4 billion people and have been used routinely since the 1960s in almost all countries throughout the world (with the exception of a few industrialized countries), many of which have decreased their use of BCG vaccination as tuberculosis rates have fallen. Despite widespread use of BCG vaccines, tuberculosis remains the leading cause of death from a curable infectious disease.[1] The World Health Organization estimates that 9 million new cases of disease and 1.5 million deaths were attributed to this organism in 2013.[2] Although most technologically advanced countries have managed to control, but not eradicate tuberculosis, the incidence of disease and infection is increasing in many poorer areas of the world. Better vaccines are needed if TB is to be eradicated.[3]

HISTORY OF BCG VACCINE DEVELOPMENT

A history of the development of BCG vaccine is summarized in Table 19.1.[4] Two French scientists—Albert Calmette, a physician, and Camille Guérin, a veterinarian—began working on a tuberculosis vaccine in 1908. The strain they selected was *Mycobacterium bovis* from a cow with tuberculous mastitis. The isolate was subcultured

Table 19.1. A brief history of the Bacille Calmette-Guérin vaccine[4]

YEAR	EVENT
1902	First isolation of *Mycobacterium bovis*
1908–1921	BCG developed from serial passage of *Nocardia* strain
1921	First human BCG vaccination
1928	League of Nations adopts BCG as standard vaccine
1929–1930	Lübeck disaster: 72 children die from oral BCG preparation contaminated with virulent strain
1939	Multiple puncture technique introduced
1947	Scarification technique introduced
1948	First International BCG Congress concluded that BCG is effective; more than 10 million vaccinations carried out
1948–1974	WHO and UNICEF campaigns; 1.5 billion vaccinations carried out
1948–1997	Yearly increase of BCG vaccination estimated to be from 50 million to almost 100 million

Adapted from Lugosi L. Theoretical and methodological aspects of BCG vaccine from the discovery of Calmette and Guérin to molecular biology: a review. *Tuberc Lung Dis.* 1992;73(5):252–261.

every three weeks for 13 years, becoming attenuated over time.

In 1948, the First International BCG Congress in Paris declared that the BCG vaccine was effective and safe, despite the lack of published controlled trials or studies. After World War II, the World Health Organization (WHO) and the United Nations International Children's Emergency Fund (UNICEF) organized campaigns to promote vaccination. By the end of 1974, more than 1.5 billion individuals had received a BCG vaccine. From 1974 to the present, BCG vaccination has been included in the WHO Expanded Programme on Immunization. Approximately 100 million children receive BCG vaccine each year, usually at birth, expanding the total number of individuals who have received BCG to more than 4 billion.

The original strain of *M. bovis* used to make BCG was maintained by serial passage at the Pasteur Institute until it was lost during World War II. Before its loss, it was distributed to dozens of laboratories in many countries. Each laboratory produced its own BCG, maintained by serial passage. Serial subculturing under different conditions resulted in many daughter BCG strains that differed widely.[5] To standardize production and stabilize vaccine characteristics, a seed lot system was adopted in the mid-1950s, and in the 1960s the WHO recommended freeze-dried storage of samples.

Strains in use today vary widely in many characteristics. Some BCG strains are considered "strong," whereas others are "weak." Case-control and cohort studies suggest that the protection against tuberculosis and the incidence of side effects differ between strong and weak strains. The strong strains have been associated with a higher rate of lymphadenitis and osteitis, especially among neonates.[6] Reduction of the vaccination dose of the strong strains reduces the incidence of lymphadenitis, probably with little effect on immediate vaccine efficacy. The use of a weaker strain is tempting for both vaccine producers and users, because immediate results without side effects ensure few problems initially. Investigators may have selected BCG strains by their desire to maximize tuberculin reactivity and minimize adenitis, which may have created the inverse of an ideal vaccine. There is no worldwide consensus about which strain of BCG is optimal for general use. In addition, the various BCG strains appear to have lost efficacy over time with serial passage.[7]

DOSAGE AND ROUTE OF ADMINISTRATION

It is generally accepted that the most accurate method of BCG vaccination is intradermal injection using a syringe and needle because the dose can be measured and the administration can be controlled. This method is recommended by the WHO and UNICEF and is used by most countries. Although many body sites can be used, the usual site for vaccination is the deltoid region of the arm. The rate of local reactions, including ulcers and lymphadenitis, is higher with the intradermal method, and administration may be difficult in newborns, the most commonly recommended age for vaccination.

Other methods of administration have been developed. Subcutaneous injection, scarification, jet injection, multipuncture, and application using bifurcated needles, have yielded highly variable and, in some cases, inadequate results. There have been no conclusive reported trials comparing the various techniques of administration for protection against tuberculosis.

The recommended dosage of BCG vaccine differs by vaccine strain and age of the recipient. Most manufacturers recommend 0.05 mL for infants and 0.1 mL for children and adults. For each strain, the dosage is adjusted to maximize the protective effect and minimize the local reactions.

Specific strain used, age, schedule, and route of administration have varied among countries and changed over time. The BCG World Atlas (http://www.bcgatlas.org/) is an online database of current and past global BCG vaccine policy and practices for 180 countries.[8] This resource catalogues the various BCG vaccination recommendations and how they have changed in different countries throughout the world over decades.

IMMUNE RESPONSES TO BACILLE CALMETTE–GUÉRIN VACCINE

Unlike most infectious diseases and commonly used vaccines that cause a measurable serological response for an average known duration, there is no serological test for protective immunity after tuberculosis infection or BCG vaccination, making the vaccine especially challenging to study.

Tuberculin skin test (TST) conversion has long been used as evidence of mycobacterial infection or as a sign of adequate response to BCG vaccine. The relationship between post-vaccination delayed hypersensitivity and protective immunity is a controversial issue, with no clear relationship established. Neither the presence nor the size of post-vaccination TST reactions reliably predict the degree of protection induced by BCG.[9]

Most of the major field trials, case-control studies and meta-analyses of BCG vaccines have demonstrated a higher level of protection against the more serious forms of tuberculosis, such as meningitis and disseminated disease, than against the more moderate forms of disease.[10] Comparison of the major BCG studies is illustrated in Figure 19.1.[3,10–37] BCG vaccination may not effectively prevent infection with *Mycobacterium tuberculosis* but presumably helps the host retard the growth of organisms at the primary site of infection and prevent massive lymphohematogenous dissemination. The duration of immunity after BCG vaccination is not known; most experts speculate that protection declines over time and is probably low to nonexistent 10–20 years after vaccination. Several studies have shown that BCG vaccine induces protection against *Mycobacterium leprae* infection that is as great as or even greater than that against tuberculosis.[38]

BACILLE CALMETTE–GUÉRIN VACCINE AND THE TUBERCULIN SKIN TEST

The BCG vaccines can have an effect on the response to the TST. Studies evaluating the proportion of previously BCG-vaccinated individuals with significant TST reactions have ranged from 0–90%. The size of the skin test reaction after BCG vaccination varies with the strain and dose of the vaccine, the route of administration, the age and nutritional status of the individual, the number of years since vaccination, and the frequency of skin testing. Some studies have found that the size of the TST reaction increases with repeated BCG vaccination, whereas others have found no such correlation (see also Chapter 6).

In a large number of studies of children who received BCG vaccine, the mean reaction to a TST ranged from 0–19 mm, although many experts believe that reactions larger than 10–15 mm after vaccination are unusual. Lifschitz[38A] found that approximately 50% of infants given BCG vaccine shortly after birth were TST-negative at six months

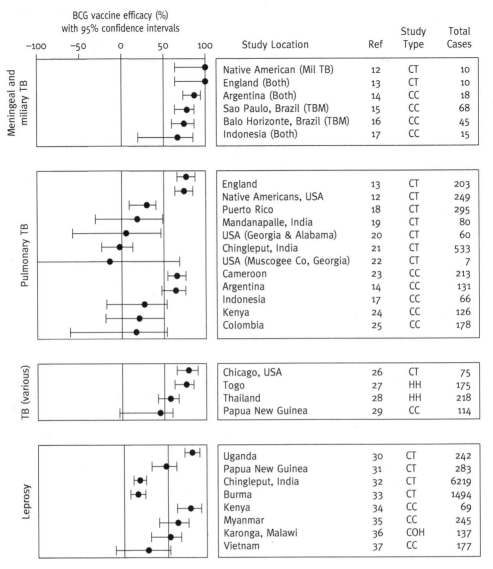

FIGURE 19.1   Estimates of Bacille Calmette-Guerin vaccine efficacy against different forms of tuberculosis (TB) and leprosy, from clinical trials (CT), case-control (CC), cohort (COH), and household (HH) studies.[11]

of age, and almost all children were TST-negative one year after vaccination. A study among West African infants found that BCG vaccination prior to one month of age was associated with more anergy to TST than vaccination after one month of age.[39] Many studies in different parts of the world have shown similar results, most demonstrating waning TST reactions over time if infection with *M. tuberculosis* has not also occurred. Some studies using interferon gamma release assays (IGRA) have called into question the belief that BCG vaccination does not cause larger TST reactions.

One study in the United States showed that up to two-thirds of BCG-vaccinated children with positive TSTs had negative IGRAs.[40] There was a trend of IGRA positivity with larger TST size, but over half of the children with TSTs over 20 mm had negative IGRAs, indicating possible false-positive TST reactions among both BCG and non-BCG vaccinated children. Until there is a reference standard, it is impossible to know if the discordance is due to false-positive TSTs or false-negative IGRAs.

Interpretation of the TST in individuals previously vaccinated with BCG may be complicated by the booster phenomenon.[41,42] The booster effect is the increase in reaction size to skin testing caused by repetitive testing in a person sensitized to mycobacterial antigens. This phenomenon is presumably caused by stimulation of a waned immunological response to mycobacterial antigens. Some experts recommend avoidance of repeated skin tests in a short period of time (less than 1 year) in persons with previous BCG vaccination, or apparent conversions of the reaction from negative to positive may be created.

Prior BCG vaccination is never a contraindication for tuberculin testing. A reaction measuring 10 mm or more in an individual who has been vaccinated with BCG may indicate infection with *M. tuberculosis*, especially if the individual has had recent contact with an infectious case or has lived in an area of the world with a high prevalence of tuberculosis. One study found that a significant TST reaction among individuals who received BCG vaccine after infancy had a positive predictive value for infection with *M. tuberculosis* of 17% among a low tuberculosis burden Canadian-born population, and 78% among recent immigrants from an area endemic for tuberculosis.[43] The probability that a TST reaction has resulted from tuberculosis infection increases:

1. as the size of the reaction increases;
2. when a patient has had contact with a person with infectious tuberculosis;
3. if the person is in a high-risk group for tuberculosis;
4. when the patient's country of origin has a high prevalence of tuberculosis; and
5. as the length of time between vaccination and tuberculin testing increases.[44]

The IGRAs, QuantiFERON-TB Gold (Cellestis, Carnegie, Australia) and T-SPOT-TB (Oxford Immunotec, Oxford, U.K.), measure interferon gamma released by T-cells stimulated by specific antigens which are found in *M. tuberculosis* but not in BCG vaccine strains. The IGRA tests, like the TST, are used to diagnose tuberculosis infection but cannot distinguish infection from disease. The major advantage of the IGRAs compared to the TST is higher specificity in persons previously vaccinated with BCG.[45] Guidelines regarding the use of the TST and IGRAs vary by region. In tuberculosis low-burden countries, the IGRA test may be preferred in individuals with BCG vaccination history

due to higher specificity. On the other hand, for children less than five years of age and in high-burden countries, the TST may be preferred for better sensitivity, especially when tuberculosis disease is suspected.

EFFICACY AND EFFECTIVENESS OF BACILLE CALMETTE–GUÉRIN VACCINES

The true effectiveness of BCG vaccines has been debated for decades. Large clinical trials conducted from the 1930s through the 1970s yielded wide-ranging and conflicting results, demonstrating efficacy ranging from 0–80% (Figure 19.1). The most recent trial, in Chingleput, India, had discouraging results and methodological difficulties that only served to continue the argument.[21,46] Since the 1980s, researchers have studied BCG efficacy using case-control, cohort, household contact, and meta-analysis study designs, but conclusions still diverge. Even with years of study and discussion, the question of how well BCG vaccines work cannot be answered definitively.

Despite the controversy, there are two areas in which BCG vaccines have shown consistent benefits: protection against disseminated tuberculosis disease and protection against leprosy. Various studies have demonstrated high levels of protection against miliary tuberculosis and tuberculous meningitis, especially among vaccinated infants (Figure 19.1). It is generally accepted that BCG vaccines are most efficacious in preventing severe childhood tuberculosis disease and reducing rates of leprosy worldwide.

Comparing the major controlled trials is difficult because they differed in a number of important aspects, including eligibility criteria, methods of disease surveillance, diagnostic criteria, vaccine strain and administration, and environmental factors. Extensive discussion comparing the controlled trials has been reviewed in previous publications.[3,47]

The randomized controlled trial is the ideal study design to address vaccine efficacy, but the lack of a simple, validated blood test for protective immunity means that the major outcome variable is usually long-term clinical observation of a large population. There is no gold standard for diagnosis of tuberculosis disease other than acid-fast stain and mycobacterial culture, which can have low sensitivity, especially among children. Also, many of these trials were conducted in developing countries in which resources for diagnosis, vaccination, follow-up, and tracking were limited. These challenges, as well as the lack of understanding of the immunology involved in protection against tuberculosis, make the design and execution of clinical trials extremely difficult.

The major controlled trials shown in Figure 19.1 demonstrated a wide range of protection from none to 80%. The largest and most recent BCG field trial was co-sponsored by the Indian Council of Medical Research, the WHO, and the U.S. Public Health Service in the Chingleput district of southern India.[21,47] The results showed no evidence of protection against pulmonary tuberculosis compared with that of placebo. Thus the world's largest BCG field trial only created more uncertainties about the efficacy of the BCG vaccines. It is not clear why there is such a wide range of results from the major controlled BCG trials. Theories attempting to explain the differences include trial methodology, variations in vaccines, concentration of NTM in the environment, host factors, regional differences in *M. tuberculosis* strains, and exogenous reinfection versus endogenous reactivation.

The lack of consensus led the WHO in the 1980s to initiate studies evaluating children who were household contacts of cases with infectious tuberculosis disease. These methods, as well as other case-control and cohort studies, yielded results similar to those of the major controlled trials, with efficacy ranging from 0% to more than 80% (Figure 19.1).

Meta-analysis has been used to evaluate the clinical effect of BCG vaccines.[10,48-50] Investigators at the London School of Hygiene and Tropical Medicine found the protective effect for meningeal and miliary disease was 86% in randomized controlled trials and 75% in case-control studies.[48] For pulmonary tuberculosis, the methods were too divergent to calculate a summary estimate. Investigators at the Harvard School of Public Health found the overall protective effect of BCG for tuberculosis disease was 50–51%.[50] The protective effect against tuberculous meningitis and disseminated disease was 64% and 72%, respectively. Among the seven prospective trials that enrolled patients randomly, the estimated protective effect was 85% for BCG vaccination at birth, 73% for vaccination at age 10 years, and 50% for vaccination at 20 years of age. Different strains of BCG were not consistently associated with more or less favorable results in the trials. Different BCG preparations and strains used in the same population gave similar levels of protection, whereas genetically identical BCG vaccines gave different levels of protection in different populations. The Harvard group also published a meta-analysis evaluating the efficacy of BCG vaccination specifically for newborns and infants.[49,50] The overall protective efficacy against all forms of tuberculosis for those vaccinated at birth or during infancy was 50% on average. Protection against death was 65%, meningitis 64%, and disseminated tuberculosis 78%.

In summary, BCG vaccination has worked well in some situations but poorly in others. Because only a small fraction of the cases in the general population of contagious, smear-positive adult pulmonary tuberculosis are potentially preventable by BCG vaccination, BCG has had little effect on the ultimate control of tuberculosis. The best use of BCG vaccines appears to be for the prevention of life-threatening forms of tuberculosis such as meningitis and disseminated disease in infants and young children. Vaccination with BCG remains the standard for tuberculosis prevention in most high-burden countries because it is available, is inexpensive, and requires only one encounter with the patient; in addition, it rarely causes serious complications, and systems for treatment of tuberculosis infection and early diagnosis and treatment of tuberculosis disease in children are lacking in many areas of the world.

SAFETY OF BACILLE CALMETTE–GUÉRIN VACCINE

For more than 70 years, BCG vaccines have been administered safely to billions of individuals throughout the world. Complications are rare, but the rate varies depending on the method of administration; the type, strength, and dose of the vaccine; and the age and immune status of the vaccinee.[51-53]

Localized adverse effects are common after BCG vaccination, but serious long-term complications are rare (Table 19.2).[53] Ninety percent to 95% of patients vaccinated with BCG develop a local reaction followed by healing cutaneous scar formation within three months, although scarring is less likely following vaccination in early infancy. The type of scar caused by BCG vaccination varies with the method of administration. Examples are shown in Figure 19.2. Individuals with tuberculosis infection often have an accelerated response to BCG vaccine characterized by induration within one to two days and scab formation and healing within 10–15 days.

Table 19.2. Estimated age-specific risks for complications after administration of Bacilli Calmette-Guérin vaccine[52]

COMPLICATION	INCIDENCE PER 1 MILLION VACCINATIONS	
	AGE <1 YR	AGE 1–20 YRS
Local subcutaneous abscess, regional lymphadenopathy	387	25
Musculoskeletal lesions	0.39–0.89	0.06
Multiple lymphadenitis, nonfatal disseminated lesions	0.31–0.39	0.36
Fatal disseminated lesions	0.19–1.56	0.06–0.72

Adapted from Lotte A, Wasz-Hockert O, Poisson N, et al. Second IUATLD study on complications induced by intradermal BCG vaccination. *Bull IUATLD*. 1988;63(2):47–59.

After cutaneous reactions, local ulceration and regional lymphadenitis are the most common complications, occurring in less than 1% of immunocompetent recipients who receive intradermal administration.[53] Local skin lesions and lymphadenitis usually occur within a few weeks to months after vaccination, but symptoms may be delayed for months in immunocompetent persons and for years in immunocompromised hosts.[54] Axillary, cervical, and supraclavicular nodes, when involved, usually are enlarged on the ipsilateral side of vaccination. The risk of suppurative lymphadenitis is greater among newborns than among older infants and children, especially when a full dose of vaccine is given; therefore, the WHO recommends using a reduced dose in infants.

The treatment of local adenitis as a complication of BCG vaccination is controversial and ranges from observation to surgical drainage to the administration of antituberculosis drugs to a combination of surgical management and medications.[55] Non-suppurative lymph nodes usually

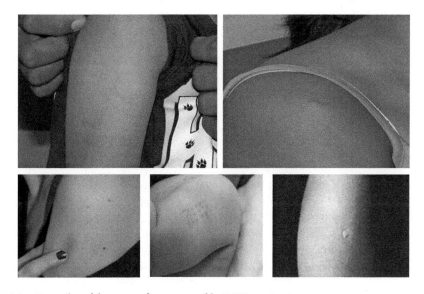

FIGURE 19.2   Examples of the types of scars created by BCG vaccination.

improve spontaneously, although resolution may take several months. Some children with lymphadenitis have responded to isoniazid and/or erythromycin.[56,57] However, a meta-analysis regarding the treatment of BCG-related adenitis found the literature lacking, concluding that treatment with oral erythromycin or antituberculosis drugs did not reduce the frequency of suppuration.[58] A Cochrane review[59] was unable to conclude if oral antibiotics (isoniazid, erythromycin, or a combination of isoniazid plus rifampin) were effective, but it found that patients might benefit from needle aspiration and possibly local instillation of isoniazid. BCG vaccine-related adenitis is a relatively rare complication with no agreed-upon standard for treatment when it occurs.

Other complications of vaccination with BCG are even less frequent. The mean risk of osteitis after BCG vaccination has varied from 0.01 per million in Japan to 300 per million in Finland.[51,60] As with lymphadenitis, osteitis rates have, on occasion, increased after introduction of a new vaccine strain into a region or country. Generalized BCG infection is extremely rare in immunocompetent patients.[61,62] A few autopsy studies of children who died of unrelated causes have demonstrated granulomas in various organs of vaccinated infants with apparently intact immune systems, suggesting that generalized nonfatal dissemination may occur in normal hosts.[63] Treatment of rare complications, including lupus vulgaris, erythema nodosum, iritis, osteomyelitis, and disseminated BCG disease, should include systemic antituberculosis medications, but pyrazinamide need not be included because all strains of BCG are resistant to this drug.

ADVERSE EVENTS IN IMMUNOSUPPRESSED INDIVIDUALS

Disseminated BCG (dBCG) disease includes BCG at a distant site combined with systemic symptoms consistent with mycobacterial disease. Until recently, fatal dBCG disease was reported at a rate of 0.19–1.56 cases per 1 million vaccinated,[53] with most cases occurring in patients with severe defects in cell-mediated immunity, such as chronic granulomatous disease, severe combined immunodeficiency, malnutrition, cancer, complete DiGeorge syndrome, interferon-γ production or receptor deficiency, or HIV infection. Studies from

France and South Africa found a higher risk of dBCG disease among HIV-infected children, with rates approaching 1% or higher.[64,65] While most dBCG disease has been reported in HIV-infected infants and young children, it has been described in an HIV-infected adult 30 years after receiving the vaccine.[66] Some studies of BCG-vaccinated infants born to HIV-infected mothers found no increased risk of serious adverse effects.[67] A systematic review of BCG vaccine-related disease in HIV-infected children analyzed articles published between 1950 and 2009 and identified a total of 69 culture- or PCR-confirmed cases, the majority from the Western Cape of South Africa.[68] Danish BCG vaccine was the most common strain reported in patients with disseminated disease; the Pasteur strain was also associated with dBCG disease. The median age of onset was eight months, with a range of 3–35 months. Of the reports that included outcome data, 81% of patients died. Survival was improved with the use of antiretroviral treatment.[69] Studies from other countries including Brazil and Thailand have not reported dBCG disease but used the Moreau and Japanese BCG vaccines, which are considered less reactogenic.[70,71] Interpretation of the different findings among studies and reports are likely to have significant implications in setting global immunization policy.

Immune reconstitution syndrome, an inflammatory disease of HIV-infected individuals associated with immunological recovery occurring after the onset of antiretroviral therapy, has been described with mycobacterial disease, including BCG vaccine strains.[72] This paradoxical reaction occurs months to years after BCG immunization and may include localized skin abscesses and regional adenitis appearing within weeks to months after initiation of antiretroviral medications. Clinicians should be aware of this possibility when treating HIV-infected individuals with prior BCG vaccination.

The efficacy of BCG vaccines in HIV-infected infants is unknown. Currently, the WHO considers HIV infection a contraindication for BCG vaccination and recommends delay of immunization in HIV-exposed infants until HIV infection has been ruled out.[73] In reality, the lack of available HIV serodiagnosis or antigen detection in many regions of the world means that in some areas, large numbers of HIV-infected infants and children are still receiving BCG vaccines. Long-term studies of these children will be important.

INDICATIONS FOR BACILLE CALMETTE–GUÉRIN VACCINE

There is disparity among nations concerning BCG vaccine schedules.[8] The official recommendation of the WHO is a single dose given in infancy. Some countries give repeated BCG vaccination during childhood as a standard schedule, and in others it is based on the absence of scar or tuberculin sensitivity. A case-control study in Brazil failed to demonstrate additional protection from a second dose of BCG vaccine given to persons younger than 20 years of age.[74] Most countries have since ceased revaccination policies and now use a single-dose schedule. Unfortunately, the optimal age (birth vs. one month of age) and schedule (single vs. multiple doses) for administration have not been firmly established, because adequate comparative trials have not been reported.

Some countries, including the United States and the Netherlands, have never recommended routine BCG vaccination, and reserve BCG vaccine for special high-risk situations, such as children exposed to multidrug-resistant tuberculosis with no options for treatment or separation from exposure. Other countries, such as the United Kingdom, have discontinued routine vaccination and recommend BCG only for infants living in high-risk areas or with high-risk individuals.[8]

In 1994, the International Union Against Tuberculosis and Lung Disease (IUATLD) suggested criteria for countries to consider when shifting from routine universal BCG vaccination to selective vaccination of high-risk groups.[75] The IUATLD recommends that BCG be discontinued only if:

1. an efficient notification system is in place; and either
2. the average annual notification rate of smear-positive pulmonary tuberculosis is less than five per 100,000; or
3. the average annual notification rate of tuberculous meningitis in children under five years of age is less than one in 10 million population over the previous five years; or
4. the average annual risk of tuberculosis infection is less than 0.1%.

As tuberculosis rates continue to decline in developed countries, trends may continue to limit BCG vaccination to selective use and lead to the discontinuation of universal immunization programs.

It is known that BCG vaccines have some efficacy against leprosy, and some countries recommend BCG vaccination for contacts of leprosy patients.[11,76] According to the WHO, widespread BCG vaccination may have contributed to the decline of leprosy in certain populations. BCG vaccines also have been shown to have some protective effect against *Mycobacterium ulcerans* disease or Buruli ulcer, a significant infectious disease in Africa that causes skin infections and osteomyelitis.[77]

The most frequent indication for use of BCG in the United States, which is unrelated to tuberculosis, is the treatment of bladder cancer by intravesicular administration, in which the vaccine has a nonspecific immunostimulant effect.

CONTRAINDICATIONS TO VACCINATION WITH BACILLE CALMETTE–GUÉRIN

Guidelines for contraindications to BCG vaccination vary among developing countries and industrialized nations, reflecting the different resources and capabilities within health services. In developed countries, BCG vaccine is contraindicated for persons with impaired immunity, including: (1) patients with HIV infection, congenital immunodeficiency, leukemia, lymphoma, or generalized malignant disease; (2) patients on suppressive corticosteroids, biological immune modifying agents, alkylating agents, antimetabolites, or radiation; or (3) patients who are pregnant.[78]

From 1987 until 2007, the WHO recommended administration of BCG vaccine to asymptomatic HIV-infected infants. Reports showing higher rates of dBCG disease among HIV-infected infants prompted the WHO in 2007 to change its policy, making HIV infection in infants a full contraindication to BCG vaccination.[73] This policy change sparked debate, mostly surrounding the challenges in identifying HIV-infected infants soon after birth.[79] The discussion continues as to whether countries with high rates of HIV and TB can practically implement effective programs for selective delay of BCG vaccination pending identification of infants infected with HIV.[80] Concerns surround the risks of delaying BCG immunization in HIV-exposed infants, most of whom will escape HIV infection but still have a high risk of exposure to tuberculosis. Successful implementation of selective vaccination strategies will depend on a number of TB and HIV program changes, including early diagnosis of HIV infection in infants, high enrollment in prevention of mother-to-child HIV transmission (PMTCT) programs, including effective antiretroviral therapy and consideration of alternative tuberculosis prevention strategies for unvaccinated infants. The BCG Working Group of the IUATLD has recommended that universal BCG immunization of infants continue in countries highly endemic for tuberculosis until it has all programs in place for implementing selective deferral of HIV-exposed infants.[80] The WHO has recognized the operational difficulties in delaying BCG vaccination. In areas where early HIV testing can be performed, the WHO recommends that BCG be deferred in HIV-exposed infants until HIV diagnostic results are available. Because low-resource areas may not have the capability to test for HIV, many HIV-infected infants are vaccinated at birth. Most studies of these infants found no significant increase in adverse reactions compared to non-HIV-infected infants vaccinated with BCG.[71]

PUBLIC HEALTH CONSIDERATIONS

For a number of reasons, it is impossible to estimate the impact of the BCG vaccines on global tuberculosis. First, the widely divergent results of the BCG vaccine trials make it difficult to estimate vaccine efficacy. Second, the reported epidemiological data on tuberculosis in the developing world are incomplete, especially for children. Third, the vaccine is primarily administered to infants and children, whereas the major worldwide burden of tuberculosis is pulmonary disease in adults. Fourth, tuberculosis increased in many countries during the 1980s and 1990s as a result of HIV as well as other factors unrelated to BCG vaccination. All of these issues make it difficult to estimate the effects of BCG vaccination programs on the epidemiology of tuberculosis.

For most infectious diseases, the expectation is that the availability of a potent vaccine can lead to the elimination of the disease from human populations, if an effective global program can be developed and implemented. Clearly, the BCG vaccines have not led to the elimination of tuberculosis from any country in the world. The distribution of these

vaccines to over 4 billion people has had little effect on the worldwide epidemiology of tuberculosis. However, it is likely that millions of cases of meningeal and disseminated tuberculosis in children have been prevented by its widespread use. Rates of leprosy, especially in Africa, also have been reduced by the use of BCG vaccination.

In most developing countries, BCG was originally introduced as an emergency measure because it was the only inexpensive tuberculosis-control measure that could be applied on a national scale. With the advent of effective and inexpensive chemotherapy, however, a two-pronged approach to tuberculosis control became possible, consisting of case finding and treatment, and BCG vaccination. Prior receipt of a BCG vaccination and chemotherapy of persons with significant TST or IGRA responses who have been close contacts of known cases are not mutually exclusive; this dual approach would prevent many cases of life-threatening disease in children and future cases of infectious reactivation disease. However, in developing countries, the impact of the current level of case finding and treatment programs on tuberculosis in young children may be small. Most transmission to children occurs before the adult source case is identified, and the short incubation period for meningeal and disseminated tuberculosis means that the time for intervention with the child has already passed. The lack of sensitive diagnostic techniques for confirming tuberculosis in children often precludes early effective treatment of their disease. Under such conditions, only effective vaccination of children can be expected to reduce the development of disease in children in a significant manner.

The WHO has recommended that a single dose of BCG vaccine be given to newborns in developing countries with a high prevalence rate of tuberculosis. This dosage schedule will have an economic impact and a short-term impact on mortality, although it probably will not contribute significantly to the control of tuberculosis. Many technologically advanced countries that have experienced great declines in the rate of tuberculosis have either already discontinued or are considering discontinuing BCG vaccination. In the United Kingdom and Sweden, cessation of a generalized BCG vaccination program has led to a slight increase in childhood and adolescent cases of tuberculosis. However, in both areas, the majority of subsequent childhood cases have been from high-risk immigrant communities whose members lived previously in regions with high rates of tuberculosis. Fairly circumscribed groups such as these could be selectively targeted for BCG immunization, as is done in the United Kingdom, or be subjected to increased surveillance and case-finding efforts.

NEW TUBERCULOSIS VACCINES

There is great need to develop new tuberculosis vaccines. There is now consensus that the BCG vaccine is ineffective in adults and that immunity generated in young children, while beneficial to some degree, wanes within a decade or so. Thus, especially given the increasing numbers of drug-resistant strains of M. tuberculosis spreading globally, innovative new vaccine approaches are badly needed. At this time, various strategies are being attempted, including different vaccines that can be given at different times and in different situations such as post-exposure vaccines.[81,82]

New Vaccines Based on BCG

1. The generation of new recombinant BCG (rBCG) vaccines uses advances in molecular technology allowing the insertion of foreign genes, or over-expression of native genes, into the BCG vaccine. The first such rBCG vaccines used over-expression of the Ag85 antigens, with increased immunogenicity. This has now further developed into the inclusion of a bacterial lysin—the idea being that this will increase macrophage apoptosis and cross-presentation of antigens—coupled with antigen over-expression. These candidates work well in animal model screening studies, but there are both safety concerns and questions regarding the long term efficacy[82A] of these candidates.

2. In prime-boost strategies, initial immunity to BCG is enhanced by boosting with a second or third inoculum. Multiple types of boosts have been tried, including protein antigens in adjuvant, DNA boosting, or viruses such as adenovirus or Modified Vaccinia Ankara (MVA). This strategy has certain attractions, including the fact that 85% of children in the world receive BCG while still very young.

One candidate, MVA85A, was recently tested in a clinical Phase-IIb trial in South Africa as a BCG-boosting vaccine.[83] In a triumph of organization, nearly 3,000 babies were studied, but while the incidence of tuberculosis in the boosted children was reduced, the difference did not reach statistical significance. Reasons for this have recently been discussed[83A], and one possibility is that the trial was conducted in a region where strains were of low fitness, making boosting of BCG statistically impossible[82A].

For practical reasons, boosting conventional BCG vaccination is the most logical current approach, but selection of candidates is still problematic and based on assay systems that are too short, thus testing the boosting of effector immunity rather than memory immunity.[84]

Other Types of Vaccine Candidates

1. Sub-unit vaccines usually consist of mixtures of proteins from M. tuberculosis, particularly proteins found in the culture filtrate. These include the Ag85 family of proteins, the RD1-associated ESAT-6 and CFP-10 proteins, and certain heat shock or chaperonin proteins such as dnaK or HspX. When delivered in TH1-inducing adjuvants, these sub-unit vaccines can induce significant protection against aerosol challenge infection. Many are now being produced as fusion proteins, including H56 (a combination of immunogenic proteins and a latency-associated antigen),[85] M72,[86] and ID93.[87] The latter is particularly promising because it also has post-exposure vaccination potential.

2. Auxotrophs and mutants are developed when one begins with a virulent strain of M. tuberculosis and attenuates it sufficiently to become safe enough to use as a vaccine. The original strategy in this area was to select for amino acid auxotrophs, with some considerable success. There remained a worry, however, that auxotrophs could revert to fully virulent bacilli in vivo, so a more recent approach has been to develop mutants by gene targeting in which at least two independent unlinked deletions are combined to produce a safe mutant. Several examples include SecA2,[88] MTBVAC,[89] and a new mutant consisting of M. smegmatis expressing several M. tuberculosis genes, shown to be particularly potent.[90]

CONCLUSION

Tuberculosis remains a leading cause of morbidity and mortality throughout the world. BCG vaccines have failed to control tuberculosis, mainly because they have little efficacy in preventing adult pulmonary disease. New vaccines are desperately needed in order to control and eventually eliminate tuberculosis. There is a great need for identification of some correlate of protective immunity in order to study new vaccine candidates effectively. Research on the optimal vaccination age, the need for booster doses, and vaccine safety in HIV-infected individuals will be important to include.

REFERENCES

1. Dye C. Global epidemiology of tuberculosis. *Lancet.* 2006 mar18;367(9514):938–940.
2. The World Health Organization. Global Tuberculosis Report, 2014. Accessed March 13, 2015. http://apps.who.int/iris/bitstream/10665/137094/1/9789241564809_eng.pdf?ua=1
3. Smith KC, Orme IM, Starke JR. Tuberculosis vaccines. In: Plotkin SA, Orenstein WA, Offit PA, eds. *Vaccines.* 6th ed. Philadelphia: WB Saunders; 2012:789–811.
4. Lugosi L. Theoretical and methodological aspects of BCG vaccine from the discovery of Calmette and Guérin to molecular biology: a review. *Tuberc Lung Dis.* 1992;73(5):252–261.
5. Osborn TW. Changes in BCG strains. *Tubercle.* 1983 Mar;64(1):1–13.
6. Kroger L, Brander E, Korppi M, et al. Osteitis after newborn vaccination with three different bacillus Calmette-Guérin vaccines: twenty-nine years of experience. *Pediatr Infect Dis J.* 1994;13(2):113–116.
7. Behr MA, Small PM. Has BCG attenuated to impotence? *Nature.* 1997;11;389(6647):133–134.
8. Zwerling A, Behr MA, Verma A, Brewer TF, Menzies D Madhukar P. The BCG world atlas: a database of global BCG vaccination policy and practices. *PLoS Med.* 2011;8(3)e1001012. doi:10.1371/journal.pmed.1001012
9. Fine PD, Sterne JA, Pönnighaus JM, Rees RJ. Delayed-type hypersensitivity, mycobacterial vaccines and protective immunity. *Lancet.* 1994;5;344(8932):1245–1249.
10. Trunz BB, Fine PEM, Dye C. Effect of BCG vaccination on childhood tuberculous meningitis and miliary tuberculosis worldwide: a meta-analysis and assessment of cost-effectiveness. Lancet. 2006 April 8;367(9517):1173–80.
11. Fine PEM, Carneiro IAM, Milstien JB, et al. Issues relating to the use of BCG in immunization programmes: a discussion document. 1999. World Health Organization, Department of Vaccines and Biologicals, Geneva.
12. Rosenthal SR, Loewinsohn E, Graham ML, Liveright D, Thorne G, Johnson V. BCG vaccination against tuberculosis in Chicago: a twenty-year study statistically analyzed. *Pediatrics.* 1961;28:622–641.
13. Hart PD, Sutherland I. BCG and vole bacillus vaccines in the prevention of tuberculosis in adolescence and early adult life. Final report to the Medical Research Council. *British Medical Journal.* 1977 10;2(6082):293–295.
14. Miceli I, de Kantor IN, Colaiacovo D, Peluffo G, Cutillo I, Gorra R, Botta R, Hom S, ten Dam HG. Evaluation of the effectiveness of BCG vaccination using the case-control method in Buenos Aires, Argentina. *Int J Epidemiol.* 1988;17(3):629–634.
15. Filho VW, de Castilho EA, Rodrigues LC, Huttly SR. Effectiveness of BCG vaccination against tuberculous meningitis: a case-control study in Sao Paulo, Brazil. *Bulletin of the World Health Organization.* 1990;68(1):69–74.
16. Camargos PAM, Guimaraes MDC, Antunes CMF. Risk assessment for acquiring meningitis tuberculosis among children not vaccinated with BCG: a case control study. *International Journal of Epidemiology.* 1988;17(1):193–197.
17. Putrali J, Sutrisna B, Rahayoe N, et al. A case-control study of effectiveness of BCG vaccination in children in Jakarta, Indonesia. Jakarta, Indonesia; November 20–25 Proceedings of the Eastern Regional Tuberculosis Conference of IUAT 1983;194–200.
18. Palmer CE, Shaw LW, Comstock GW. Community trials of BCG vaccination. *American Review of Tuberculosis and Pulmonary Disease.* 1958;77(6):877–907.
19. Frimodt-Moller J, Thomas J, Parthasanathy R. Observations on the protective effect of BCG vaccination in a south Indian rural population. *Bull World Health Organ.* 1964;30:545–574.
20. Comstock G, Palmer C. Long-term results of BCG vaccination in the southern United States. *Am Rev Respir Dis.* 1966;93(2):171–183.
21. Tripathy SP. Fifteen-year follow-up of the Indian BCG prevention trial. *IJTLD.* 1987;62:69–73.
22. Comstock G, Shaw L. Controlled trial of BCG vaccination in a school population. *Public Health Rep.* 1960;75(7):583–594.
23. Blin P, Delolme HG, Heyraud JD, Charpak Y, Sentilhes L. Evaluation of the protective effect of BCG vaccination by a case-control study in Yaounde, Cameroon. *Tubercle.* 1986;67(4):283–288.
24. Orege PA, Fine PEM, Lucas SB, Obura M, Okelo C, Okuku P. Case control study of BCG vaccination as a risk factor for leprosy and tuberculosis in Western Kenya. *Int J Lepr Other Mycobact Dis.* 1993;61(4):542–549.
25. Shapiro C, Cook N, Evans D, et al. A case-control study of BCG and childhood tuberculosis in Cali, Colombia. *Int J Epidemiol.* 1985;14(3):441–446.
26. Stein SC, Aronson JD. The occurrence of pulmonary lesions in BCG-vaccinated and unvaccinated persons. *Am Rev Tuberc.* 1953;68(5):695–712.

27. Tidjani O, Amendome A, ten Dam HG. The protective effect of BCG vaccination of the newborn against childhood tuberculosis in an African community. *Tubercle.* 1986;67(4):269–281.

28. Padungchan S, Konjanart S, Kasiratta S, Daramas S, ten Dam HG. The effectiveness of BCG vaccination of the newborn against childhood tuberculosis in Bangkok. *Bull World Health Organ.* 1986;64(2):247–258.

29. Murtagh K. Efficacy of BCG [letter]. *Lancet.* 1980;1(8165):423.

30. Stanley SJ, Howland C, Stone MM, Sutherland I. BCG vaccination of children against leprosy in Uganda: final results. *J Hyg (Camb).* 1981;87(2):235–248.

31. Bagshawe A, Scott GC, Russell DA, Wigley SC, Merianos A, Berry G. BCG vaccination in leprosy: final results of the trial in Karimui, Papua New Guinea. *Bull World Health Organ.* 1989;67(4):389–399.

32. Tripathy SP. The case for BCG. *Ann Nat Acad Med Sci (India).* 1983;19(1):11–21.

33. Lwin K, Sundaresan T, Gyi MM, et al. BCG vaccination of children against leprosy: fourteen-year findings of the trial in Burma. *Bull World Health Organ.* 1985;63(6):1069–1078.

34. Orege PA, Fine PEM, Lucas SB, Obura M, Okelo C, Okuku P. Case control study of BCG vaccination as a risk factor for leprosy and tuberculosis in Western Kenya. *Int J Lepr Other Mycobact Dis.* 1993;61(4):542–549.

35. Bertolli J, Pangi C, Frerichs R, Halloran ME. A case-control study of the effectiveness of BCG vaccine for preventing leprosy in Yangon, Myanmar. *Int J Epidemiol.* 1997;26(4):888–895.

36. Pönnighaus JM, Fine PE, Sterne JAC, et al. Efficacy of BCG vaccine against leprosy and tuberculosis in northern Malawi. *Lancet.* 1992;339(8794):636–639.

37. Thuc NV, Abel L, Lap VC, et al. Protective effect of BCG against leprosy and its subtypes: a case control study in Southern Viet Nam. *Int J Lepr Other Mycobact Dis.* 1994;62(4):532–538.

38. Rodrigues LC, Kerr-Pontes LRS, Frietas MVC, Barreto ML. Long lasting BCG protection against leprosy. *Vaccine.* 2007;25(39–40):6842–6844.

38A. Lifschitz M. The value of the tuberculin skin test as a screening test for tuberculosis among BCG-vaccinated children. *Pediatrics.* 1965;36(4):624–627.

39. Garly ML, Balé C, Martins CL, et al. BCG vaccination among West African infants is associated with less anergy to tuberculin and diphtheria-tetanus antigens. *Vaccine.* 2001;20(3–4):468–474.

40. Cruz AT, Starke JR. Relationship between tuberculin skin test (TST) size and interferon gamma release assay (IGRA) result: when should clinicians obtain IGRAs in children with positive TSTs? *Clin Pediatr (Phila).* 2014;53(12):1196–1199. doi: 10.1177/0009922813515743. [Epub 2013 Dec 23.]

41. Sepulveda RL, Ferrer X, Latrach C, Sorensen RU. The influence of Calmette-Guérin bacillus immunization on the booster effect of tuberculin testing in healthy young adults. *Am Rev Respir Dis.* 1990;142(1):24–28.

42. Sepulveda RL, Burr C, Ferrer X, Sorensen RU. Booster effect of tuberculin testing in healthy 6-year-old school children vaccinated with Bacillus Calmette-Guérin at birth in Santiago, Chile. *Pediatr Infect Dis J.* 1988;7(8):578–581.

43. Menzies R, Vissandjee B. Effect of bacilli Calmette-Guérin vaccination on tuberculin reactivity. *Am Rev Respir Dis.* 1992;145(3):621–625.

44. Young TK, Mirdad S. Determinants of tuberculin sensitivity in a child population covered by mass BCG vaccination. *Tuberc Lung Dis.* 1992;73(2):94–100.

45. Sollai S, Galli L, deMartino M, Chiappini E. Systematic review and meta-analysis on the utility of interferon-gamma release assays for the diagnosis of *Mycobacterium tuberculosis* infection in children: a 2013 update. *BMC Infect Dis.* 2014;14(Suppl 1)S6. doi: 10.1186/1471-2334-14-S1-S6. [Epub 2014 Jan 8.]

46. Tuberculosis Prevention Trial: Trial of BCG vaccines in South India for tuberculosis prevention: first report. *Bull World Health Organ.* 1979;57(5):819–827.

47. Comstock GW. Field trials of tuberculosis vaccines: how could we have done them better? *Control Clin Trials.* 1994;15:247–276.

48. Rodriques LC, Diwan VK, Wheeler JG. Protective effect of BCG against tuberculous meningitis and miliary tuberculosis: a meta-analysis. *Int J Epidemiol.* <YEAR?>22:1154–1158.

49. Colditz GA, Berkey CS, Mosteller F, et al. The efficacy of bacillus Calmette-Guérin vaccination of newborns and infants in the prevention of tuberculosis: meta-analyses of the published literature. *Pediatrics.* 1995;96:29–35.

50. Colditz GA, Brewer TF, Berkey CS, et al. Efficacy of BCG vaccine in the prevention of tuberculosis: meta-analysis of the published literature. *JAMA.* 1994;271:698–702.

51. Lotte A, Wasz-Hockert O, Poisson N, Dumitrescu N, Verron M, Couvet E. BCG complications: estimates of the risks among vaccinated subjects and statistical analysis of their main characteristics. *Adv Tuberc Res.* 1984;21:107–193.

52. Victoria MS, Shah BR. Bacillus Calmette-Guérin lymphadenitis: a case report and review of the literature. *Pediatr Infect Dis J.* 1985;4(3):295–296.

53. Lotte A, Wasz-Hockert O, Poisson N, et al. Second IUATLD study on complications induced by intradermal BCG vaccination. *IJTLD.* 1988;63(2):47–59.

54. Reynes J, Perez C, Lamaury I, Janbon F, Bertrand A. Bacille Calmette-Guérin adenitis 30 years after immunization in a patient with AIDS [letter]. *J Infect Dis.* 1989;160(4):727.

55. Caglayan S, Yegin O, Kayean K, Timocin N, Kasirga E, Gun M. Is medical therapy effective for regional lymphadenitis following BCG vaccination? *Am J Dis Child.* 1987;141(11):1213–1214.

56. Hanley SP, Gumb J, MacFarlane JT. Comparison of erythromycin and isoniazid in treatment of adverse reactions to BCG vaccination. *BMJ (Clin Res Ed).* 1985;290(6473):970.

57. Murphy PM, Mayers DL, Brock NF, Wagner KF. Cure of bacille Calmette-Guérin vaccination abscess with erythromycin. *Rev Infect Dis.* 1989;11(2):335–337.

58. Goraya JS, Virdi VS. Treatment of Calmette-Guérin bacillus adenitis: a meta-analysis. *Pediatr Infect Dis J.* 2001;20(6):632–634.

59. Cuello-Garcia CA, Perez-Gaxiola G, Jimenez Gutierrez C. Treating BCG-induced disease in children. *Cochrane Database Syst Rev.* [Internet] 2013;31;1. Available from:http://www.mrw.interscience.wiley.com/Cochrane/clsysrev/articles/CD008300/frame.html. doi:10.1002/14651858.CD008300.pub2

60. Kroger L, Korppi M, Brander E, et al. Osteitis caused by bacillus Calmette-Guérin vaccination: a retrospective analysis of 222 cases. *J Infect Dis.* 1995;172(2):574–576.

61. Casanova JL, Blanche S, Emile JF, et al. Idiopathic disseminated bacille Calmette-Guérin infection: a French national retrospective study. *Pediatrics.* 1996;98(4 Pt 1):774–778.

62. Thamthitiwat S, Marin N, Baggett HC, et al. Mycobacterium bovis (bacille Calmette-Guerin) bacteremia in immunocompetent neonates following vaccination. *Vaccine.* 2011;29(9):1727–1730.

63. Trevenen CL, Pagtakhan RD. Disseminated tuberculoid lesions in infants following BCG. *CMJ.* 1982;127(6):502–504.

64. Besnard M, Sauvion S, Offredo C, et al. Bacillus Calmette-Guérin infection after vaccination of human immunodeficiency virus-infected children. *Pediatr Infect Dis J.* 1993;12(12):993–997.

65. Hesseling AC, Marais BJ, Gie RP, et al. The risk of disseminated bacille Calmette-Guérin (BCG) disease in HIV-infected children. *Vaccine.* 2007;25(1):14–18.

66. Armbruster C, Junker W, Vetter N, Jaksch G. Disseminated bacille Calmette-Guérin infection in an AIDS patient 30 years after BCG vaccination [letter]. *J Infect Dis.* 1990;162(5):1216.

67. Thaithumyanon P, Thisyakorn U, Punnahitananda S, Praisuwanna P, Ruxrungtham K. Safety and immunogenicity of bacillus Calmette-Guérin vaccine in children born to HIV-1 infected women. *Southeast Asian J Trop Med Public Health.* 2000;31(3):482–486.

68. Azzopardi P, Bennett CM, Graham SM, Duke T. Bacille Calmette-Guerin vaccine-related disease in HIV-infected children: a systematic review. *Int J Tuberc Lung Dis.* 2009;13(11):1331–1334.

69. Nuttall JJ, Davies MA, Hussey GD, Eley BS. Bacillus Calmette-Guérin (BCG) vaccine-induced complications in children treated with highly active antiretroviral therapy. *Int J Infect Dis.* 2008;12(6):e99–e105.

70. Fernandes RD, de Araujo LC, Medina-Acosta E. Reduced rate of adverse reactions to the BCG vaccine in children exposed to the vertical transmission of HIV infection and in HIV-infected children from an endemic setting in Brazil. *Eur J Pediatr.* 2009;168(6):691–696.

71. World Health Organization: Use of BCG vaccine in HIV-infected infants. *Wkly Epidemiol Rec.* 2010;85:29–36.

72. Puthanakit T, Oberdorfer P, Punjaisee S, Wannarit P, Sirisanthana T, Sirisanthana V. Immune reconstitution syndrome due to bacillus Calmette-Guerin after initiation of antiretroviral therapy in children with HIV infection. *Clin Infect Dis.* 2005;41(7):1049–1052.

73. World Health Organization. Revised BCG vaccination guidelines for infants at risk for HIV infection. *Wkly Epidemiol Rec.* 2007;82(21):193–196.

74. Dantas OM, Ximenes RA, de Albuquerque MdeF, et al. A case-control study of protection against tuberculosis by BCG revaccination in Recife, Brazil. *Int J Tuberc Lung Dis.* 2006;10(5):536–541.

75. International Union Against Tuberculosis and Lung Disease. Criteria for discontinuation of vaccination programmes using bacille Calmette Guérin (BCG) in countries with a low prevalence of tuberculosis. *Tuberc Lung Dis.* 1994;75(3):179–180.

76. Düppre NC, Camacho LA, da Cunha SS, et al. Effectiveness of BCG vaccination among leprosy contacts: a cohort study. *Trans R Soc Trop Med Hyg.* 2008;102(7):631–648.

77. Portaels F, Aguiar J, Debacker M, et al. Mycobacterium bovis BCG vaccination as prophylaxis against Mycobacterium ulcerans osteomyelitis in Buruli ulcer disease. *Infect Immun.* 2004;72(1):62–65.

78. Centers for Disease Control and Prevention. The role of BCG vaccine in the prevention and control of tuberculosis in the United States: a joint statement by the Advisory Council for the Elimination of Tuberculosis and the Advisory Committee on Immunization Practices. *MMWR Recomm Rep.* 1996;45(RR-4):1–18.

79. Hesseling AC, Caldwell J, Cotton MF, et al. BCG vaccination in South African HIV-exposed infants: risks and benefits. *SAMJ.* 2009;99(2):88–91.

80. Hesseling AC, Cotton MF, Fordham von Reyn C. Consensus statement on the revised World Health Organization recommendations for BCG vaccination in HIV-infected infants. *Int J Tuberc Lung Dis.* 2008;12(12):1376–1379.

81. Orme IM. Vaccine development for tuberculosis: current progress. *Drugs.* 2013 Jul;73(10):1015–1024. http://dx.doi.org/10.1007/s40265-013-0081-8

82. Orme IM. Tuberculosis vaccines: types and timings. *Clin Vaccine Immunol.* 2015;22(3):249–257. http://dx.doi.org/10.1128/CVI.00718-14

82A. Henao-Tamayo M, Shanley CA, Verma D, Zilavy A, Stapleton MC, Furney SK, Podell B, Orme IM. The Efficacy of the BCG Vaccine against Newly Emerging Clinical Strains of Mycobacterium tuberculosis. *PloS One.* 2015;10:e0136500. http://dx.doi.org/10.1371/journal.pone.0136500

83. Tameris MD, Hatherill M, Landry BS, et al.; Team MATS. Safety and efficacy of MVA85A, a new tuberculosis vaccine, in infants previously vaccinated with BCG: a randomised, placebo-controlled phase 2b trial. *Lancet.* 2013;381(9871):1021–1028. http://dx.doi.org/10.1016/S0140-6736(13)60177-4

83A. McShane H, Williams A. 2014. A review of preclinical animal models utilised for TB vaccine evaluation in the context of recent human efficacy data. Tuberculosis (Edinburgh, Scotland) 94:105–110. http://dx.doi.org/10.1016/j.tube.2013.11.003

84. Henao-Tamayo M, Ordway DJ, Orme IM. 2014. Memory T cell subsets in tuberculosis: what should we be targeting? *Tuberculosis (Edinb).* 2014;94(5):455–461. http://dx.doi.org/10.1016/j.tube.2014.05.001

85. Andersen P, Kaufmann SH. 2014. Novel vaccination strategies against tuberculosis. *CSH Perspect Med.* 2014;4:a018523. http://dx.doi.org/10.1101/cshperspect.a018523

86. Day CL, Tameris M, Mansoor N, et al. Induction and regulation of T-cell immunity by the novel tuberculosis vaccine M72/AS01 in South African adults. *Am J Respir Crit Care Med.* 2013;188(4):492–502. http://dx.doi.org/10.1164/rccm.201208-1385OC

87. Bertholet S, Ireton GC, Ordway DJ, et al. A defined tuberculosis vaccine candidate boosts BCG and protects against multidrug-resistant Mycobacterium tuberculosis. *Sci Translat Med.* 2010;2(53):53ra74. http://dx.doi.org/10.1126/scitranslmed.3001094

88. Hinchey J, Lee S, Jeon BY, et al. Enhanced priming of adaptive immunity by a proapoptotic mutant of Mycobacterium tuberculosis. *J Clin Invest.* 2007;117(8):2279–2288. http://dx.doi.org/10.1172/JCI31947

89. Arbues A, Aguilo JI, Gonzalo-Asensio J, et al. Construction, characterization and preclinical evaluation of MTBVAC, the first live-attenuated M. tuberculosis-based vaccine to enter clinical trials. *Vaccine.* 2013;31(42):4867–4873. http://dx.doi.org/10.1016/j.vaccine.2013.07.051

90. Sweeney KA, Dao DN, Goldberg MF, et al. A recombinant Mycobacterium smegmatis induces potent bactericidal immunity against Mycobacterium tuberculosis. *Nature Med.* 2011;17(10):1261–1268. http://dx.doi.org/10.1038/nm.2420

20

MYCOBACTERIUM BOVIS (NON-BCG) IN CHILDREN

Jeffrey R. Starke

HIGHLIGHTS OF THIS CHAPTER

- Human disease caused by *Mycobacterium bovis* is uncommon but underdiagnosed because of the difficulty of distinguishing this bacterium from *Mycobacterium tuberculosis* in most clinical laboratories.
- Transmission of *M. bovis* to children is mainly through the ingestion of unpasteurized dairy products, although person-to-person airborne transmission has been documented.
- The clinical manifestations of *M. bovis* disease in children are mainly extrapulmonary, affecting the cervical lymph nodes and the alimentary tract.
- While *M. bovis* is inherently resistant to pyrazinamide, it is usually susceptible to isoniazid and rifampin, although the recommended length of treatment for disease is nine months.
- The most important measures to reduce human disease caused by *M. bovis* are those used to control the disease in animals, particularly cattle.

MYCOBACTERIUM BOVIS is a member of the *Mycobacterium tuberculosis*-complex and is the main cause of tuberculosis in cattle and a large number of domesticated and wild mammal species.[1] In the last several decades, *M. bovis* has accounted for a small proportion (0.5–7.2%) of all patients with bacteriologically confirmed tuberculosis disease in industrialized countries.[1,2] The true incidence of infection and disease in humans caused by *M. bovis* is probably underestimated, because most of the tests used to detect *M. tuberculosis* are also positive when *M. bovis* is the infecting organism, and most microbiology laboratories—especially those in resource-constrained countries—lack the sophistication to differentiate *M. bovis* from other members of the *M. tuberculosis*-complex. Although there is historical evidence that *M. bovis* does not establish itself in humans as readily as *M. tuberculosis* does, the organism is infectious for humans and poses a considerable zoonotic risk.[1,3,4] Person-to-person transmission also has been documented.[5]

MICROBIOLOGY

M. bovis has most of the characteristics shared with other members of the *M. tuberculosis*-complex. The organism is an aerobic, non-spore-forming, non-motile, and slightly curved or straight rod (0.2–0.6 μm by 1.0–10 μm), has a complex cell wall containing mycolic acids, and a genome with a high guanine plus cytosine (G+C) content. Its high-lipid cell wall structure makes it difficult to stain with dyes routinely used in bacteriology, such as the Gram stain. When stained with special procedures (e.g., Ziehl-Neelsen staining), they are not easily decolorized, even by acid alcohol, hence they are referred to as acid-fast or acid/alcohol fast. The organism displays greater than 99.95% nucleotide sequence similarity with *M. tuberculosis*. It has a doubling time close to 24 hours, compared to 20–45 minutes for most bacteria, and takes three to four weeks to form colonies on solid media. *M. bovis* is aerobic and grows best in an atmosphere enriched with 5–10% carbon dioxide (CO_2) when using conventional solid media. Its growth is also enhanced by fatty acids, which may be provided in the form of egg yolk or oleic acid. Although optimal growth temperatures vary widely among different mycobacterial species, *M. bovis* grows best at 35–37°C.

Discrimination between *M. bovis* and *M. tuberculosis* by methods based on molecular markers is not straightforward because of their 99.5% similarity at the nucleotide level and identical 16S rRNA sequences.[1] Advanced techniques such as multiplex-PCR based on simultaneous detection of *pncA* 169C>G change in *M. bovis* and IS6110 present in *M. tuberculosis* can distinguish between the organisms,[5] but advanced techniques such as this are rarely available to the clinician. Tests such as GeneXpert MTB/RIF do not distinguish between the species. The most common distinguishing feature is that isolated pyrazinamide (PZA) resistance is inherent in *M. bovis* but is quite rare in *M. tuberculosis*. However, many laboratories do not routinely perform PZA resistance testing; as a result, many country's notification systems for human tuberculosis do not distinguish cases caused by different species within the *M. tuberculosis*-complex.

TRANSMISSION AND EPIDEMIOLOGY

The first documented cases of tuberculosis disease in animals and humans occurred over a century ago.[6,7]

Only a small number of so-called "maintenance" or "reservoir" host species, most notably domestic cattle, self-sustain infection with *M. bovis* without exposure to other species.[8] By far the most common mode of transmission to humans has been through the ingestion of milk from diseased cows, but other natural modes of transmission from animals to humans, including exposure to infected aerosols, center on contact with wildlife (non-human primates, badgers, possums, deer), farm animals (cattle, pigs, goats) or domesticated animals (cats, dogs) that are infected.[2,9] As a result, farmers, veterinarians, abattoir workers, meat inspectors, animal handlers, hunters, and gamekeepers are at increased risk for disease caused by *M. bovis*. Cases of pulmonary or disseminated disease in dogs or cats may pose a zoonotic and animal health risk when their keepers elect to treat rather than euthanize the diseased pet.[10]

The early medical literature contains a small number of reports of suspected person-to-person transmission of *M. bovis*.[1] These were considered to be largely sporadic events until it was noticed that adults infected with HIV were more likely to develop tuberculosis caused by *M. bovis* and infect other people, especially if they lived in close contact with infected cattle.[11,12] In 2005, a cluster of six human tuberculosis cases (five pulmonary that were acid-fast sputum smear-positive, one meningitis) caused by *M. bovis* occurred among individuals who frequented the same bar in the West Midlands of the United Kingdom; while the first case had a zoonotic link, the subsequent five cases did not, and the DNA fingerprints of the organisms from these patients were indistinguishable, implying that person-to-person transmission, presumably by the airborne route, had occurred.[6] Four of the five secondary cases had underlying conditions that are known to predispose to tuberculosis disease. This specific cluster occurred in the midst of a general increase in the recognition of tuberculosis cases caused by *M. bovis* in this region.

Tuberculosis caused by *M. bovis* and *M. tuberculosis* cannot be distinguished clinically, radiographically, or pathologically in individual patients.[13] Human tuberculosis caused by *M. bovis* has been described all over the world. *M. bovis* caused as many as 25% of cases of human tuberculosis in developed countries in the late nineteenth and early twentieth centuries. The pasteurization of milk and the testing and culling of infected cattle in developed countries have resulted in steep decreases in the incidence of *M. bovis* tuberculosis so that only 1–2% of human tuberculosis cases currently are caused by *M. bovis*.[9] The disease is often sporadic, although clusters have been detected. In New York City in the period from 2001–2004, an investigation of 35 cases of geno-typically confirmed cases of human *M. bovis* tuberculosis implied that foodborne transmission had occurred within the United States, because there was a lack of evidence for airborne person-to-person transmission and none of the patients under 5 years of age (one of whom died from peritoneal tuberculosis) had a history of international travel.[14]

The CDC conducted a study of *M. bovis* infections in the United States from 1995–2005 and select cases from 1993–2003 using genetic typing of organisms and available clinical information.[15] Of 11,860 tested isolates of the *M. tuberculosis*-complex, 165 (1.4%) were *M. bovis*. Patients not born in the United States, Hispanic patients, children under 15 years of age, patients living with HIV, and patients with extrapulmonary disease each had an adjusted odds ratio in favor of having *M. bovis* versus *M. tuberculosis*. Of the Hispanic patients, 29 of 32 (91%) had extrapulmonary disease, and the median age was 9.5 years. However, certain geographic regions and communities have much higher rates. In California, the percentage of tuberculosis cases attributable to *M. bovis* increased from 3.4% in 2003 to 5.4% in 2011; multivariate analysis showed that Hispanic ethnicity, extrapulmonary disease, diabetes, and immunosuppressive conditions, including HIV, were independently associated with *M. bovis* disease.[16] From 2001–2005, *M. bovis* accounted for nearly 10% of culture-positive tuberculosis cases in San Diego, California, including 54% of those from children under 15 years of age and 8% of those from adults.[17] Nearly all (97%) case-patients were Hispanic, and the majority had an epidemiological link to another country where disease caused by *M. bovis* was more common. Studies of children in this area have implied that transmission probably was from consumption of unpasteurized, contaminated dairy products, for several reasons: (1) the near absence of *M. bovis* disease among children less than 12 months of age; (2) a high percentage of extra-pulmonary disease in children, particularly abdominal disease; and (3) an association between positive tuberculin skin test (TST) or interferon-gamma release assay (IGRA) results and the consumption of unpasteurized dairy products.[17–19]

Extensive study of the epidemiology of *M. bovis* infections has also been conducted in Latin America.[20,21] From 1970 to 2007, only 4 of 10 Latin American countries reported bacteriologically confirmed cases of *M. bovis* disease. In Argentina during this time, 0.34% to 1.0% of the tuberculosis cases were caused by *M. bovis*. Rates were even lower in countries that had robust programs to prevent infection and disease in cattle. However, in one region of Mexico, 13.8% of isolates from patients with tuberculosis were found to be *M. bovis*.[22] Not surprisingly, at that time only 30% of the 7 million liters of milk annually produced in Mexico was pasteurized, and *M. bovis* was found to be prevalent in cattle in some parts of the country.[21–23] Muller et al.[24] performed a systematic review of relevant literature published from 1992–2012 concerning *M. bovis*-induced disease in humans. They found that, on average, 0.4% of tuberculosis cases in Europe were caused by *M. bovis*, although higher percentages—but never above 2.3%—were found for specific populations and settings. There is concern about the incidence of disease caused by *M. bovis* in Africa because the disease is common in cattle, but effective disease control, including milk pasteurization and slaughterhouse meat inspection, is largely absent.[12] Of course, the situation there is likely to be exacerbated by co-infection with HIV. Data from Africa are sparse, with a median of 2.8% (range of 0–37.7%) of human tuberculosis cases caused by *M. bovis*. While the reported rates of disease caused by *M. bovis* were low in the Western Pacific, no data were found for any country in southeast Asia.[24]

CLINICAL PRESENTATION AND DIAGNOSIS

The clinical presentations of disease caused by *M. bovis* are indistinguishable from those caused by *M. tuberculosis*. In the California study, 38% of adults with disease caused by *M. bovis* had only extrapulmonary manifestations, while 40% had only pulmonary manifestations, and 22% had both.[16] In other studies, as many as 50% of adults with documented *M. bovis* tuberculosis present with adult-type pulmonary disease, including upper lobe infiltrates, often in a fibronodular pattern, and cavities.[25] Many affected adults have the same underlying conditions that predispose to disease caused by *M. tuberculosis* including diabetes, malignancy and HIV infection. However, adults with underlying immunosuppressive conditions more often present with extrapulmonary findings. In a recent study from Argentina, 93% of the adult patients had a least one risk factor for a zoonotic infection, including occupational exposure (65%), consumption of unpasteurized dairy products (4%), and living in a rural agricultural area (31%).[26] Pulmonary disease was present in 100% of the adults with occupational exposure, emphasizing the importance of airborne transmission. Among the adults with pulmonary disease, the most common manifestations were cough (84%), sputum production (84%), weight loss (80%), fever (64%), malaise (56%), night sweats (32%), hemoptysis (28%), dyspnea (28%), and headache (8%). The chest radiograph showed alveolar infiltrates (50%), cavities (38%), a miliary pattern (8%), and pleural effusion (8%). The tuberculin skin test was positive in only 35% of the patients who were tested. Ziehl-Neelsen stain of the sputum was positive for acid-fast bacilli in 77% of cases.

Children can present with pulmonary disease caused by *M. bovis*, and the manifestations are the same as for disease caused by *M. tuberculosis*. Young children get the manifestations of primary pulmonary tuberculosis, and intrathoracic lymphadenopathy dominates the pathological, radiographic and clinical picture. Children discovered soon after infection may have clearly discernable lymphadenopathy in the chest but few to no clinical symptoms. When symptoms occur, they are most commonly cough, fever, weight loss, and malaise. Adolescents may develop either primary-type tuberculosis or adult-type disease with the usual manifestations.

The majority of children with *M. bovis* tuberculosis have extrapulmonary manifestations that correlate with the route of transmission, which is most often from ingestion of contaminated dairy products. In California, 87% of the children with confirmed *M. bovis* disease had only extrapulmonary manifestations, and an additional 5% had both pulmonary and extrapulmonary disease.[16] The most common disease is scrofula or disease of the cervical lymph nodes. In the Middle Ages it was believed that royal touch, the touch of the sovereign of England or France, could cure diseases due to the divine right of kings, a capacity known in the medicine of that time as adenochirapsology; as a result, scrofula became known as the "King's Evil." This practice was continued in England until the early 1700s, when it was stopped by King George I. Scrofula caused by *M. bovis* presents in the same way as disease caused by *M. tuberculosis*. The onset is usually insidious, although it is occasionally explosive. The anterior cervical chain is most often affected, and the disease can be either unilateral or bilateral. The lymph nodes enlarge but usually remain painless and only minimally tender. As the disease progresses, the nodes invade surrounding tissues, particularly the skin, causing scrofuloderma. The disease may progress and cause a thinning and red-purple tingeing of the skin. Eventually, one or more sinus tracts may develop from the node to the skin, causing drainage. Occasionally, when many nodes are involved, there can be massive necrosis and drainage from the sinus tract(s). Secondary infection can complicate the picture and make diagnosis more challenging. Supraclavicular lymphadenitis can complicate pulmonary disease.

The second most common extrapulmonary site for disease caused by *M. bovis* is the alimentary tract. It is not unusual for several members of the same family, who ingested the same contaminated animal products, to present with symptoms of abdominal disease within a short period of time. This may result in a true enteritis, which should be considered in any child presenting with nonspecific constitutional symptoms and longstanding abdominal complaints, and may be present from weeks to months. Although the majority of these children will present with chronic or acute-on-chronic onset of symptoms, a few children present with an apparent acute abdomen, often mimicking an acute appendicitis or intestinal obstruction. The most common symptoms are abdominal pain, abdominal distension, fever, failure to thrive or loss of weight, malnutrition, abdominal mass, ascites, diarrhea or constipation, and peripheral lymphadenopathy. Less frequent symptoms are vomiting, gastrointestinal hemorrhage, and hematochezia. Imaging studies may reveal fibrin strands, loculations and debris, bowel wall thickening, or a mass composed of bowel loops, adherent omentum, and lymphadenopathy. Focal lesions can sometimes be seen in the liver or spleen. In longstanding disease, calcifications throughout the abdomen may be apparent.

M. bovis can cause disseminated disease in young and immunocompromised children, with the typical features of miliary tuberculosis. Meningitis is an uncommon complication, and the clinical and radiographic presentations, as well as the findings in CSF, are the same as for tuberculous meningitis. Cutaneous lesions are rare in children because they usually require direct contact with infected animal tissues.

Microbiological diagnosis of *M. bovis* disease requires isolation and adequate testing of the infecting organism. Generally available tests to detect

M. tuberculosis, such as microscopy, PCR, and GeneXpert MTB/RIF, will also be positive when *M. bovis* is the cause of disease. Similarly, the TST and IGRA tests are often positive.

MANAGEMENT

Infection with *M. bovis* precedes the development of disease, but there is no available test that distinguishes infection caused by *M. bovis* from that caused by *M. tuberculosis*. As a result, most children asymptomatically infected with *M. bovis* are presumed to have tuberculosis infection and are managed accordingly.

There have been no randomized controlled trials for the treatment of disease caused by *M. bovis*, so the optimal treatment has not been determined. The major feature that distinguishes *M. bovis* is its inherent resistance to PZA. The vast majority of strains of *M. bovis* are susceptible to isoniazid (INH), rifampin (RMP), and ethambutol (EMB), so the usual initial regimens used for tuberculosis disease should be effective against disease caused by *M. bovis*.[27] However, because PZA is ineffective, treatment with INH and RIF must be given for a minimum of nine months. Isoniazid-resistant and MDR strains of *M. bovis* have been found but are uncommon. In San Diego, California, 7% of the *M. bovis* isolates were resistant to INH, and 1% were resistant to RIF, percentages that were similar to those for isolates of *M. tuberculosis* in the same community.[27] In this same study, treatment completion rates were similar for patients with disease caused by *M. bovis* and *M. tuberculosis*, but the death rate was higher in patients with *M. bovis*, probably because of a stronger association with HIV infection in the adult patients, and only one patient relapsed.[27]

PREVENTION

The most important measures to reduce human disease caused by *M. bovis* are those used to control the disease in animals, particularly cattle. Animal vaccination, periodic testing, and culling from the herds the animals that are infected are the critical measures. Whenever possible, children should not ingest unpasteurized animal products, particularly in settings where animal control is lacking. Ironically, although the BCG vaccines were derived from a strain of *M. bovis*, it has never been demonstrated that BCG vaccines are protective for humans

against infection or disease caused by *M. bovis*. In addition, the effectiveness of treatment with INH for asymptomatic infection caused by *M. bovis* may be inferred but has not been demonstrated.

REFERENCES

1. De la Rua-Domenech R. Human *Mycobacterium bovis* infection in the United Kingdom: incidence, risks, control measures and review of the zoonotic aspects of bovine tuberculosis. *Tuberculosis*. 2006;86:77–109.
2. Collins CH. The bovine tubercle bacillus. *Br J Biomed Sci*. 2000;57:234–240.
3. Ashford DA, Whitney E, Raghunathan P, Cosivi O. Epidemiology of selected mycobacteria that infect humans and other animals. *Rev Sci Tech*. 2001;20(1):325–337.
4. Francis J. Control of infection with the bovine tubercle bacillus. *Lancet*. 1950;258:34–39.
5. Spositto FLE, Campanerut PAZ, Ghiraldi LD, et al. Multiplex-PCR for differentiation of *Mycobacterium bovis* from *Mycobacterium tuberculosis*-complex. *Braz J Microbiol*. 2014;45(3):841–843.
6. Evans JT, Smith EG, Banerjee A, et al. Cluster of human tuberculosis caused by *Mycobacterium bovis*: evidence for person-to-person transmission in the UK. *Lancet*. 2007;369:1270–1276.
7. Pritchard DG. A century of bovine tuberculosis 1888–1988: conquest and controversy. *J Comp Pathol*. 1988;9:357–399.
8. Cousins DV. *Mycobacterium bovis* infection and control in domestic livestock. *Rev Sci Tech*. 2001;20(1):71–85.
9. O'Reilly LM, Daborn CJ. The epidemiology of *Mycobacterium bovis* infections in animals and man: a review. *Tubercle*. 1995;76(Suppl 1):1–46.
10. Monies RJ, Cranwell MP, Palmer N, Inwald J, Hewinson RG, Rule B. Bovine TB in domestic cats. *Vet Rec*. 2001;146:407–408.
11. Cosivi O, Grange JM, Daborn CJ, et al. Zoonotic tuberculosis due to *Mycobacterium tuberculosis* in developing countries. *Emerg Infect Dis*. 1998;4(1):59–70.
12. Ayele WY, Neill SD, Zinsstag J, Weiss MG, Pavlik I. Bovine tuberculosis: an old disease but a new threat to Africa. *Int J Tuberc Lung Dis*. 2004;8(8):924–937.
13. Grange J. *Mycobacterium bovis* infections in human beings. *Tuberculosis*. 2001;81:71–77.
14. Centers for Disease Control and Prevention. Human tuberculosis caused by *Mycobacterium bovis*—New York City, 2001–2004. *MMWR*. 2005;54:605–608.

15. Hlavsa MC, Moonan PK, Cowan LS, et al. Human tuberculosis due to *Mycobacterium bovis* in the United States, 1995–2005. *Clin Infect Dis.* 2008;47:168–175.

16. Gallivan M, Shah N, Flood J. Epidemiology of human *Mycobacterium bovis* disease, California, USA, 2003–2011. *Emerg Infect Dis.* 2015;21(3):435–443.

17. Rodwell TC, Moore M, Moser KS, Brodine SK, Strathdee SA. Tuberculosis from *Mycobacterium bovis* in binational communities, United States. *Emerg Infect Dis.* 2008;14:909–916.

18. Dankner WM, Davis CE. *Mycobacterium tuberculosis* as a significant cause of tuberculosis in children residing along the United States–Mexico border in the Baja California region. *Pediatrics.* 2000;105(6):E79.

19. Besser RE, Pakiz B, Schulte JM, Alvarado S, Zell ER, Kenyon TA. Risk factors for positive Mantoux tuberculin skin tests in children in San Diego, California: evidence for boosting and possible foodborne transmission. *Pediatrics.* 2001;108:305–310.

20. De Kantor IN, Ambroggi M, Poggi S, et al. Human *Mycobacterium bovis* infection in 10 Latin American countries. *Tuberculosis.* 2008;88:358–365.

21. De Kantor IN, LoBue PA, Thoen CO. Human tuberculosis caused by *Mycobacterium bovis* in the United States, Latin America and the Caribbean. *Int J Tuberc Lung Dis.* 2010;14(11):1369–1373.

22. Perez-Guerrero L, Milian-Suazo F, Arriaga-Diaz QC, Romero-Torres C, Escartin-Chavez M. Molecular epidemiology of cattle and human tuberculosis in Mexico. *Salud Publica Mex.* 2008;50:286–289.

23. Milian-Suazo, Salman MD, Ramirez C, Payeur JB, Rhyan JC, Santillan M. Identification of tuberculosis in cattle slaughtered in Mexico. *Am J Vet Res.* 2000;61:86–89.

24. Muller B, Durr S, Alonso S, et al. Zoonotic *Mycobacterium bovis*–induced tuberculosis in humans. *Emerg Infect Dis.* 2013;19(6):899–908.

25. Dankner WM, Waecker NJ, Essey MA, Moser K, Thompson M, Davis CE. *Mycobacterium bovis* infections in San Diego: a clinicoepidemiologic study of 73 patients and a historical review of a forgotten pathogen. *Medicine.* 1993;72(1):11–37.

26. Cordova E, Gonzalo X, Boschi A, et al. Human *Mycobacterium bovis* infection in Buenos Aires: epidemiology, microbiology and clinical presentation. *Int J Tuberc Lung Dis.* 2012;16(3):415–417.

27. LoBue PA, Moser KS. Treatment of *Mycobacterium bovis* infected tuberculosis patients: San Diego County, California, United States, 1994–2003. *Int J Tuberc Lung Dis.* 2005;9(3):333–338.

21

PUBLIC HEALTH AND PROGRAMMATIC ISSUES FOR CHILDHOOD TUBERCULOSIS

Jeffrey R. Starke

HIGHLIGHTS OF THIS CHAPTER

- Children often benefit from family-centered care, which aids in case detection, adherence to treatment, and determination of drug susceptibility for the child with tuberculosis infection or disease.
- When children with tuberculosis are discovered via passive case finding, it is more difficult to establish the correct diagnosis, they tend to be sicker and more difficult to treat with more complications, and for 70% of cases, the drug-susceptibility pattern of their tuberculosis will be unknown.
- Contact investigation is the ultimate form of active case finding and targeted testing that finds children before serious disease has developed.
- Accurate case reporting of both clinical and confirmed cases of childhood tuberculosis is critical to understanding the epidemiology of tuberculosis in a community, and to ensuring adequate resources for the pediatric patients.
- Directly observed therapy is an integral part of the management of childhood tuberculosis disease and should be considered in all cases.
- Although young children with tuberculosis are rarely contagious, their caregivers may also have tuberculosis disease that has not yet been diagnosed.
- Prevention of childhood tuberculosis can be a useful quality measure for tuberculosis programs.

DESPITE THE availability of the BCG vaccines, inexpensive and safe treatment for tuberculosis infection, and curative therapy for tuberculosis disease, current estimates are that between 600,000 and 1 million children develop tuberculosis disease every year and 74,000 HIV-uninfected children annually die from this curable disease (there are no formal estimates for the number of HIV-infected children who die with or from tuberculosis).[1-2] Sophisticated models suggest that over 53 million children are living with tuberculosis infection in just the 22 highest-burden countries.[3] Each case of childhood tuberculosis—and particularly each death—represents a potential failure of the public health system and, arguably, the failure to eliminate tuberculosis remains the biggest public health failure in human history. One of the major factors contributing to this situation is the failure to include the needs of children and adolescents when designing and implementing tuberculosis programs. There are many reasons why children have been neglected (Box 21.1).

Children with tuberculosis often come from families that are poor, lack knowledge about the disease, and live in communities with limited access to health services.[4] These problems are often magnified for families who have recently migrated or are refugees from countries with high rates of tuberculosis. Many children in these circumstances suffer from malnutrition and other neglected health problems that increase the likelihood that tuberculosis infection will progress to disease. These families often settle in communities with higher than average tuberculosis rates, adding to the possible exposures of the children to infection and disease.

Box 21.1. Ten Reasons Why Childhood Tuberculosis Has Been Neglected

1. Inadequate data for cases and contacts
2. Difficulty with the microbiological confirmation of disease
3. Children are rarely contagious (public health "dead end")
4. Perception from policy makers that treating adults is enough
5. Misplaced faith in the BCG vaccines
6. National tuberculosis programs fail to address children and their needs
7. Lack of family-centered care and contact investigation
8. Perceived (inaccurate) lack of scientific study and scrutiny
9. Lack of industry support for drug formulations and new diagnostic tests for children
10. Inadequate attention and advocacy by pediatricians and child health experts

---

A major reason for the relative neglect of children in tuberculosis programs is the difficulty in confirming the diagnosis through currently available microbiological testing. Even in resource-rich countries, the diagnosis is most often established through indirect means, including the presence of symptoms, a positive test of infection (tuberculin skin test [TST] or interferon-gamma release assay [IGRA]), an abnormal chest radiograph (pulmonary disease) or physical examination (extrapulmonary disease), and a history of recent contact to a contagious tuberculosis case. This difficulty with diagnosis was compounded by the decision several decades ago to rely on acid-fast sputum-smear microscopy to diagnose tuberculosis in tuberculosis programs in resource-poor countries. Because microscopy of any available sample from a child with tuberculosis is positive in less than 10% of cases, the decision to rely on microscopy ensured that the detection and reporting of childhood tuberculosis cases would be woefully inadequate. While this result was unintentional, it illustrates why it is important that the needs of children be represented when public health strategies are formed and decisions are made.

The control of tuberculosis among children depends on the integrity and proper functioning of a public health system and tuberculosis program. This chapter will review several aspects of the public health aspects of childhood tuberculosis and emphasize potent and inexpensive strategies that could decrease the burden of disease in a relatively short period of time.

FAMILY-CENTERED CARE

There is a tendency to view tuberculosis as a disease of the individual, and the phrase "patient-centered care" is often used to emphasize that tuberculosis patients often have many other needs and barriers to effective care that must be addressed for treatment to be successful.[5] However, the impact of tuberculosis extends beyond the individual to the entire family, and there are two main reasons to think of tuberculosis in the context of families. First, having a family member with tuberculosis often creates a variety of other stresses and problems for the children (Box 21.2). Many adults with milder forms of tuberculosis do not perceive treatment of the disease to be as immediately important as other problems, such as staying employed and providing food and shelter for the family. Having a family member

CASE FINDING

Passive versus Active Case Finding

Passive case finding occurs when patients present themselves to a healthcare provider because they are experiencing symptoms and desire treatment. In this regard, the patient is "sick," meaning that he not only is experiencing an illness but recognizes that he needs help and treatment. Children can have tuberculosis disease—defined by an abnormal chest radiograph or physical examination and mild or no symptoms—but not be sick in the sense of seeking care. By the time a child is experiencing enough symptoms that his family seeks care, the tuberculosis is often quite extensive or severe, as in the case of meningitis. However, somewhat paradoxically, tuberculosis in children can be difficult to diagnose and especially to confirm with passive case-finding because the microbiological tests—especially the more rapid tests—are frequently negative, and the clinician often lacks the knowledge that the child has been exposed recently to a person with contagious tuberculosis.

Active case finding occurs when a clinician or program seeks out individuals who are at high risk of having tuberculosis infection or disease and evaluates them appropriately.[9,10] The obvious advantages of active case finding are the ability to find children who have been recently exposed or infected by a person with contagious tuberculosis so that prevention of disease can be undertaken, or finding a child with early tuberculosis disease who can be treated before disease has advanced. The tests that support the diagnosis of tuberculosis in a child, such as the TST or IGRA and chest radiograph, have a much higher positive predictive value when it is known that the child has been exposed recently to tuberculosis. In other words, a history of recent contact with a tuberculosis case improves the accuracy of diagnosis. However, it is important to conduct active case finding with a considered and systematic approach to ensure efficiency and to prevent overwhelming an already stressed tuberculosis program.[10] Another form of active case finding is asking about possible tuberculosis exposure when evaluating a child for pneumonia. This can be incorporated into community-based programs for mothers and children such as Integrated Management of Childhood Illness (IMCI) and Integrated Community Case Management (ICCM) by simply asking, "Is anyone in the family or household currently being treated

---

Box 21.2. Economic and Social Burdens for Children When There Is Tuberculosis in the Family

- Medication costs for the family
- Cost of hospitalization or institutional treatment
- Redirection of resources away from other needs
- Lost earnings for the family (especially if the primary wage-earner has tuberculosis)
- Withdrawal from school to care for other children or earn money
- Stigmatization and discrimination
- Creation of orphans if one or both parents dies from tuberculosis

---

with tuberculosis often causes financial hardship for the family; in many countries, patients have to pay for their medications, and many patients spend time in the hospital with a resulting loss of wages while having to cover the costs of care.[6] Older children may be pulled from school to earn extra money, especially if the person with tuberculosis is the main wage-earner. Tuberculosis in some countries continues to cause stigma and discrimination that are often experienced by other family members. For treatment of the individual to be successful, all of these difficulties need to be addressed and the family needs to be supported. Finally, the World Health Organization (WHO) estimates that there are almost 10 million children who have be orphaned by the loss of one or both parents who died from tuberculosis.[7]

Second, from a public health perspective, it is advantageous to extend the attention from the patient to family members and other individuals with a high risk of recent infection and rapid progression to disease. As the incidence of tuberculosis in the United States declined in the 1960s, it became apparent that tuberculosis infection and disease existed in what Katherine Hsu called "pools"; that an enormous proportion of cases were found in these pools; and that there was a relative scarcity of tuberculosis between pools.[8] She compared children with tuberculosis infection or disease to "sensitive Geiger counters," as such a child was indicative of an adjacent case of contagious tuberculosis.

for tuberculosis?" The most developed form of active case finding is the contact investigation.

Contact Investigation

The contact investigation is the process of conducting an epidemiological investigation around a documented or suspected case of possibly contagious tuberculosis, known as a source case.[8,11] Contacts are individuals who are at risk of acquiring infection with *M. tuberculosis* because they have "shared the air" with the source case. The degree of risk is dependent on the degree of contagiousness of the source case (Table 21.1), the frequency and duration of exposure, and the characteristics of the environment where the exposure took place.[12] Environmental

Table 21.1. Clinical, radiographic and environmental features indicative of potentially contagious tuberculosis

CATEGORY	FEATURE
Clinical	Presence of cough
	Productive cough
	Laryngeal involvement
	Draining skin or soft tissue lesion(s)
	Inappropriate treatment or early in treatment
	Unknown drug resistance
Radiographic	Cavitary lesion(s)
	Apical lung segment involvement
Microbiological	Acid-fast sputum smear-positive microscopy
Environmental	Exposure in indoor spaces with poor ventilation
	Recirculating air with droplet nuclei
	Inadequate cleaning of contaminated equipment or handling of specimens
	Undergoing airway instrumentation

factors are extremely important, because even a potentially contagious person may not transmit the organism in a well-ventilated setting. The risk of transmission is higher when the volume of air is low, the ventilation is poor, and the air is recirculated. Most houses, even in resource-rich settings, do not provide much protection from transmission; this factor, along with the fact that many contagious patients spend the most time with their families, explains why the household is the place where many children acquire the organism. In the United States, 2–3% of household contacts already have developed tuberculosis disease by the time they are evaluated. On average, 30–50% of household contacts have tuberculosis infection, although this can vary between 0% and 100%, depending on the source case and the environment. Of course, transmission can occur in other places in the community that have the same environmental characteristics.[13]

There are several important reasons for conducting a contact investigation:

1. Identifying other individuals who already have developed tuberculosis disease and referring them for evaluation and treatment

2. Identifying individuals who have been exposed to the source case, to prevent infection or the development of disease (especially in young and immunocompromised children, who tend to develop disease rapidly)

3. Identifying individuals who already have tuberculosis infection and will benefit from treatment

4. Ensuring access to medical evaluation and treatment for the exposed and infected individuals

5. Identifying environmental factors that may be contributing to transmission of the organism

6. Linking a child to a known case of culture-confirmed tuberculosis (with drug-susceptibility results) is the only way to determine the drug-susceptibility profile of the strain of *M. tuberculosis* for 70% of children with tuberculosis disease and 100% with tuberculosis infection; this is particularly important in settings where drug-resistant tuberculosis is occurring[14,15]

7. Preventing tuberculosis disease in children is highly cost-saving for both the family and the local healthcare system, including the tuberculosis program

Especially when children or adolescents are among the contacts, it is imperative that the contact investigation begin as soon as possible to prevent rapid development of disease. The first step is to interview the person thought to have tuberculosis to determine who they have been near and where they have gone during the period of time they were probably contagious. In most cases, this time is considered to be two to three months before the patient states the symptoms began. An assessment of risk is made to identify the contacts most likely to be affected, based on their individual risk factors and the environment where the contact occurred. In general, the highest risk is among household contacts, and they are evaluated first. The investigation typically utilizes history-taking, assessment of symptoms, and, where available, a test of infection, either the TST or an IGRA. If investigation of the closest contacts reveals an infection rate that exceeds what is expected for the population in general, the investigation proceeds to the next level of contacts, which are often persons who "shared the air" with the source case in a place of work, hospital or clinic, school, church, social establishment, or other indoor setting. The investigation stops when a level of contacts is found to have no more infection than is found in the community.

In settings where the TST and IGRA are not available, the contact investigation should still occur but is usually focused on just the household. Adults and children with symptoms compatible with tuberculosis should be referred for further evaluation.[16] Asymptomatic children less than five years of age or with immunocompromising conditions, especially HIV infection, should receive six months of isoniazid (unless the source case is found to have isoniazid-resistant tuberculosis, in which case the treatment of contacts should be adjusted accordingly).[17]

There is little doubt that in most tuberculosis high-burden countries, where children would benefit the most, the contact investigation is rarely performed, and treatment is often not offered.[18] There are many potential reasons for this observation, such as: limited resources within the tuberculosis program; poor recognition of the importance of this activity to preventing childhood tuberculosis; false perception that treating with a single drug is never appropriate; lack of coordination with other child health services; and inadequate education and training of clinicians in the tuberculosis program and the community.

Another related concept is the "reverse contact investigation." This occurs when a child is found to have tuberculosis infection or disease, and the process works backwards to try to identify the source case and other individuals with infection or disease.[19] When these investigations have been performed in the United States, the percentage of household contacts with tuberculosis infection and disease has been, unsurprisingly, similar to that found in contact investigations.

Targeted Case Finding

Targeted testing is the identification and evaluation of children who are at increased risk of having tuberculosis infection or disease. The ultimate form of targeted testing is the contact investigation, but the concept can be applied in other situations.[20,21] In tuberculosis high-burden settings, many children with tuberculosis are either misdiagnosed as having some other infection or condition, or are missed entirely. Two obvious places to look for children with tuberculosis are facilities or programs that manage children with HIV infection and malnutrition.

Children with untreated HIV infection are at high risk of developing tuberculosis disease after infection. Unfortunately, a survey of pediatric antiretroviral treatment programs in Africa, Asia, the Caribbean, and Central and South America documented low utilization of tuberculosis diagnostic and screening services in these programs.[22] Although sputum microscopy and chest radiography were available to all programs, among the 146 children diagnosed with tuberculosis during the study period, chest radiography was used in 86%, sputum microscopy in 52%, induced sputum microscopy in 26%, culture in 17%, and GeneXpert MTB/RIF in only 8%. Only 86% of the sites provided treatment for tuberculosis, and 30% never provided isoniazid preventive treatment to HIV-infected children. Clearly, there are many missed opportunities to detect and treat tuberculosis among the children in these clinics. Studies have shown that HIV-infected pregnant women are at risk of transmitting both HIV and tuberculosis to their infants. Although the WHO recommends integration of tuberculosis services into the Prevention of Mother-To-Child Transmission of HIV (PMTCT), programs, and several antenatal programs have demonstrated this to be feasible and productive,[23,24] this integration is inadequate or lacking in most of these programs in countries with a high tuberculosis burden.

In countries with a high tuberculosis burden, malnutrition in children is a predictor of tuberculosis disease and worse outcomes.[25,26] Pulmonary tuberculosis in young malnourished children often presents as pneumonia, but the correct diagnosis may not be considered until the disease is far advanced. A study in a Bangladesh hospital that investigated causes of pneumonia in severely malnourished children under five years of age found that 405 of 1,482 (27%) children had respiratory symptoms and an abnormal chest radiograph, and tuberculosis was confirmed microbiologically in 7% and clinically in 16%.[27] Most of the cases did not have a known source case or a positive TST. Unfortunately, tuberculosis screening at nutritional rehabilitation centers is often lacking. A study of one such center in Karnataka, India, found that a standardized tuberculosis diagnostic algorithm was followed for only 37% of the children; the study authors also identified operational challenges, including non-availability of a pediatrician, nonfunctioning radiographic equipment, use of an inferior TST solution, and poor training of the staff.[28]

Tuberculosis programs should work with other child health programs in the community to determine where children with tuberculosis might be found, and the best methods to identify, evaluate, and treat them.

CASE REPORTING AND RECORDING

Other chapters in this book (e.g., Chapter 5) have emphasized the difficulties in determining accurately the exact magnitude of childhood tuberculosis due to incomplete reporting and recording of cases. The diagnostic challenges for childhood tuberculosis have been discussed throughout this book. In addition, children diagnosed with tuberculosis are not always reported to national surveillance systems because of the lack of linkages among individual pediatricians, pediatric hospitals, and national tuberculosis programs. In addition, data from national surveys that include children are limited, and some surveys still do not fully disaggregate data by age. Many countries lack vital registration systems in which deaths from tuberculosis are reported and disaggregated by age. As a result, there is tremendous disparity in the proportion of total tuberculosis cases that are attributable to children among countries. For example, according to results reported to the WHO for 2013, less than 1% of total tuberculosis cases were children under 15 years of age in China and Cambodia, compared with 12% in South Africa and 11% in Afghanistan.[1] These differences cannot be explained simply by population distribution or other epidemiological factors. The model used by WHO estimates that 45% of childhood tuberculosis cases go unreported, while other models have predicted that 65% are unreported in high-burden countries.[1,3]

Accurate and complete reporting of childhood tuberculosis cases is critical for several reasons. Both tuberculosis and child health programs may not pay adequate attention to childhood tuberculosis if the number of reported cases is far below the actual burden. Allocation of resources depends on case numbers, and both tuberculosis and child health programs, and other funding sources such as foundations and nongovernmental organizations (NGOs), will not provide adequate support if the case numbers are inaccurately low.[4] The rate of childhood tuberculosis can be an important quality indicator for the tuberculosis program (see below). Reporting accurate numbers is also important for community and professional support and education.

Little attention has been paid to the reporting of tuberculosis infection in children, defined either through testing or by using recent close exposure (contact) as a surrogate. Most childhood tuberculosis experts recommend that a registry of tuberculosis contact and/or infection be kept and the children in it followed to ensure they receive adequate evaluation and complete treatment. Reconciling a registry for exposure/infection with one for disease will be informative for determining the effectiveness of the overall tuberculosis program.

ADHERENCE TO TREATMENT AND DIRECTLY OBSERVED THERAPY

The medical, ethical, and societal issues surrounding tuberculosis treatment are different from those in most other infections and diseases. Tuberculosis is one of the few diseases treated in the public health sector that requires long-term treatment. For most diseases, adherence to treatment is an issue for just the patient. However, for tuberculosis, adherence has broader implications: a patient with pulmonary tuberculosis who is non-adherent can relapse, their organism can develop drug resistance, and the patient can transmit the resistant *M. tuberculosis* through the air to other persons. Effective treatment is complicated, requiring several drugs that have a variety of possible adverse effects be taken for many months. There are many factors that can adversely affect adherence with tuberculosis treatment (Box 21.3).[29-36] The reasons for poor adherence usually are not only multifaceted and complex, but may result from characteristics and health beliefs of individual patients and families and the quality of the social and economic environment in which they live.

Studies have shown that physicians' predictions for which patients will be non-adherent with treatment are accurate in fewer than 50% of cases.[37] In one study for tuberculosis treatment, physicians identified only 32% of non-adherent patients and incorrectly identified 8% of adherent patients as non-adherent.[38] Patients' self-reporting is notoriously unreliable because of issues such as forgetfulness, unwillingness to admit that medications were not taken, and desire to please the medical provider. However, there is some evidence that patients with a variety of medical conditions who have had experience with a treatment regimen can predict their own level of adherence in the future and that careful questioning by providers may yield better predictions about adherence.[39-41]

There are several reasons why adherence to treatment can be a particularly important problem for children. Some children—especially if found via active case finding—have few or mild symptoms, and the family's perceived need for treatment may be low. Also, these mildly ill children will not show much improvement while taking the medications, so the family does not get the positive feedback of an improving clinical course. The inability to microbiologically confirm most cases of childhood tuberculosis may create doubt in the family about whether tuberculosis is the correct diagnosis. Many children with tuberculosis come from socially disadvantaged families where the presence of multiple caregivers is common, which can lead to inconsistency in medication administration to the child. An important practical problem is that very few antituberculosis medications are available in pediatric formulations; young children in particular may have difficulty taking the required volumes and forms of medications that often involve crushing pills or making suspensions. Finally, treating tuberculosis requires communication with both the adult family members and the child; it is important that the child's questions be answered and fears addressed in an age-appropriate manner so the child will cooperate with treatment.

A variety of measures have been used to support adherence to treatment.[32,33] The most important may be education of the child and family, both at diagnosis but also periodically during the treatment regimen. One study showed that 15–20 minutes of education can yield two months of unbroken clinic appointments and improved treatment adherence.[42]

Box 21.3. General Factors That Adversely Affect Patient Adherence

- Patients begin to feel better (and think they no longer need treatment)
- Greater number of medications
- Higher frequency of drug administration
- Longer duration of treatment
- Lack of clear instructions for taking medications
- Adverse effects from medications—perceived or actual
- High cost of treatment—direct and indirect costs
- Poor packaging of drugs
- Poor tolerance of drug-taking—form, size, taste, texture
- Lack of transportation
- Unpleasant clinic conditions
- Language barriers with clinic staff
- Difficult interactions with the clinician
- Long lag time between referral and appointment
- Lack of family/friend support

It is important to identify the specific barriers to treatment that the child and family might have so they can be addressed at the beginning of treatment. Also helpful is the provision of incentives—things that enhance the desirability of treatment such as toys and books—and enablers—things such as food, bus tokens, or access to other medical services that actually help the patient and family overcome barriers to care. Tailoring incentives and enablers to individual families seems to offer more benefit than general approaches.

Certain characteristics of the treatment regimen may help promote adherence. The parents should be asked about aspects of their work and daily living activities that could hinder or assist in the administration of the medication to the child. Reminders and the use of "self-rewards" for the child or the family can be effective. Adherence is often enhanced if families link giving medication with something else they do every day, such as eat a meal or go to sleep at night. Clinicians can assist families by asking questions that allow them to come up with practical, realistic, and success-producing strategies of their own.

In spite of the best efforts of the clinician, family, and patient, significant barriers to successful treatment of tuberculosis in children often remain. In response, the concept of directly observed therapy (DOT) has been developed.[43] Although the administration of medication is the centerpiece, true DOT programs offer a package of ideas and services that enhance treatment and make it easier for the family and child. There are many different ways of administering medications under DOT. Some believe that parents administering medication to a child is DOT, but most DOT programs do not consider this to be adequate. Numerous studies have shown that DOT, defined as the administration of medication by a healthcare worker or other third party (non-family member), significantly improves adherence to tuberculosis treatment. In some cases, the person who administers DOT travels to the patient's home and in others the patient has to go to a specific location, often a clinic. In the United States and some other countries, DOT is considered to be the standard of care for treating adults and children with tuberculosis disease. DOT is also utilized for some children with tuberculosis exposure or infection who are considered to be at high risk of rapid progression to disease. However, whether universal DOT is necessary is quite controversial, and in some settings it is reserved for patients with demonstrated non-adherence or with retreatment tuberculosis. Programs are also developing novel ways to enhance adherence and conduct DOT using less personnel time, such as the use of cellphone video and webcams, sending text medication reminders to patients and parents, and using electronic medication monitors.

INFECTION CONTROL AND CHILDHOOD TUBERCULOSIS

It has long been held that only rare children with pulmonary tuberculosis can transmit the organism to others, and there are a number of reasons why children are less contagious than adults.[44,45] First, children usually have paucibacillary disease, leading to low rates of acid-fast smear-positive specimens. Second, young children are less likely to have cavitary lesions, due, in part, to less mature immune responses. Third, prepubertal children have a less forceful cough than adults and the cough is less likely to be productive, leading to decreased aerosolization. Fourth, childhood tuberculosis is more likely to be extrapulmonary in nature than disease in immunocompetent adults. Finally, children may be less contagious on a public health level simply because they have more circumscribed social networks than adults.

It is difficult to tell in a community setting if children with tuberculosis are contagious, because they are usually in contact with the same people as the adult or adolescent from whom they acquired the infection, and determining individual contributions to transmission is difficult. The most useful data to determine which children should be considered potentially contagious have come from institutions that care for children. In the early 1900s, Wallgren[46] and other investigators in Europe noticed that when an adult with tuberculosis was working in an orphanage, many of the children developed tuberculosis, but when a young child in the orphanage had pulmonary tuberculosis, none of the other children developed the disease. Data from children's hospitals in the United States have demonstrated very low rates of tuberculosis infection among healthcare workers in contact with children with tuberculosis.[47,48] Only rare cases of massive transmission have been associated with a child under 10 years of age. In one report, 20% of the close contacts of a nine-year-old boy with cavitary tuberculosis and acid-fast-positive sputum smears developed tuberculosis infection and no other cases of tuberculosis were reported in this area.[49] A nine-year old boy in England had extensive pulmonary lesions but acid-fast-negative sputum smears; however, the rate of positive TSTs in his classmates was statistically higher than among other students at his school (79% vs. 35%, $p < 0.01$).[50] Both children had characteristics of pulmonary tuberculosis that are more typical of adult-type disease.

Nosocomial transmission of *M. tuberculosis* from infants and children has been reported rarely. These cases have often been associated with several common variables: older adolescents, a child with cavitary or other high-inoculum pulmonary disease (including children who are acid-fast smear-positive), and children undergoing airway instrumentation procedures. There are several case reports of healthcare worker infection after exposure to a congenitally infected infant with miliary disease.[51,52] These infants often have a very high organism burden and tuberculosis is not initially suspected, resulting in delayed infection-control precautions. As a general rule, any child with radiographic or symptomatic features of adult-type tuberculosis should be treated as contagious (Table 21.1). One study identified several predictors of acid-fast sputum smear-positivity in adolescents: cough of more than four weeks' duration (adjusted odds ratio [aOR]: 13.8), involvement of the superior segment of the lower lobes (aOR: 12.6), and cavitary lesions (aOR: 7.7).[53] However, nosocomial transmission from healthcare workers and other adults to children in healthcare facilities is more common than transmission from children to adults.[54] For example, infection has been documented in patients of pediatricians and a newborn-nursery nurse, from breastfeeding mothers or other hospital visitors. An alternative nosocomial route of transmission has been reported for children receiving chemotherapy solutions that were cross-contaminated with the BCG vaccine used to treat bladder cancer.[55]

Preventing the Transmission of *M. tuberculosis* in Healthcare Settings

Various organizations have made recommendations for the prevention of transmission of *M. tuberculosis* in healthcare facilities, and a complete review is beyond the scope of this chapter.[56]

Recommendations are broken down into administrative, environmental, and personal respiratory protection, in that order of importance. Most transmission can be prevented by developing policies and procedures that limit the likelihood that a patient with contagious tuberculosis will go unrecognized. Administrative measures reduce risk of exposure to patients who potentially have tuberculosis, by screening for risk factors, delineating factors requiring isolation, integrating the laboratory and local health departments into the infection-control team, training healthcare workers on tuberculosis prevention, and appropriate cleaning of equipment. Environmental measures minimize the number of areas in which exposure can occur by using ventilation and other measures, such as high-efficiency particulate air (HEPA) filters and ultraviolet light, to decrease transmission and reduce the concentration of bacilli in the air. In resource-constrained settings where the cost of providing negative-pressure and HEPA-protected environments is prohibitive, clinics and hospitals can be designed to take advantage of movement of air via natural ventilation enhanced by the use of open windows and strategically placed extractor fans. Personal respiratory protection measures further decrease the risk of transmission in these protective areas by the use of appropriately fitting masks and respirators in the rooms of potentially contagious patients.

Unfortunately, studies have shown that these protective measures often are not fully applied in children's institutions, even in resource-rich countries. A tuberculosis infection-control survey of 195 U.S. pediatric facilities (both free-standing children's hospitals and hospitals with pediatric units) showed that, despite almost universal isolation of children with cavitary lesions and positive acid-fast sputum smears, there was considerable variation in number of in-hospital contact investigations done, reasons for discontinuing isolation, visitation policies, and methods of screening visitors for tuberculosis. While 88% of institutions reported a sufficient number of negative-pressure inpatient rooms, only 42% had isolation rooms in outpatient areas, and over 30% of facilities used simple surgical masks, not the recommended N95 respirators, for high-risk surgical and endoscopy procedures.[48] An observational study showed that adherence with infection control practices by visitors and healthcare workers caring for children with suspected tuberculosis was low.

Screening Family Members of Children with Suspected Tuberculosis

The diagnosis of tuberculosis in a child is a sentinel event, as this usually represents recent community transmission. Because families have different thresholds for seeking care for their children and for themselves, and because children often present with more severe symptoms than do adults, the child may be the first one in the family diagnosed with tuberculosis. Especially for young children, there is a high likelihood that an adult who accompanies or visits the child in the hospital is the one with undiagnosed disease. In two consecutive series of patients at Texas Children's Hospital, 15% and 17%, respectively, of adults accompanying children with suspected tuberculosis had as-yet-undiagnosed pulmonary tuberculosis that was detected when the hospital performed chest radiographs on these adult visitors.[57,58] This case rate of 15,000–17,000 per 100,000 is one of the highest found in any tuberculosis screening program. By doing this screening, many cases of tuberculosis in adults were immediately referred for treatment, the diagnosis of tuberculosis in the child was strengthened by finding a source case, and the hospital prevented possible nosocomial transmission from the adult case. To address the issue of contagious visitors, the hospital's policy now limits children with suspected tuberculosis to two visitors who undergo chest radiography at the hospital's expense. Thus, the unit of infection control for childhood tuberculosis is not the patient, but the family. As a result, no healthcare worker at this hospital who cared for a tuberculosis patient became infected, and this strategy was more high-yield and cost-efficient than periodic screening of all healthcare workers for tuberculosis infection.

There are virtually no data about transmission of *M. tuberculosis* within children's healthcare facilities in tuberculosis high-burden areas, but it almost certainly occurs. Limited availability and high cost of chest radiographs probably would preclude use of this strategy in most resource-poor settings, but, at a minimum, adult visitors—especially those for children with suspected tuberculosis—can be screened for symptoms of tuberculosis and, when appropriate, referred immediately for further evaluation. Periodic evaluation of healthcare workers in children's facilities, at least by symptom screening and history of contact, is also important as one

contagious person could affect an enormous number of vulnerable children.

CHILDHOOD TUBERCULOSIS AS A QUALITY MEASURE

Young children develop tuberculosis disease fairly rapidly after infection, which brings good news and bad news. The "bad news" is that transmission of *M. tuberculosis* rapidly puts many children at risk for developing severe disease. However, the "good news" is that rapid intervention after transmission has occurred can prevent a large proportion of childhood tuberculosis cases. The concept of "preventable childhood tuberculosis" can be thought of as a quality measure for tuberculosis programs. Except for cases when the child with tuberculosis presents before or at the same time as the contagious case, many cases of childhood tuberculosis could be prevented.

For several decades, the WHO and many other organizations have recommended the evaluation and treatment of children less than five years of age and all immunocompromised children who are close contacts of adult tuberculosis patients, usually focusing on the family and the household. Symptomatic children should be referred for evaluation of disease. Asymptomatic children should be given six months of isoniazid (assuming the source case has drug-susceptible disease) to prevent progression to disease.[17] Providing these measures, in addition to BCG vaccine where it is used routinely, will prevent a large proportion of tuberculosis cases in children and adolescents. Unfortunately, most high-burden countries have never put this intervention into place—a missed opportunity to prevent childhood tuberculosis. Most high-burden countries do not report or have a registry for close contacts, so it is impossible to determine if they are being appropriately identified and treated. Creating these measures and providing treatment to childhood contacts would prevent a large proportion of childhood tuberculosis cases.

Resource-rich countries have tried to put these measures in place via the contact investigation. In these countries, tests of infection and chest radiography are commonly used as part of the investigation. However, when these procedures are not carried out properly, preventable childhood tuberculosis cases still occur. Several studies have estimated that 30–50% of childhood tuberculosis cases in resource-rich settings could be prevented, and have examined the reasons why they are not.[59,60] Among the reasons are:

1. the adult source case is never reported to the tuberculosis program (is cared for in the private sector);
2. there is a delay in evaluation of the contacts because of lack of personnel or other resources;
3. treatment for the contacts is not offered;
4. the source case has isoniazid-resistant tuberculosis and the child's treatment is not changed; or
5. the family refuses treatment.

A recent tragic event in my clinic occurred with a healthy 15-month-old child who was a known household contact of an adult with acid-fast sputum smear-positive tuberculosis. The child had a normal physical exam, a negative TST, and a normal chest radiograph, and he was to be placed on directly observed isoniazid therapy to prevent disease. Unfortunately, the child's family moved from one health jurisdiction to another without notification, he did not receive the treatment, and three months later he developed severe tuberculous meningitis.

If one truly believes that a case of childhood tuberculosis is a sentinel event, as is so often stated, it seems logical that every case of childhood tuberculosis should be investigated to determine if it could have been prevented and if there are any systematic weaknesses in the tuberculosis program that allowed it to occur. Of course, this would be nearly impossible to carry out in a high-burden setting, but should be a routine practice in low-burden settings where the true patterns of transmission are exposed. However, more robust detection, reporting, recording, and analysis of childhood tuberculosis cases will give all tuberculosis programs, in both high- and low-burden settings, much more insight into the effectiveness of their overall activities and should suggest new and novel strategies to detect and prevent the disease in children and adults in their jurisdictions.

REFERENCES

1. World Health Organization. *Global TB Report, 2014*. Geneva: World Health Organization; 2014.
2. Jenkins HE, Tolman AW, Yuen CM, Becerra M. Incidence of multidrug-resistant tuberculosis disease in children: systematic review and global estimates. *Lancet*. 2014;383(9928):1572–1579.
3. Dodd PJ, Gardiner E, Coghlan R, Seddon JA. Burden of childhood tuberculosis in 22 high-burden countries: a mathematical modelling study. *Lancet Global Health*. 2014;2:453–459.
4. World Health Organization. *Roadmap for Childhood Tuberculosis—Towards Zero Deaths*. Geneva; 2013.
5. Grant R. Patient-centred care: is it the key to stemming the tide? *Int J Tuberc Lung Dis*. 2013;17(10–Suppl 1):S3–S4.
6. Ukwaja KN, Modebe O, Igwenyi C, Alobu I. The economic burden of tuberculosis care for patients and households in Africa: a systematic review. *Int J Tuberc Lung Dis*. 2012;16(6):733–739.
7. World Health Organization. *Global TB Report, 2013*. Geneva: World Health Organization; 2013.
8. Hsu, KHK. Contact investigation: a practical approach to tuberculosis eradication. *Am J Public Health*. 1963;53(11):1761–1769.
9. Anger HA, Proops D, Harris TG, et al. Active case finding and prevention of tuberculosis among a cohort of contacts exposed to infectious tuberculosis cases in New York City. *Clin Infect Dis*. 2012;54(9):1287–1295.
10. Uplekar M, Creswell J, Ottmani S-E, Weil D, Sahu S, Lonnroth K. Programmatic approaches to screening for active tuberculosis. *Int J Tuberc Lung Dis*. 2013;17(10):1248–1256.
11. Fox GJ, Barry SE, Britton WJ, Marks GB. Contact investigation for tuberculosis: a systematic review and meta-analysis. *Eur Respir J*. 2013;41:140–156.
12. Ling D-L, Liaw Y-P, Lee C-Y, Lo H-Y, Yang H-L, Chan P-C. Contact investigation for tuberculosis in Taiwan contacts aged under 20 years in 2005. *Int J Tuberc Lung Dis*. 2011;15(1):50–55.
13. Brooks-Pollock E, Becerra MC, Goldstein E, Cohen T, Murray MB. Epidemiologic inference from the distribution of tuberculosis cases in households in Lima, Peru. *J Infect Dis*. 2011;203:1582–1589.
14. Shah AN, Yuen CM, Heo M, Tolman AW, Becerra MC. Yield of contact investigations in households of patients with drug-resistant tuberculosis: systematic review and meta-analysis. *Clin Infect Dis*. 2014;58(3):3981–391.
15. Laniado-Laborin R, Cazares-Adame R, Volker-Soberanes M-L, et al. Latent tuberculosis infection prevalence among paediatric contacts of drug-resistant and drug-susceptible cases. *Int J Tuberc Lung Dis*. 2014;18(5):515–519.
16. Triasih R, Robertson CF, Duke T, Graham SM. A prospective evaluation of the symptom-based screening approach to the management of children who are contacts of tuberculosis cases. *Clin Infect Dis*. 2015;60(1):12–18.

17. World Health Organization. *Rapid Advice: Treatment of Tuberculosis in Children.* Geneva: World Health Organization; 2010.

18. Shivaramakrishna HR, Frederick A, Shazia A, et al. Isoniazid preventive treatment in children in two districts of South India: does practice follow policy? *Int J Tuberc Lung Dis.* 2014;18(8):919–924.

19. Puryear S, Seropola G, Ho-Foster A, et al. Yield of contact tracing from pediatric tuberculosis cases in Gaborone, Botswana. *Int J Tuberc Lung Dis.* 2013;17(8):1049–1055.

20. Dowdy DW, Azman AS, Kendall EA, Mathema B. Transforming the fight against tuberculosis: targeting catalysts of transmission. *Clin Infect Dis.* 2014;59(8):1123–1129.

21. Pediatric Tuberculosis Collaborative Group. Targeted tuberculin skin testing and treatment of latent tuberculosis infection in children and adolescents. *Pediatrics.* 2004;114(4–Suppl):1175–1201.

22. Ballif M, Renner L, Dusingize JC, et al. Tuberculosis in pediatric antiretroviral therapy programs in low- and middle-income countries: Diagnosis and screening practices. *J Pediatr Infect Dis Soc.* 2014;4(1):30–38.

23. Uwimana J, Jackson D. Integration of tuberculosis and prevention or mother-to-child transmission of HIV programmes in South Africa. *Int J Tuberc Lung Dis.* 2013;17(10):1285–1290.

24. Kancheya N, Luhanga D, Harris JB, et al. Integrating active tuberculosis case finding in antenatal services in Zambia. *Int J Tuberc Lung Dis.* 2014;18(12):1466–1472.

25. Chisti MJ, Ahmed T, Pietroni MAC, et al. Pulmonary tuberculosis in severely-malnourished or HIV-infected children with pneumonia: a review. *J Health Popul Nutr.* 2013: 31(3):308–313.

26. Jaganath D, Mupere E. Childhood tuberculosis and malnutrition. *J Infect Dis.* 2012;206:1809–1815.

27. Chisti MJ, Graham SM, Duke T, et al. A prospective study of the prevalence of tuberculosis and bacteraemia in Bangladeshi children with severe malnutrition and pneumonia including an evaluation of Xpert MTB/RIF assay. *PloS One.* 2014;9(4):e93776.

28. Bhat PG, Kumar AMV, Naik B, et al. Intensified tuberculosis case finding among malnourished children in nutritional rehabilitation centres in Karnataka, India: missed opportunities. *PloS One.* 2013;8(2):e84255.

29. Guernsey BG, Alexander MR. Tuberculosis: Review of treatment failure, relapse and drug resistance. *Am J Hosp Pharm.* 1978;35:690–698.

30. Sbarbaro JA. Compliance: inducements and reinforcements. *Chest.* 1979;76(Suppl):750–756.

31. Anderson RJ, Kirk LM. Methods of improving patient compliance in chronic disease states. *Arch Intern Med.* 1982;142:1673–1675.

32. Snider DE, Hutton MD. *Improving Patient Compliance in Tuberculosis Programs.* Atlanta, GA: Centers for Disease Control; 1986.

33. Cuneo WD, Snider DE Jr. Enhancing patient compliance with tuberculosis therapy. *Clin Chest Med.* 1989;10:375–380.

34. Sbarbaro JA. The patient–physician relationship: Compliance revisited. *Ann Allergy.* 1990;64:325–332.

35. Ormerod LP, Prescott RJ. Inter-relations between relapses, drug regimens and compliance with treatment in tuberculosis. *Respir Med.* 1991;85:239–242.

36. Menzies R, Rocher I, Vissandjee B. Factors associated with compliance in treatment of tuberculosis. *Tubercle Lung dis.* 1993;74:32–37.

37. Musklin AI Appel FA. Diagnosing patient noncompliance. *Arch Intern Med.* 1977;137:318–321.

38. Wardman AG, Knox AJ, Muers MF. Profiles of noncompliance with anti-tuberculous therapy. *Br J Dis Chest.* 1988;82:285–289.

39. Kaplan RM, Simon HJ. Compliance in medical care: reconsideration of self-predictions. *Ann Behav Med.* 1990;12:66–71.

40. Stewart M. The validity of an interview to assess a patient's drug taking. *Am J Prev Med.* 1987;3:95–100.

41. Steele DJ, Jackson TC, Gutmann MC. Have you been taking your pills? The adherence-monitoring sequence in the medical interview. *J Fam Pract.* 1990;30:294–299.

42. Seesha MA, Aneja KS. Problem of drug default and role of "motivation." *Indian J Public Health.* 1982;26:234–243.

43. Sumartojo E. When tuberculosis treatment fails. A social behavioral account of patient adherence. *Am Rev Respir Dis.* 1993;142:1311–1320.

44. Cruz AT, Starke JR. A current review of infection control for childhood tuberculosis. *Tuberculosis.* 2011;91(supplement):S11–S15.

45. Marais BJ, Gie RP, Schaaf HS, Beyers N, Donald PR, Starke JR. Childhood pulmonary tuberculosis: old wisdom and new challenges. *Am J Respir Crit Care Med.* 2006;173:1078–1090.

46. Wallgren AJ. On the contagiousness of childhood tuberculosis. *Acta Paediatr Scand.* 1937;22:229–234.

47. Christie CD, Constantinou P, Marx ML, Willke MJ, Marot K, Mendez FL. Low risk for tuberculosis in a regional pediatric hospital: nine-year study of community rates and the mandatory employee tuberculin skin test program. *Infect Control Hosp Epidemiol*. 1998;19:168–174.

48. Kellerman SE, Simonds D, Banerjee S, Towsley J, Stover BH, Jarvis W. APIC and CDC survey of *Mycobacterium tuberculosis* isolation and control practices in hospitals caring for children. Part 2: Environmental and administrative controls. *Am J Infect Control*. 1998;26:483–487.

49. Curtis AB, Ridzon R, Vogel R, McDonough S, Hargreaves J, Ferry J. Extensive transmission of *Mycobacterium tuberculosis* from a child. *N Engl J Med*. 1999;341:1491–1495.

50. Paranjothy S, Elsenhut M, Lilley M, Bracebridge S, Abubaker L, Mulla R. Extensive transmission of *Mycobacterium* from a 9-day old child with pulmonary tuberculosis and negative sputum smear. *Br Med J*. 2008;337:e1184.

51. Reynolds DL, Gillis F, Kitai I, Deamond SL, Silverman M, King SM. Transmission of *Mycobacterium tuberculosis* from an infant. *Int J Tuberc lung Dis*. 2006;10:1051–1056.

52. Lee LH, LeVea CM, Graman PS. Congenital tuberculosis in a neonatal intensive care unit: case report, epidemiological investigation, and management of exposures. *Clin Infect Dis*. 1998;27:474–477.

53. Wong KS, Huang YC, Lai SH, Chiu CY, Huang YH, Lin TY. Validity of symptoms and radiographic features in predicting positive AFB smears in adolescents with tuberculosis. *Int J Tuberc Lung Dis*. 2010;14:155–159.

54. Fisher KE, Guaran R, Stack J, et al. Nosocomial pulmonary tuberculosis contact investigation in a neonatal intensive care unit. *Infect Control Hosp Epidemiol*. 2013;34(7):754–756.

55. Waecker NJ Jr., Stefanova R, Cave MD, Davis CE, Dankner WM. Nosocomial transmission of *Mycobacterium bovis* bacilli Calmette-Guerin to children receiving cancer therapy and to their health care providers. *Clin Infect Dis*. 200;30:356–362.

56. Centers for Disease Control and Prevention. Guidelines for preventing the transmission of *Mycobacterium tuberculosis* in healthcare settings. *MMWR*. 2005;54:1–141.

57. Munoz FM, Ong LT, Seavy D, Medina D Correa A, Starke JR. Tuberculosis among adult visitors of children with suspected tuberculosis and employees at a children's hospital. *Infect Control Hosp Epidemiol*. 2002;23:568–572.

58. Cruz AT, Medina D, Whaley EM, Ware KM, Koy TH, Starke JR. Tuberculosis among families of children with suspected tuberculosis and employees at a children's hospital. *Infect Control Hosp Epidemiol*. 2011;32:188–190.

59. Nolan RJ Jr. Childhood tuberculosis in North Carolina: a study of the opportunities for intervention in the transmission of tuberculosis to children. *Am J Public Health*. 1986;76:26–30.

60. Mehta JB, Bentley S. Prevention of tuberculosis in children: missed opportunities. *Am J Prev Med*. 1992;8(5):283–286.

22

THE ROADMAP FOR CHILDHOOD TUBERCULOSIS

Stephen M. Graham and Anne Detjen

HIGHLIGHTS OF THIS CHAPTER

The 10 Essential Steps in the Roadmap

1. Include the needs of children and adolescents in research, policy development and clinical practices.
2. Collect and report better data, including data on prevention.
3. Develop policy guidance, training and reference materials for healthcare workers.
4. Foster local expertise and leadership.
5. Do not miss critical opportunities for intervention.
6. Engage key stakeholders.
7. Develop integrated family-centered and community-centered strategies.
8. Address research gaps.
9. Meet funding needs for childhood tuberculosis.
10. Form coalitions and partnerships to improve tools for diagnosis and treatment.

THE ROAD TO THE ROADMAP

The past decade has seen increasing attention to the challenges and needs related to tuberculosis in children. Initial efforts by a small group of childhood tuberculosis experts with support of the International Union Against Tuberculosis and Lung Disease (IUATLD) and the World Health Organization (WHO) led to the formation of the Stop TB Partnership's Childhood TB Subgroup in 2003. The subgroup has since provided input to multiple tuberculosis control initiatives by WHO, ensuring that childhood tuberculosis was visible and included in national as well as global agendas. It has led the effort to develop WHO's *Guidance for National Tuberculosis Programmes* (NTPs) on the management of tuberculosis in children that was first published in 2006 and recently updated in 2014,[1] to revise dosage recommendations for first-line anti-tuberculosis medications in young children,[2] to include childhood tuberculosis representation in tuberculosis-control strategic planning and policy at global and regional levels, to provide technical support to NTPs, to facilitate research, and to develop capacity for technical expertise in tuberculosis-endemic countries.

In 2011, the first international meeting in over 50 years on childhood tuberculosis was held in Stockholm, co-facilitated by the European Centers for Disease Control and the WHO Stop TB Partnership. This meeting was attended by a wide range of stakeholders, including community representation with children who had been treated for tuberculosis, and civil society organizations along with professional advocacy groups. The need for stronger and more effective advocacy on behalf of children and families affected by tuberculosis was highlighted, and the resulting "Call to Action for Childhood TB" was posted on the WHO website, which has since been signed by over 1,000 individuals and organizations.[3] As a result, the WHO's annual *Global Tuberculosis Report* included estimates of the global burden of tuberculosis in children for the first time in 2012.[4]

The new focus on the challenges of tuberculosis in children by a wider range of expertise and stakeholders served to highlight the many wide gaps along the continuum from global and national policy to the provision of effective management and prevention at all levels of care, including at the community level. It also highlighted the fact that almost no funding was being sought by NTPs to address the needs of tuberculosis in children, and that there was very limited investment in research needs. Despite the obvious need, children were rarely being included in either novel research of diagnostics or treatment, or operational research to address the wide policy–practice gaps.

The increasing attention to the needs of tuberculosis control in children coincided with the broadening of the WHO's global tuberculosis-control strategy since 2006 beyond a public health strategy aimed at reducing transmission, to increasing case-finding and prevention of all cases, including among vulnerable populations such as children. There also was increasing recognition that more integrated approaches to addressing tuberculosis were necessary. The WHO post-2015 global tuberculosis strategy, which was endorsed by the World Health Assembly in 2014, provides an unprecedented opportunity to address many of the major gaps and priorities for childhood tuberculosis.[5]

It was in this context of political opportunity and recognition of the many diverse challenges that members of the Child TB Subgroup recognized the need to develop an overarching guidance document, or "Roadmap."

THE DEVELOPMENT OF THE ROADMAP

The development of this roadmap was led by core team members of the Stop TB Partnership's Childhood TB Subgroup. A major achievement was the engagement, support and input during the process by key organizations: WHO, IUATLD, the U.S. Centers for Disease Control and Prevention (CDC), the Treatment Action Group (TAG), the U.S. Agency for International Development (USAID), and the United Nations Children's Fund (UNICEF). During the process of developing the roadmap, key challenges were identified:

- Increasing numbers of NTPs in tuberculosis-endemic countries were attempting to address the previous neglect of tuberculosis in children by updating national guidelines as a first step, but required guidance about how to move forward with implementation to address the wide policy–practice gap. A framework for NTPs to address childhood tuberculosis was required.
- Children with tuberculosis do not primarily present to tuberculosis services that are administered by the NTP, but rather to child health services that manage children with a wide range of illnesses. Tuberculosis in children often causes symptoms that overlap with other common causes of child morbidity and mortality, such as pneumonia or malnutrition. There was a clear need to more actively engage the maternal and child health sector in understanding the presentations of tuberculosis in children and tuberculosis control strategies for children, consistent with WHO's post-2015 tuberculosis-control strategy.
- Tuberculosis needed to be considered in the broader context of child survival. The countries with the highest infant and child mortality rates are also often tuberculosis-endemic countries, and infants and young children (<5 years) are at the highest risk for severe tuberculosis.[6] The estimates of deaths from tuberculosis in children are limited by a lack of vital registration data

from many high-incidence countries, and by the fact that there are virtually no available data of the contribution of tuberculosis to deaths in HIV-infected children. Furthermore, there are recent data suggesting that tuberculosis is underdiagnosed as a cause or comorbidity in children with severe pneumonia, severe malnutrition, or meningitis, and may be a larger contributor to under-five deaths than has been recognized.[7-10] The facts that infants and young children are rarely sputum acid-fast smear-positive, and that they are not a common source of ongoing transmission of *Mycobacterium tuberculosis,* underlie why childhood tuberculosis has been neglected in the public health approach to tuberculosis control. However, the need to pay attention to childhood tuberculosis becomes more compelling when it is considered as a common cause of childhood morbidity and mortality in high-mortality settings, especially as almost all tuberculosis-endemic countries regard the reduction of infant and under-five mortality as a national health priority.

- The importance of integration of training and management for childhood tuberculosis with other relevant programs for maternal, child, and adolescent health is crucial, and input was provided by a wide range of stakeholders during the development of the roadmap. The endorsement by UNICEF meant that a major provider that primarily focuses on global child health officially recognized the importance of tuberculosis in children.
- The accurate diagnosis of childhood tuberculosis continues to be the central challenge to progress, not just for improved care and outcomes, but also for improved estimates, quality of research, and more effective advocacy. As current diagnostic tools are inadequate, continued efforts to develop improved diagnostics and to optimize the use of currently available tools are critical priorities.
- Multi-drug resistant tuberculosis (MDR-TB) is now a major global public health challenge, and the burden of MDR-TB in children is likely to reflect that of the wider population. Although case detection, effective management, and prevention of MDR-TB are as relevant and important for children as for adults, the burden of MDR-TB in children has received significantly less attention.
- Adolescents (10–19 years) needed to be more explicitly included within the "child" tuberculosis

agenda. Adolescence is a vulnerable age group, not only at increased risk of developing (often smear-positive) tuberculosis, but also with unique needs for case detection and effective management. These needs, which include access to diagnosis and care, treatment supervision, and adherence, are not necessarily specific to tuberculosis but are common challenges for adolescent health in general. Adolescents often need to negotiate a transitional stage between pediatric and adult health services, and adolescent care traditionally has developed as an extension of child health services.

THE LAUNCH OF THE ROADMAP

World TB Day focused on tuberculosis in children for the first time in 2012, and the group developing the roadmap produced an advocacy document to highlight ongoing efforts to increase attention to the many needs for childhood tuberculosis, both within the tuberculosis community and within the broader maternal and child health community.[11] On October 1, 2013, the *Roadmap for Childhood Tuberculosis—Towards Zero Deaths* was launched in Washington, D.C., in a broadly publicized event that was covered by more than 150 media outlets.[12]

THE CONTENT: TEN KEY ACTIONS TOWARDS ZERO DEATHS FROM CHILDHOOD TUBERCULOSIS

At the core of the roadmap are 10 priority actions to comprehensively address the issues around child and adolescent tuberculosis (Figure 22.1). These are actions that are as relevant at regional and national levels as they are at the global level.[13]

1. Include the Needs of Children and Adolescents in Research, Policy Development, and Clinical Practices

The post-2015 global tuberculosis control strategy is built on three core pillars of public health: (1) integrated, patient-centered tuberculosis care and prevention; (2) bold policies and supportive systems; and (3) intensified research and innovation.[5] The intention is to move from the traditional vertical (disease-specific programs) approach of tuberculosis control to a more horizontal approach that

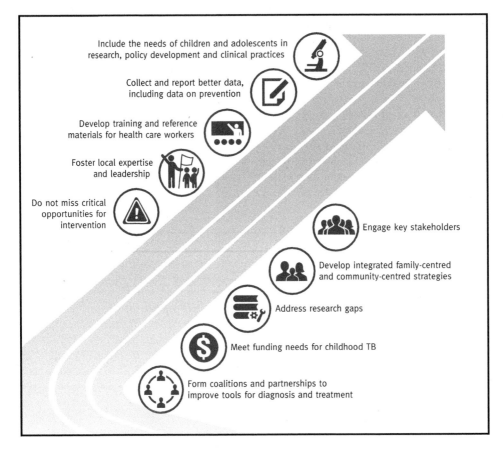

FIGURE 22.1   Ten key priorities towards zero deaths.

From: *Roadmap for Childhood Tuberculosis.* WHO; 2013.

includes the wider health sector through integrated activities, community engagement, and collaborative partnerships. This provides the necessary platform to engage the broader child and adolescent health community in tuberculosis control. There is increased emphasis on active case-finding and prevention through contact screening, an activity that is particularly relevant for child contacts. Innovative research for improved diagnostics and case-detection in children with tuberculosis is a critical need. Adolescents have been explicitly included in recognition of the specific unmet needs of this vulnerable age group.

This strategy recognizes the need for country-specific solutions to reach the targets of 95% reduction of tuberculosis deaths and 90% reduction in the tuberculosis incidence rate by 2035. It is important that countries, while developing their strategies, create a framework that addresses childhood tuberculosis as outlined in Figure 22.2, and ensure that the needs of children and adolescents with tuberculosis are included in all three pillars.

2. Collect and Report Better Data, Including Data on Prevention

More accurate and comprehensive data of the burden of tuberculosis and treatment outcomes in children and adolescents are absolutely critical within a framework for strengthening tuberculosis control in children (Figure 22.2). Data provide a foundation for situational analysis, for identifying gaps and priorities, for monitoring and evaluation of progress and implementation, for planning and procurement of diagnostics and drugs, as well as being a necessary tool for effective advocacy and for funding needs for this vulnerable population.

As outlined in Chapter 5, global data on the true burden of tuberculosis in children are

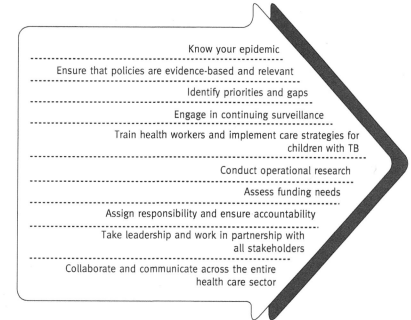

FIGURE 22.2   A framework for improving childhood tuberculosis activities within National Tuberculosis Control Programs.

From: *Roadmap for Childhood Tuberculosis*, WHO; 2013.

generally challenged by under-recording and under-reporting by NTPs of children diagnosed with tuberculosis; by uncertainties of diagnostic accuracy, given that most cases in young children are diagnosed clinically without microbiological confirmation; and by major uncertainties in the numbers of children with tuberculosis that are not detected or diagnosed. The wide range of annual disease estimates published by the WHO and other groups in 2014 (from 500,000–1,000,000 children) reflect these challenges and emphasize the need for better data to estimate the true burden.[14-16] At country level, robust baseline data that might be used to set national targets as outlined in the post-2015 strategy, or to identify gaps and priorities for implementation, often do not exist. It is crucial, therefore, that children be included in all tuberculosis surveillance activities. All childhood cases should be registered with the NTP, including data on age, disease type, HIV status, and treatment outcome. Children are also being diagnosed and treated for tuberculosis in the private sector without being registered with the NTP; this is likely to vary among settings,

but the numbers are completely unknown.[17] An important reason for a lack of data on the burden of disease in adolescents is that this age group (10–19 years) overlaps with two of the routinely reported age groups of 5–14 years and 15–24 years. The WHO Global TB Program is currently supporting efforts to define the burden of adolescent tuberculosis.

Tuberculosis-related mortality is an extremely important burden-of-disease indicator that is the major target for the post-2015 strategy and for which there also are inadequate data for children and adolescents. The 2013 WHO estimate of 80,000 tuberculosis-related deaths in children did not include tuberculosis-related deaths in HIV-infected children and was extrapolated from vital registration data from a limited number of tuberculosis-endemic countries.[16] Vital registration data require pre-mortem diagnosis, but tuberculosis-related mortality is highest in the youngest children presenting with severe disease such as pneumonia, meningitis, or severe malnutrition; when seen in the context of primary and secondary care facilities, the contribution of tuberculosis may not be recognized or reported.[17,18]

As contact screening and management, including provision of treatment for eligible contacts, are more widely implemented by NTPs, there is a need to routinely record and report data for monitoring and evaluation purposes. A number of countries such as Viet Nam have already developed registers for quarterly reporting as community-based contact screening is implemented.[13]

3. Develop Policy Guidance, Training, and Reference Materials for Healthcare Workers

The WHO published revised guidance on the management of tuberculosis in children in 2014, based on best available current evidence.[1] The guidelines included new recommendations on a range of issues, including the use of GeneXpert MTB/RIF assay in children and drug dosages and regimens. NTPs in resource-limited, tuberculosis-endemic settings are increasingly developing national guidelines for childhood tuberculosis, adapted for local context, epidemiology, and health system capabilities. To support the implementation of such guidelines, there is inevitably a need for training and training tools, such as for health workers based at the peripheral levels of health care where most children with tuberculosis and child contacts are initially evaluated and managed.

Decentralization of services and skills to manage childhood tuberculosis is an important step for implementation, as management of the disease has traditionally been concentrated within the tertiary care facilities in many settings. Health workers at the primary and secondary care levels need to have the confidence to manage most cases of childhood tuberculosis and to know when to refer to the next level of care. Training in childhood tuberculosis should not be provided as a stand-alone activity, but rather integrated within existing training and pre-service curricula such as those related to maternal and child health, integrated management of childhood illness, HIV care, or NTP reviews.

The WHO and IUATLD have developed generic material to support training and clinical practice that can be adapted to country contexts and integrated into routine training and supervision activities by NTPs and other maternal and child health programs (Table 22.1). In addition, there is a great need for information, education, and communication material that support engagement of the community and the community-based health workers on childhood tuberculosis management and prevention.

4. Foster Local Expertise and Leadership

The challenges of supporting NTPs to address childhood tuberculosis, and of building partnerships between the NTP and the maternal and child health sector, require committed leadership and expertise with a range of skills. The model of the "child tuberculosis working group" was established at the global level in 2003, and has since expanded to be widely representative. There are now efforts to establish a similar model at the regional level, such as with the establishment of the WHO Western Pacific Region's Taskforce on Child TB in 2014, which includes representation from both the tuberculosis control and maternal and child health sectors.[13] While some NTPs have identified a member of staff as the focal person for child tuberculosis, there is still a need to develop national child tuberculosis working groups with broad national representation and expertise to support training, implementation, operational research, and advocacy in order to create sustainable activities and structures.

The establishment of a working group and identification of child tuberculosis champions were identified by NTPs in the African region as important initial steps to improve services for children (Box 22.1). National pediatric associations have an important role to play in supporting the NTPs by educating pediatricians and developing consensus to adopt and implement guidelines, including those in the private sector. Medical and nursing colleges in tuberculosis endemic countries must include education about childhood tuberculosis epidemiology and management in the pre-service training curricula. Ultimately, health providers at different levels of the system involved in the care of children should be aware of their role in the prevention, diagnosis, management, and monitoring of tuberculosis in children.

5. Do Not Miss Critical Opportunities for Intervention

There are numerous opportunities for intervention in the continuum from exposure of a child to *M. tuberculosis* to possible disease development and

Table 22.1. Childhood tuberculosis guidance documents and training materials

RESOURCE	AVAILABLE AT:
Guidance for National Tuberculosis Programs on the Management of Tuberculosis in Children, 2nd ed. WHO; 2014.	http://whqlibdoc.who.int/hq/2006/WHO_HTM_TB_2006.371_eng.pdf?ua=1
Desk Guide for Diagnosis and Management of TB in Children (IUALTD; 2010, revised 2014). The guide is aimed at health workers at the district or more peripheral level of care. It is available in English and French.	http://www.theunion.org/what-we-do/publications/technical/desk-guide-for-diagnosis-and-management-of-tb-in-children
Sentinel Project on Pediatric Drug-Resistant TB: Management of Multidrug-Resistant Tuberculosis in Children: A Field Guide. 2nd ed. 2014.	http://sentinelproject.join25.org/wp-content/uploads/2014/10/sentinel_field_guide_second_edition_20141-2.pdf
WHO/IUATLD Childhood TB Training Toolkit. The toolkit targets the national TB program and health workers that manage sick children and/or TB cases of any age in the community or at the more peripheral level of health care—primary health care facilities and district hospitals. It consists of ten modules covering a range of topics from epidemiology, diagnosis, and treatment, to managing childhood TB in the community.	http://www.who.int/tb/challenges/Child_TB_Training_toolkit_web.pdf?ua=1
IUATLD's Centre for Childhood TB provides access to free online courses as well as resources to address childhood TB. IUATLD/WHO online course: Childhood TB for healthcare workers. This 6-module interactive, case-based course targets primary and secondary-level health care workers.	https://childhoodtb.theunion.org/
IUATLD. *Diagnostic Atlas of Intrathoracic Tuberculosis in Children: A Guide for Low-Income Countries.* 2003.	http://www.theunion.org/what-we-do/publications/technical/english/pub_diagnostic-atlas_eng.pdf

cure (Figure 22.3 and Table 22.2). Again, many of these interventions will require the support of child health services. The starkest example of the wide policy–practice gap in childhood tuberculosis is the screening and management of children who are close contacts of sputum acid-fast smear-positive cases.[19] This practice is almost universal policy, based on evidence accumulated over 50 years, and it has huge potential to increase early case detection and provide effective prevention for at-risk contacts; however, it is rarely implemented in high-burden, resource-limited settings where it would have the highest impact.

6. Engage Key Stakeholders

Collaboration and communication among stakeholders at all levels, globally and locally, and across disciplines is essential to successfully implementing and sustaining childhood tuberculosis interventions. Already mentioned above was the engagement of UNICEF in the development of the roadmap. Each NTP has a number of non-governmental organizations (NGOs) that are already involved in the provision of tuberculosis and tuberculosis/HIV case detection and care that are potentially important partners for addressing childhood tuberculosis.

Box 22.1. Steps to Improve the Diagnosis and Care of Children with TB Identified by National Tuberculosis Control Programs from Eastern and Southern Africa, Kigali, Rwanda, 2010

- Adapt international strategies and develop national guidelines for diagnosing and treating children with TB.
- Operationalize the guidelines addressing childhood TB.
- Identify someone to champion the cause of children with TB.
- Establish a working group on childhood TB at each national TB program, and identify a person at the program who will develop links with pediatricians and national pediatric associations.
- Provide training about childhood TB, and incorporate it into continuing education on TB and TB/ HIV co-infection.
- Incorporate activities to address childhood TB into annual plans and five-year strategic plans.
- Ensure that national TB programs incorporate activities addressing childhood TB into their budgets.
- Include data on TB in children in routine reporting and in reviews of national TB programs.
- Develop and implement operational research to determine the constraints and barriers to diagnosing and treating children.
- Implement research aimed at improving the diagnosis and treatment of children with TB and the care of children who are contacts of someone with TB.

From: *Roadmap for Childhood Tuberculosis*, WHO; 2013.

While advocacy groups are increasingly making a crucial contribution, important stakeholders that are often overlooked are the communities, families, and individuals with tuberculosis along with civil society organizations and community-based NGOs. Vulnerable populations such as children require champions that are recognized within their communities. In addition, the language used to communicate the issues and aspirations has usually reflected the traditional medical model, but there are many misunderstandings and misconceptions that require clarification through the use of clear messages that avoid technical language.

7. Develop Integrated Family-Centered and Community-Centered Strategies

While it is self-evident that integrated strategies are required for effective provision of care for families living with tuberculosis (and including comorbidities such as HIV infection or diabetes) and for education of health workers and communities, the actual implementation of integrated activities in the field remains challenging. There needs to be political will and leadership shown by the relevant disease-control programs and health sectors, but the implementation also requires a range of governmental and non-governmental stakeholders that work at the community care level, along with support from the communities themselves (Table 22.3).

An important example of a currently wide policy–practice gap that could be addressed by strengthening integrated family-centered and community-centered is the screening and management of household contacts of people diagnosed with tuberculosis.[19] To do this has been almost universal policy for decades, has a strong evidence base showing the potential impact for both increased active case-finding and prevention of tuberculosis in children, but is rarely implemented.[20–23] The WHO guidelines published in 2006, consistent with the recent edition,[1] introduced a simple symptom-based screening approach to child contact management so that this could be implemented by community-based health workers and directly observed therapy (DOT) providers at the most peripheral level. Recent studies from Indonesia provide further support for this approach.[23,24] When implemented at the large health facility level, there is very poor uptake of treatment of contacts, given

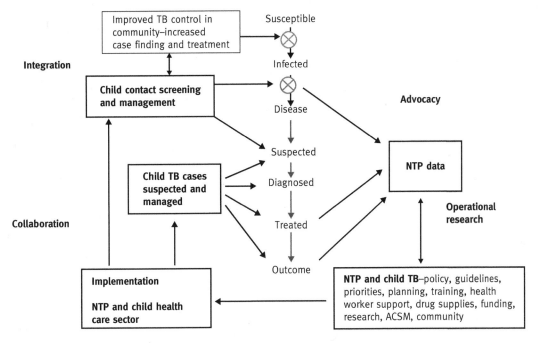

FIGURE 22.3   Interventions that target stages in the continuum from susceptibility to disease outcomes in children with tuberculosis.

From: Graham SM, *Int J Infect Dis.* 2014.[13]

the challenges of access.[24] A more decentralized approach at the community and family level, as is now being implemented in Viet Nam, has a much better uptake rate. Innovative approaches are needed; for example, through collaboration with often-existing community-based health structures to refer and cross-refer patients. Besides contact screening, community-based providers are ideally placed to play a role in treatment support and adherence counseling to patients and their families, advocacy efforts, and infection-control measures.

Maternal and child health programs and family-centered programs are also ideal entry points for detecting presumed tuberculosis cases and improving awareness and screening by healthcare workers. Existing community platforms such as integrated community case management (iCCM) or the integrated management of childhood illness (IMCI) provide an important opportunity for the integration of basic tuberculosis interventions (Figure 22.4).[25] The WHO and UNICEF recently adapted, and are piloting, iCCM materials for community health workers, including simple

tuberculosis interventions such as asking about close contacts of children with cough, malnutrition, and/or HIV infection.[26] Other opportunities for systematic screening for symptoms include antenatal and postnatal care, care for children and adolescents living with HIV, or nutritional rehabilitation units managing malnourished children. This is an important area for operational research.

8. Address Research Gaps

"Intensified research and innovation" is one of the three pillars of the post-2015 global tuberculosis-control strategy, as it is acknowledged that novel diagnostics and therapeutics that perform better than current tools are required in order to achieve the ambitious targets set for 2050. The Stop TB Partnership recently published an International Roadmap for TB Research that sets out priorities.[27] These priorities are as important for children as for adults. While it is recognized that a much improved diagnostic tool for young children is a major priority, the Roadmap identifies a range of current challenges for research:

Table 22.2. Transitions in tuberculosis and opportunities for intervention

STAGE	OPPORTUNITY FOR INTERVENTION
Susceptible, exposed	**PREVENT INFECTION** Improve TB control in the community Improve infection control
Infected	**PREVENT DISEASE** Implement screening for children who are contacts of someone with TB Manage the care of children who are contacts of someone with TB Provide preventive therapy to all children younger than five years and all HIV-infected children Record and report delivery of isoniazid preventive therapy (IPT)
Sick, accessed care, recognized	**DIAGNOSE DISEASE** Suspect TB in children who are contacts of someone with TB or who have typical signs and symptoms Recognize typical signs and symptoms of TB at all levels of the healthcare system Ensure that capabilities exist to diagnose TB at least to a secondary level of care Recognize danger signs, such as respiratory distress or severe malnutrition, and refer to the appropriate level of care Ensure that referral systems are in place for children identified by health care providers, as well as to refer complicated cases or very sick children to a higher level of care
Treatment completed, cured, outcome	**SUPPORT CHILDREN AND THEIR FAMILIES** Ensure that treatment follows national guidelines Ensure that appropriate medicines are available, including those for drug-resistant TB Provide care for HIV infection Develop or implement strategies to improve treatment completion rates and prevent loss to follow-up Record outcomes
Register, record, report	**REPORT ACCURATE DATA, MONITOR AND EVALUATE SERVICES, ENGAGE IN ADVOCACY AND OPERATIONAL RESEARCH** Ensure that all healthcare workers know that they are responsible for registering all children with TB

From: *Roadmap for Childhood Tuberculosis*, WHO; 2013.

Epidemiology

- Better-define the burden of disease in women, adolescents and children; this includes conducting nationwide inventory surveys to measure the under-reporting and, if possible, the under-diagnosis of childhood tuberculosis.

- Improve recording and reporting systems to capture all tuberculosis cases, and report data disaggregated by age and sex.
- Improve the understanding of variations in the dynamics of tuberculosis in different settings, and the social, environmental, and biological drivers of the transmission of *M. tuberculosis* in different settings.

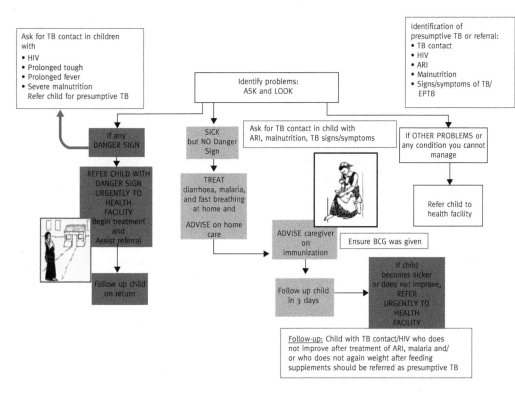

FIGURE 22.4 Caring for the sick child in the community: potential tuberculosis-related actions.[25]

- Conduct evaluations to understand better the epidemiology of tuberculosis and Tuberculosis/HIV co-infection in adolescents.

Fundamental Research

- Characterize human tuberculosis using modern biochemical, clinical, and epidemiological approaches, and address issues specific to improving the understanding of the disease in children.
- Better understand the host–pathogen interaction; this includes improving our understanding of the immune system in children in relation to its responses to mycobacterial infection at different ages.
- Apply discovery science to identify biomarkers that better differentiate the various stages of the disease spectrum and distinguish between infection and disease in children.

Development of New Diagnostics

- Evaluate new diagnostics, and determine whether they are useful for confirming the diagnosis of tuberculosis in children.

- Develop diagnostics suitable for use with pediatric samples.
- Develop point-of-care diagnostics for use in children.

Development of New Anti-Tuberculosis Medicines

- Identify the optimal doses for children of all ages of new and existing anti-tuberculosis medicines and regimens.
- Identify the optimal treatment duration and dosing of rifampicin-based treatment for children.
- Identify aspects of the design of clinical trials that can be tailored specifically for studies in children in regards to endpoints, sample size, inclusion criteria, and at what point studies should assess the use of new anti-tuberculosis medicines in children.
- Determine whether new and existing medicines for which data on safety or toxicity in children are missing are suitable for use in children.

Table 22.3. Key stakeholders and their roles in addressing childhood tuberculosis

STAKEHOLDERS	MAIN ROLES
POLICY-MAKERS	
Global policy-makers	• Collaboratively address childhood TB across disciplines by providing leadership and guidance • Develop policies, strategies, and guidelines for the management of childhood TB that are based on the best evidence • Provide support so that activities aimed at addressing childhood TB can be adopted at the national level; support may include training, tools, data-collection systems, technical support, and the monitoring and evaluation of activities • Help define research needs for childhood TB and TB/HIV co-infection
National policy-makers (including national TB-control programs as well as other relevant stakeholders)	• Provide high-level support throughout a country to assist in the scaling up of childhood TB services • Develop a framework to address TB in women and children that includes collaboration among national disease-control programs (e.g., among those addressing TB, HIV, and maternal and child health) and national leaders in children's health care • Include childhood TB in the strategic plans and budgets of national TB programs • Ensure that guidelines on caring for children with TB or HIV, or both, are adopted and implemented; ensure that data on childhood TB are collected, reported, and recorded; and that staff have appropriate training • Support or perform operational research to improve activities aimed at addressing childhood TB (see additional information for Researchers below)
RELEVANT NATIONAL HEALTHCARE PROGRAMS	
Maternal and child health services	• Ensure that children and pregnant women are screened, diagnosed, and treated for TB; this is especially important for HIV-infected women • Give TB-preventive therapy when indicated • Provide appropriate care for neonates exposed to TB • Engage community health services in TB control activities, such as contact tracing • Record and report TB cases to the national TB program
HIV services	• Ensure antenatal screening is implemented for HIV and TB • Ensure that all children exposed to or infected with HIV are regularly screened for TB • Provide preventive therapy to HIV-infected children according to national guidelines • Ensure that all children exposed to or infected with HIV are screened for TB, and diagnosed and treated promptly
Health education institutions	• Ensure that childhood TB is adequately discussed in the standard curricula for all levels of health workers • Incorporate information on childhood TB into continuing training, in keeping with national guidelines
Stakeholders	Main roles

Table 22.3. Continued

STAKEHOLDERS	MAIN ROLES
SPECIFIC HEALTH ACTORS	
Private healthcare sector	• Ensure that children with TB are managed according to national guidelines • Report all children with a diagnosis of TB to the national TB program
Community-based organizations and nongovernmental organizations	• Support local programs according to capacity. This may include supporting initiatives aimed at increasing community education and awareness, or providing contact tracing, preventive therapy, TB diagnosis, and treatment or referral • Provide technical assistance and training if appropriate
Community leaders	• Promote TB education and awareness • Help the community understand TB and its treatment to decrease the stigma associated with the disease • Support case-finding efforts and adherence to treatment • Promote the empowerment of children and families affected by TB by engaging them to help the community better understand the disease
Researchers	• Develop child-friendly, point-of-care diagnostics • Develop child-friendly formulations of anti-TB medicines • Develop improved or novel vaccines, or both • Continue work to fill the many knowledge gaps that exist
Advocacy groups	• Promote education and awareness • Help the community understand TB and its treatment to decrease the stigma associated with the disease • Advocate for resource mobilization • Provide input into national and international policy-making

From: *Roadmap for Childhood Tuberculosis.* WHO; 2013.

Development of New Vaccines

• Define suitable clinical endpoints and immunological markers for vaccine trials in children.
• Improve clinical trials of vaccines in infants and children by conducting pre- vaccine epidemiological studies in order to standardize protocols, assays, and methodological and clinical parameters.
• Develop improved vaccines for prime-boost vaccination that are safe and efficacious in preventing tuberculosis in children (including in those living with HIV), and define optimal conditions for their use in children, including defining the best ages for vaccination.

Operational and Public Health Research

• Strengthen the recording and reporting of tuberculosis; improve global estimates of childhood tuberculosis (including drug-resistant tuberculosis in children); promote case-based electronic recording and reporting systems that can facilitate the compilation and analysis of data disaggregated by age.
• Advocate for and promote the development and establishment of vital registration systems that have national coverage.
• Determine the best approaches for identifying children who have been exposed to tuberculosis and determine how best to provide treatment for children who are contacts of someone

with tuberculosis and for children who are HIV-infected.

- Develop an evidence base for treatment of children infected with drug-resistant tuberculosis.
- Improve collaboration among tuberculosis services and other child-care services to increase case-finding.
- Within the general context of healthcare services and efforts to expand community-based care, address issues specific to children in terms of case-finding, screening, access to diagnostics, access to treatment and the delivery of treatment, interactions between tuberculosis and HIV programs, and infection control. Answer the following questions:
  - How can collaboration between tuberculosis and HIV services in maternal and child health settings be improved?
  - How can programs to prevent mother-to-child transmission of HIV be used to ensure that both HIV-infected and HIV-uninfected women receive appropriate tuberculosis screening during pregnancy?
- Identify the unique needs and concerns of adolescents; pilot test, evaluate, and scale up optimal approaches to addressing tuberculosis and Tuberculosis/HIV co-infection among adolescents.
- Investigate how to optimize tuberculosis case-finding in children and adolescents; determine how to best measure the impact of intensive or enhanced case-finding on mortality and other outcomes.
- Determine the value of tuberculosis screening strategies in antenatal care programs, HIV programs, and maternal and child health programs; determine ways in which screening can be operationalized.
- Develop and evaluate models for implementing sustainable collaboration with all private and public providers of tuberculosis care and control services. Evaluate how pregnant women and children are being or will be addressed during the roll-out and scaling up of the use of new diagnostic tests and new treatment or preventive regimens.

Since the development of the research agenda and publication of the Roadmap, many of the above-mentioned issues are being addressed and contributing to the evidence base for childhood tuberculosis, to the development of improved diagnostics and therapeutics, and to informing best practices for implementation. Research requires funding investment, and while it is encouraging that research funding for childhood tuberculosis is increasing, the amount invested in 2013 was still only one-quarter of projected requirements.[28]

9. Meet Funding Needs for Childhood Tuberculosis

Of the total 7.7 billion USD needed between 2011 and 2015 for research and development of new tools to prevent, diagnose, and treat tuberculosis, 200 million USD needed to be spent on pediatric research and development.[12] However, only about a quarter of this amount had been spent by midpoint of the timeline: 25,318,577 USD (Figure 22.5).[28] This figure does not include the funding needed at the programmatic level to implement sustainable child tuberculosis interventions. NTPs in the past have not included funding for childhood tuberculosis activities in their budgets, but there is now a much wider recognition that costs for childhood tuberculosis need to be included in strategic plans, concept notes, and budgets. The lack of reliable estimates of the burden of childhood disease in many tuberculosis-endemic countries make accurate projection of the program costs difficult, with gross underestimates in some countries leading to little or no funding for childhood tuberculosis. Expert input was provided during the development of the roadmap to estimate the current funding required annually in order to implement current policy and practice for childhood tuberculosis globally. Preliminary analyses estimated that between $84 and $319 are needed per case, totaling only 80 million USD globally per year.[12]

10. Form Coalitions and Partnerships to Improve Tools for Diagnosis and Treatment

Creative collaborations among industry, academia, major governmental and non-governmental organizations, as well as donors are crucial in order to address the needs for improved diagnosis and treatment of tuberculosis, including drug-resistant disease. The paucibacillary nature of tuberculosis in infants and young children, as well as the specific difficulty of adequate specimen collection, are recognized challenges for improved diagnostics for this important age group. An accurate blood-based

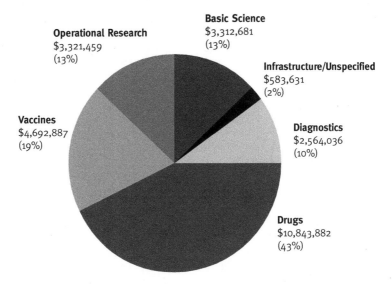

Operational Research
$3,321,459
(13%)

Basic Science
$3,312,681
(13%)

Infrastructure/Unspecified
$583,631
(2%)

Diagnostics
$2,564,036
(10%)

Vaccines
$4,692,887
(19%)

Drugs
$10,843,882
(43%)

FIGURE 22.5   Childhood tuberculosis research & development funding by research category, 2013.

From: Treatment Action Group. *2014 Report on Tuberculosis Research Funding Trends*, 2005–2013.

point-of-care test would be a major step forward, and there is a current research focus on biomarkers for diagnosis that is showing early promise.[29,30] It is also important that evaluations of new diagnostics and therapeutics adhere to standardized protocols and classifications for reporting of findings as closely as possible, with well-defined study populations that include standardized measures of disease severity.[31,32]

For the first time in decades, there are several new drugs for tuberculosis and MDR-TB in various stages of development. These drugs should be evaluated in children following phase II studies once their safety profile is established.[33] This enables the determination of optimal dosages in young children using pharmacokinetic data, early development of child-friendly formulations, and the inclusion of children in the initial approval process. The pragmatic needs of NTPs for implementation and procurement for children also must be considered prospectively in order to reduce the risks of confusion, as recently happened following the changes to recommended dosages for first-line anti-tuberculosis drugs in children.[34] The Global Alliance for TB Drug Development is a not-for-profit organization that is working closely with other partners to provide more child-friendly formulations for children.

The increasing global burden of MDR-TB is a major challenge that requires a strong, coordinated, and collaborative response that is currently being led by the Sentinel Project with the Stop TB Partnership Childhood TB subgroup. Most children with MDR-TB are not being detected or diagnosed, and there is a lot of uncertainty among health workers about the management of MDR-TB in children and of treatment for MDR-TB contacts of all ages.[15,35,36] Multi-country research collaborations are underway to ensure that children are included in the evaluation of new regimens for MDR-TB infection and disease.

CONCLUSION

Tuberculosis is an important challenge for child health in tuberculosis-endemic countries that is now being recognized globally, regionally, and nationally. The opportunities for interventions to prevent, detect, and cure tuberculosis in children are growing and must be grasped. Leadership, technical support, and advocacy from the child health sector, in collaboration with community-based healthcare providers and civil society, is critical to support tuberculosis control programs, as was recognized by Edith Lincoln more than 50 years ago. The Roadmap for Childhood Tuberculosis identifies the challenges and opportunities, and provides guidance for a range of relevant stakeholders to engage collaboratively to reduce the burden of tuberculosis in children.

REFERENCES

1. World Health Organization. *Guidance for National Tuberculosis Programmes on the Management of Tuberculosis in Children*. 2nd ed. Geneva: WHO; 2014.

2. World Health Organization. *Rapid Advice: Treatment of Tuberculosis in Children*. Geneva: WHO; 2010.

3. Sandgren A, Cuevas LE, Dara M, et al. Childhood tuberculosis: progress requires an advocacy strategy now. *Eur Respir J*. 2012;40:294–297.

4. World Health Organization. *Global Tuberculosis Report*. Geneva: WHO; 2012.

5. World Health Organization. Global strategy and targets for tuberculosis prevention, care and control after 2015. Available at http://apps.who.int/gb/ebwha/pdf_files/EB134/B134_12-en.pdf?ua=1. 2014. Accessed January 26, 2015.

6. Marais BJ, Gie RP, Schaaf HS, et al. The natural history of childhood intra-thoracic tuberculosis: a critical review of literature from the pre-chemotherapy era. *Int J Tuberc Lung Dis*. 2004;8:392–402.

7. Chisti MJ, Graham SM, Duke T, et al. A prospective study of the prevalence of tuberculosis and bacteraemia in Bangladeshi children with severe malnutrition and pneumonia including an evaluation of Xpert MTB/RIF assay. *PLoS One*. 2014;9:e93776.

8. Graham SM, Sismanidis C, Menzies HJ, Marais BJ, Detjen AK, Black RE. Importance of tuberculosis control to address child survival. *Lancet*. 2014;383:1605–1607.

9. Nantongo JM, Wobudeya E, Mupere E, et al. High incidence of pulmonary tuberculosis in children admitted with severe pneumonia in Uganda. *BMC Pediatr*. 2013;13:16.

10. Oliwa J, Karumbi J, Marais B, Madhi S, Graham SM. Tuberculosis and childhood pneumonia in tuberculosis endemic settings—common, cause or consequence? A review of the evidence. *Lancet Respir Med*. 2015;3:235–243.

11. World Health Organization. *No More Crying No More Dying. Towards Zero TB Deaths in Children*. Geneva: WHO; 2012.

12. World Health Organization. *Roadmap for Childhood Tuberculosis—Towards Zero Deaths*. Geneva: WHO; 2013.

13. Graham S, Grzemska M, Brands A, *et al.* Regional initiatives to address the challenges of tuberculosis in children: perspectives from the Asia-Pacific region. *Int J Infect Dis*. 2015;32:166–169.

14. Dodd PJ, Gardiner E, Coghlan R, Seddon JA. Burden of childhood tuberculosis in 22 high-burden countries: a mathematical modelling study. *Lancet Glob Health*. 2014;2:e453–e459.

15. Jenkins HE, Tolman AW, Yuen CM, et al. Incidence of multidrug-resistant tuberculosis disease in children: systematic review and global estimates. *Lancet*. 2014;383:1572–1579.

16. World Health Organization. *Global Tuberculosis Report*. Geneva: WHO; 2014.

17. Lestari T, Probandari A, Hurtig AK, Utarini A. High caseload of childhood tuberculosis in hospitals on Java Island, Indonesia: a cross sectional study. *BMC Public Health*. 2011;11:784.

18. Drobac PC, Shin SS, Huamani P, et al. Risk factors for in-hospital mortality among children with tuberculosis: the 25-year experience in Peru. *Pediatrics*. 2012;130:e373–e379.

19. Hill PC, Rutherford ME, Audas R, van Crevel R, Graham SM. Closing the policy-practice gap in the management of child contacts of tuberculosis cases in developing countries. *PLoS Med*. 2011;8:e1001105.

20. Triasih R, Robertson CF, Duke T, Graham SM. A prospective evaluation of the symptom-based screening approach to the management of children who are contacts of tuberculosis cases. *Clin Infect Dis*. 2014;60:12–18.

21. Graham SM, Triasih R. More evidence to support screening of child contacts of tuberculosis cases: if not now, then when? *Clin Infect Dis*. 2013;57:1693–1694.

22. Jaganath D, Zalwango S, Okware B, et al. Contact investigation for active tuberculosis among child contacts in Uganda. *Clin Infect Dis*. 2013;57:1685–1692.

23. Triasih R, Rutherford M, Lestari T, Utarini A, Robertson CF, Graham SM. Contact investigation of children exposed to tuberculosis in South East Asia: a systematic review. *J Trop Med*. 2012;2012:301808.

24. Rutherford ME, Ruslami R, Anselmo M, et al. Management of children exposed to *Mycobacterium tuberculosis*: a public health evaluation in West Java, Indonesia. *Bull World Health Organ*. 2013;91:932–941A.

25. Detjen A, Gnanashanmugam D, Talens A. A framework for integrating childhood tuberculosis into community-based child health care. CORE group/Paris: International Union Against Tuberculosis and Lung Ddisease, 2013.

26. World Health Organization. Caring for newborns and children in the community, adaptation for

high HIV or TB settings. Available at http://www.who.int/maternal_child_adolescent/documents/newborn-child-community-care/en/. 2014. Accessed January 26, 2015.

27. World Health Organization, Stop TB Partnership. An international roadmap for tuberculosis research. Available at http://www.stoptb.org/assets/documents/resources/publications/technical/tbresearchroadmap.pdf. 2011. Accessed January 26, 2015.

28. Treatment Action Group. Tuberculosis research and development. 2014 report on tuberculosis research funding trends, 2005–2013. Available at http://www.treatmentactiongroup.org/sites/g/files/g450272/f/201410/TAG_2014_TB_Funding_Report.FINAL_.pdf. Accessed January 26, 2015.

29. Anderson ST, Kaforou M, Brent AJ, et al. Diagnosis of childhood tuberculosis and host RNA expression in Africa. *N Engl J Med*. 2014;370:1712–1723.

30. Portevin D, Moukambi F, Clowes P, et al. Assessment of the novel T-cell activation marker-tuberculosis assay for diagnosis of active tuberculosis in children: a prospective proof-of-concept study. *Lancet Infect Dis*. 2014;14:931–938.

31. Graham SM, Ahmed T, Amanullah F, et al. Evaluation of tuberculosis diagnostics in children: 1. Proposed clinical case definitions for classification of intrathoracic tuberculosis disease. Consensus from an expert panel. *J Infect Dis*. 2012;205(Suppl 2):S199–S208.

32. Wiseman CA, Gie RP, Starke JR, et al. A proposed comprehensive classification of tuberculosis disease severity in children. *Pediatr Infect Dis J*. 2012;31:347–352.

33. Donald PR, Ahmed A, Burman WJ, et al. Requirements for the clinical evaluation of new anti-tuberculosis agents in children. *Int J Tuberc Lung Dis*. 2013;17:794–799.

34. Detjen A, Mace C, Perrin C, Graham SM, Grzemska M. The adoption of revised dosage recommendations for childhood TB in countries with different childhood TB burden. *Public Health Action*. 2012;1:1–28.

35. Becerra MC, Swaminathan S. Commentary: a targets framework: dismantling the invisibility trap for children with drug-resistant tuberculosis. *J Public Health Pol*. 2014;35:425–454.

36. Seddon JA, Perez-Velez CM, Schaaf HS, et al. Consensus statement on research definitions for drug-resistant tuberculosis in children. *J Pediatr Infect Dis Soc*. 2013;2:100–109.

Index

clarithromycin
pharmacokinetics and general pharmacological
characteristics of, 279, 271t, 269t
clavulanate
pharmacokinetics and general pharmacological
characteristics of, 279, 271t, 269t
clofazimine
in childhood TB management, 342
pharmacokinetics and general pharmacological
characteristics of, 279, 274t, 270t, 269t
close contact
defined, 233t
CMI. *see* cell-mediated immunity (CMI)
CNGTST. *see* combined nasogastric-tube-and-string-test
(CNGTST)
CNS. *see* central nervous system (CNS)
collapse
in childhood TB, 59, 56t
combination antiretroviral therapy (cART)
delayed access to
HIV infection/TB coinfection in infants, children, and
adolescents related to, 247–248
determination of appropriate regimen, 255–256
in HIV infection management, 246
TB development while on, 255
in TB management in HIV–infected infants, children, and
adolescents, 253–257
initiation of, 254
combined nasogastric-tube-and-string-test (CNGTST)
in intrathoracic childhood TB diagnosis, 160
complete DiGeorge syndrome (CDGS), 32
complication(s)
defined, 126
Comptes Kendus de la Societé de Biologie, 2
computed tomography (CT)
of abdominal TB, 187, 136–137, 137f, 136f
of chest
in childhood TB evaluation, 116–120, 119f, 118f
of intrathoracic childhood TB, 152
of peripheral lymphadenitis, 180
of spinal TB, 181
of TBM, 206, 129–132, 129f–134f
of tuberculous arthritis, 185
concentration(s)
critical, 22–23
congenital tuberculosis
defined, 233t
consolidation
bronchopneumonic
in childhood TB, 59–60, 56t
caseating
in childhood TB, 60, 56t
contact(s)
close
defined, 233t
TB
history of, 249
contact investigation
case finding–related, 384–385, 384t
contact lens staining
drug-susceptible childhood TB management and
treatment of, 321
conversion
defined, 86
in *M. tuberculosis* infection diagnosis, 86–87
corticosteroids
in childhood TBM management, 212
in drug-susceptible childhood TB management, 315, 318f

in TB management in HIV–infected infants, children, and
adolescents, 256
Cotton, M.F., 245
cough
chronic
differential diagnosis of, 161, 161t–164t
cranial nerve enhancement
TBM and, 132, 134f
critical concentrations, 22–23
CRRS. *see* Chest Radiograph Reading and Recording
System (CRRS)
CSF. *see* cerebrospinal fluid (CSF)
CT. *see* computed tomography (CT)
culture
in childhood TB diagnosis, 20–22
culture filtrate protein 10 (CFP-10), 85–86, 86f
cutaneous tuberculosis, 188–194, 192f–194f, 190t–191t
classification of, 188–189, 190t–191t
clinical presentation of, 189–193, 192f–194f, 190t–191t
diagnosis of, 193–194
miliary, 192
pathogenesis of, 188–189, 190t–191t
CXR. *see* chest radiography (CXR)
cycloserine
pharmacokinetics and general pharmacological characteristics of,
278, 273t, 270t, 269t

dactylitis
tuberculous osteomyelitis and, 185
delamanid (DLM)
in childhood TB management, 342, 265
EMA on, 342
"De L'Hérédité parasitaire del la tuberculose humaine," 2
Demers, A-M, 13
diagnostic imaging
of childhood TB, 109–146
abdominal TB, 134, 136–138, 136f–137f
appearances on, 111–127 (*see also specific modality, e.g., chest
radiography (CXR)*)
chest US, 120, 121f, 120f
clinician-led interpretation *vs.* telereading in, 110
CNS TB, 127–134, 127f–135f (*see also* central nervous system
(CNS) tuberculosis, diagnostic imaging of)
complications-related, 121–125, 123f–125f
CT of chest in, 116–120, 119f, 118f
CXR in, 109–116, 112f–117f
intrathoracic TB, 152, 156t–158t, 154f–155f
looking outside of chest, 110–111
MDCT in, 117–118
MRI, 120–121, 123f, 122f
musculoskeletal TB, 138–144, 139f–143f
progression-related, 121–125, 123f–125f
PTB, 109–110
radiology department *vs.* point of care in, 110
rationale for, 109–110
soft-tissue TB, 144, 144f
strategies for improved, 110–111
urogenital TB, 138, 138f
US in, 110–111
of HIV/TB coinfection, 125–127, 126f
of IRIS, 125–127, 126f
in TB diagnosis in HIV–infected infants, children, and
adolescents, 253
in TBM diagnosis, 206, 208f, 207f
diffusion weighted imaging (DWI)
of abdominal TB, 137
in childhood TB evaluation, 121, 123f
DiNardo, A., 79

immunity from, 32–35, 35f
nontuberculous (*see* nontuberculous mycobacteria (NTM))
mycobacterial culture
   in childhood PTB diagnosis, 101–102
mycobacterial immunity, 32–35, 35f
   B-cell function and, 32–35, 35f
   control of
      neutrophils in, 36–37
   HIV prevention in, 33
   T-cell function and, 32–35, 35f
mycobacteria other than TB (MOTT), 14
Mycobacterium bovis, 375–380
   CDC on, 377
   in children, 375–380
   clinical presentation of, 377–379
   described, 375
   diagnosis of, 377–379
   epidemiology of, 376–377
   in humans *vs.* animals, 375
   management of, 379
   microbiology of, 376
   M. tuberculosis vs.
      TB caused by, 376–377
   prevention of, 379
   transmission of, 376–377
Mycobacterium spp.
   members of, 14
Mycobacterium tuberculosis
   described, 1
   immune responses in containing, 32
   immune responses induced by, 31
   M. bovis vs.
      TB caused by, 376–377
   mechanisms of, 15
   primary infection with, 14–15
      complications associated with, 15
   resistance to drugs (*see* drug-resistant
      tuberculosis (DR-TB); multidrug-resistant
      tuberculosis (MDR-TB))
   sputum from, 15
   transmission of, 14
      prevention in healthcare settings, 389
Mycobacterium tuberculosis complex (MTBC), 14
   members of, 14
Mycobacterium tuberculosis infection
   ARTI in, 85
   burden of, 72, 70
   course of, 80, 80f
   diagnosis of, 79–96
      future tests in, 89, 91–92
      IGRAs in, 69, 85–92, 90t, 91f, 86f
      imaging in, 109–146 (*see also* diagnostic imaging, of
         childhood TB)
      immunological tests in, 81, 82f
      NTM in, 84
      perspective on, 89, 91–92
      reversion, conversion, and boosting in, 86–87
      risk factors associated with, 80
      screening questions in, 81, 82t
      tests in, 81–92, 68–69 (*see also specific tests*)
      TST in, 81–92, 83f, 84t, 90t, 91f, 82f
   epidemiology of, 80–81, 82f
   responses to
      spectrum of, 80, 80f
   risk factors for, 80–81
   test performance in, 80–81, 82f
   transmission of, 80
Myers, J.A., 8

NAATs. *see* nucleic acid amplification tests (NAATs)
NALC (N-acetyl-L-cysteine)-NaOH (sodium hydroxide)
      method, 18
nasopharyngeal aspirate (NPA)
   in childhood PTB diagnosis, 99
National Institutes of Clinical Excellence, United Kingdom
   on INH and RMP for childhood TB infection, 294
National Tuberculosis Control Programs (NTPs)
   framework for improving childhood TB activities within,
      399–400, 399f
NAT2. *see* N-acetyltransferase 2 (NAT2)
natural killer (NK) cells
   in immune response to TB, 38
nausea
   drug-susceptible childhood TB management and
      treatment of, 319–321
necrotizing cavitating pneumonia
   PTB and
      CXR of, 116, 117f
neonate(s)
   defined, 233t
   TB-exposed, 234–235, 235f
      defined, 233t
   TB in, 231–243
      infection control for, 240–241
      terminology related to, 233t
Neuland, W., 7
neuritis
   optic
      drug-susceptible childhood TB management and, 322
neutrophil(s)
   in *M. tuberculosis* control, 36–37
newborn(s). *see* neonate(s)
Nicol, M.P., 97
NK cells. *see* natural killer (NK) cells
NNRTIs. *see* non-nucleoside reverse transcriptase inhibitors (NNRTIs)
nodular lung disease
   intrathoracic TB and, 169, 167t
nodular tuberculids, 193, 194f
non-nucleoside reverse transcriptase inhibitors (NNRTIs)
   in TB management in HIV–infected infants, children, and
      adolescents, 255–256
non-severe disease
   defined, 127
nontuberculous mycobacteria (NTM), 14
   in *M. tuberculosis* infection diagnosis, 84
nontuberculous mycobacterial (NTM) lymphadenitis
   TB *vs.*, 223
nose
   TB of, 195–196
NPA. *see* nasopharyngeal aspirate (NPA)
NRTIs. *see* nucleoside reverse transcriptase inhibitors (NRTIs)
NTM. *see* nontuberculous mycobacteria (NTM)
NTPs. *see* National Tuberculosis Control Programs (NTPs)
nucleic acid amplification tests (NAATs)
   in childhood PTB diagnosis, 102–103, 104b, 102b
   in childhood TB diagnosis, 19–20
   in intrathoracic childhood TB diagnosis, 160–161
   in TBM diagnosis, 206
nucleoside reverse transcriptase inhibitors (NRTIs)
   in TB management in HIV–infected infants, children, and
      adolescents, 255–256
nutritional support
   in drug-susceptible childhood TB management, 319

OA-TB. *see* osteoarticular tuberculosis (OA-TB)
ocular tuberculosis
   in adolescents, 219–220, 219t

ofloxacin
  pharmacokinetics and general pharmacological characteristics of, 277–278, 273t, 270t, 269t
optic neuritis
  drug-susceptible childhood TB management and treatment of, 322
Orme, I.M., 359
osteoarticular tuberculosis (OA-TB), 180–186, 182f, 183t, 184t, 185f, 181t
  chronic tuberculous rheumatism, 185
  pathogenesis of, 181
  sites of, 181t
  spinal TB, 181–183, 182f, 183t, 181t
  tuberculous arthritis, 183–185, 185f, 184t
  tuberculous osteomyelitis, 185–186
osteomastoiditis
  tuberculous
    diagnostic imaging of, 143–144, 143f
osteomyelitis
  tuberculous, 185–186

Pagel, W., 7
pain
  abdominal
    drug-susceptible childhood TB management and, 319–321
pan-arteritis
  inflammatory
    TBM and, 131, 133f
papulonecrotic tuberculids, 193, 194f
para-aminosalicylate (PAS)
  pharmacokinetics and general pharmacological characteristics of, 278–279, 274t, 270t, 269t
paradoxical IRIS
  in TB management in HIV–infected infants, children, and adolescents, 254–255, 255t
paraplegia
  spinal tuberculosis and, 182
Parrot, J.M-J, 2, 3f
Parrot's Law, 2
PAS. see para-aminosalicylate (PAS)
Pasteur Institute
  on BCG vaccines, 360, 360t
pathology
  of TB, 13–29
patient (child)-centered care
  in drug-susceptible childhood TB management, 322
PCR tests. see polymerase chain reaction (PCR) tests
Perez-Velez, C.M., 147
pericardial disease
  intrathoracic TB and, 172–173
pericardial effusion
  intrathoracic TB and, 172–173
pericarditis
  tuberculous, 125, 125f
perinatal period
  defined, 233t
perinatal tuberculosis, 232, 236–238, 237f
  defined, 233t
peripheral lymphadenitis, 178–180, 179t, 178t
  in adolescents, 219, 219t
  bacteriology and histology of, 180
  clinical presentation of, 179–180
  diagnosis of, 179–180
  differential diagnosis of, 179t
  imaging of, 180
  overview of, 178–179
  pathogenesis of, 179

peritonitis
  tuberculous, 186
PHA. see phytohemagglutinin (PHA)
Phemister's triad, 183
phenotypical testing methods
  in drug resistance determination in childhood PTB, 104
phytohemagglutinin (PHA), 86
Pinto, L.M., 116
Pirquet, C., 5–6
pleural disease
  in childhood TB, 60–61, 56t–57t
  intrathoracic TB and, 171
pleural effusion
  in childhood PTB, 111
  in childhood TB, 60–61, 56t–57t
  in intrathoracic childhood TB, 171
pleurisy
  tuberculous, 125, 125f
PMTCT programs. see prevention of mother-to-child transmission (PMTCT) programs
pneumonia(s)
  acute
    PTB related to, 251
  intrathoracic TB and, 170, 167t
  necrotizing cavitating
    PTB and, 116, 117f
polymerase chain reaction (PCR) tests
  in childhood PTB diagnosis, 102
Poncet's disease, 185
post-mortems
  TB in age of, 1–4, 3f
postnatal tuberculosis, 232
  defined, 233t
PPD. see purified protein derivative (PPD)
PPD-S, 81
pre-chemotherapy era
  pioneers in childhood TB from, 48, 53f
pregnancy
  anti-TB drugs during, 238–240, 239t
  TB in, 231–235, 233t, 232f, 234f–236f
    clinical presentation of, 234, 234f
    diagnosis of, 233–234
    infection control for, 240–241
    prevalence of, 232
    risk factors for, 232–233
    terminology related to, 233t
prematurity
  defined, 233t
"pre-tuberculous" child
  history of, 7–8
prevention of mother-to-child transmission (PMTCT) programs, 246
  BCG vaccines–related, 368
PREVENT TB study
  of Tuberculosis Trials Consortium
    on INH and RPT for childhood TB infection, 301, 298, 295–296, 296t
primary (Ghon) complex, 14
primary pulmonary infection
  in childhood TB, 48, 53–55, 55f, 56t, 54f
    timetable of, 48, 53–55, 55f, 56t, 54f
programmatic issues
  childhood TB–related, 381–393 (see also childhood tuberculosis, public health and programmatic issues related to)
protein-energy malnutrition
  compromised CMI related to, 40
prothionamide

streptomycin (SM)
  in children
    mechanisms of action, dosage, and adverse effects of, 320*t*
string test
  in childhood PTB diagnosis, 100
  in intrathoracic childhood TB diagnosis, 160
substance abuse
  TB among adolescents and, 224–225
sub-unit vaccines
  for TB, 369
Swaminathan, S., 311

TAG. *see* Treatment Action Group (TAG)
TB. *see* tuberculosis (TB)
TBM. *see* tuberculous meningitis (TBM)
T cell(s)
  CD4
    in immune response to TB, 33–34
  regulatory
    in immune response to TB, 38–39
telereading
  in diagnostic imaging of childhood TB, 110
Terplan, K., 4
thalidomide
  in childhood TBM management, 213
The Pathogenesis of Tuberculosis, 5
thioridazine
  in childhood TB management, 342
throat
  TB of, 195–196
thrombocytopenia
  drug-susceptible childhood TB management and
    treatment of, 321
tracheobronchial disease
  intrathoracic TB and, 169, 167*t*
"tram-track sign"
  in bronchiectasis, 123
transcriptomics
  in M. tuberculosis infection diagnosis, 91–92
Treatment Action Group (TAG)
  in *Roadmap for Childhood Tuberculosis–Towards
    Zero Deaths*, 396
T-SPOT-TB, 363
TST. *see* tuberculin skin test (TST)
tuberculids, 192–193, 194*f*, 193*f*
  nodular, 193, 194*f*
  papulonecrotic, 193, 194*f*
tuberculin
  discovery of, 5–7, 6*f*
tuberculin skin test (TST)
  BCG vaccines and, 361
  in childhood TB diagnosis, 69
  in intrathoracic childhood TB diagnosis, 153, 152
  in *M. tuberculosis* infection diagnosis, 81–92, 83*f*, 84*t*, 90*t*, 91*f*, 82*f*
    described, 81–82, 83*f*
    factors diminishing reactivity to, 83–84, 83*t*
    with IGRAs, 89, 91*f*, 90*t*
    interpretation of, 84–85, 85*t*
    variability of results of, 81–83, 83*f*
  in TB diagnosis in HIV–infected infants, children, and
    adolescents, 252–253
tuberculoma(s), 204–205, 205*f*
tuberculosis (TB). *see also* neonate(s); tuberculous meningitis
    (TBM); *specific types, sites, and target groups, e.g.,*
    genitourinary tuberculosis
  abdominal, 134, 186–188, 136–138, 136*f*–137*f* (*see also*
    abdominal tuberculosis)
  in adolescents, 219–229 (*see also* adolescent(s))

"adult"
  characteristics of, ix
bone lesions caused by
  diagnostic imaging of, 141–143, 142*f*
in children (*see* childhood tuberculosis)
CNS (*see* central nervous system (CNS) tuberculosis; central
    nervous system (CNS) tuberculosis in children; tuberculous
    meningitis (TBM))
confusing language of, x
congenital
  defined, 233*t*
cutaneous, 188–194, 192*f*–194*f*, 190*t*–191*t* (*see also* cutaneous
    tuberculosis)
defined, 218
in developing communities, ix
diagnosis of
  laboratory tests in, 15–24
disease progression in, 232
drug-resistant (*see also* drug-resistant tuberculosis (DR-TB))
  in children, 329–358 (*see also* drug-resistant tuberculosis
    (DR-TB) in children)
drug-susceptible
  in children, 311–328 (*see also* drug-susceptible tuberculosis in
    children)
of ear, nose, and throat, 195–196
elimination of
  WHO on, 80
epidemiology of, 246, 8–9, 67–68, 8*f*
extrapulmonary
  FAS in, 111
extrathoracic (*see* extrathoracic tuberculosis; extrathoracic
    tuberculosis in children)
genitourinary
  in adolescents, 219, 219*t*
in HIV–infected infants, children, and adolescents, 245–261 (*see
    also* HIV infection; HIV/TB coinfection)
HIV infection with (*see* HIV/TB coinfection)
immune response to
  components in, 32, 37–39, 33*f*
incidence of, 69, 67
infectious
  in adults, ix
intestinal, 186
intrathoracic (*see* intrathoracic tuberculosis; intrathoracic
    tuberculosis in children)
introduction, 67–68
of kidney/urinary tract, 194–195
latent, 6
lymph node, 186
microbiology of, 13–29
mortality data, 359, 8–9, 67–69, 8*f*
  history of, 6, 6*f*
  ICD-10 on, 69
musculoskeletal
  diagnostic imaging of, 138–144, 139*f*–143*f* (*see also*
    musculoskeletal tuberculosis, diagnostic imaging of)
mycobacteria other than, 14
mycobacteriology/taxonomy of, 13–14
in neonates and infants, 231–243 (*see also* infant(s); neonate(s))
NTM lymphadenitis *vs.*, 223
ocular
  in adolescents, 219–220, 219*t*
organs affected by, 150, 151*t*
osteoarticular, 180–186, 182*f*, 183*t*, 184*t*, 185*f*, 181*t* (*see also*
    osteoarticular tuberculosis (OA-TB))
pathogenesis of, 14–15, 14*f*
pathology of, 13–29
perinatal, 232, 236–238, 237*f*

tuberculous pericarditis, 125, 125f
tuberculous peritonitis, 186
tuberculous pleurisy, 125, 125f
tuberculous pseudo-abscesses, 204–205, 205f
tuberculous rheumatism
    chronic, 185
tuberculous spondylitis
    diagnostic imaging of, 138–140, 140f, 139f
tuberculous verrucosa cutis, 189, 192f
Tuli, S.M., 183, 184t
"two-step testing," 86
Tygerberg Children's Hospital
    first-line treatment regimens for childhood TBM at, 207, 209t

UIFNγ. see unstimulated interferon-gamma (UIFNγ)
ultrasound (US)
    of abdominal TB, 187, 136, 136f
    chest
        in childhood TB evaluation, 120, 121f, 120f
    in childhood PTB diagnosis, 110–111
    in intrathoracic childhood TB diagnosis, 152
    of urogenital TB, 138
UNICEF. see United Nations International Children's Emergency
        Fund (UNICEF)
United Nations International Children's Emergency Fund
        (UNICEF)
    on BCG vaccines, 360, 360t
    in Roadmap for Childhood Tuberculosis–Towards Zero Deaths, 396
United States Public Health Service (USPHS)
    on INH for childhood TB infection, 286–287
unstimulated interferon-gamma (UIFNγ)
    in intrathoracic childhood TB diagnosis, 158, 153
urinary lipoarabinomannan (LAM)
    in childhood PTB diagnosis, 103
urinary tract
    TB of, 194–195
        diagnosis of, 195
        pathogenesis of, 195
urine
    in childhood PTB diagnosis, 99–100
urogenital tuberculosis
    diagnostic imaging of, 138, 138f
US. see ultrasound (US)
U.S. Agency for International Development (USAID)
    in Roadmap for Childhood Tuberculosis–Towards Zero Deaths, 396
USAID. see U.S. Agency for International Development (USAID)
USPHS. see United States Public Health Service (USPHS)

vaccine(s)
    auxotrophs, 369
    BCG (see Bacille Calmette-Guérin (BCG) vaccines)
    for childhood TB
        research gaps in, 407
    MTBVAC, 369
    mutants, 369
    MVA85A, 369

new, 369
    rBCG, 369
    SecA2, 369
    sub-unit, 369
van Toorn, R., 201
verrucosa cutis
    tuberculous, 189, 192f
Villemin, J-A, 2
visceral tuberculosis, 187
VOCs. see volative organic compounds (VOCs)
volative organic compounds (VOCs)
    detection of
        mass spectroscopy in, 92
vomiting
    drug-susceptible childhood TB management and
        treatment of, 319–321
von Pirquet, C., 47, 5–6, 8f

Wallgren, A.J., 48, 53f
Weiner, M., 301
Whitelaw, A.C., 13
Whittaker, E., 31
WHO. see World Health Organization (WHO)
WHO Expanded Programme on Immunization
    on BCG vaccines, 360, 360t
WHO Global TB Program, 399
World Health Assembly, 396
World Health Organization (WHO)
    on adolescents, 217
    on anti-TB drugs, 264
    on BCG vaccines, 368, 367, 360, 360t
    on childhood TB management, 383
    on childhood TB prevalence, 201
    on DR-TB in children, 330
    first-line treatment regimens for childhood TBM of, 207, 209t
    on IGRAs in M. tuberculosis infection diagnosis, 89
    on RMP for childhood TB infection, 292
    in Roadmap for Childhood Tuberculosis–Towards Zero Deaths,
        395–396
    on TB, 68
    on TB elimination by 2050, 80
    on TB infection, 284
    on TB in women, 231
    on TB treatment guidelines, 312
    on Xpert in childhood PTB diagnosis, 102–103, 104b, 102b

XDR-TB. see extensively drug-resistant tuberculosis (XDR-TB)
Xpert
    in childhood PTB diagnosis
        WHO on, 102–103, 104b, 102b
    in drug resistance determination in childhood PTB, 104–105
x-ray(s)
    discovery of, 5–7, 6f

Zar, H.J., 97